HUMAN ANATO

A Dissection Ma

HUMAN ANATOMY
A Dissection Manual

Sujatha Kiran PhD
Professor and Head
Department of Anatomy
and
Academic Vice Principal
MNR Medical College
Sangareddy, Andhra Pradesh, India

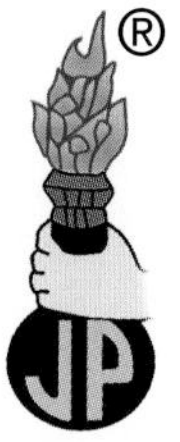

JAYPEE BROTHERS MEDICAL PUBLISHERS (P) LTD
New Delhi • Panama City • London

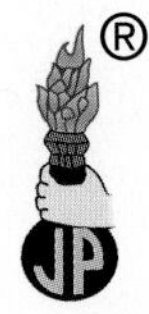

Jaypee Brothers Medical Publishers (P) Ltd

Headquarter

Jaypee Brothers Medical Publishers (P) Ltd
4838/24, Ansari Road, Daryaganj
New Delhi 110 002, India
Phone: +91-11-43574357
Fax: +91-11-43574314
Email: jaypee@jaypeebrothers.com

Overseas Offices

JP Medical Ltd,
83 Victoria Street London
SW1H 0HW (UK)
Phone: +44-2031708910
Fax: +02-03-0086180
Email: info@jpmedpub.com

Jaypee-Highlights Medical Publishers Inc
City of Knowledge, Bld 237, Clayton
Panama City, Panama
Phone: 507-317-0160
Fax: +50-73-010499
Email: cservice@jphmedical.com

Website: www.jaypeebrothers.com
Website: www.jaypeedigital.com

Inquiries for bulk sales may be solicited at: jaypee@jaypeebrothers.com

Publisher: Jitendar P Vij
Publishing Director: Tarun Duneja
Cover Design: Seema Dogra

Human Anatomy: A Dissection Manual

First Edition: **2012**

ISBN 978-93-5025-015-0

Printed at: Ajanta Offset & Packagings Ltd., New Delhi

Dedicated to

My Father
Sri Pendyala Nageswara Rao

Preface

Anatomy is the study of structure of the human body. The gross anatomy describes the structures as they are seen in the body. To study them, dissections are performed on the cadaver.

Human anatomy conventionally is studied as regional anatomy. The body is divided into six to seven regions and the structures located in a particular region are described in dissection manuals and standard textbooks.

The dissection manual is a practical guide in the dissection hall to unfold the position, relations and functions of the structures seen. This book is written with a view that a single body is given to a set of students for the whole year. In this dissection manual the regional division of the body follows the order of upper limb, thorax, abdomen, pelvis and perineum, lower limb, head and neck and brain. This helps in following the continuity of structures, particularly at the junctional zones by dissection.

Each regional chapter starts with an introductory note. This gives an outline of arrangement of structures in that part and their functional specialization. This is followed by smaller segments of dissection regions. Each region describes the structures seen in that particular region with a pictorial depiction. This carries information needed to identify the structure in the body.

Living and surface anatomy is incorporated at places to make the student understand the correlation between the structures that are seen in the cadaver and the functions they perform in the living.

This book is primarily for undergraduate students and is also useful to postgraduate students for quick revision. After seeing and identifying the structures, the students are expected to read the details from a standard textbook.

Sujatha Kiran

Acknowledgments

The life of this book lies in the well-created diagrams. As an author, I could conceive each and every diagram. But to be able to draw on a computer is totally a different art. I could not venture to publish a book of this dimension due to lack of skilled artists to support me.

I thank Shri Jitendar P Vij, Chairman and Managing Director, M/s Jaypee Brothers Medical Publishers (P) Ltd for accepting to publish this book, Mr Tarun Duneja (Director-Publishing) for taking special interest in this book and for designing the cover page. I profusely acknowledge the work of Mr Sanjay Chauhan and the team members: Mr Ram Murti, Mr Arun Sharma, Mr Sukhdev Prasad, Mr Rakesh Verma, Mr Deepak Gupta and Mr Manoj Pahuja, the computer animation specialists of Jaypee Brothers Medical Publishers to have poured life into the diagrams. They showed me the first diagram sometime in 2009. The team worked relentlessly for more than two years to complete all these diagrams. They all sat with me and corrected the figures with utmost care and dedication. I also thank Mr KK Raman (Production Manager) and Mr Shakiluzzaman (Proofreader) for taking special care to complete the book in record time.

I would like to thank Mr Ravi Kiran, my husband, who is totally responsible for my ascent in my career, and he is my guiding force and supporter to this endeavor.

Contents

CHAPTER 1

GENERAL INTRODUCTION

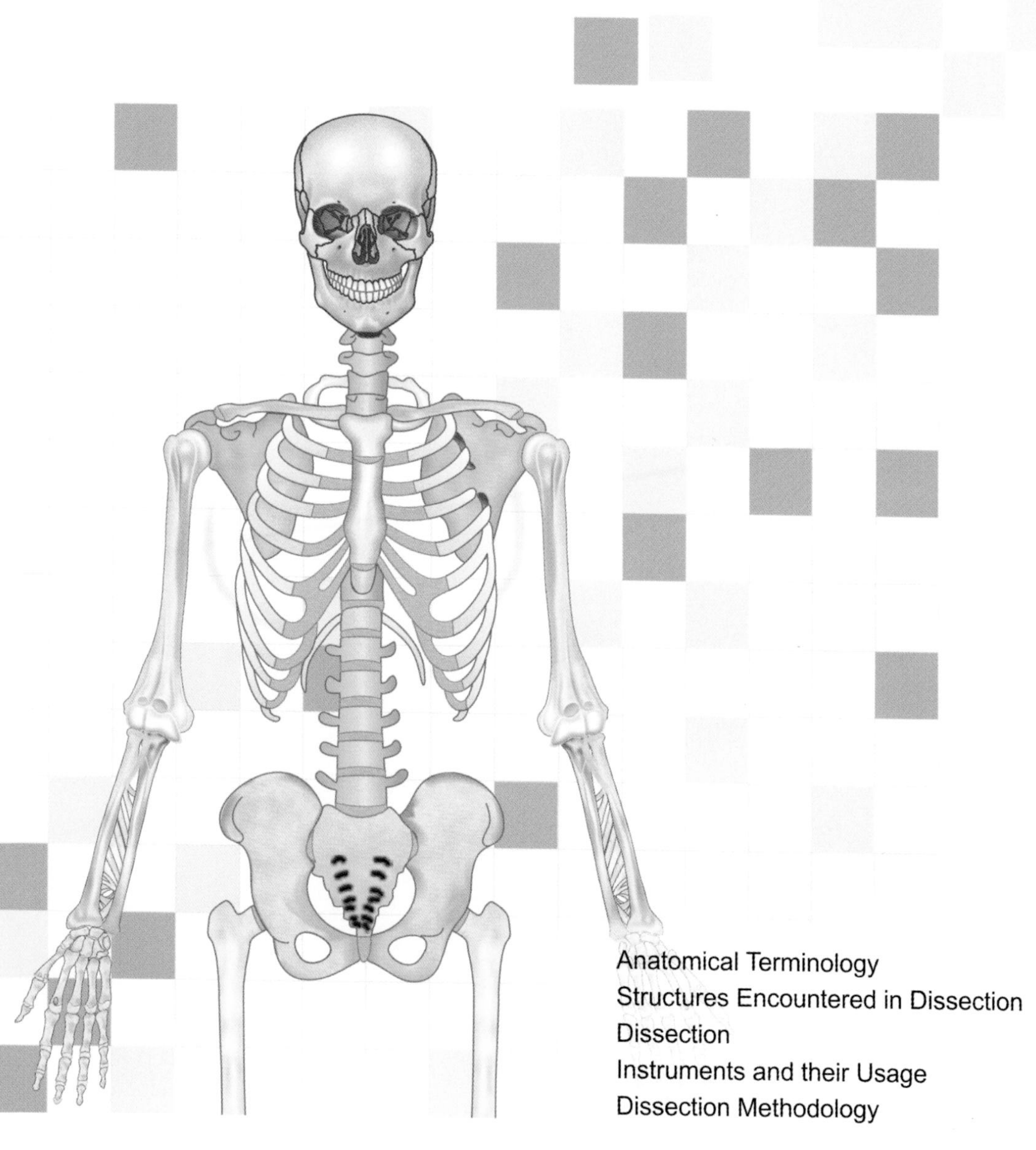

- Anatomical Terminology
- Structures Encountered in Dissection
- Dissection
- Instruments and their Usage
- Dissection Methodology

ANATOMICAL TERMINOLOGY

The human body is obtained after death after clearing all the legal formalities. Now the cadaver is properly embalmed with appropriate embalming fluid and well preserved. All the human beings have the same structure, but can still differ. These differences are called variations. Each and every structure in the body is named. These names are coined, generally with some meaning and are universally accepted by the scientists of this field. This chapter explains the structures that are encountered in the dissection and the common terminology used.

ANATOMICAL POSITION

Anatomical position (Fig. 1) is described as one where the person stands upright with the upper limbs hanging by the sides and the palms facing forwards. All the structures within the body are described as they lie in the anatomical position, though in reality the body lies horizontal on the table.

ANATOMICAL TERMS

Anatomical terms are the names used to identify the structures in the body. Try to study and practice the following terms.

Median: Denotes the midline of the body. This is a definitive term. All the other terms are relative.

Superficial: Nearer to the skin, e.g. the veins are superficial to the deep fascia.

Deep: Away from the skin, e.g. the veins are deep to the skin.

Superior/cephalic: Nearer to the head, e.g. eyes are superior to the nose.

Inferior/caudal: Nearer to the tail, e.g. the diaphragm is caudal to the heart.

Anterior/ventral: Nearer to the front, e.g. the heart is ventral to the vertebrae.

Dorsal/posterior: Towards the back, e.g. the vertebrae lie posterior to the heart.

Medial: Nearer to the midline, e.g. the trachea lies medial to the lungs.

Lateral: Away from the midline, e.g. the lungs lie lateral to the trachea.

External: Nearer to the outside, e.g. the pericardium lies external to the heart.

Internal: Nearer to the inside, e.g. the heart lies internal to the pericardium.

Proximal: Nearer to the body, e.g. the arm lies proximal to the forearm.

Distal: Away from the body, e.g. the forearm lies distal to the arm.

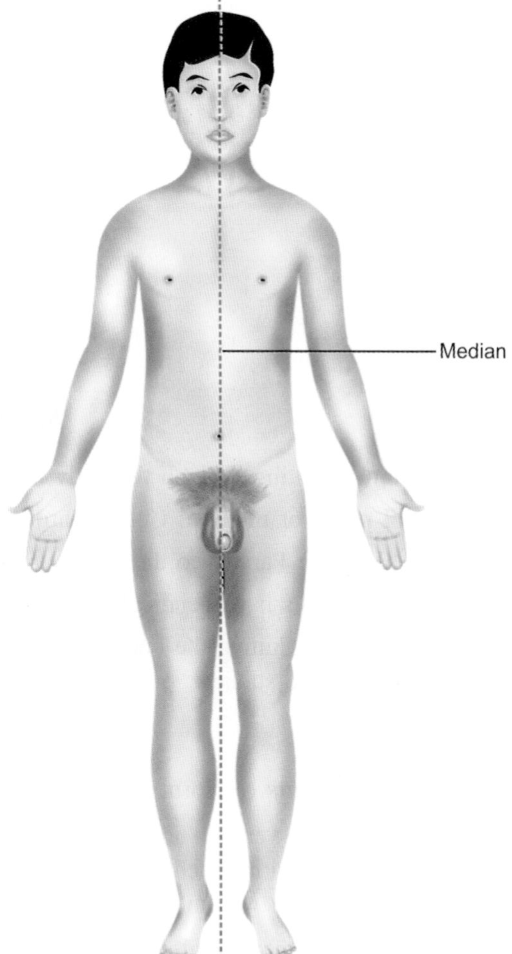

FIGURE 1 Anatomical position

Radial, ulnar, tibial, fibular are the terms used to denote the structures nearer to those bones, e.g. ulnar artery—the artery related to the bone ulna.

Superolateral, inferomedial, anteroinferior, posterosuperior are the terms used to depict an accurate position of a structure in the body, e.g. the subclavian artery lies posterosuperior to the subclavian vein.

Palmar means towards the palm of the hand, e.g. the palmar aponeurosis lies in the palm of the hand.

Plantar means towards the sole of the foot, e.g. the plantar aponeurosis lies in the sole of the foot.

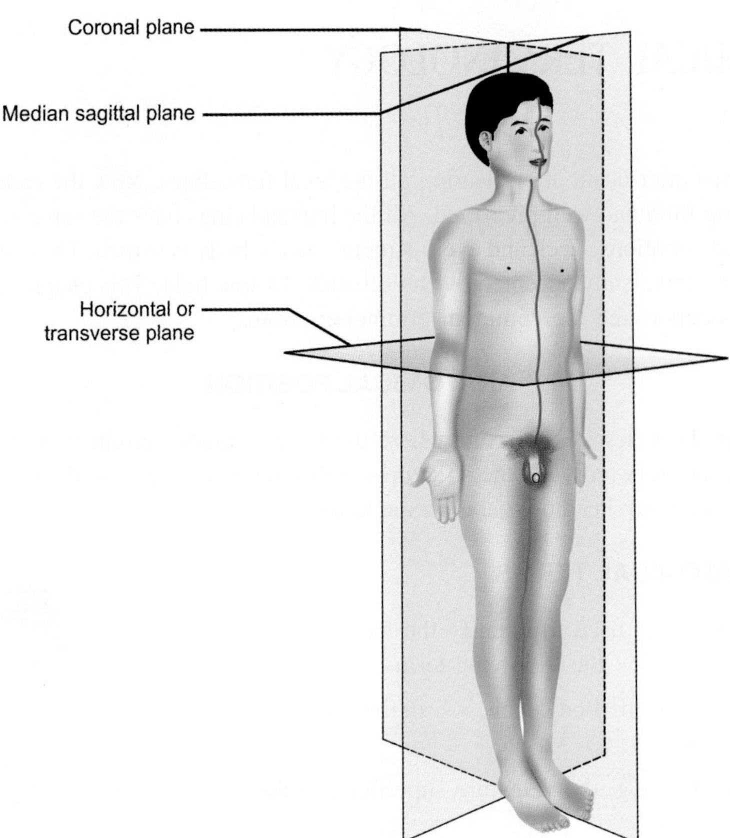

FIGURE 2 Anatomical planes

ANATOMICAL PLANES (Fig. 2)

Sagittal plane: Cutting through the body anteroposteriorly.

Midsagittal plane or **median:** Cutting through the body exactly in the midline.

Parasagittal plane: Parallel to the sagittal plane.

Coronal plane: This is perpendicular to the sagittal plane – cutting the body from one side to the other.

Transverse plane: Cutting the body horizontally—this is generally used to study the organs for diagnostic purposes like MRI, ultrasound studies.

TERMS OF MOVEMENTS

Terms of movements (perform them on your body and appreciate).

Flexion is when two ventral surfaces/anatomical or embryological approximate, flexion is also described as closing up of an angle, e.g. forearm touching the arm at the elbow joint. In lower limb back of the leg touching the back of the thigh is flexion. Here two embryological ventral surfaces approximate each other.

Extension is when two dorsal surfaces approximate or opening up of an angle, e.g. bringing arm and forearm into a straight line. In lower limb bringing the thigh and leg into straight line is extension.

Abduction is going away from the midline, e.g. the upper limb moving away from the body, in relation to the movement of the fingers, the imaginary midline passes through the middle of the middle finger, move the fingers away from the middle finger. The hand moving away from the body or moving towards the radial side is called radial deviation.

Adduction bringing the part nearer to the midline, e.g. bringing the upper limb nearer to the body, move the fingers of the hand, back to touch the middle finger. When the hand moves towards the body it is called adduction or ulnar deviation.

Internal/medial rotation—where the ventral surface of the part turns medially, e.g. turn the hand to the back, holding the humerus in your hand, feel the humerus turning around a vertical axis.

External/lateral rotation is where the ventral surface of the part turns laterally, e.g. turn the hand out by holding the humerus. This is a rotation around a vertical axis.

Protraction is where a part moves bodily forwards, e.g. move the shoulder forwards.

Retraction is where a part moves backwards, e.g. bracing the shoulders.

Supination is where the palm lies in normal anatomical position, when the body is put on the table facing forwards it is said that the body is in supine position.

Pronation is where the palm faces backwards or where the body is put on the table with face touching the table.

Dorsiflexion is used only in relation to foot. When the foot moves towards the front of leg it is called dorsi-flexion.

Plantar flexion is when the foot is lifted off the ground with the sole facing backwards.

Circumduction is where the part moves in a circular motion creating a cone, e.g. move the upper limb totally in a circular motion.

Opposition is a special movement of the thumb, where the thumb touches the other fingers.

STRUCTURES ENCOUNTERED IN DISSECTION

This chapter explains the structures you encounter as you do your dissection.

SKIN

Skin is the organ which covers the body totally. While doing the dissection you will realize number of specializations within the skin. The skin over the palms and soles is very thick and is connected to the deeper fascia by means of thick connective tissue septa and the gaps between the septa is filled with fat. So it is difficult to pull the skin of the palms and soles. It is devoid of hair follicles, sebaceous glands and arrectores pilorum muscle. Skin of the scalp is also connected to the deeper fascia by connective tissue septa. Skin of the scalp, the pubic region and the axillary region is heavily laden with hair follicles, sebaceous glands and sweat glands. The skin on the ventral aspect of the body is lighter and thinner, can easily be pulled from the underneath fascia. Pull it and see. Skin on the back is darkly colored, thick and firmly attached to the deeper fascia. While reflecting the skin you have to keep these features in mind. See the skin flexure creases near the wrist, elbow, knee etc. These are due to constant folding of the part and pull of the connective tissue beneath. Observe dermal ridges and flexor creases on the palmar and plantar skin. These are genetically determined and are formed within the intrauterine life itself. The study of these is called dermatoglyphics. The dermal ridge patterns are unique to each individual. This is used in forensic study.

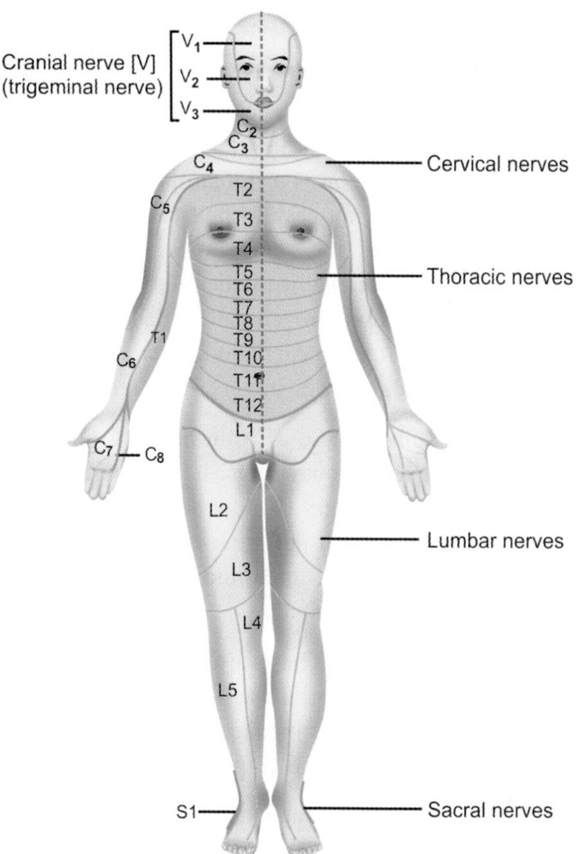

FIGURE 3 Dermatomes

Nerve supply of the skin (Fig. 3): The skin develops from dermatome part of the somite. As it develops it drags the nerve supply along with it. So the nerve supply of the skin denotes from which somatic segment it is derived. This arrangement is definitive throughout the body. Knowledge of this pattern is very much essential to diagnose the damage to a particular spinal nerve.

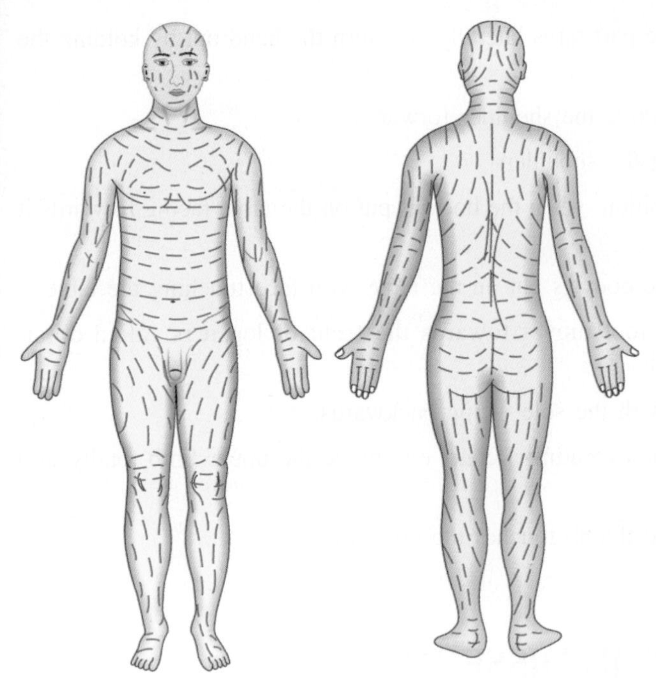

FIGURE 4 Langer's line

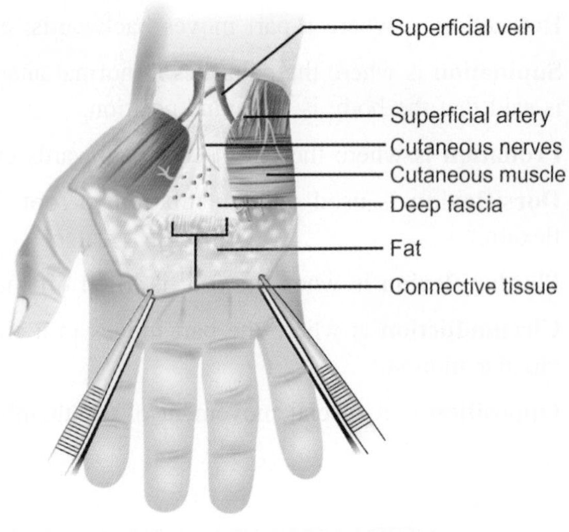

FIGURE 5 Superficial fascia

Langer's line (Fig. 4): Skin is the first structure to be cut in any operation. The collagen fibres beneath the skin follow a definitive pattern. If collagen fibres are cut across, they form a thick scar in wound repair. Instead, if a cut is made along the fibre direction, during wound repair there will be minimal scar formation. So the knowledge of the arrangement of collagen fibres beneath the skin is very much essential for a surgeon. This arrangement of collagen fibres beneath the skin is called Langer's lines.

SUPERFICIAL FASCIA (Fig. 5)

As you reflect the skin the next structure you encounter is the superficial fascia. It is the connective tissue deep to the skin. The arrangement of tissue is variable in different parts of the body. In most of the places it is loose and yielding. Try to pull the skin on your forearm. The area on which the skin slides is the superficial fascia. Note that on the back of your body it is not easy to pull the skin, because the connective tissue here is dense connective tissues. Note that in the palms, soles and scalp skin is very thick. That is because the connective tissue here connects the skin to the deep fascia beneath, and is divided into number of fat laden compartments. This forms a thick cushion in these regions. The superficial fascia is generally filled with fat. The amount of fat present varies from person to person. Even in a very thin person, the gluteal region, anterior abdominal wall and greater omentum are heavily laden with fat. The cutaneous blood vessels and nerves traverse through the superficial fascia.

Cutaneous veins: These are thin bluish to black tubes seen in the superficial fascia. At the time of death the arteries undergo a wave of contraction and push the blood into the venous system. It gets stagnated there and gives a black coloration. Make a tight fist and see the veins on the back of your hand. These appear greenish in color. They form a superficial prominent definitive system of veins in the upper limb and lower limb. These are generally made use to draw blood and inject fluids into the body. In other parts of the body they accompany the medium and small sized arteries as venae comitantes.

Cutaneous arteries: These are very fine arteries. They are always accompanied by venae comitantes. These are veins accompanying the arteries. The cutaneous arteries are small and difficult to identify unless they are injected with red lead. Nowadays this practice of injecting the arteries is discontinued. Generally the cutaneous arteries are identified by identifying their venae comitantes.

Cutaneous nerves: Cutaneous nerves generally accompany cutaneous vessels in the body. In the limbs, cutaneous nerves pierce the deep fascia at definitive places, traverse long distance, branch and supply a big area of skin. These are sensory nerves. They carry cutaneous sensations like pain, touch pressure type of sensation from skin.

Lymphatics: These are very thin vessels and difficult to trace. The lymph nodes into which the lymphatics drain are definitive in their position. These can be easily identified along with the drainage vessels. The nodes appear deep brown in color and oval to round in appearance.

Cutaneous muscles: These are muscles present within the dermis of the skin. These are smooth muscle fibres called arrectores pilorum muscle. They cannot be identified in dissection but they can be seen under microscope. The panniculus carnosus group of muscles is a subcutaneous sheet of muscle. They are inserted into the skin and can move it. So in places where they are present you have to take a great care while reflecting the skin, e.g. muscles of facial expression, dortos muscle of scrotum and palmaris brevis of palm.

DEEP FASCIA

The thick white glistening protective sheet that you see deep to the superficial fascia is the deep fascia. It is made of collagen fibres. The collagen fibres are longitudinally arranged in limbs where it covers the musculature. At many a places it is thick and gives attachment to muscles, e.g. fascia lata of thigh gives attachment to gluteus maximus and tensor fascia lata muscle. It is a thick owen structure when it tries to protect the tendons crossing the bones. Here it is called a retinaculum, e.g. flexor retinaculum, peroneal retinaculum. The deep fascia sends in septa, to separate different functional groups of muscles. This can be easily identified by pulling the deep fascia outwards while reflecting the fascia.

SKELETAL MUSCLE

Once you reflect the fascia the reddish brown muscle mass you see is skeletal muscle. It is under voluntary control. All these muscles have at least one bony attachment. Generally they extend from one bone to the other, crossing a joint or more than one joint. But the muscles over the face get attached from the bone to the skin. They move the skin of the face and are called muscles of facial expression. They belong to the panniculus carnosus group of muscles. This is the muscle sheet which lies beneath the skin in carnivores and help them to shrug. For the muscles of tongue the distal attachment is mucous membrane, the muscles of eyeball the distal attachment is sclera.

Arrangement (Fig. 6): The muscles form the major bulk in limbs; they are arranged in compartments as functional groups, e.g. the flexors of the arm occupy the anterior compartment. The compartments are separated from each other by septa. Each compartment has its own set of neurovascular bundle which supplies blood and nerves. The neurovascular bundle is supported by loose connective tissue, which you need to clean to identify the branches. The nerve enters the muscle bellies on its under surface.

Fibre arrangement: In skeletal muscle, the muscle fibres are cylindrical in shape. They are covered by connective tissue. The muscle fibres reach the bone through this connective tissue. The force generated by the muscle fibres reach the bone through this connective tissue fibres called Sharpey's fibres. The proportion of connective tissue and muscle fibres is variable. The sartorius is ***muscular*** throughout its extent, the flexor muscles of forearm have long tendons, anterior abdominal muscles are replaced by big aponeurosis near their insertion. The arrangement of muscle fibre to the connective is variable. The muscle acquires their shape based on the connective tissue. They can be ***strap muscles*** when fibres are parallel and connective tissue is less, e.g. sartorius; ***spindle shaped*** or ***fusiform,*** when the muscle fibres from a belly in the center and reach the bone through ends, e.g. biceps, digastrics; ***unipennate*** where

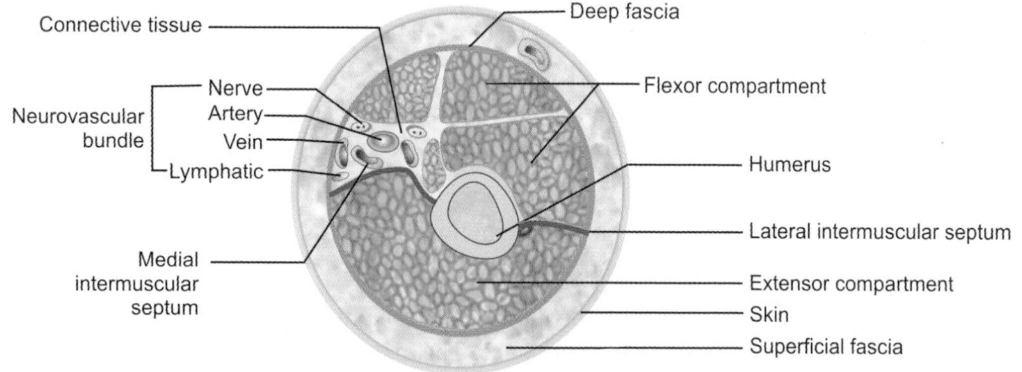

FIGURE 6 Skeletal muscle arrangement section through arm

all the muscle fibres get attached to a tendon from one side, e.g. flexor pollices longus; ***bipennate*** where muscle fibres get attached to a central tendon from two sides, e.g. dorsal interossei; ***multipennate*** where the muscle fibres are short and get attached to number of central tendons which unite together to from a big tendon near the insertion, e.g. deltoid; is ***circumpennate*** arrangement, where all fibres converge from all sides to a central tendon, e.g. tibialis anterior.

Nomenclature: Muscles are named for convenience of understanding based on number of parameters. They are named based on ***shape***—deltoid (triangular), quadratus (quadrangular). Rhomboideus (diamond shaped) teres (rounded) lumbrical (worm like) ***size***—major (big), minor (small), longus (long), brevis (short), latissimus (broad); depending upon ***number of heads***—biceps (two heads), triceps (three heads), quadriceps (four heads), digastric (two bellies); based upon ***position***—superficialis (nearer to skin), profundus (deeper to the skin), externus (near to outside); based on ***location***—anterior (infront), dorsal/posterior (back), lateralis (external side), superior (nearer to the head), inferior (nearer to the tail), interosseous between the bones, pectoralis (over the chest), brachialis (in the arm), femoris (in the thigh), oris (in the mouth), oculi (in relation to the eye); depicting the ***attachment***—sternocleidomastoid (from sternum to mastoid process), based on ***action***—flexor (performs flexion), extensor (performs extension), abductor (performs abduction), adductor (performs adduction), supinator (performs supination), pronator (performs pronation); and a combination of any of the above, e.g. flexor carpi radialis brevis—a small muscle which performs flexion of the carpal bones on the radial side.

Living anatomy: Muscle testing is a common practice to assess the damage of a muscle. As they are in groups it is difficult to assess a single muscle damage. But a group performance can easily be assessed. If a person is asked to perform a movement against resistance the muscle will stand out, e.g. try to approximate the forearm to the arm by pushing the forearm with the other hand. The biceps of the arm will stand out, as it is a flexor of the forearm at the elbow joint. In the dissection hall try to test as many muscles as possible.

Muscle action: Many factors come into play when a muscle contracts to bring about a particular action. To understand this one should be familiar with axis. The axis is the least mobile line or plane in a joint while performing a movement. Any muscle which crosses the axis exactly perpendicular will have the best powerful action, as they move away from the center the action will be weaker. Based upon this factor a muscle can be described as ***prime mover,*** e.g. biceps is a prime mover for flexion of forearm on arm at elbow. The muscles which help this prime mover are called ***agonists,*** e.g. brachialis and pronator teres are agonists to perform flexion. The muscles which cross the axis on the opposite side of the agonists are ***antagonists,*** e.g. the triceps which brings about extension of the forearm at elbow is an antagonist to biceps. When an action is to be performed against gravity both progravity and antigravity muscles perform the action. It is like putting a break to a car when we are riding on a slope. It is called paying out rope action, e.g. lowering a heavy weight to the ground. Here both biceps and triceps contract. When both agonists and antagonists contract to bring about an intricate powerful movement it is said that they are ***synergists,*** e.g. while making a fist both flexors and extensors of the hand contract.

Biomechanics: Kinesiology is the subject which deals with the biomechanics of the joints. Here only basics are mentioned for understanding the muscle movement. Each muscle generates a force when contracts. This force is passed on to the bone through Sharpey's fibres. A combination of all forces generated by all the muscles result in the net movement produced at a particular joint. The point of insertion is the fulcrum.

Spurt force: When a muscle is inserted into a part nearer to the joint, and when it contracts it pulls the distal segment. This moves with a greater range. This is spurt force, e.g. the biceps which is inserted into the proximal part of the radius, causes the range in flexion of the forearm.

Shunt force: When a muscle is inserted into a distal segment of the bone it pushes the proximal part backwards and creates shunt (like locos) force, e.g. the pronator teres, brachioradialis by pushing the radius towards the elbow joint they create a stabilizing force.

Spin force: When a muscle spirals or runs transversely and gets attached to a convexity, it produces a spin force. It produces a rotatory movement (like spinning a cricket ball), e.g. infraspinatus at the shoulder joint and pronator teres between radius and ulna.

Soleal pump: This is a special feature seen in soleus. Veins form a plexus within the soleus muscle of the leg. It functions as a peripheral heart and aids in the venous return.

Sesamoid bone: These are bones which develop in the muscles. When a muscle or a tendon crosses a joint too closely, it replaces the capsule and develops bone within its substance. This prevents friction and wearing away of the muscle. These can be bony or cartilaginous, e.g. patella or knee cap in the tendon of quadriceps femoris muscle (feel it), number of sesamoid bones in tendons of sole.

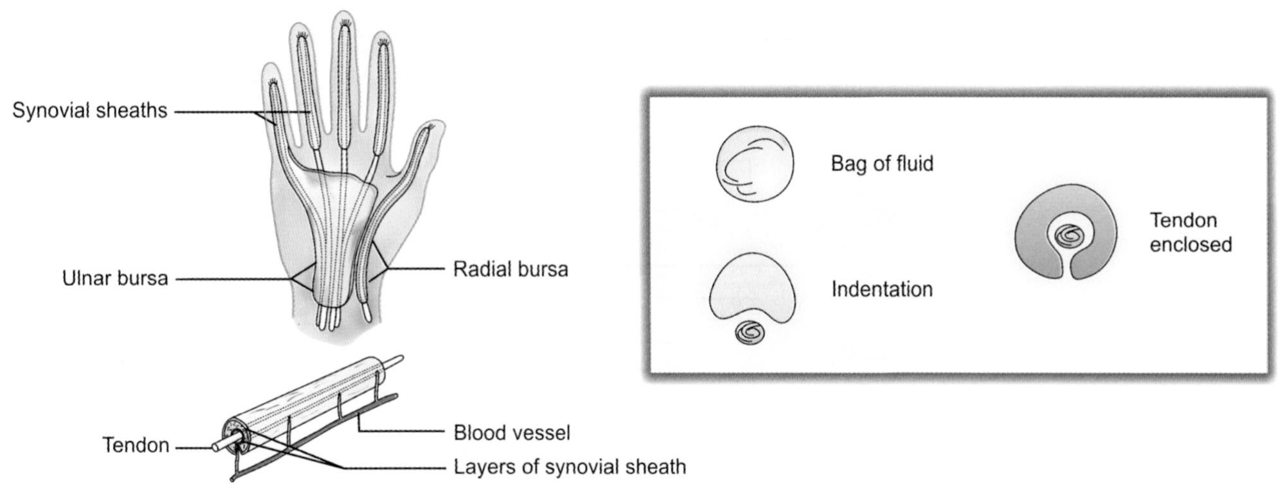

FIGURE 7 Formation of synovial sheath diagrammatic representation

Synovial sheaths (Fig. 7): When tendons pass over bones and joints they are protected by synovial sheaths. These are bags of connective tissue filled with fluid. This pre vents friction of the tendons over the bones, e.g. flexor sheaths of long tendons of fingers.

Bursa: Number of muscles are separated from the nearby bone by bags of synovial fluid called bursa. This gives a play for the muscles, e.g. subscapular bursa.

Nerve supply: Though conventionally it is said that motor nerve, supplies a muscle and it brings about contraction, in reality both motor and sensory nerves supply the muscle fibres. The motor nerve initiates the contraction of muscle, whereas sensory fibres carry proprioceptive/stretch sensations from the muscle. The receptor here is called muscle spindle. The knowledge of this is essential to initiate contraction.

***Motor unit*:** Each nerve has number of fibres and each nerve fibre supplies as many as 100 muscle fibres. This is called a motor unit, so stimulation of each nerve fibre initiates a contraction of 100 muscle fibres. More and more muscle fibres will be involved in contraction depending upon the force required in contraction.

Hilton's law: The nerve which supplies a group of muscles that act on a joint will give a branch to supply the joint. These are sensory fibres and carry stretch sensations from tendons, capsule and ligaments.

The spindle shaped muscles are generally supplied in the center and into their bellies, e.g. biceps. In muscles where the fibres are spread out, the nerve has a long course and it gives branches along the length of the muscle, e.g. accessory nerve to trapezius. Generally all the muscles are supplied on their ventral aspects.

Blood supply: The medium sized arteries accompanied by venae comitantes supply the muscles along with the nerves. It is called a neurovascular bundle. The tendons are supplied by arteries which supply the joints. When the tendons are too long they have their own neurovascular bundle, e.g. vincula longa and brevia of flexor digitorum superficialis and profundus.

CARDIAC MUSCLE

The ***cardiac muscle*** is a specialized muscle specific for heart. It runs in layers to control the contraction of different chambers.

SMOOTH MUSCLE

Smooth muscle is involuntary musculature, present in the internal organs. Generally they are arranged in layers. They produce peristaltic movement in gastrointestinal tract, and the uterine musculature expels the fetus during parturition.

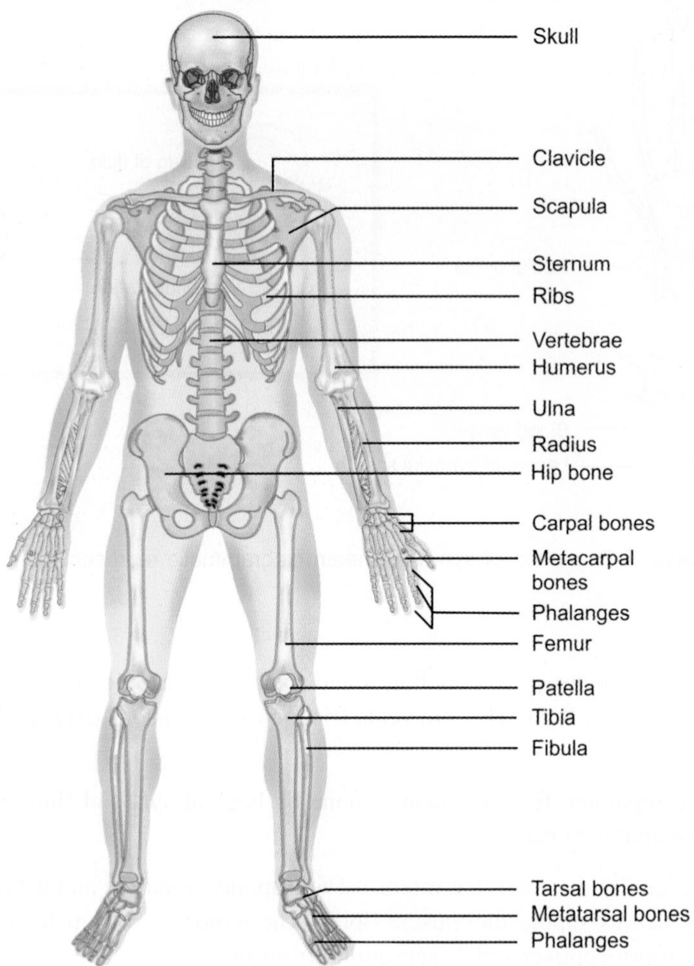

FIGURE 8 Skeleton

BONE

The muscles are attached to bones. The next structure you would come across in the body is bone. The study of bones is called osteology. It is a big field and only the details needed for dissection is covered in this book.

The bones form the framework of our body. The dried bones taken out of a human body are articulated into a skeleton with the help of screws, wires and corks. It is essential to go to a skeleton and study the bones, to understand the location of the joints and the position of muscle attachment. You need to see the direction of muscle fibres to understand their actions.

Skeleton (Fig. 8): Go to a skeleton and see the arrangement of bones. The central axis of the body is made up of the vertebral column. The skull, the ribs and the pelvis form the axial skeleton, the bones of the limbs form the skeleton of the appendages, the appendicular skeleton.

Shapes of the bones: Note that the bones are of different shapes and sizes. Observe the bones on the vault of the skull, scapula and hip bone, they are ***flat bones.*** See the bones forming the base of the skull and the vertebrae, they are ***irregular bones***. See the bones of the limbs and ribs, they are ***long bones,*** they have a shaft and two articular ends. Look at the carpals and tarsals, they are ***short bones.*** See a midline cut skull, you can see number of cavities within the bone, they are ***pneumatic bones.***

Contours of the Bones

While doing dissection you can appreciate that the bones present two parts, the part which gives attachment to muscles and ligaments, and the other part which takes part in the formation of joints.

Intra-articular parts: These are the parts which contribute to the joint formation and are smooth, and show different shapes. ***Head*** is rounded structure, present towards the ends of the bones, e.g. head of femur, head of humerus. ***Neck*** is the part that follows the head, e.g. neck of the humerus, neck of the mandible. ***Condyles*** are semicircular bulges at the ends of the bones, e.g. femoral condyles, tibial condyles. ***Trochlea*** is a pulley shaped elevation, e.g. trochlea on humerus. Eminence is a central elevation, e.g. intercondylar eminence on tibia. This is the elevated area between the two tibial condyles.

Markings due to muscle pull: The part of the bone which gives attachment to muscles and ligaments raise elevations due to the pull of the muscles, and are given different names**.** ***Trochanter*** is a big elevations on the bone, e.g. greater trochanter and lesser trochanter of femur. Tubercles, tuberosity, protuberance, supracondyles are the words commonly used to denote small elevation, e.g. greater and lesser ***tubercle*** of humerus, ischial ***tuberosity,*** deltoid tuberosity, external occipital ***protuberance,*** medial and lateral ***epicondyles*** of humerus. Sometimes they cause linear elevations and the words used are crest, ridge, line, e.g. iliac crest, supracondylar ridge, gluteal lines. Irregular projections are named as processes, spines, e.g. ***coronoid process*** on mandible, ***olecranon process, spine*** of the scapula. Depressions on the bone are named as pit or ***fovea, fossa,*** e.g. pit on the head of the femur, olecranon fossa.

Blood and nerve supply of bones: When you carefully observe the bone you will see number of small foraminae. They are all vascular foramina for the entry of blood vessels and nerves. The biggest of the foramina is the ***nutrient foramen,*** generally seen in the middle of a bone. See the nutrient foramen of the femur in the middle of it, and see the ***vascular foramina*** near the neck of the femur.

Periosteum: When you try to see the articulated skeleton, it is devoid of periosteum so you will see it rough. But when you observe the bone on the cadaver you will note it to be glistening, it is due to the periosteum. It is the covering on the bone, and helps the Sharpey's fibres to penetrate.

JOINTS

The area where one or more bones approximate is a joint. The joints are classified based on the tissue that unites them **(Fig. 9).**

FIBROUS JOINTS: Here the bones are united by fibrous tissue. Go to an articulated skeleton and see how they are articulated. Look at the skull and note that it is made up of number of bones. But the bones look inseparable. These are united by connective tissue and are called ***sutures***.

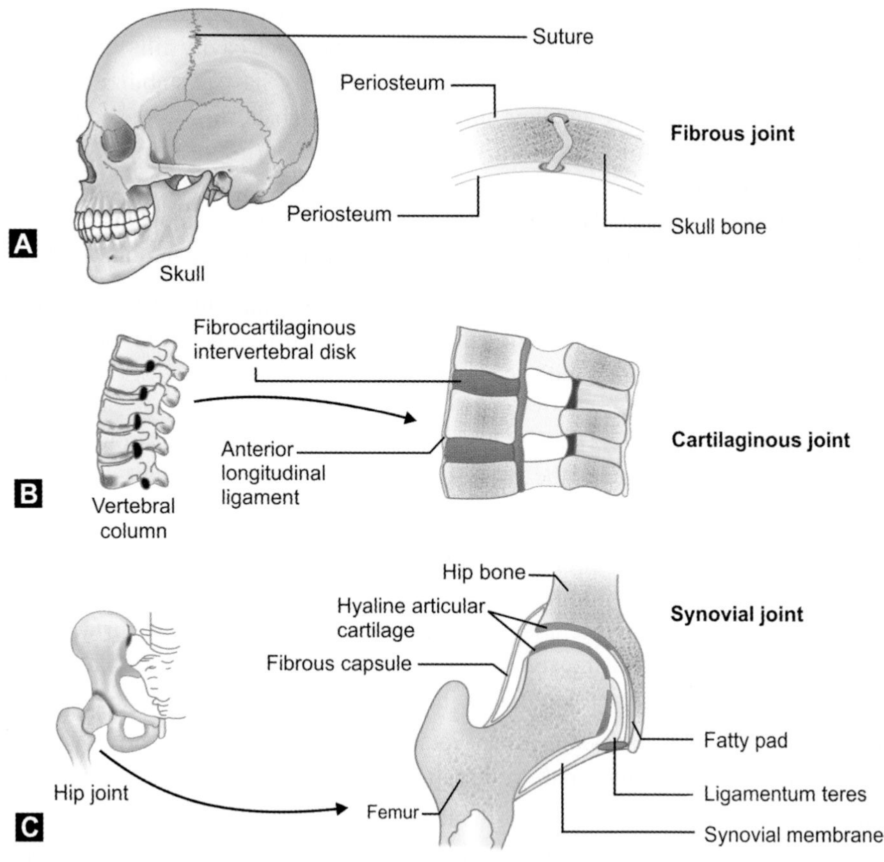

FIGURE 9 Joints

Sutures: Depending upon, how the bones overlap they are described as ***simple sutures,*** e.g. between two maxillae; ***serrate suture*** is where the opposing surfaces interlock with serrations or waves, e.g. sagittal suture; ***dentate suture*** is where opposing surface look like teeth, e.g. lambdoid suture; ***squamous suture*** is where the bones overlap and are united together, e.g. squamous suture. ***Syndesmosis*** is where the bones are united by identifiable amount of connective tissue, e.g. lower end of tibia and fibula, interosseous membrane connecting radius and ulna and tibia and fibula. ***Gomphosis*** is a specific word used for the teeth fixation into the mandible or maxilla. It is a peg and socket joint.

CARTILAGINOUS JOINT: Here the approximated bones are united together by cartilage.

Primary cartilaginous joint: During development, the bone is laid as a cartilaginous model. Ossification centers develop in this to form the diaphysis (shaft) and the epiphysis (ends). The cartilage which remains between the ossifying centers is hyaline cartilage and is temporary. This is a primary cartilaginous joint. In certain places like the costal cartilages it remains throughout life.

Secondary cartilaginous joint/symphysis: Here the cartilage that unites two bones is fibrocartilage. It is present in the midline of the body. It acts like a cushion, e.g. intervertebral disc, symphysis pubis (in articulated skeleton it is represented by corks).

SYNOVIAL JOINT: It is one where the bones are separated and are lubricated by a synovial fluid. The first structure you see in a synovial joint is the capsule and associated ligaments.

Capsule: It is the thick fibrous structure which connects the bones together. The thickness of the capsule is variable. In number of places even muscles are directly inserted into the capsule, e.g. rotator cuff of shoulder joint. Once you open the joint cavity you will feel the sticky substance, the synovial fluid, secreted by the synovial membrane. The ***synovial membrane*** is very thin, secretory, and lines the capsule and gets reflected on to the nonarticulating bony surfaces. The synovial fluid prevents friction.

Intra-articular structures: The articular part of the bone appears smooth and glistering as it is covered by the articular cartilage. Number of joints have intra-articular structures within their joint cavities performing different functions. Positioning of ***intra-articular cartilage*** separates the joint cavity into two compartments. This results in functional separation of the joint into two joints, and permits two different types of movements, e.g. articular disc in temporomandibular joint; elevation and depression is performed in upper compartment and rotation is performed in lower compartment. Move your jaw and feel it. Presence of fat in the joint cavity fills the incongruities of the bony surfaces, e.g. knee joint. Sometimes ***tendons*** pass through the joint. They have a stabilizing effect, e.g. long head of biceps in the shoulder joint. The fat and the tendons in the joint, though lie inside the joint cavity, lie out side the synovial membrane. This prevents the structures from getting damaged during movement.

Blood vessels and nerves are fine branches which enter the joint. They are generally branches derived from the nearby muscular branches. In many a joints the blood vessels form an anastomotic plexuses around the joint and fine branches enter from here to supply the joint, e.g. anastomosis around knee by genicular vessels.

Bursae: Muscles cross the joints closely. So there is every possibility for the muscle to get damaged due to friction. This is prevented by positioning bags of synovial fluid called bursae positioned between the muscle and capsules/bone. In many a places these bursae are continuous with the joint cavity, e.g. knee joint.

CLASSIFICATION OF SYNOVIAL JOINTS: The bones move against each other around an axis, the least mobile line or plane. The shape of the bone determines the type of movement feasible at a joint. Based upon these factors the synovial joints are further classified.

Plane synovial joint—is one without an axis. Look at articulations of carpal bones. You will note that they all have plane surfaces, they slide over each other.

Uniaxial condylar joint—is one where movement is produced around one axis, and the surface of the bone is condylar. Look at the phalanges. See the bulging heads received into the flattened bases. They are like hinges of a door, and are also called hinge joints. Movement takes place around the transverse axis and the movement is flexion and extension.

Uniaxial pivot joint—here the bony surfaces are pivots rotating on a vertical axis. Move your hand to a prone and supine position by holding the radius is your hand. You realize it is moving in a circular fashion.

Biaxial ellipsoid joint—here the articular surfaces are oval in outline, and produce movement both in transverse and anterior posterior axis. Look at the wrist joint of an articulated skeleton. Perform the movement on your hand. You can perform flexion and extension, and abduction and adduction.

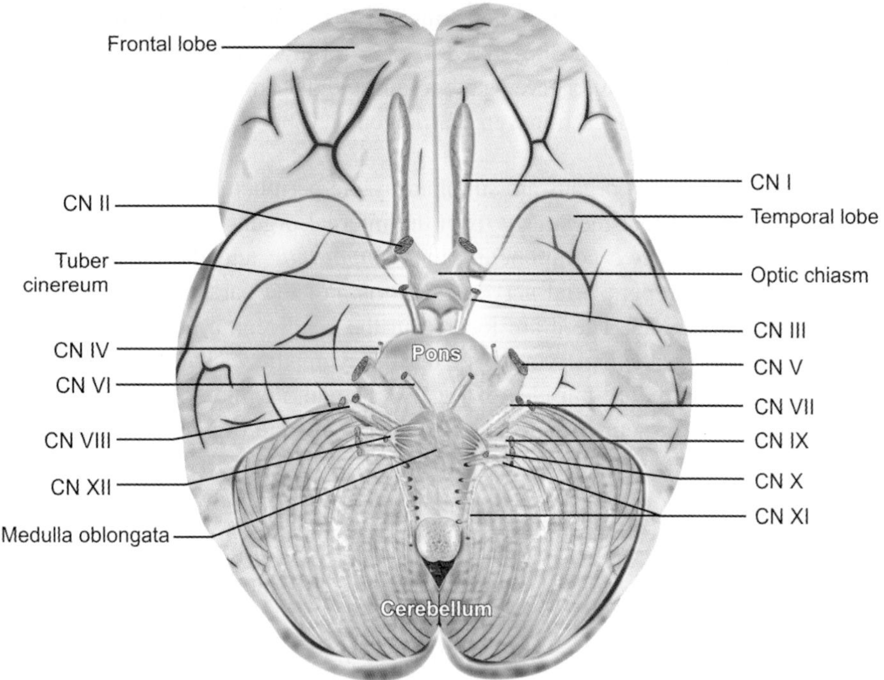

FIGURE 10 Cranial nerves

Biaxial sellar joint—here the bones are reciprocally concavo-convex. Movement is possible around two axes. Look at the articulation of trapezium and the base of the first metacarpal bone. Flexion and extension, abduction and adduction are feasible here. Move your thumb and appreciate the movement.

Polyaxial ball and socket joint—here movement is possible in all directions around all possible axes. Look at the articulations at the hip joint. The rounded head of the femur fits into a cup shaped acetabulum. Move the hip joint and see.

NERVES

You will see nerves in every part of your dissection. They are white thread like structures. The nerves conduct impulses from and to different parts of the body.

Even though functionally they carry fibres of different modalities structurally they look the same. The nerves arise from the central nervous system, the brain and the spinal cord. They are named cranial and spinal nerves respectively. Once they leave the central nervous system, the nerves that you see in the dissection belong to peripheral nervous system. The nerves get organized in definitive patterns to reach the different parts of the body.

The **cranial nerves (Fig. 10):** The nerves you see in the head and neck mainly come from the brain and are cranial nerves. They are twelve in number and supply all the sense organs, the associated musculature and other internal organs.

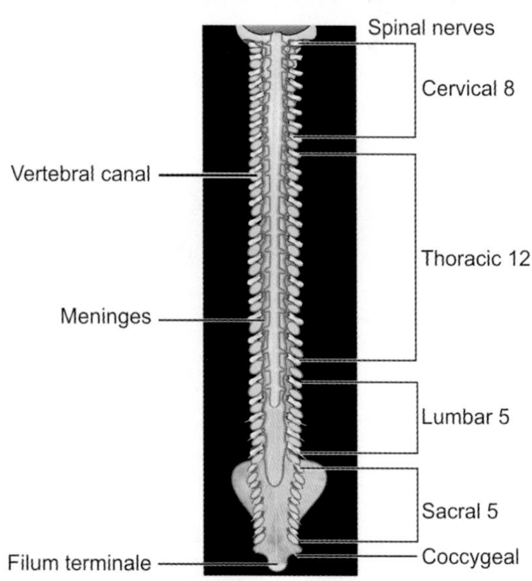

FIGURE 11 Spinal cord

The **spinal nerves (Fig. 11)** are connected to the spinal cord. They are thirty one pairs of them and are segmental in arrangement. They are mixed nerves, they have both motor and sensory parts. The spinal nerves, as soon as they leave the vertebral canal join the blood vessels and form neurovascular bundles. The ***muscular branches*** are predominantly motor branches, enter the muscle bellies and supply the muscles. They do have few sensory branches which carry the stretch sensation from the muscles and tendons. The ***articular*** branches carry sensations from the joints. The ***cutaneous*** *nerves* are sensory nerves supplying the skin. The named cutaneous nerves pierce the deep fascia, branch to supply the skin. Near the skin they are very fine branches and are difficult to locate. The ***vascular branches*** are the fine branches to supply the blood vessels that they accompany.

Nerve plexuses: The upper and lower limbs are outpouchings of the ventral segment of the body. They are supplied by the anterior ramus of the spinal nerves. As they have to pass through narrow passages, they arrange themselves into a plexiform arrangement. In the limbs the nerves have a longitudinal arrangement, e.g. brachial plexus and lumbar plexus. In the trunk region the nerves have a transverse arrangement.

Autonomic nervous system: The internal organs are supplied by the peripheral part of the autonomic nervous system. They are mixed nerves. The sensation that they carry from the internal organs is the stretch sensation. The motor part of the autonomic nervous system has two components, the ***sympathetic*** and the ***parasympathetic***. The autonomic motor nerves have relay ganglia in the peripheral nervous systems. For the parasympathetic nervous systems there are called peripheral parasympathetic ganglia. These are located in the head region, e.g. ciliary ganglion, pterygopalatine ganglion. The relay ganglia of the sympathetic nervous system is the sympathetic chain. It is segmental and is paravertebral in position. They supply glands and smooth muscles of organs. The autonomic nervous system forms nerve plexuses, accompany the blood vessels and form neurovascular bundles and enter the organs through the hila, e.g. aortic plexus hepatic plexus **(Fig. 12)**.

BLOOD VESSELS

The blood vessels form a distribution network in the body. The ***heart*** is the organ which controls the blood vascular system **(Fig. 13)**. The ***aorta*** begins from the left ventricle of the heart, and gives branches to all parts of the body. These are ***arteries*** and carry oxygenated nutritive blood. They end in ***capillaries*** at cellular level. The ***veins*** begin from the capillaries and carry waste products from the cells and reach the right atrium of the heart as superior and inferior vena cava. The deoxygenated blood thus brought to heart is sent to lungs for purification through pulmonary circulation.

You will see blood vessels throughout your dissection. At the time of death the arteries undergo a wave of contraction. So whatever blood is present in the arteries is pushed into the veins. The blood that gets stagnated, gets solidified there and appears bluish to blackish in color. In a cadaver the fine veins look collapsed but can be easily identified due to this coloration in the veins. The arteries look like thin plastic tubes. They show a bulge and when cut, show a clear cavity within. The big arteries like aorta are accompanied by big veins like inferior vena cava. All the small and medium sized arteries are accompanied by two veins called venae comitantes. In the superficial fascia, they are very fine and are called cutaneous vessels. Near the joints the arteries form alternative anastomic channels. These are fine vessels derived

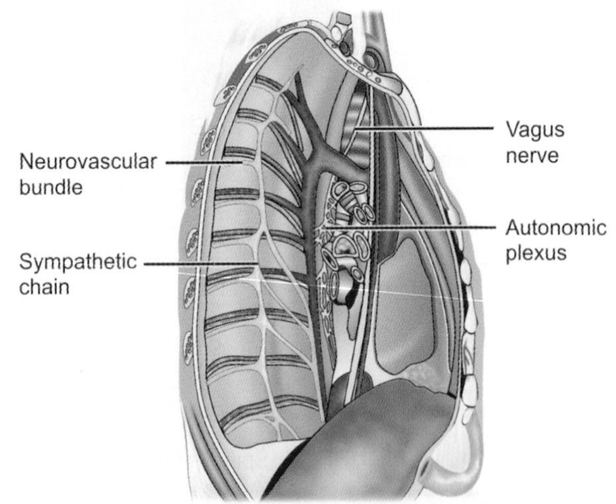

FIGURE 12 Autonomic nervous system

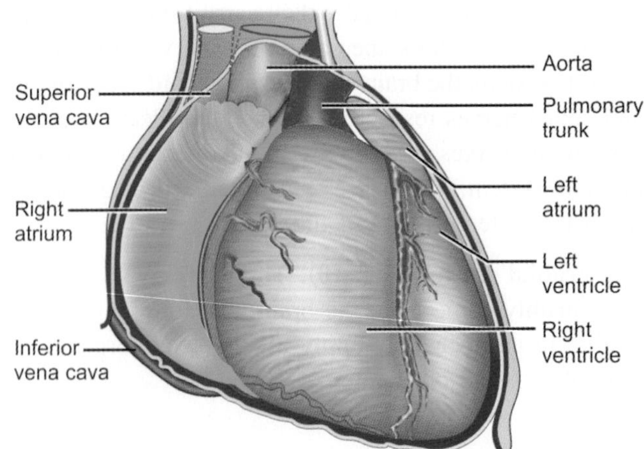

FIGURE 13 Heart

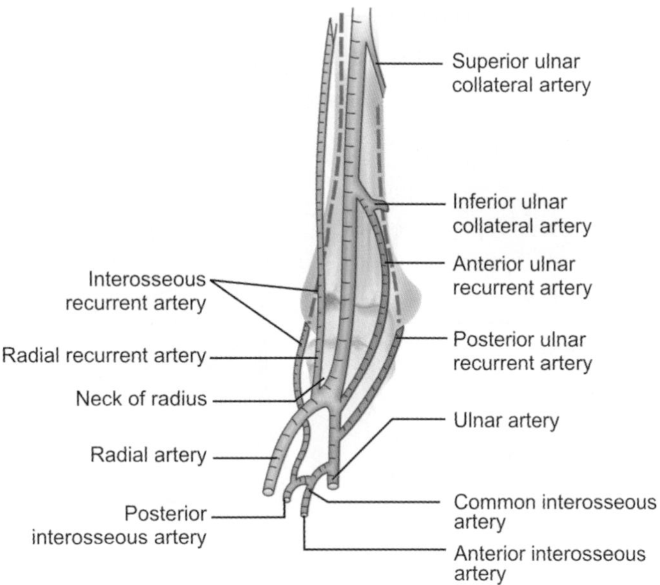

FIGURE 14 Collateral circulation/arterioarterial anastomosis

from the nearby blood vessels. This is called ***collateral circulation/arterioarterial anastomosis*** **(Fig. 14)**. The blood vessels that reach the brain, heart and retina of the eye are ***end arteries***, they do not anastomose with the neighboring vessels.

Functionally the arteries are divided into elastic arteries, muscular arteries and capillary plexus. ***Elastic arteries*** are vessels nearest to the heart. They expand when the heart contracts and the blood is pumped into it, e.g. aorta, carotid arteries. ***Muscular arteries*** or distribution arteries—these are the medium sized arteries. They control the blood flow to any particular organ as per the need. They have more muscle in their walls, e.g. superior mesenteric, obturator artery. ***Capillary plexus***—the arteries are closed tubes. But when the blood vessels reach the cells they form a capillary plexus. At this level the blood plasma oozes out of the capillaries and forms the tissue fluid, in which each and every cell is bathed. The veins and lymph start from the capillary plexus. You can easily see the capillary plexus, by pressing the fingertip. Note that it becomes red in color. That is the tissue fluid that is seen beneath the skin.

Vascular sheaths: The blood vessels when they pass through narrow passages drag connective tissue sheaths with them. In such circumstances, the sheath over the arteries is thicker and the sheath over the veins is thinner, e.g. axillary sheath. At times the lymphatics occupy a special compartment, e.g. femoral sheath.

The ***veins*** begin at the capillary plexus and leave as veins which accompany the arteries. They form ***venae comitantes*** around small and medium sized arteries. They are named veins in relation to big arteries, e.g. femoral artery accompanied by femoral vein. Valves are present in all the veins which drain against gravity and those veins which drain towards gravity have no valves, e.g. external jugular vein internal jugular vein. Many a veins form a ***plexiform arrangement***, e.g. pterygoid plexus, pampiniform plexus of veins. In the brain they are located in the thick dura mater and are called ***venous sinuses***. In limbs and head and neck the veins form a superficial and deep system of veins. The superficial set of veins is subcutaneous in location and is not accompanied by arteries, e.g. external jugular vein, great saphenous vein and cephalic vein. These can be easily identified in people who are fair. In them it can be seen as green bulging structures. These are made use of, to inject intravenous fluids and to withdraw blood for diagnostic purposes.

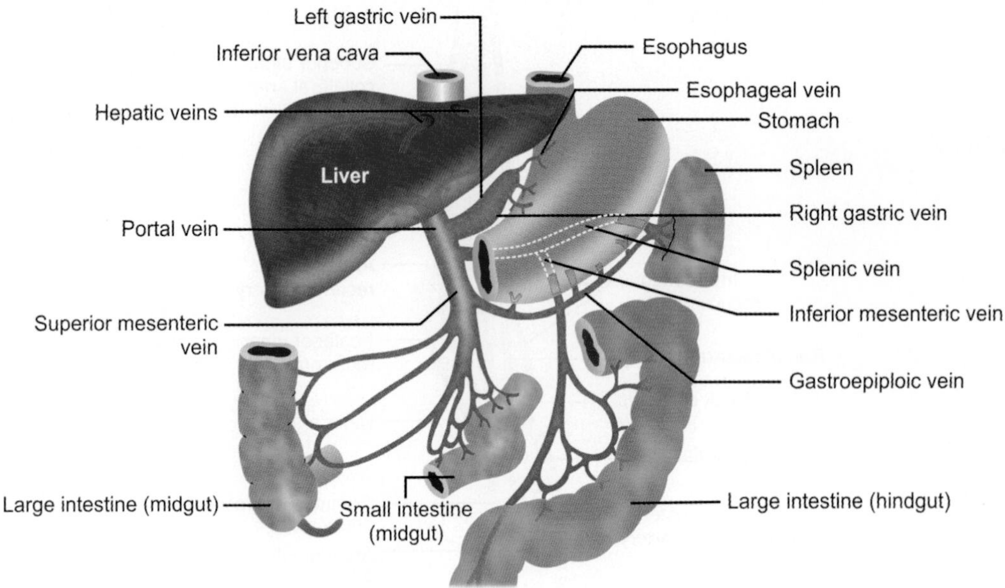

FIGURE 15 Portal system

Portal system (Fig. 15): At few places in the body the veins which begin in the capillaries form bigger veins by receiving more tributaries but again break into capillary network. This is a function based arrangement, e.g. the portal vein. This forms in the walls of the gastrointestinal system, drains the nutritive material from here and carries it to the liver for storage where it further breaks down into capillaries. It is called the portal vein. Such portal systems are present in the kidney as well as near the pituitary gland.

Neurovascular bundle: All the structures in the body are supplied by arteries, veins, lymphatics and nerves. They reach the muscles and the organs as a single unit called neurovascular bundle. They are medium sized arteries and are accompanied by two veins called venae comitantes. In a muscle they enter the center of the muscle belly, or they run along the length of the muscle. In an organ they enter the organ at a port called porta or hilum, e.g. hilum of kidney, porta hepatis. In gastrointestinal tract it runs along the length of the organ.

Lymphatics (Fig. 16): Millions and millions of cells in the body are bathed in tissue fluid. The arterial blood gets the nutrition and seeps out into the tissue fluid at the arterial end of the capillary, the waste products get into circulation at the venous end of the capillary. So the tissue fluid is an exudate of the blood. The lymphatic channels begin at the tissue fluid. These channels drain the bigger molecule which cannot enter back into the venous circulation. It is difficult to locate them in the gross anatomy dissection, as they have very thin walls. The lymphatic channels accompany the blood vessels.

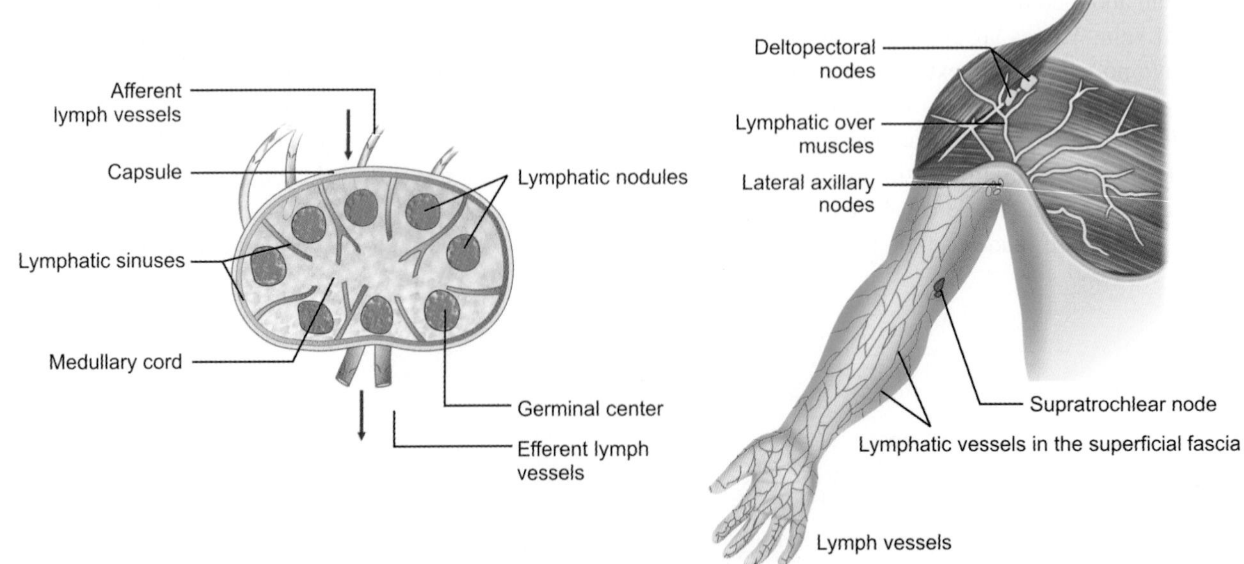

FIGURE 16 Lymphatics

Lymph nodes: The lymphatic channels pass through lymph nodes at strategic points in the body. These identify the foreign bodies and initiate the antibody reaction. These are part of immune system in the body. Ultimately, the lymph reaches back into the venous system.

The lymph, the cerebrospinal fluid, the urine and the fluid in the anterior and posterior chamber of the eye, all are filtrates of the blood only. All these form a part of the circulatory system of the body.

INTERNAL ORGANS

Each of the internal organ has its own size, shape and location. The organs are kept in bags of fluid, e.g. the ***pericardium, peritoneum.*** They protect the organs from getting rubbed off during movement. The internal organs are further protected in bony cases, e.g. brain in skull, eyeballs in orbit. The thorax lodges the heart and lungs and the abdomen lodges parts of the gastrointestinal system and urinary system.

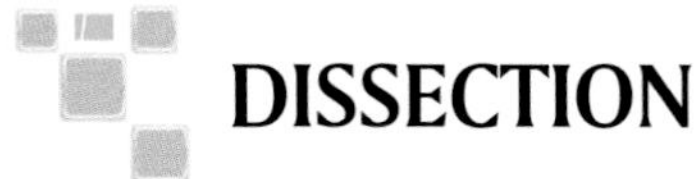

DISSECTION

While undertaking dissection we follow regional method. We expect one cadaver is given to a batch of students for the academic year. The body is divided into six parts – the upper limb, thorax, abdomen, lower limb, head and neck and central nervous system, and it is dissected in that order.

Upper limb and lower limb: The skeleton with the bones and joints forms the framework of limbs. The muscles which act on the joints are arranged in functional groups and kept in compartments along with its neurovascular bundle. The compartments are separated by septa and all the groups are wrapped by deep fascia and covered by skin.

Thorax and abdomen: Together forms the trunk. Here the skeleton forms an external protective covering. The organs are located in its interior. The organs are kept in specialized compartments, well protected by bags of fluid.

Head and neck: In this region, the head, neck and the back are dealt. The head is the part of communication with the external world. It has a concentration of sense organs and brain and structures associated with them. All these sense organs and the brain are protected in bony cases. The respiratory and digestive systems begin here.

The neck is a passageway for the organs of respiration and digestion which communicate with external world, and the neurovascular bundle where the blood vessels ascend up and the cranial nerves descend down. Back is the part located posterior to the axis, the vertebral column, it is muscular in nature. The vertebral canal lodges the spinal cord.

Central nervous system: It constitutes the brain and spinal cord. It is made up of cell bodies of neurons which form the gray nuclear matter and axons and dendrites which form the tracts. In gross anatomy, it is not possible to identify the individual details. The formalin hardened brain and spinal cord are soft structures. Here we cut the organ with special brain knife and stain with special stain to bring out the differentiation between the nuclei and fibres.

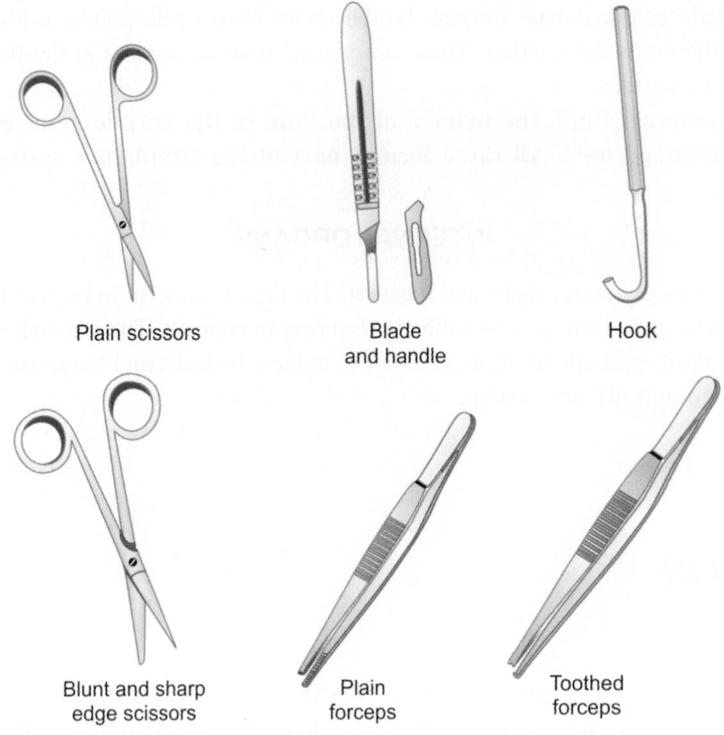

FIGURE 17 Instruments

INSTRUMENTS AND THEIR USAGE

The cadaver is your subject and your teacher. The dissection manual and the instruments are your tools to learn this ocean of material. Choose your instruments correctly, use them properly, identify the structures correctly, perform and learn their functions properly **(Fig. 17)**.

Scalpel with blade: Here two to three sizes are available. You may buy at least two sizes, a bigger size to cut the skin, a smaller blade to cut small structures. The blades may get blunt very fast, so always keep extra blades in hand.

Scissors: Again you need more than one pair of scissors. A 6" blunt and sharp scissors is useful for cutting muscles. A 4" both sharp edge scissors is very much essential to cut smaller structures like tendons, blood vessels and fascia.

Forceps: You need small 4" forceps to hold fine nerves and arteries, a medium 6" plain forceps to do most of the dissection, and a 6" or 8" toothed forceps to hold the skin during skin reflection.

Hook: A single hook is necessary to lift the blood vessels and nerves and a double hook is essential to lift the muscles and organs.

Probe: A long probe or long needles are useful in tracing the fine structures without damaging them.

Chistle, hammer, small saw, brain knife are required for dissections. Generally, these are available in the dissection hall.

DISSECTION METHODOLOGY

Before you begin, you should be familiar with area of dissection. You should read the chapter before hand and be aware of what to expect in your dissection. Make correct ***incision lines*** with a white wet chalk piece. Put your first skin reflection line along the skin marking. Use a sharp blade and make a fine cut slowly and gradually through the thickness of the dermis. In ***skin reflection,*** you are separating the dermis of the skin from the hypodermis and superficial fascia. You have to use the toothed forceps to pull the skin and hold the blade in a slant and keep putting water as you are reflecting the skin. This will hydrate the connective tissue and make it more yielding. If you are not careful there is more chance of removing the structures in chunks. The structures in the ***superficial fascia*** are generally masked by fat. The fat is variable in different parts of the body and in different people. Identifying structures in superficial fascia is time consuming and is not essential to identify all the structures. The ***deep fascia*** has many modifications. You should learn to observe all the features before you cut it. Once you cut the deep fascia all the structures, the muscles, vessels, nerves, tendons joints etc. just unfold. All of them are surrounded by the loose connective tissue, the packing material of our body. The ***loose connective tissue*** yields when you hydrate it. It is essential to hydrate the parts during dissection. Your responsibility is to clean this loose connective tissue and identify the structures. Once you open the deep fascia do not use the scalpel. Use the forceps, the scissors and the back of the handle to separate the tissue and remove it. ***Muscles*** are big and appear brown in color. Use your hand especially while separating the muscles, testing the muscles and holding the bigger blood vessels. Always hold the ***blood vessels and nerves*** proximally and use the forceps to clear the connective tissue and trace the branches. While removing the ***internal organs*** you need to use the twine and make two knots, cut the organ between the knots. This prevents leakage of the contents. You may use saw, chistle and hammer while removing the brain from the cranial cavity and performing other dissections on the skull.

The dissection schedule of each region is designed in such a way that you penetrate into the body methodically and understand the interrelationship of the structures within a particular area. As you are dissecting, support your study by performing/feeling or locating the structures on a living body. Simultaneously, study the osteology and X-rays/CT scans.

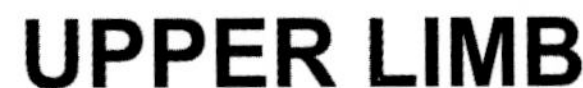

CHAPTER 2

UPPER LIMB

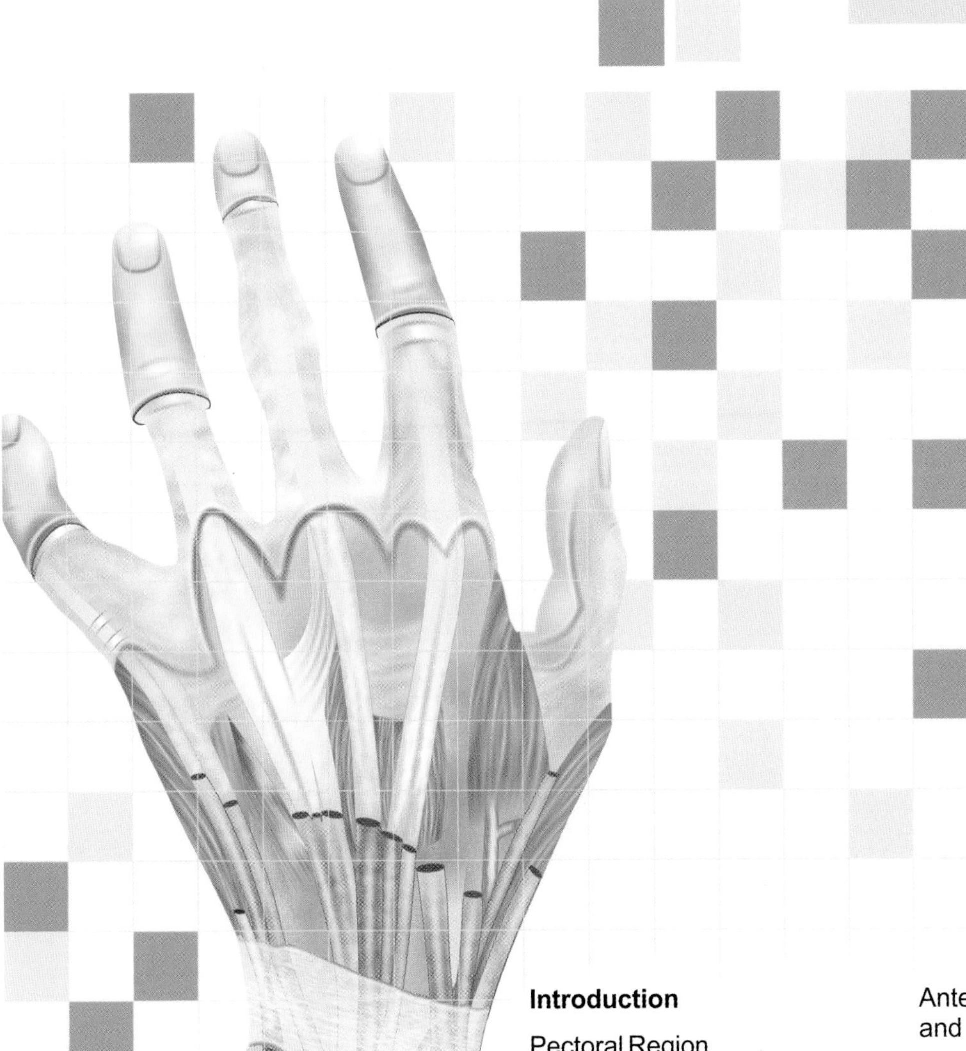

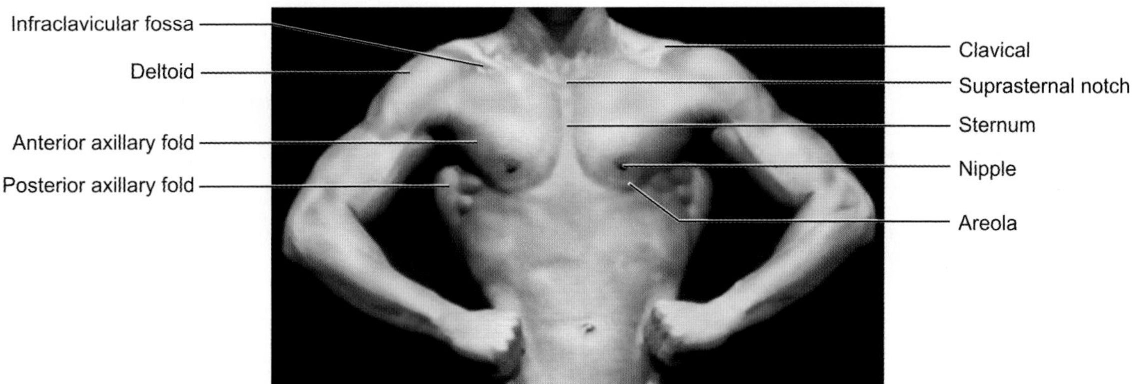

FIGURE 3 Surface anatomy

SURFACE ANATOMY (Figs 3 and 4)

Identify the suprasternal notch, in the midline. Feel the ***sternum*** and the ***clavicle*** which are subcutaneous. The ribs though not subcutaneous are palpable. Try to identify them. Put your finger below the clavicle. The space that you can identify is the first intercostal space. The rib felt immediately below is the ***second rib***. Count the other ribs from this level onwards. The ***anterior axillary fold*** is a muscular fold formed by the pectoralis major muscle. Identify the ***infraclavicular fossa;*** this is a depression below the middle of the clavicle and between the bulging ***pectoralis major***, and the ***deltoid*** muscles. Feel the ***posterior axillary fold***. It is formed by the latissimus dorsi.

Nipple and areola: Identify the nipple over the fourth intercostal space, and the colored areola surrounding it. This is the position in the adult males. The nipple lodges the lactiferous ducts. These are the ducts of the mammary gland. The gland is rudimentary in males and is well developed in adult females.

Go to a female body and study the extent. Note that it extends from the lateral border of the sternum to the midaxillary line, and superoinferiorly from second to sixth ribs. It is conical in young females to pendulus in old. The position of the areola and the nipple are variable in females depending on the state of breast. Note that the areola is surrounded by fine hairs.

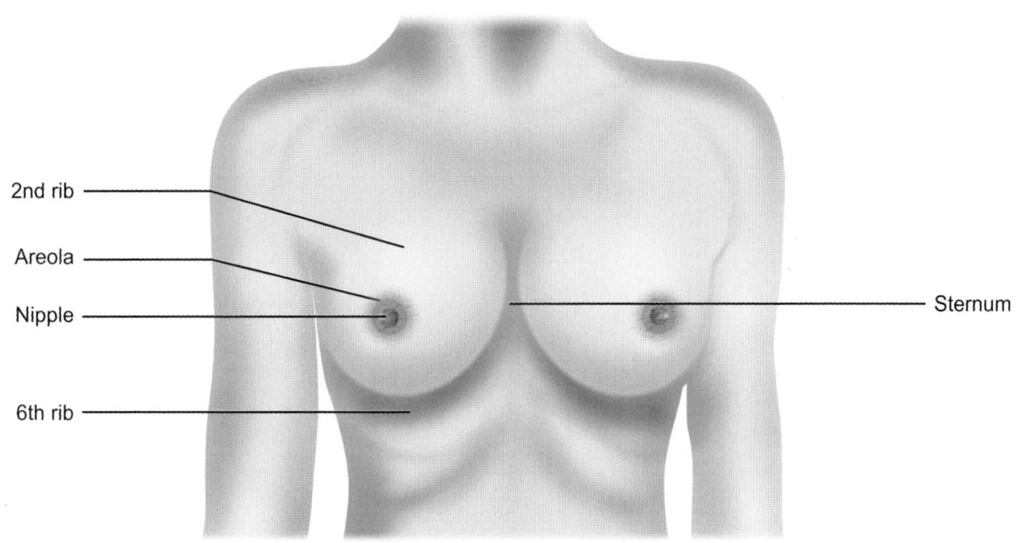

FIGURE 4 Surface anatomy

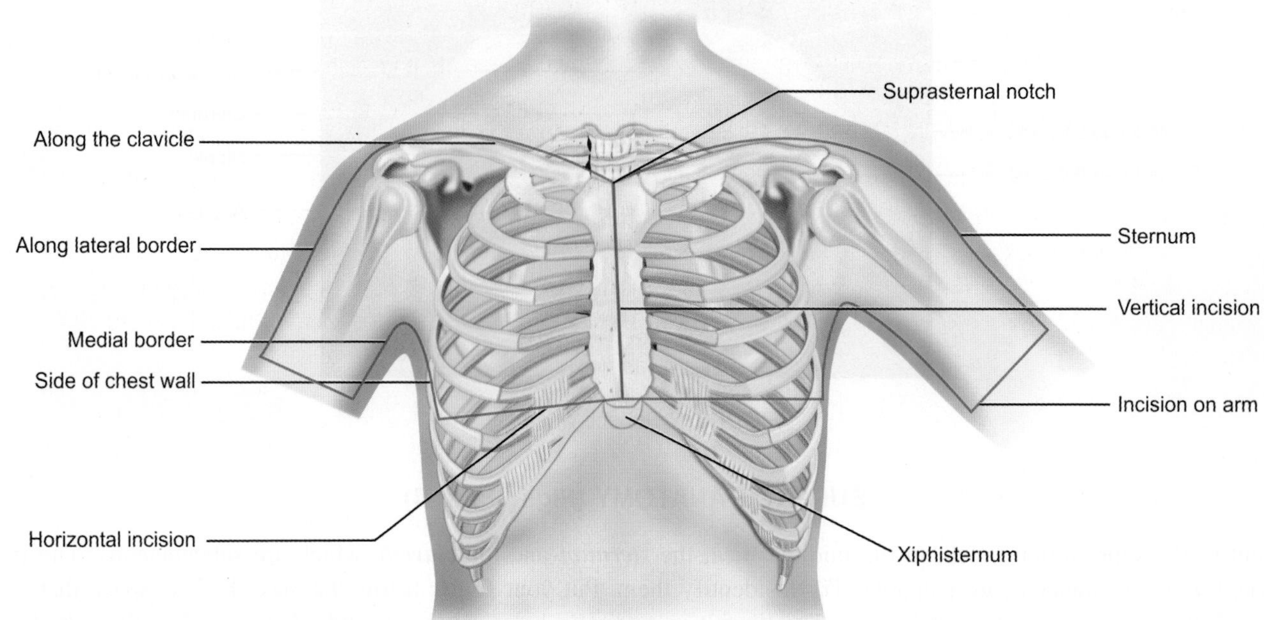

FIGURE 5 Skin incision—pectoral region

SKIN INCISION (Fig. 5)

Dissection: As per the figure make the following incisions.

Make a vertical incision from suprasternal notch to the xiphisternum in the midline; a horizontal incision from the suprasternal notch along the clavicle to the acromian process; a vertical incision from the acromian process, along the lateral border of the arm to the middle of the arm; horizontal incision from the xiphisternum to the side of the chest wall as far as you can reach; a horizontal incision along the middle of the arm from lateral to medial border; a vertical incision along the posterior wall of axilla to join the lower horizontal incision on the chest wall as well as the arm.

With the above incision the total skin in front of the chest wall, axilla and anterior aspect of the arm will be removed. Skin in this area is very thin. Reflect and remove the total skin with a sharp scalpel. In the female body retain the nipple and areola.

SUPERFICIAL FASCIA

The superficial fascia is occupied by the mammary gland, cutaneous vessels and nerves.

BREAST/MAMMARY GLAND (Figs 6 and 7)

Go to a female body and study the organ. The mammary gland is a modified sweat gland located within the superficial fascia. In adult females, it has got around twenty lobes radiating from the nipple. The glandular tissue in each lobe is drained by the lactiferous duct, which opens on the nipple. The lobes are separated by septa and the interstices of the gland is filled by fat. In an adult female, it is made up of only duct system. During pregnancy and lactating time the mammary gland increases in size by developing glandular tissue and becomes functional. A small part of the breast tissue, called axillary tail of Spence pierces through the deep fascia and reaches the axilla.

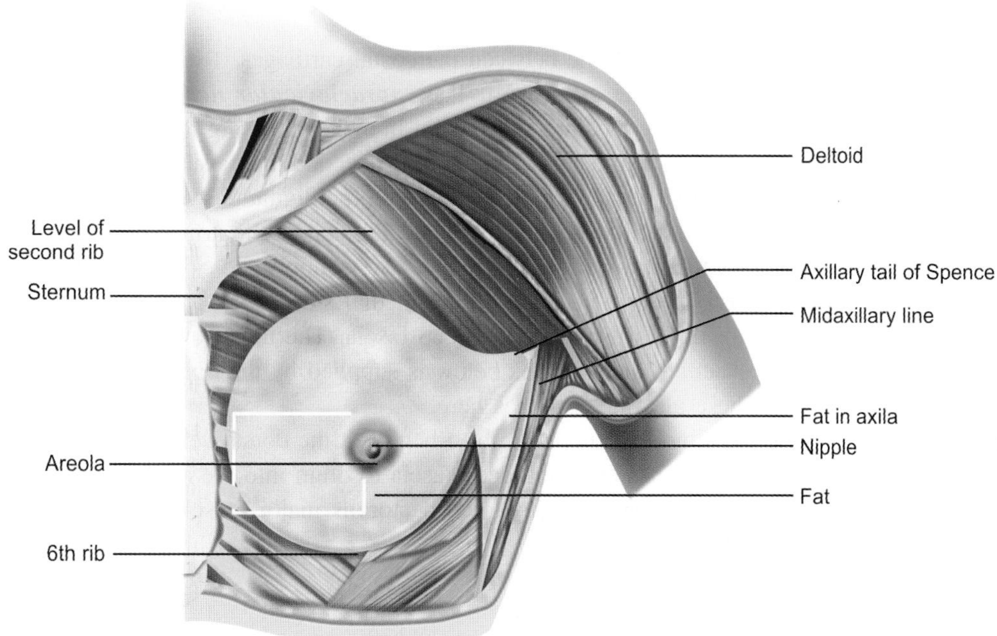

FIGURE 6 Breast/mammary gland

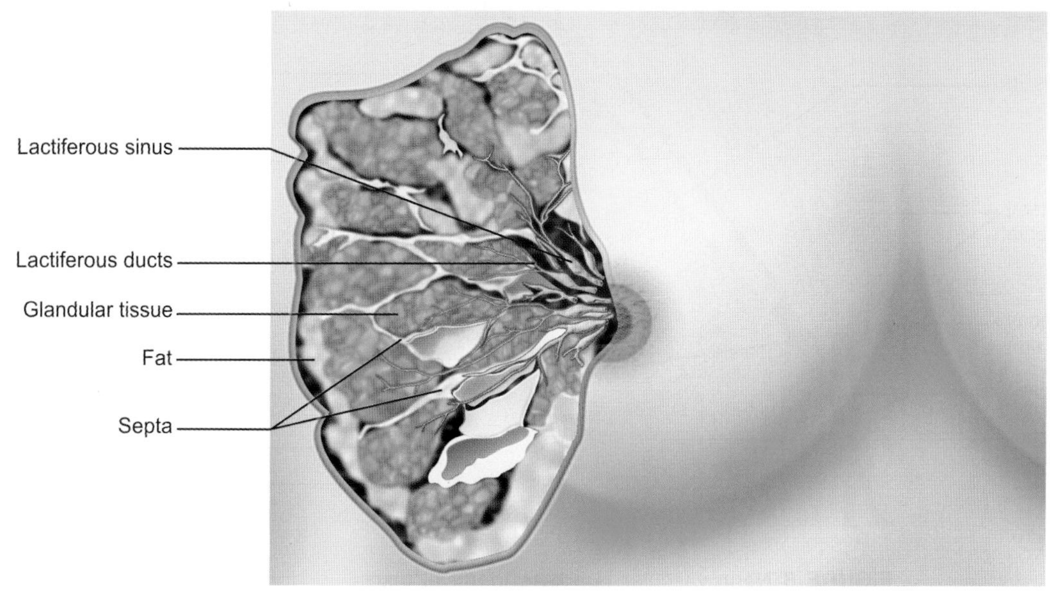

FIGURE 7 Breast/mammary gland

Blood supply: The gland is supplied by the perforating branches of the internal thoracic, intercostal arteries and the branches of the lateral thoracic artery. The veins drain into the corresponding veins.

The lymphatic drainage of the mammary gland is of great importance due the common occurrence of cancer in this gland. Read it from a standard textbook.

Dissection: Carefully try to dissect the fat away from the breast tissue. You can identify the duct pattern and the septae. You can see the breast tissue reaching the deep fascia. Separate it from the deep fascia and remove it. While doing so note its deeper relations, the pectoralis major and the serratus anterior muscles which form its floor. Try to trace the fine blood vessels leaving the breast. Identify the cutaneous vessels and nerves on the chest wall, in the axillary floor and the lateral side of the arm.

NEUROVASCULAR BUNDLE (Fig. 8)

The ***anterior cutaneous nerves and blood vessels*** lie between the costal cartilages, 1 cm lateral to the sternum. They supply the anteromedial side of the skin of the chest wall. The ***supraclavicular nerves*** are very thin and are not accompanied by arteries. They are lateral, intermediate and medial branches crossing the clavicle. All these branches may not be seen clearly. They supply the skin of the chest wall up to the second intercostal space. The ***lateral cutaneous vessels*** and ***nerves*** lie along the midaxillary line. Identify them between the digitations of serratus anterior. The second and third lateral cutaneous nerves cross the axilla and reach the medial side of the arm. The second joins the medial cutaneous nerve of the arm and is called ***intercostobrachial nerve***. They supply the skin along the lateral side of the chest wall. The ***medial cutaneous nerve of the arm*** is along the medial side of the arm. It supplies the skin on the medial side of the arm. Try to identify this as it pierces the deep fascia. The upper end of the skin over the arm is supplied by the lateral supraclavicular nerves, and the area below is supplied by the ***upper lateral cutaneous nerve of arm,*** branches of the radial nerve. These are fine branches here.

Cephalic vein is the big superficial vein of the upper limb. It begins at the dorsal venous arch of the dorsum of the hand, traverses the forearm and arm, where it pierces the deep fascia to drain into the axillary vein. Identify this vein in the deltopectoral groove, the groove between the deltoid and pectoralis major muscle **(Fig. 8).**

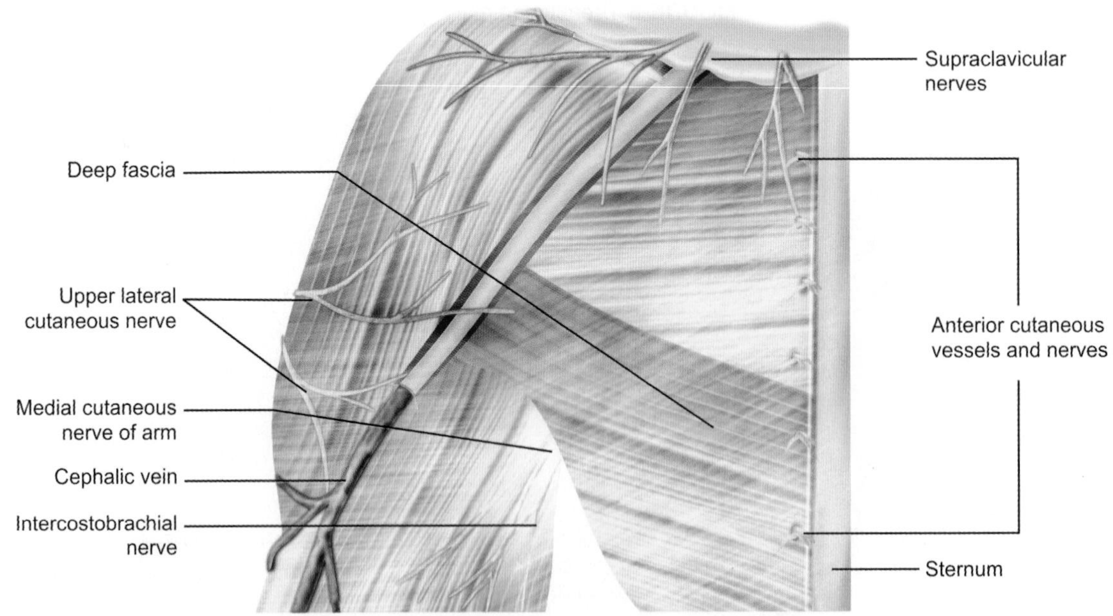

FIGURE 8 Neurovascular bundle–superficial fascia

DEEP FASCIA

Identify the white glistening deep fascia here. It covers the pectoralis major muscle where it is called ***pectoral fascia,*** it covers the deltoid, it covers the arm pit between the anterior and posterior axillary folds where it is called the ***axillary fascia,*** on a deeper aspect it covers the pectoralis minor and the subclavius muscle where it is called the ***clavipectoral*** *fascia*.

PECTORALIS MAJOR (Fig. 9)

Dissection: Remove the white fascia, the pectoral fascia that overlies the pectoralis major muscle.

Note that it is a big fan-shaped muscle covering the full area of the anterior aspect of the chest and forms the anterior axillary fold. Identify the origin of the muscle on the body and study the same on the skeleton—it has a ***clavicular origin*** from the medial half of the anterior surface of the clavicle, a ***sternal origin*** from the lateral part of the anterior aspect of the sternum, a ***costal origin*** from the anterior aspect of the upper six costal cartilages and an ***aponeurotic origin*** from the upper aspect of the external oblique aponeurosis. All the fibres converge to form the anterior wall of the axilla. Note that the clavicular fibres descend down and form the superficial lamina near axilla. The lower fibres run upwards and form the deep lamina and the fibres in-between remain between the two **(Fig. 9).**

Pectoralis major is supplied by medial and lateral pectoral nerves. They reach the muscle on its undersurface. Study the action of the muscle by performing the action against resistance. Perform flexion and note the contraction of clavicular fibres. Perform extension and note the contraction of sternocostal fibres. Suspend yourself from parallel bars and raise the body slowly, notice the contraction of the total muscle. The fibres cross the shoulder joint in front, so can rotate the humerus medially. It is flexor, extensor, antigravity muscle and a medial rotator.

Dissection: Cut the pectoralis major by a vertical incision near the insertion. Identify the lower border of the muscle throughout its extent. Clear the fat and connective tissue and lift the muscle with the back of your scalpel along the inferior border. Detach the muscle from its costal and clavicular origin and lift it towards the lateral side. While doing so note the nerve supply reaching the undersurface, the nerve that pierces through the pectoralis minor is the **medial pectoral nerve**. It may pierce the minor through the middle or nearer to the insertion. Trace the **lateral pectoral nerve**. It pierces the clavipectoral fascia above the pectoralis minor.

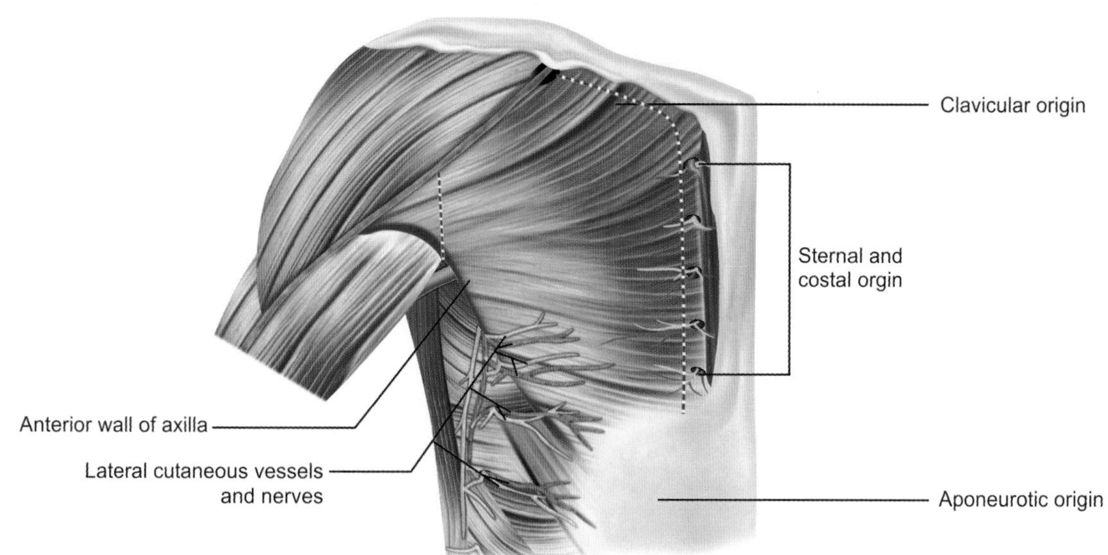

FIGURE 9 Pectoralis major

STRUCTURES UNDER COVER OF PECTORALIS MAJOR (Figs 10 and 11)

The area from the undersurface of the clavicle to the floor of the axilla is occupied by a thick fascia. It encloses ***subclavius muscle,*** forms ***clavipectoral fascia*** between the subclavius muscle and pectoralis minor, encloses ***pectoralis minor*** muscle and extends as the ***suspensory ligament*** to the floor of the axilla.

Dissection: Remove the cut part of the pectoralis major muscle and see the structures under cover of it. While doing so keep a small part of the muscle along with the nerve supply.

Identify the ***clavicle***. See the ***subclavius*** muscle through the fascia. It encloses the muscles and is attached to the two lips of the groove into which the subclavius muscle is attached (identify this on a dry bone). Note that this fascia stretching between the subclavius and the pectoralis minor muscle. This is called ***clavipectoral fascia***. Note the ***thoracoacromial artery*** coming out piercing this membrane. Trace its four branches, the pectoral, the acromial, the deltoid and the clavicular. They supply the areas as per their name. See the ***lateral pectoral nerve*** piercing the clavipectoral fascia and accompanying the thoracoacromial artery. Identify the ***deltopectoral groove,*** the gap between the pectoralis major and deltoid muscle. Note the ***cephalic vein*** in the deltopectoral groove. Note its point of dipping in through the clavipectoral fascia, near the infraclavicular fossa. See the ***pectoralis minor*** muscle glistening through the fascia. Here the fascia splits and encloses it. See the thick fascia below the pectoralis minor muscle to the floor of the axilla. It is called the ***suspensory ligament***. It pulls the skin of the armpit and raises it.

Dissection: Remove the deep fascia and identify the muscles.

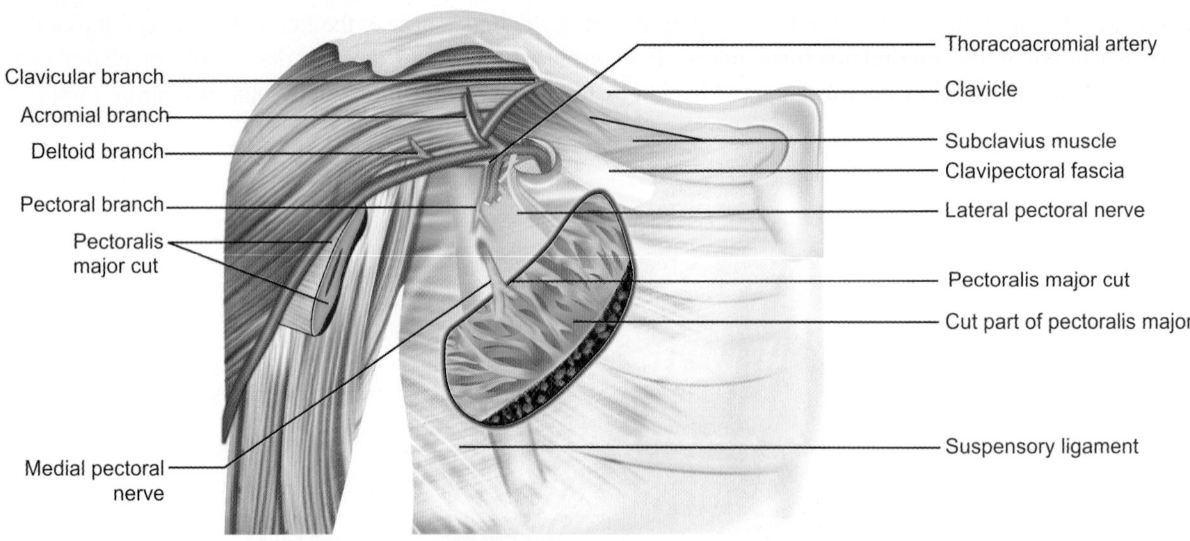

FIGURE 10 Structures under cover of pectoralis major

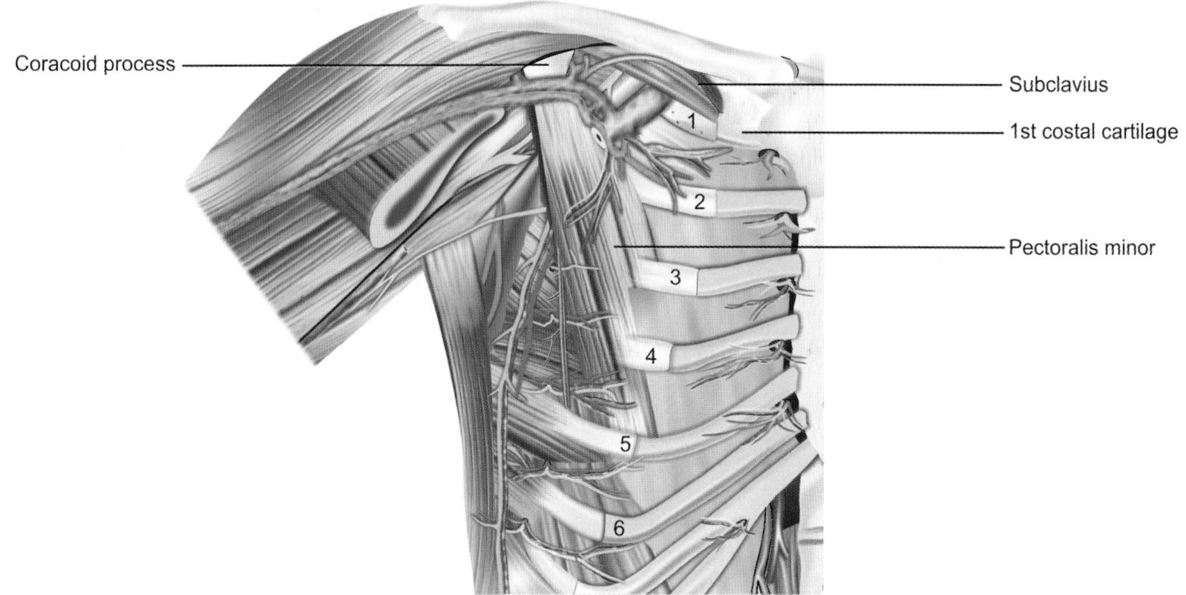

FIGURE 11 Subclavius and pectoralis minor

Subclavius muscle: This is a muscle of pectoral girdle. See the subclavian groove on the inferior surface of the clavicle. This gives insertion to the subclavius muscle. See the 1st costal cartilage and the first rib junction. See the subclavius muscle extending from here to the undersurface of the clavicle. This muscle is supplied by nerve to subclavius, coming from the neck region (this will be seen in the head and neck dissection). The subclavius is a depressor of the clavicle.

Pectoralis minor muscle: It arises from the outer surface of 2, 3, 4 or 3, 4, 5th ribs near their anterior angles. Trace this triangular muscle to its insertion into the coracoid process. Look for its nerve supply from the medial pectoral nerve. Pectoralis minor is a girdle muscle and it depresses the girdle.

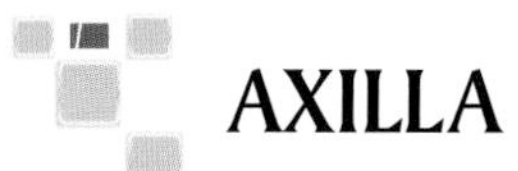

AXILLA

BOUNDARIES: The arrangement of the pectoral girdle on the chest wall creates a gap between the bones. It is described as a truncated area called the axilla. The ***anterior wall*** of the axilla is formed by the pectoralis major, the pectoralis minor, the subclavius, the clavipectoral fascia and the suspensory ligament (pectoral region). The ***posterior wall*** is formed by the scapula, the subscapularis muscle, the teres major and the latissimus dorsi muscle. The ***medial wall*** is formed by the upper five ribs and its intercostal spaces, covered by the serratus anterior muscle. The ***lateral wall*** is formed the part of the humerus between the anterior and posterior walls. This is called intertubercular sulcus and lodges the long head of biceps and coracobrachialis muscle. The ***apex*** is formed by the outer border of the first rib, the superior border of the scapula and the posterior surface of the clavicle. The ***floor*** is formed by the axillary fascia that stretches between the pectoralis major and latissimus dorsi muscle. The neurovascular bundle of the upper limb enters the apex of the axilla, passes along its length and continues on into the arm.

CONTENTS: The axillary artery, axillary vein, axillary lymph nodes and the infraclavicular part of the brachial plexus form the contents of the axilla. The position of pectoralis minor is taken advantage in describing the axillary contents. Here the axillary artery forms the central part. The axillary artery is divided into three parts for descriptive purposes. The part from the outer border of first rib to the upper border of the pectoralis minor, the part behind the pectoralis minor and the part between the pectoralis minor and the lower border of teres major. The brachial plexus is located around the axillary artery. Here it presents two parts, the cords stage and the branches stage. The cord stage of the brachial plexus lies around the first and second parts of axillary artery and the branches are related to the third part of axillary artery. The axillary vein is the most superficial structure in the axilla and the axillary lymph nodes are spread throughout the axilla.

The ***axillary lymph nodes*** are small black nodule like structures seen within the fat of the axilla. They are classified and studied according to the positions that they occupy. They are called ***pectoral group*** in the anterior wall, ***subscapular group*** along the posterior wall ***lateral group*** along the axillary vessels, the ***central group*** accompanies the axillary vein and ***apical group*** is located near the apex of the axilla. They drain the lymph from the upper limb, breast and the back. As you are cleaning, try to identify their position.

Dissection: Remove the fat along with the lymph nodes from the axilla and identify the following structures with the pectoralis minor *in situ*.

AXILLARY CONTENTS – 1 (Fig. 12)

Here you will see the superficial structures, proximal and distal to the pectoralis minor.

Locate the ***intercostobrachial nerve*** in the lateral aspect of the second intercostals space. This nerve is the lateral cutaneous branch of the second intercostal nerve. Trace it to the medial cutaneous nerve of arm to which it joins. The ***medial cutaneous nerve of the arm*** is the most superficial nerve seen in the medial aspect of the arm. You may note, the nerve piercing the deep fascia of the arm. This lies between the axillary vein and the skin. The ***axillary vein*** is the big prominent superficial structure seen here. Identify the axillary vein, the bluish, most superficial structure. It is formed at the outer border of the teres major muscle, by the basilic vein and the venae commitantis of the brachial artery. It receives all the tributaries accompanying the branches of the axillar artery. It also receives the cephalic vein near its termination. Pull the axillary vein towards you and locate two nerves—the ***medial cutaneous nerve of forearm*** a thinner superficial nerve and the ***ulnar nerve*** and thicker deeply placed nerve. These two nerves run between axillary vein and axillary artery. Locate the ***axillary artery*** which lies deep to the axillary vein. Note the ***median nerve*** on the axillary artery. It is formed by two roots called the medial and lateral roots. See them, the medial root comes from the medial cord and lateral from the lateral cord of brachial plexus. Trace the lateral root of the median nerve upwards. It joins the thick, laterally located nerve, the ***musculocutaneous nerve***. The lateral root of median nerve and the musculocutaneous nerve are terminal divisions of the ***lateral cord***. Locate this lateral cord which is a thick nerve related to the lateral aspect of the second part of the axillary artery. Pull the medial root of the median nerve and trace it up to the medial cord which lies medial to the second part of the axillary artery.

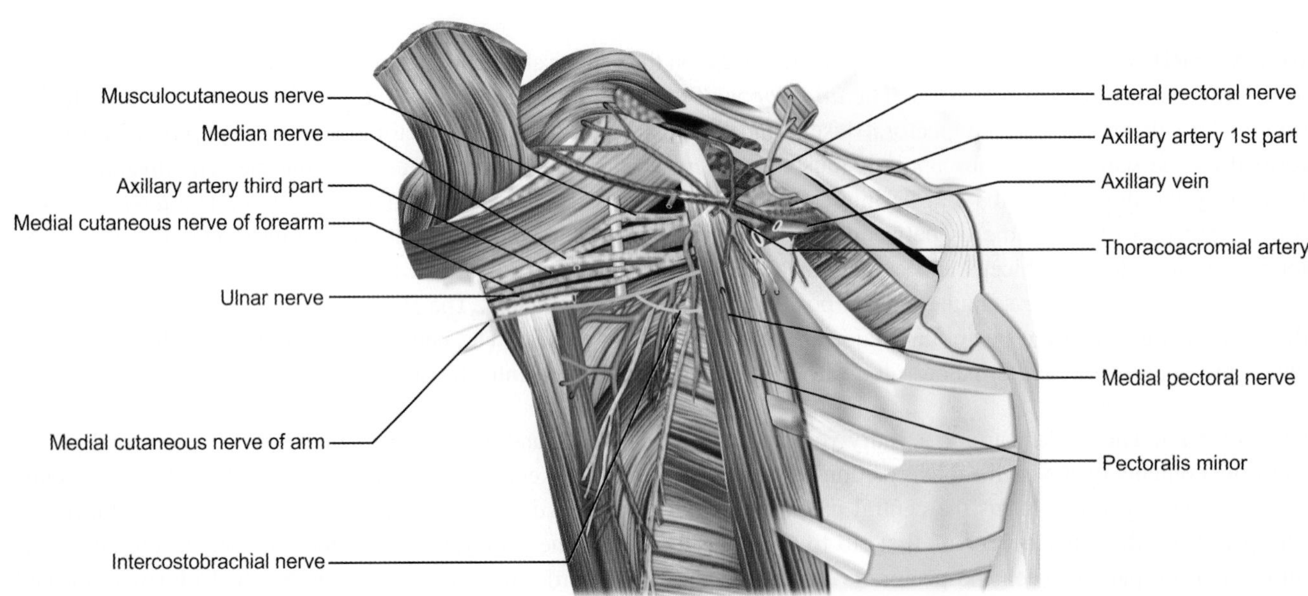

FIGURE 12 Axillary contents–1

THE AXILLARY ARTERY: See the three parts of the axillary artery. See the ***thoracoacromial artery*** along the upper border of the pectoralis minor and the ***lateral thoracic artery*** along its lower border. These two branches are given off from the second part of the axillary artery behind the pectoralis minor. The thoracoacromial artery moves upwards and the lateral thoracic artery moves downwards. The thoracoacromial artery is the artery of supply to the anterior wall, deltoid and acromian process. The ***lateral thoracic artery*** is the artery of supply to the medial wall of axilla and the mammary gland. The lateral thoracic artery runs vertically down along the outer border of pectoralis minor accompanied by the long thoracic nerve and supplies the serratus anterior muscle.

Dissection: Detach the pectoralis minor from its origin and reflect it towards its insertion. You can cut and remove the muscle leaving a small part attached to the coracoid process. Cut and remove part of the axillary vein to identify the following. Cut the thoracoacromial artery and the lateral thoracic artery.

AXILLARY CONTENTS – 2 (Fig. 13)

Here you will see the structures lying in a deeper plane, deep to the pectoralis minor.

See the first part of the axillary artery. This gives off a small artery called the ***superior thoracic artery*** and supplies the upper part of thorax. The second part of the axillary artery lies deep to the pectoralis minor muscle. See the cut ends of the ***thoracoacromial artery*** and the ***lateral thoracic artery***. Clean the 3rd part of the axillary artery between the pectoralis minor and the teres major. Identify three branches given off from this. The big artery that is seen on the ventral aspect of the posterior wall is the ***subscapular artery*** which goes to the back along the lateral border of the scapula to reach the back of the scapula to participate in the subscapular anastomoses. After giving off the ***circumflex scapular artery*** it continues down as the ***thoracodorsal artery***/artery to latissimus dorsi to supply the latissimus dorsi muscle. Identify two more arteries given off from the third part of the axillary artery. The ***anterior circumflex humeral artery*** is given off from the lateral aspect of the axillary artery. Locate this artery and note that it disappears under cover of the biceps muscle. Feel the neck of the humerus and note the ***posterior circumflex humeral artery***. This is given off from the lateral part of axillary artery along with the anterior circumflex humeral artery but this is deeper in position and bigger in size, note that it leaves the axilla to reach the posterior aspect of the arm along the posterior surface of the neck of the humerus.

Axillary artery branches are variable. If they are not seen in their normal positions, it means that they have a variable origin.

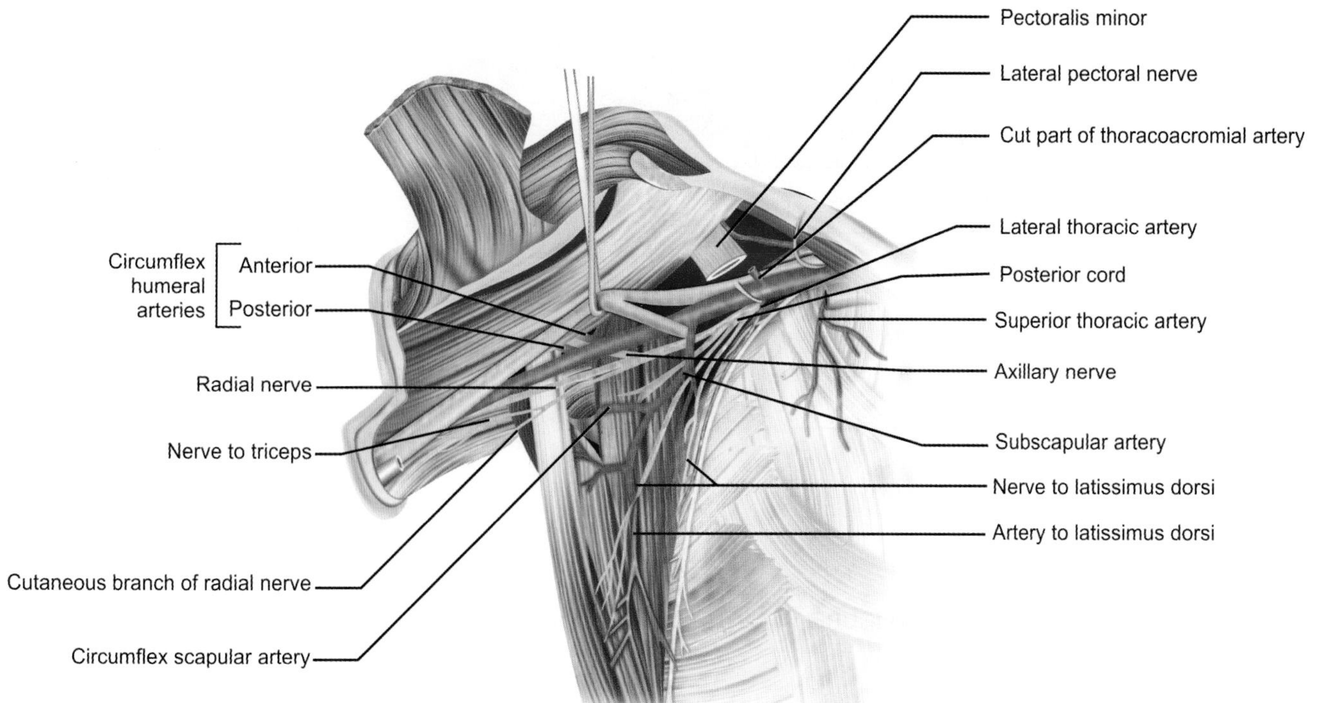

FIGURE 13 Axillary contents–2

Retrace the cut part of the ***lateral pectoral nerve to the lateral cord.*** Retrace the ***medial pectoral nerve*** into the medial cord. Pull the nerves laterally and clean and locate the thick ***axillary nerve*** accompanying the posterior circumflex humeral artery. This nerve lies posterior to the third part of the axillary artery and in front of the musculature of the scapula. Locate a second thick nerve lying deep to the axillary artery. It is the ***radial nerve.*** Trace these two nerves proximal to the second part of the axillary artery and note the thick ***posterior cord.*** Note that the radial nerve gives off two cutaneous and two muscular branches before entering into the spiral groove—the ***lower lateral cutaneous nerve* of arm, *posterior cutaneous nerve of arm*** and the ***nerve to the medial head and long heads of triceps muscle.*** Note that these nerves along with radial nerve leave the axilla between the muscles. Trace three nerves from the posterior cord, the nerve to the ***latissimus dorsi/thoracodorsal nerve,*** the ***lower subscapular nerve*** and the ***upper subscapular nerve.*** Trace them to the respective muscles. The upper subscapular nerve is given quite high up from the cord and immediately enters the subscapularis muscle. Pull the arm forward and locate this nerve entering into the muscle or it can be seen in a later dissection

MEDIAL AND POSTERIOR WALL (Fig. 14)

Dissection: Clean the connective tissue between the chest wall and the ventral aspect of the posterior axillary wall and note the following structures.

MEDIAL WALL: Identify the ***serratus anterior*** muscle arising by eight slips from the outer surfaces of the 1st rib to the eighth rib near its anterior angles (conform its origin on a skeleton). It winds round the chest wall and reach the back to get inserted into the medial border of the scapula. It acts on the pectoral girdle as a protractor. Identify the *long* ***thoracic nerve*** seen on the external surface of the serratus anterior muscle. This supplies the serratus anterior muscle (the insertion will be seen in the dissection of the back).

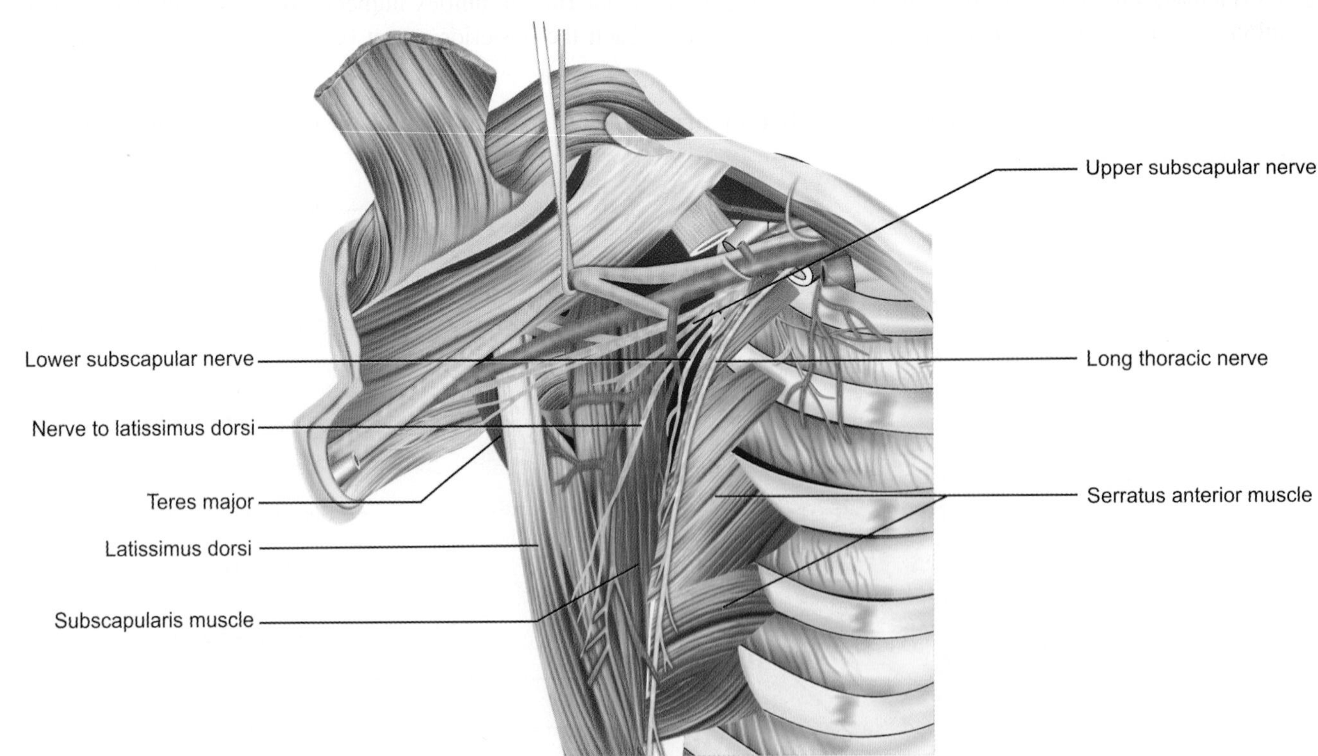

FIGURE 14 Medial and posterior wall of axila

POSTERIOR WALL: The ***latissimus dorsi*** muscle forms the lateral aspect of the posterior axillary wall. The part that is seen here is the insertion aspect and the origin of this muscle is seen on the back of the trunk. Reidentify the ***thoracodorsal nerve***/nerve to latissimus dorsi and the ***thoracodorsal artery,*** the artery supplying the latissimus dorsi. The ***subscapularis*** muscle occupies the ventral aspect of the scapula, see this muscle. The ***lateral border of the scapula*** can be felt between the latissimus dorsi and subscapularis muscle. The ***teres major muscle***—this is a muscle of the scapular region. It forms the posterior axillary fold along with the latissimus dorsi. In fact, the latissimus dorsi winds round and lies ventral and medial to the teres major.

STERNOCLAVICULAR JOINT (Fig. 15)

This is a plane synovial joint between the large medial end of clavicle and the shallow notch on the superolateral angle of the manubrium sterni and the superior surface of the first costal cartilage. Identify this joint on the cadaver as well as on the skeleton. This is the only articulation of the upper limb with the trunk as the scapula is suspended by musculature to the trunk. The clavicle acts as strut to keep the scapula in position and transmits the forces from the upper limb to the trunk.

Dissection: Clean the anterior aspect of the joint. Identify the medial end of the clavicle, the superolateral angle of manubrium sterni and the first costal cartilage. The **capsule** connects ends of both the bones. Identify the capsule on the anterior aspect. Slit it to see the interior of the joint. Identify the ***articular disc*** inside. It is a fibrocartilaginous circular plate attached to the capsule peripherally. Identify the ***costoclavicular ligament*** extending from the first costal cartilage and the first rib to the inferior surface of the clavicle near its medial end. It is a very thick powerful ligament. The total disarticulation of the joint will be done in the head and neck dissection after studying the structures arising from the upper part of the clavicle.

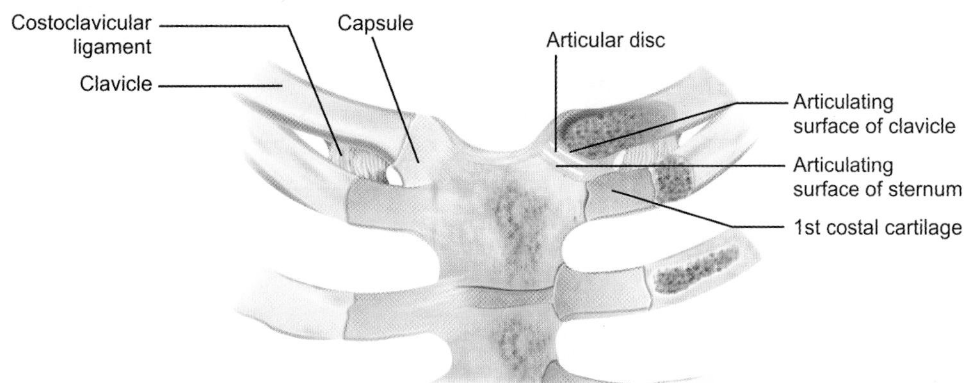

FIGURE 15 Sternoclavicular joint

Movements: As there is an articular disc separating the joint into two joint cavities though it is a plane synovial joint it permits flexion, extension, elevation, depression and rotation. The details will be discussed along with the girdle movements.

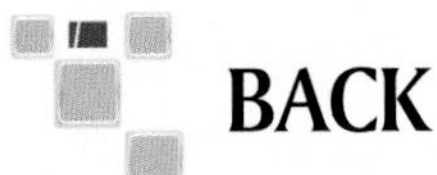

BACK

The girdle bone scapula is connected to the trunk by musculature. This is generally described as back. The scapula has a lot of freedom of movement, as it has no articulation with the trunk. The scapula gives attachment to musculature, which crosses the shoulder joint and gets attached to the humerus. This musculature moves the humerus at the shoulder joint. This is called the scapular region (this will be studied after disarticulating the limb).

SKELETON (Fig. 16)

Go to an articulated skeleton and identify the bony prominences on the posterior aspect. Identify the ***spines*** of the vertebrae in the midline. See and count the thoracic vertebrae. Appreciate the curvature of the thoracic cage. Note the position of the ***scapula*** on the thoracic cage. Feel the ***medial border, superior border, lateral border, lateral angle, the spine, the acromian process and the inferior angle*** of the scapula. Note that the spine of the scapula lies opposite to the 3rd vertebral spine and the inferior angle of the scapula lies opposite to the 7th thoracic spine.

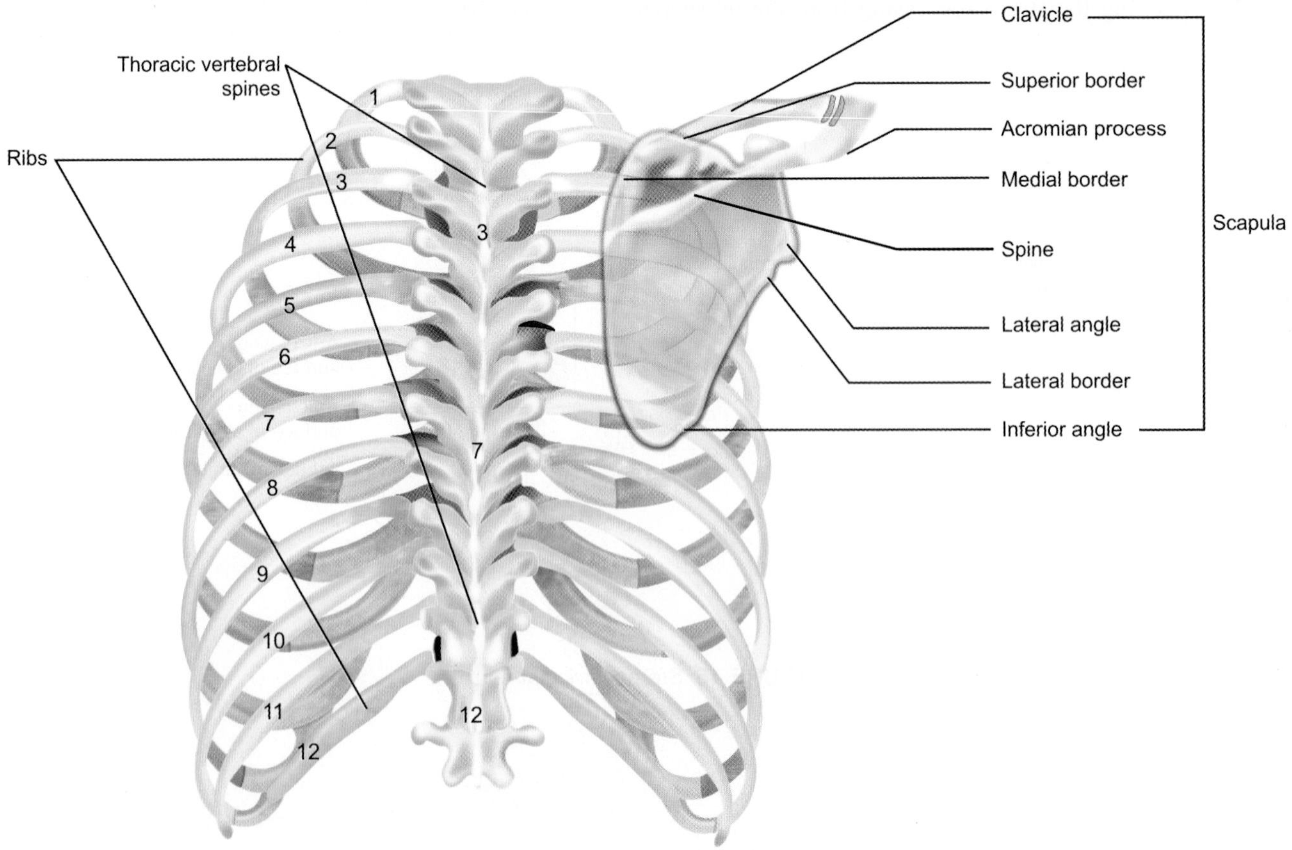

FIGURE 16 Skeleton–back

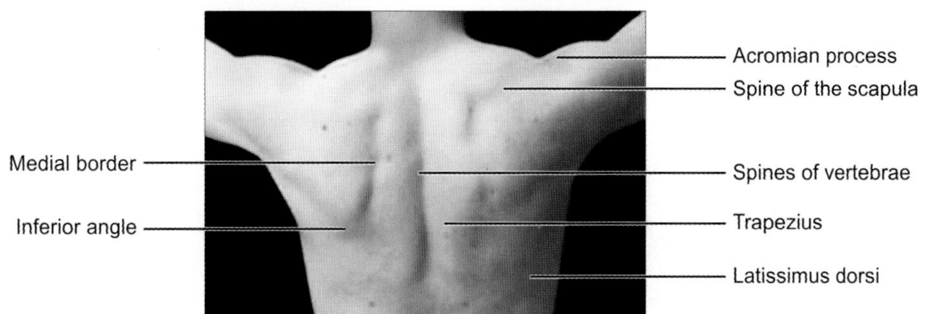

FIGURE 17 Surface anatomy–back

SURFACE ANATOMY (Fig. 17)

Feel the vertebral spines. Feel the scapula. Run your fingers along the medial border, inferior angle, lateral border, the spine and the acromian process of the scapula. Do hyperabduction and see the rotation of the scapula on the thoracic cage. You can see the trapezius and latissimus dorsi.

SKIN INCISION (Fig. 18)

Dissection: Make a vertical incision from the 7th cervical spine to the eighth thoracic spine. Make two horizontal incisions—the upper one from the first spine to the lateral side to join the reflection of skin done on the anterior aspect to the clavicle, the lower one from the 8th thoracic vertebral spine, to the skin reflection on the anterior aspect of the trunk. Reflect the total skin and discard. Note that the skin in this region is thick compared to the ventral surface of the body. Remove the skin on the posterior aspect of the arm until its middle. Clean the superficial fascia from lateral to medial side in the exposed area. While cleaning the fascia note the exposed muscles. The muscles on the lateral side are the scapular muscles, originating from the scapula and the muscle exposed on the medial side is part of the trapezius. The latissimus dorsi muscle occupies the inferolateral part.

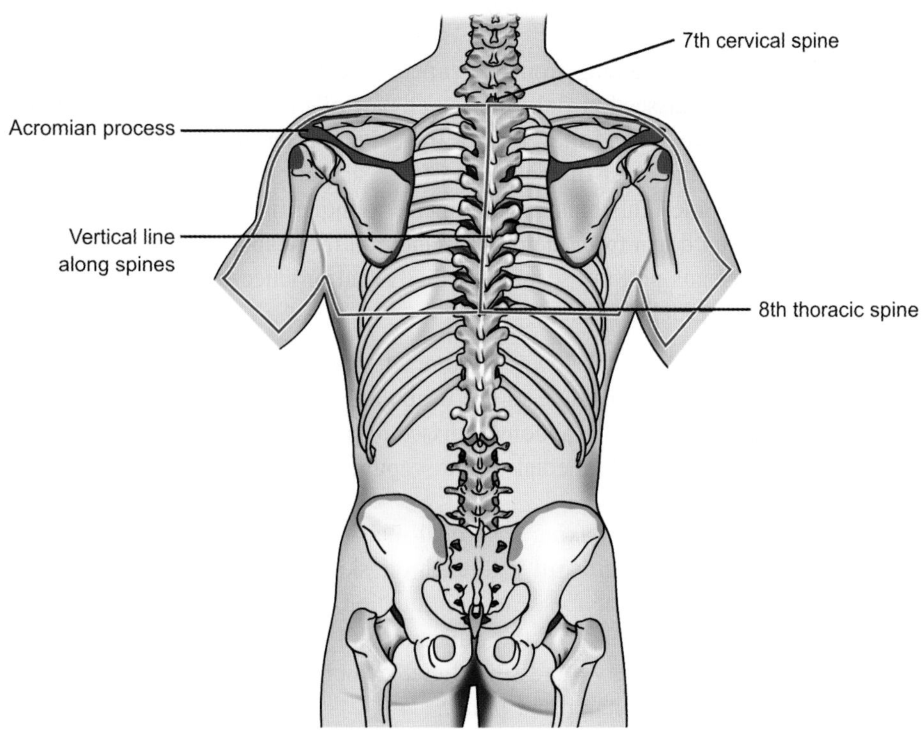

FIGURE 18 Incision–back

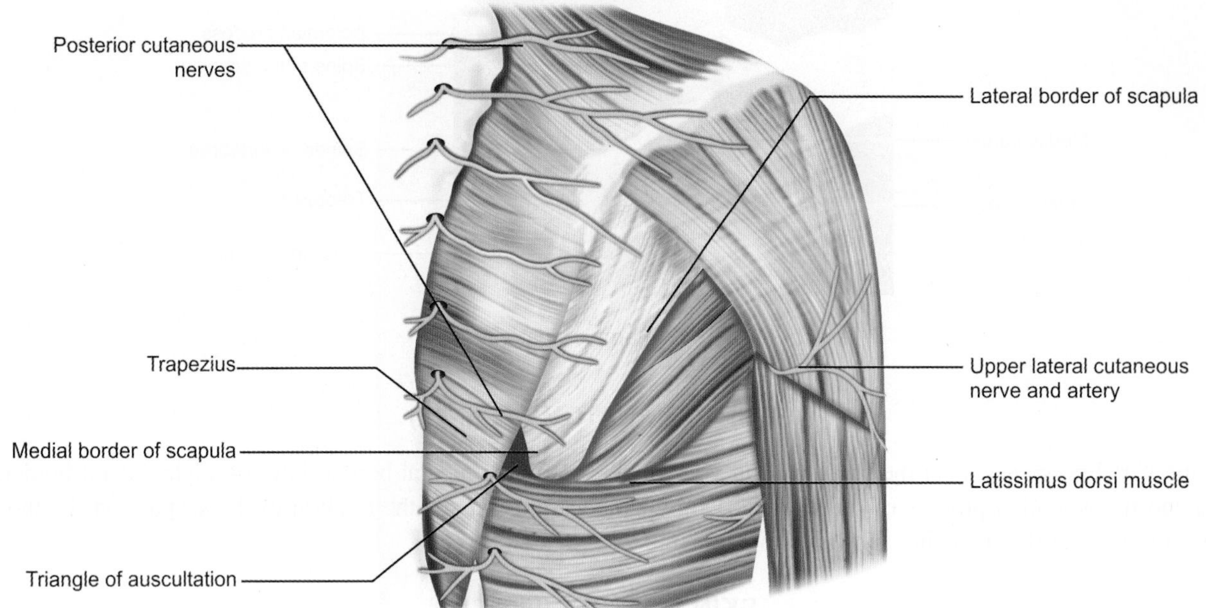

FIGURE 19 Superficial structure–back

SUPERFICIAL STRUCTURES (Fig. 19)

Cutaneous structures: Look for the ***posterior cutaneous nerves.*** They pierce the deep fascia lateral to the vertebral spines and supply the skin a finger breadth from the vertebral spines to the lateral side. Look for the ***upper lateral cutaneous nerve of the arm***. It is the cutaneous part of the axillary nerve.

Triangle of auscultation: Identify the trapezius, latissimus dorsi and the medial border of scapula. The triangular area between these three is called triangle of auscultation. As the muscles are thin here it is easy to hear the internal sounds, so is called triangle of auscultation.

Trapezius: This is a triangular muscle stretching from the superior nuchal line and external occipital protuberance to the last thoracic spine. In the present dissection only the lower part of the muscle is visible. It is aponeurotic at its origin. When muscles of both sides are viewed they form a trapezium so the name trapezius. Trace the muscle to its insertion into the superior border of the crest of the spine of the scapula; medial border of acromian and superior border of the lateral 1/3rd of the clavicle. This muscle has superior oblique fibres, middle horizontal fibres and inferior oblique fibres. The superior fibres run down from their origin and pull the scapula superiorly and causes elevation. The middle horizontal fibres of the trapezius pull the scapula medially and produce retraction. The inferior, oblique fibres pull the scapula downward and cause depression.

Latissimus dorsi: It has a wide origin from the lower six thoracic spines, from the thoracolumbar fascia, iliac crest, lower three or four ribs and from the inferior angle of the scapula. Identify its origin from the inferior angle of the scapula (the remaining parts will be seen in the abdomen dissection). The whole muscle converges laterally to form the posterior wall of the axilla. Cut the muscle medial to the scapular origin.

Dissection: Cut through the trapezius by making a vertical incision nearer to its origin up to the 8th thoracic spine. Lift up the muscle from below upwards till you reach the skin incision. On the lateral side detach it from its insertion. It is helpful to keep the muscle to see its continuation while doing the neck dissection. As you are reflecting the muscle, clean the undersurface of the trapezius and identify the neurovascular bundle entering into the trapezius. They are accessory nerve and superficial branch of the transverse cervical artery. See the next layer of muscles, the rhomboideus major and minor.

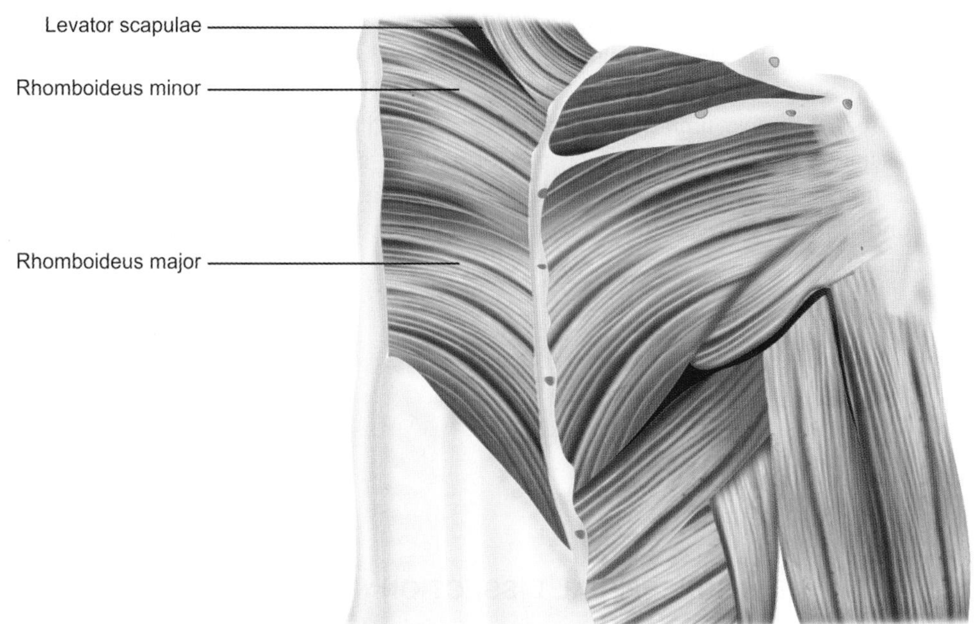

FIGURE 20 Rhomboideus major and minor

DEEP STRUCTURES (Fig. 20)

Rhomboideus major and minor (Fig. 20): These form the deeper group of musculature and are retractors of scapula. Clean the muscles stretching between the spines and the medial border of scapula. They are the rhomboideus minor from 1st to 3rd thoracic spines to the scapula opposite to its spine, the rhomboideus major from 3rd to 4th thoracic spines to the medial border of the scapula from the point below the spine to the inferior angle.

Dissection: Cut through both the muscles vertically one inch away from the origins. Reflect the muscle laterally towards their insertion.

Clean the undersurface of the muscles nearer to their insertions and note the neurovascular bundle entering into the muscles. They are ***dorsal scapular nerve and deep branch of transverse cervical artery***. These two muscles pull the scapula medially and upwards and cause ***retraction***.

DISARTICULATION OF THE UPPER LIMB

The upper limb is attached to the trunk by its anterior, posterior and medial walls. The muscles, pectoralis major, pectoralis minor anteriorly, trapezius, rhomboideus major, minor posteriorly are already detached.

Dissection: Now note the insertion of levator scapulae muscle along the medial border between the spine of the scapula and the superior angle. Total muscle will be seen in the neck dissection. Cut it near the scapula. Run your fingers along the superior border of the scapula. Near the lateral end you will feel the insertion of the omohyoid muscle and the suprascapular vessels and nerves near the notch. Cut through both at this region.

Lift the body to the side and trace the serratus anterior muscle. Note that it extends from the chest wall to the scapula. Here the muscle is inserted into the ventral aspect of the medial border of the scapula. Note that the upper fibres from the upper two ribs run horizontally to reach the upper ½ of scapula, digitations from 3rd and 4th ribs reach the lower ½ of scapula and the remaining lower 4 slips reach the inferior angle of scapula. Note that the function of the muscle is to keep the scapula in contact with the chest wall. It is also a protractor as it slides the scapula over the chest wall. During protraction, the upper limb is thrust forward along with the scapula (perform this action and feel the medial border of the scapula).

Dissection: With a scissors cut the serratus anterior one inch away from its insertion into the medial border of the scapula. Saw through the clavicle at the junction of medial 2/3rd of the clavicle with lateral 1/3rd, i.e. the gap between the origins of pectoralis major and deltoid. Detach the clavicular part of the trapezius from its upper surface. This frees the upper limb in all directions except within the axilla.

Tie the neurovascular bundle near the second part of axillary artery (i.e. under cover of pectoralis minor muscle) with twine thread by 2 knots, one near the other. The ties should be at the distal end of the cords proximal to their division. Cut between the knots and remove the now detached upper limb with the scapula and its attached muscle.

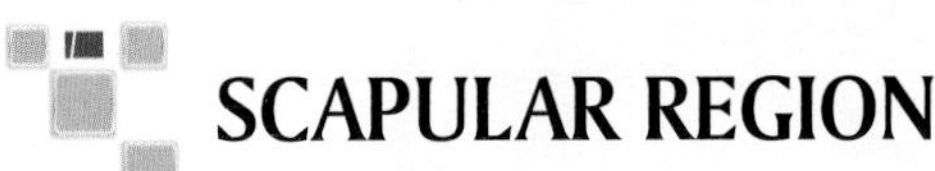

SCAPULAR REGION

SUPERFICIAL DISSECTION (Fig. 21)

Dissection: Clean the connective tissue over the deltoid muscle on the lateral aspect of arm.

Deltoid muscle: This forms the lateral bulge on the arm and it is a powerful abductor. On the free upper limb locate the lateral 1/3rd of clavicle, lateral border of acromion, lower border of spine of scapula. Note the muscle deltoid arising from all the above parts. Deltoid is a multipennate powerful antigravity muscle. The anterior fibres from clavicle run downwards and laterally and will produce flexion, the middle fibres run downwards from the acromian process and are abductors. The scapular fibres run downwards and forwards and produce extension. All the fibres converge on the lateral aspect of the middle of the humerus.

Dissection: Cut through the muscle one inch away from its origin, from front to back and pull the muscle towards its insertion. While doing so observe the axillary nerve and the posterior circumflex humeral artery. This is the neurovascular bundle for the deltoid muscle. See it running on the deeper aspect of the deltoid from posterior to anterior end.

Muscles of Back of Scapula: The ***supraspinatus*** is a triangular muscle seen above the spine. It takes origin from the medial 2/3rd of the supraspinous fossa. See the ***infraspinatus*** muscle arising from the medial 2/3rd of the infraspinus fossa. Identify the ***teres minor*** muscle arising from the upper 2/3rd of the posterior aspect of the lateral border of scapula.

Insertion: Note that the above three muscles get inserted into the greater tubercle of the humerus by merging into the capsule of shoulder joint. Identify the ***teres major*** muscle arising from the lower 1/3rd of the posterior aspect of the lateral border of the scapula. Note that this muscle goes forward to the medial lip of the intertubercular sulcus. Feel the infraglenoid tubercle on the upper end of the lateral border of the scapula. This gives origin to the ***long head of triceps*** muscle. This muscle is seen deep to the teres minor and superficial to the teres major muscle.

The quadrangular space*:** It is bounded above by teres minor, inferiorly by the teres major, medially by the long head of triceps and laterally by the neck of the humerus. The ***axillary nerve is one of the terminal divisions of the posterior cord of brachial plexus. Note it in the quadrangular space and see its origin once again in the axilla from the posterior cord: note the ***nerve to teres minor*** in the quadrangular space. It is a branch of the axillary nerve here. See its entry into the lower border of the teres minor. The ***posterior circumflex humeral artery*** is seen in the quadrangular space along with the axillary nerve. Reconfirm its emergence from the 3rd part of the axillary artery. Note its branches entering into the deltoid muscle and the one winding round the neck of the humerus to anastomose with the anterior circumflex humeral artery. Note the ***upper lateral cutaneous nerve of arm*** which winds round the posterior border of the lower part of the deltoid muscle. As the name signifies it is cutaneous to the upper part of the lateral aspect of the skin of the arm.

The triangular space*:** It is bounded by teres minor above, teres major below and long head of the triceps laterally. See the ***circumflex scapular artery in the triangular space, reconfirm its origin from the subscapular artery. After supplying the teres major and minor its passes deep to the infraspinatus.

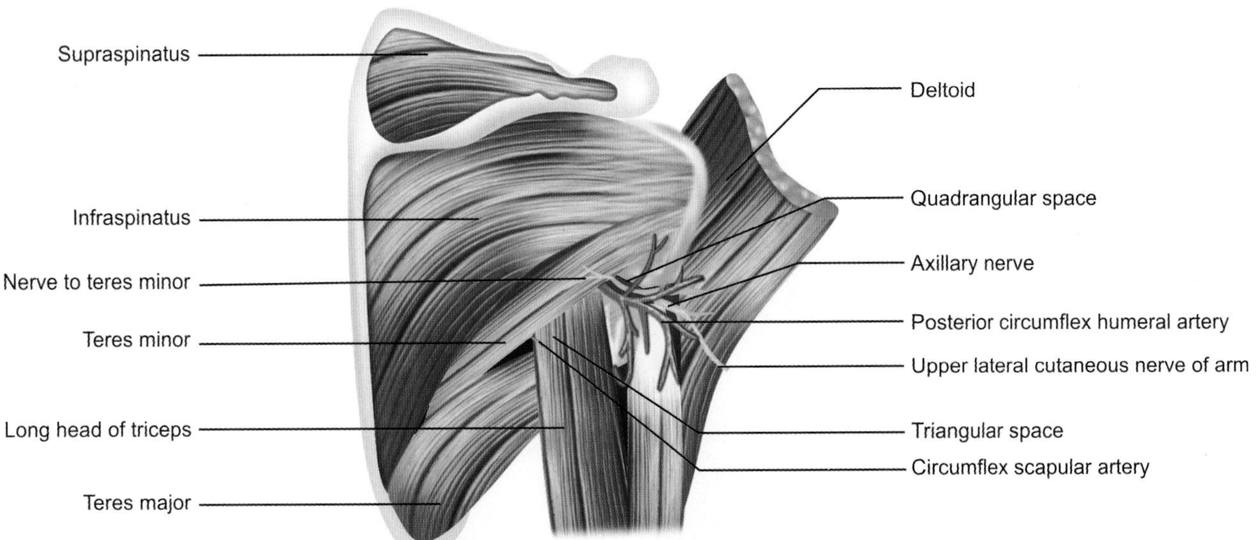

FIGURE 21 Scapular region–superficial dissection

DEEP DISSECTION (Fig. 22)

Dissection: Cut through the supraspinatus, infraspinatus and the teres minor by a vertical incision from the suprascapular notch to the lateral border of the scapula. Pull the muscles to the insertion.

Identify the ***suprascapular artery*** superior to ***suprascapular ligament.*** It is a branch of the subclavian artery and will be dissected in the neck dissection. It descends deep to the supra- and infraspinatus muscles to anastomose with circumflex scapular artery.

Anastomosis: This is a pathway for anastomosis between the 3rd part of the subclavian artery to the 3rd part of the axillary artery.

Locate the ***suprascapular*** *nerve* deep to the suprascapular ligament. It is a branch of the upper trunk of brachial plexus. This will be seen in the dissection of the neck. Note the point of entry of this nerve into the deep surface of supra- and infraspinatus muscles.

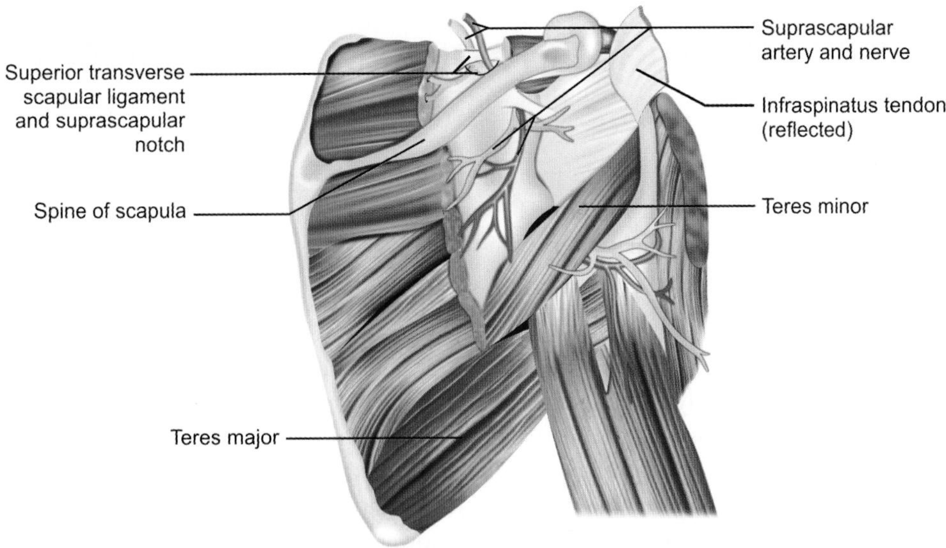

FIGURE 22 Scapular region–deep dissection

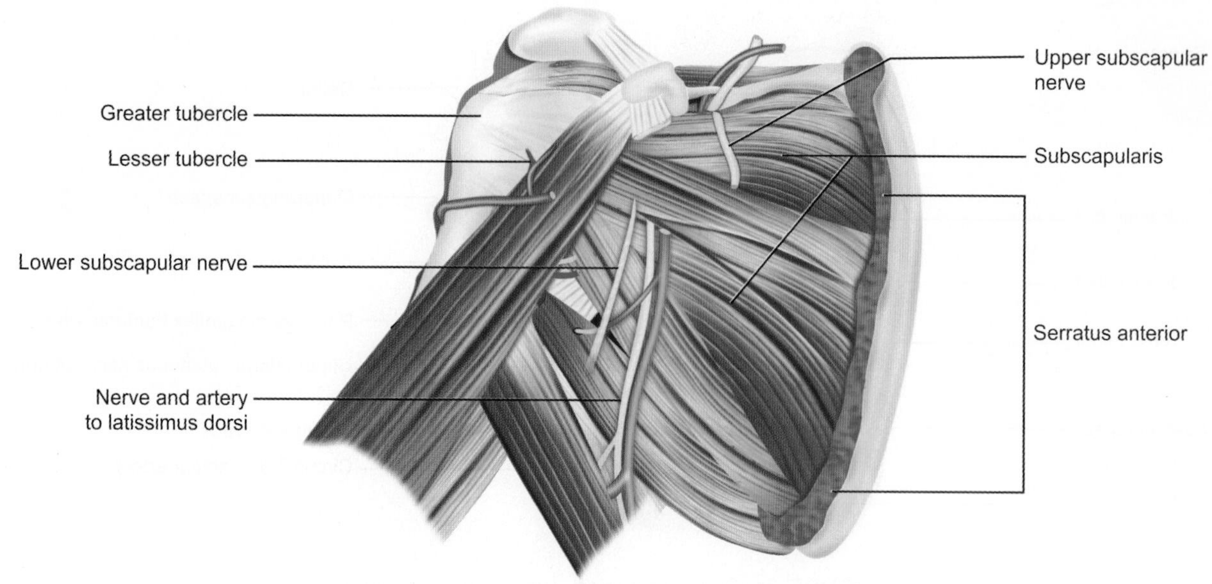

FIGURE 23 Subscapular region

SUBSCAPULAR REGION (Fig. 23)

Turn the arm with the costal surface facing up. Reidentify the following structures—See insertion of ***serratus anterior*** along the ventral aspect of the medial border. See the origin of ***subscapularis muscle*** from the costal surface of the scapula. Identify the same on the bone and note the bony ridges it raises on the bone. See the origin of the ***latissimus dorsi*** muscle from the inferior angle of the scapula. Locate the ***posterior cord*** of brachial plexus. Trace the small ***upper subscapular nerve*** which enters the subscapularis muscle near the lateral angle of the scapula. Identify the ***nerve to latissimus dorsi,*** the long branch descending down over the ventral aspect of the scapula to reach the ventral aspect of the latissimus dorsi muscle. See the ***lower subscapular nerve*** entering the ventral aspect of the muscle near its middle. Reidentify the ***subscapular artery*** and its branch accompanying the nerve to latissimus dorsi. Feel the ***lesser tubercle*** and note that the subscapularis muscle merges with the capsule of the shoulder joint.

ANTERIOR COMPARTMENT OF ARM AND CUBITAL FOSSA

The anterior compartment is the part which lies in front of the humerus, between the medial and lateral intermuscular septae. It lodges the flexors of the arm and forearm. The nerve of this compartment is the musculocutaneous nerve. The artery of this compartment is the brachial artery.

SKELETON (Fig. 24)

Skeleton of the arm is formed by the ***humerus.*** See it on an articulated skeleton. Identify its ***head.*** It is 2/3rds of a circle and faces posteriorly and medially. Note its articulation with the flat glenoid fossa of the scapula. Identify the narrow ***anatomical neck*** immediately beyond the head. See the ***greater tubercle, lesser tubercle*** and the ***intertubercular sulcus*** on the lateral aspect. Note that the upper part of the ***shaft*** of the humerus is rounded in shape, the lower half is triangular in shape. At the junction between the upper and lower part note the laterally located deltoid tuberosity. See medial and lateral ***supracondylar ridges.*** Identify the enlarged lower end, the medial ***trochlea*** and the laterally located rounded ***capitulum.*** In an articulated skeleton, see the articulation of the humerus with the forearm bones, radius and ulna. The bend of the elbow where the humerus articulates with the radius and ulna, forms the cubital fossa. So at this

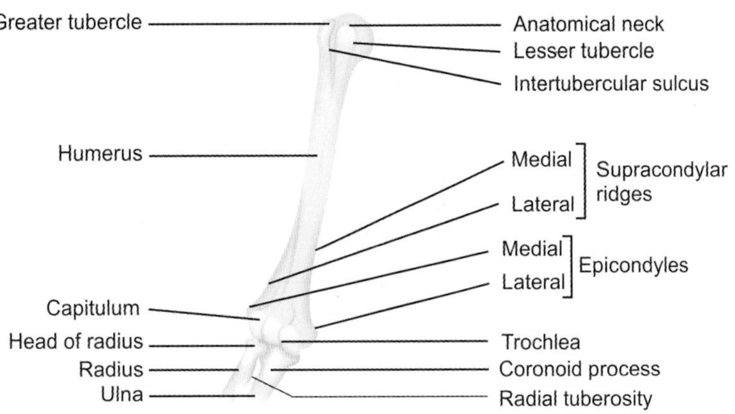

FIGURE 24 Skeleton—arm and cubital fossa

stage see the upper ends of the radius and ulna and their articulation with the humerus. The upper end of ***ulna*** is beak shaped and presents two processes. They are posterior ***olecranon process*** and anterior ***coronoid process.*** They clasp the trochlea of the humerus. Move the ulna over the humerus and see the sliding of the bone. Note that during extreme flexion and extension they fit into the coronoid fossa and olecranon fossa of the humerus. See the roughened depression on the anterior aspect of the coronoid fossa. This is for the insertion of the brachialis muscle.

The upper end of the ***radius*** forms the ***head.*** This articulates with the capitulum of the humerus whereas the circumference of the head articulates with the notch on the ulna. Identify the ***neck*** below the head. Note the radial tuberosity facing the medial side. This gives attachment to the biceps brachii muscle.

SURFACE ANATOMY (Fig. 25)

Make a tight first rotate the forearm and identify the following muscles. Feel the ***biceps brachii*** in the anterior aspect of the arm. Note its tendon near the elbow. Note that the ***flexor musculature*** forms the medial bulge and the ***extensor musculature*** forms the lateral bulge at the junction of the arm and forearm. The ***cubital fossa*** is the depression between the two.

Feel the subcutaneous ***medial epicondyle*** on the medial side and the ***lateral epicondyle*** on the lateral side. See the greenish prominent ***median cubital vein*** at the bend of the elbow. Apply deep pressure and feel the pulsations of the ***branchial artery*** medial to the biceps tendon in the cubital fossa. Trace it up and you can feel its pulsations on the medial side of the arm.

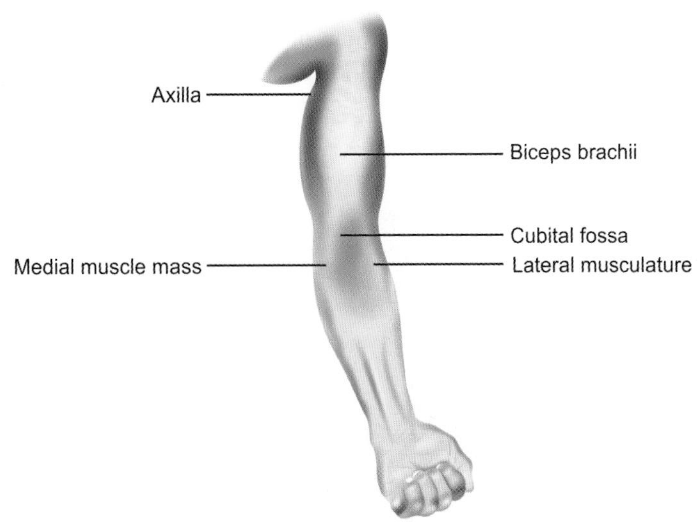

FIGURE 25 Surface anatomy

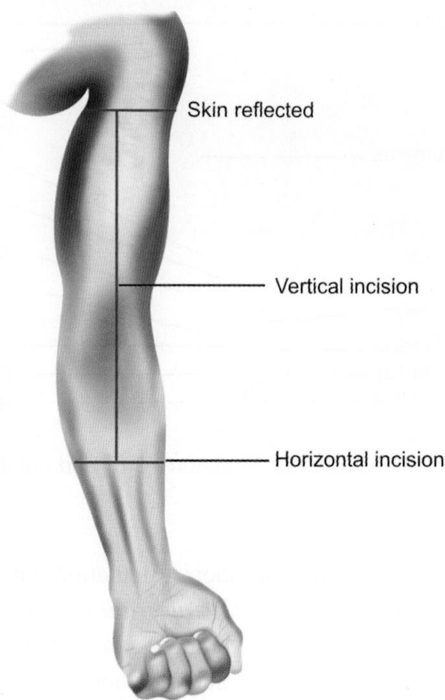

FIGURE 26 Skin incision

SKIN INCISION (Fig. 26)

Dissection: Make a vertical incision from the middle of the arm to middle of forearm. Make a horizontal incision in the middle of the forearm. Skin here is thin. Carefully reflect the flaps to the lateral and medial side. The two flaps can be cut along the sides.

CUTANEOUS STRUCTURES (Fig. 27)

Identify the veins at the bend of the elbow. See the ***cephalic vein*** on the lateral side and see its continuation into the deltopectoral groove. See the ***basilic vein*** on the medial side. This continues up to join the venae comitantis of the brachial artery to form the axillary vein. The median cubital vein connecting the cephalic and basilic vein lies on the firm bicipital aponeurosis and is used for intravenous injections.

Note: ***The lateral cutaneous nerve of forearm,*** the continuation of the musculocutaneous nerve accompany the cephalic vein near the bend of the elbow and the ***medial cutaneous nerve of forearm*** from the medial cord of brachial plexus accompany the lower part of basilic vein.

Deep fascia: It is white glistening, thick sheet here. Note the tendon of biceps sends an expansion into the deep fascia on the medial side below the bend of the elbow. This is one of the insertions of the biceps muscle called ***bicipital aponeurosis***. It helps in tightening the medial side of the forearm.

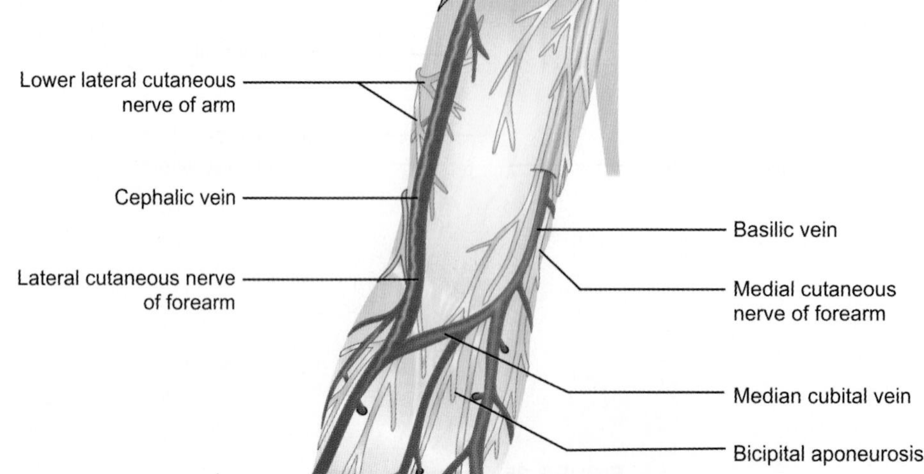

FIGURE 27 Cutaneous structures—arm and cubital fossa

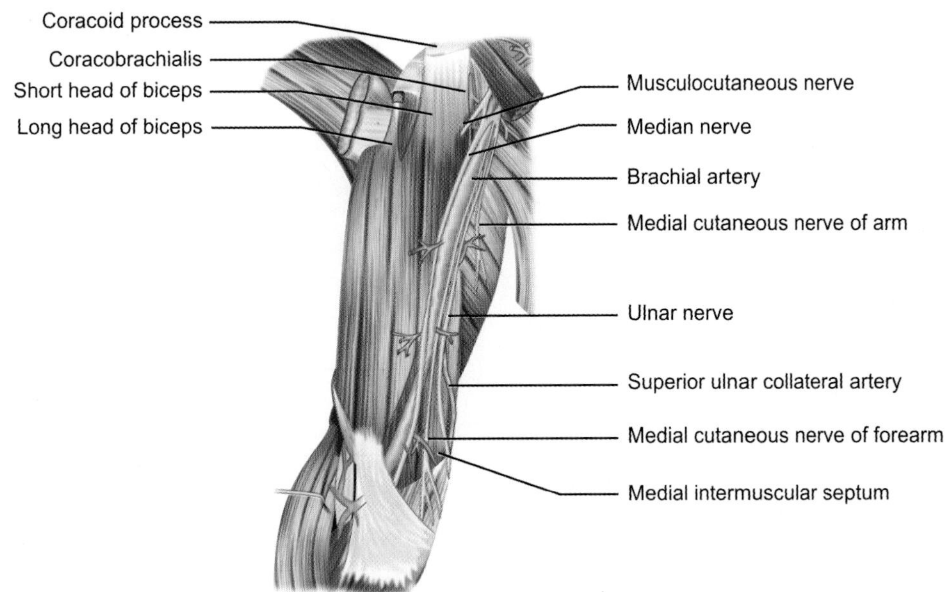

FIGURE 28 Anterior compartment of arm–superficial structures

SUPERFICIAL STRUCTURES (Fig. 28)

Dissection: Make a vertical incision similar to the skin incision and reflect the deep fascia to either side. While reflecting in the lower side, see the lateral and medial intermuscular septa stretching from the deeper aspect of the deep fascia stretching on to the medial and lateral superior condylar lines. Identify these bony lines on the humerus.

Trace the axillary structures along the arm to the forearm. Identify the ***axillary artery*** and trace it down into the forearm. Beyond the lower border of the teres major the artery is called ***brachial artery.*** Note that the artery is on the medial side of the arm anterior to the brachialis and medial to the biceps brachii muscle. The ***ulnar nerve*** lies medial to the brachial artery up to the medial intermuscular septum. It leaves the anterior compartment above the medial intermuscular septum accompanied by the ***superior ulnar collateral artery***—trace these two structures up to the medial epicondyle. Ulnar nerve has no branch in the arm. Reidentify the ***median nerve*** formed by two roots in front of the axillary artery. Trace it down up to the bend of the elbow. Note that the nerve gradually crosses the artery and lies medial to the artery at the bend of the elbow.

MUSCLES OF ANTERIOR COMPARTMENT

Biceps brachii: This is the superficial muscle in this compartment. It has two heads, the short head arises from the coracoid process along with the coracobrachialis, and the long head arises from the supraglenoid tubercle of the scapula, crosses across the head of the humerus (this is intracapsular and cannot be identified at this stage) travels down between the greater and lesser tubercles of the humerus joins the short head and forms the bulk of the muscle (identify the bony parts on the skeleton, and note the direction of the muscle). In the lower part of the arm it becomes tendinous and enters the cubital fossa. Note its insertion into the radial tuberosity. The superficial part of the muscle sends an aponeurotic insertion into the deep fascia on the medial side of forearm.

Dissection: Cut the biceps brachii near its center and reflect the cut parts up and down. Cut the bicipital aponeurosis nearer to its tendon.

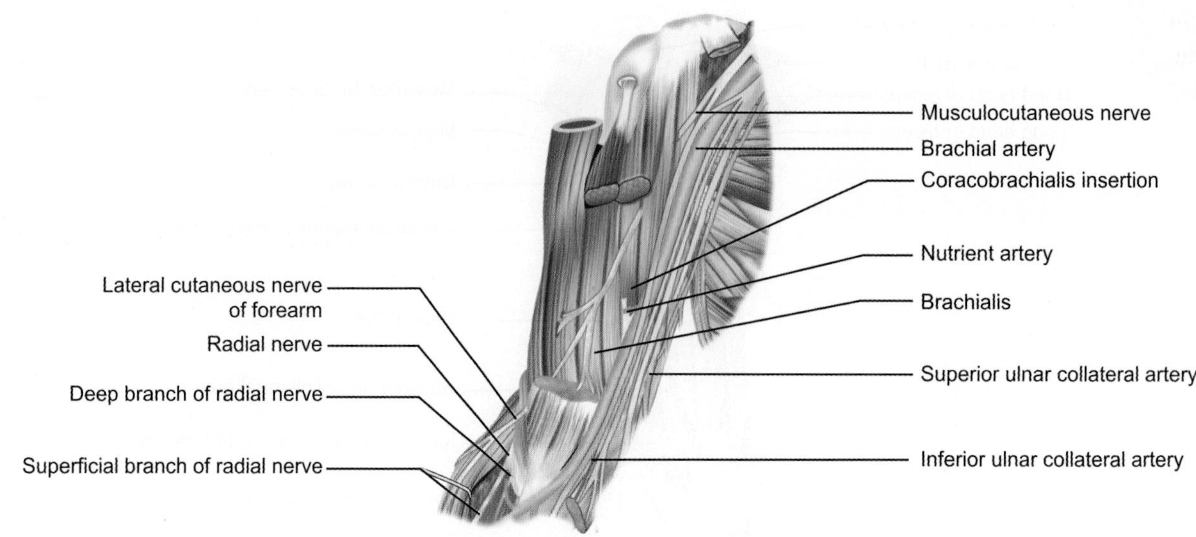

FIGURE 29 Anterior compartment of arm–deep structures

DEEP STRUCTURES (Fig. 29)

Coracobrachialis: Identify this small muscle extending from the coracoid process to the middle of the medial border of humerus. See the musculocutaneous nerve passing through this muscle. This is a rare phenomenon where a nerve passes through the muscle. This is due to the fact that in the lower forms this is a composite muscle made up of two heads and the nerve was passing between the two heads and it continues to remain in the same position.

Brachialis: This is the deeper muscle which takes origin from the anterior aspect of the humerus and extends up, to the area between the insertions of deltoid and coracobrachialis. Note its position on the anterior aspect of the humerus, trace it down to its insertion into the tubercle on the anterior aspect of coronoid process of ulna.

Nerve supply: Identify the musculocutaneous nerve entering into the coracobrachialis. It passes through the muscle and after coming out of the coracobrachialis it supplies the biceps brachii and the brachialis muscle. Further it becomes the cutaneous nerve called lateral cutaneous nerve of forearm. It pierces the deep fascia and accompanies the cephalic vein into the forearm. This was identified along with the cephalic vein among the superficial structures.

Actions: The long head of the biceps brachii holds the head of the humerus against the glenoid cavity, especially during abduction of the arm. The short head of biceps and the coracobrachialis are flexors of the arm at the shoulder joint. The biceps brachii and the brachialis are flexors of the forearm at the elbow joint. The biceps is also a supinator of the forearm at the radioulnar joints.

Brachial artery: This is the artery of the arm and it gives off the following branches.

Dissection: Pull the artery medially and identify the following branches.

Profunda brachii artery: It is the first and biggest of the branches, given off on its posterior aspect and leaves the compartment below the teres major to reach the posterior compartment of arm. ***Nutrient artery*** is a small branch entering into the humerus lateral to the insertion of coracobrachialis. Identify the position of the nutrient foramen on the humerus. ***Superior ulnar collateral artery*** is the branch which leaves above the medial intermuscular septum to accompany the ulnar nerve. ***Inferior ulnar collateral artery*** is a small branch which reaches the anterior aspect of the medial epicondyle. ***Muscular branches*** accompany the musculocutaneous nerve branches into the muscles.

The radial nerve: It leaves the axilla to reach the back of the arm, reenters the front of the arm above the lateral intermuscular septum. ***Trace it down between the brachialis and the brachioradialis muscles.*** Here note that the brachialis muscle is supplied both by the musculocutaneous as well as the radial nerve. It is a composite muscle by development.

CUBITAL FOSSA

In the lower part of the anterior compartment of the arm the musculature of the forearm ascends up to get attached to the humerus. On the medial side locate the ***pronator teres*** muscle**.** It is the muscle arising from the medial intermuscular septum and the medial supracondylar ridge. This is the first muscle of the flexor compartment of the forearm muscles. On the lateral side locate the ***brachioradialis*** and ***extensor carpi radialis longus*** muscles. It arises from the lateral intermuscular septum and the lateral supracondylar ridge.

The insertion of brachialis and biceps brachii into the forearm bones and the migration of the forearm muscles into the arm create a gap between the muscle masses and through this the neurovascular bundle enters the forearm. This creates a triangular depression at the bend of the elbow. It is called cubital fossa.

Dissection: Clean the deep fascia from this region and identify and define this area.

BOUNDARIES (Fig. 30)

Superior boundary is an imaginary line joining the medial and lateral epicondyle. Identify them. ***Medial boundary*** is formed by the pronator teres muscle. This is the most lateral muscle of the flexor group of musculature. ***Lateral boundary*** is formed by the brachioradialis. This is the most anterior muscle of the extensor group of musculature.

Floor and contents will be studied in the forearm dissection.

Collateral circulation at elbow is an area where branches of the brachial artery anastomose with the branches of radial and ulnar arteries. Near their union they are too thin. These branches enlarge in case of need.

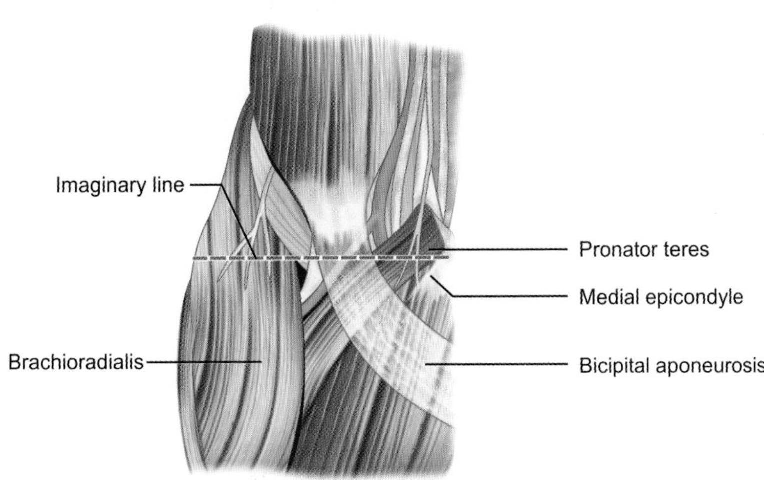

FIGURE 30 Cubital fossa

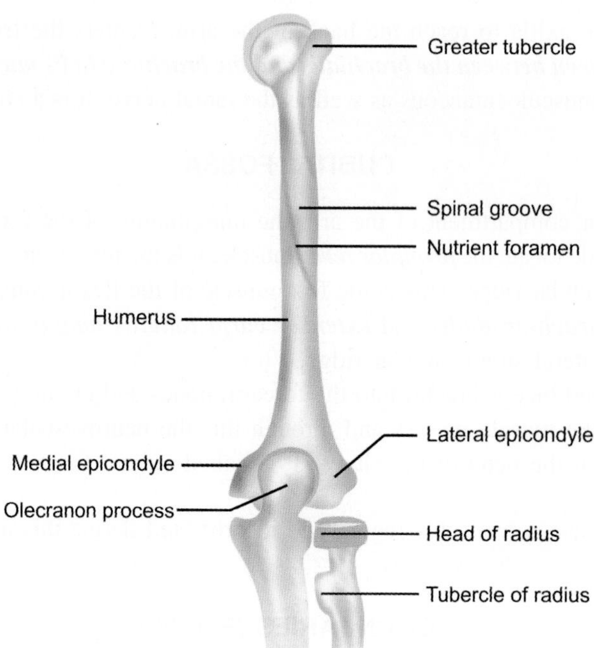

FIGURE 31 Skeletal–back of the arm

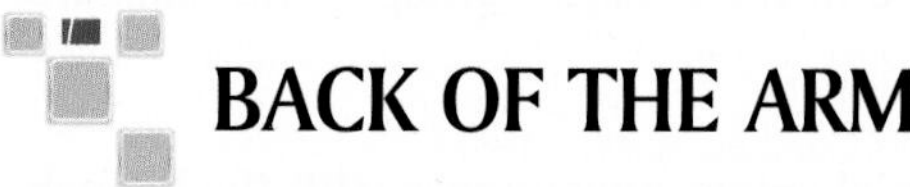

BACK OF THE ARM

The back of the arm is the extensor compartment of the arm. It has only one muscle - the triceps. As the name indicates it has three heads of origin. The nerve of this compartment is the radial nerve and the artery of this compartment is the profunda brachii artery.

SKELETON (Fig. 31)

The arm is made up of ***humerus.*** Look at the back of the humerus in an articulated skeleton. Identify the ***radial groove*** near its middle, on the back of the humerus. In the lower end identify the ***trochlea*** and the ***olecranon fossa*** above it. See the ***medial epicondyle*** projecting beyond the ***lateral epicondyle.*** Realize that the capitulum is not seen at the back.

The ulna: See the prominent olecranon process on the posterior aspect of the upper end of the ulna. This fits into the olecranon fossa of the humerus.

SURFACE ANATOMY (Fig. 32)

Feel the medial and lateral epicondyles once more. Identify the most prominent olecranon process in the midline. It is the posterior part of the ulna and is subcutaneous. See the muscle mass on the back. It is due to the triceps muscle.

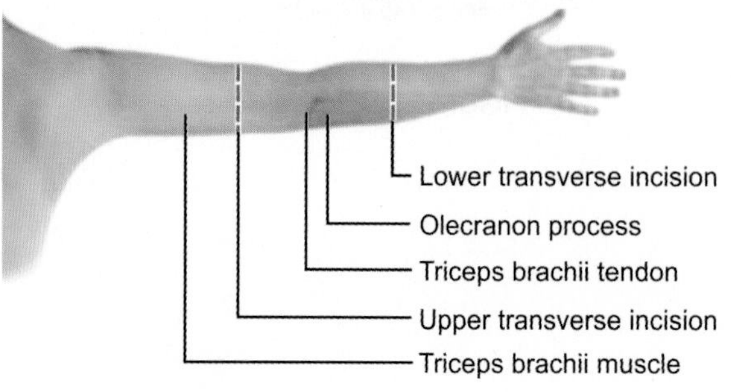

FIGURE 32 Surface anatomy and skin incision

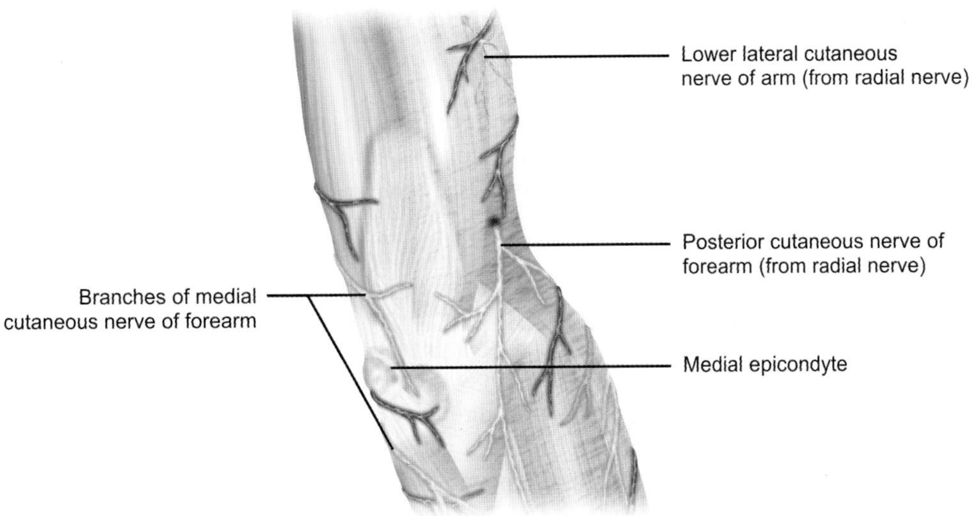

FIGURE 33 Cutaneous structures

SKIN INCISION

Dissection: Make a transverse skin incision in line with the anterior incision near the middle of forearm. Inferiorly make another transverse incision near the middle of the forearm in line with the anterior incision. Reflect the total skin from the back.

CUTANEOUS STRUCTURES (Fig. 33)

The ***lower lateral cutaneous nerve of the arm*** is a branch of radial nerve, locate it on the lower aspect of the lateral side. The ***posterior cutaneous nerve of the arm*** runs along the middle of the posterior aspect of the arm. It is a branch of the radial nerve. Trace them back to the radial nerve. They are given off while the radial nerve is in the axilla. There are no identifiable veins on the posterior aspect. Trace the terminal branches of the medial cutaneous nerve of the forearm into the forearm.

Dissection: Identify the deep fascia and clean the triceps muscle, while doing so retain the cutaneous nerves. The whole back is covered by one single muscle, the triceps.

SUPERFICIAL DISSECTION OF BACK OF ARM (Fig. 34)

The ***triceps*** has three heads of origin. You have already identified the ***long head*** arising from the infraglenoid tubercle of the scapula. The ***lateral head*** has an oblique origin from the superior border of the spiral groove and the ***medial head*** from the lower part of the shaft of humerus on its posterior aspect. Note its origin on the humerus. Note that the long and medial heads soon join. Trace the muscle to its insertion into the top of the olecranon process of ulna. Perform

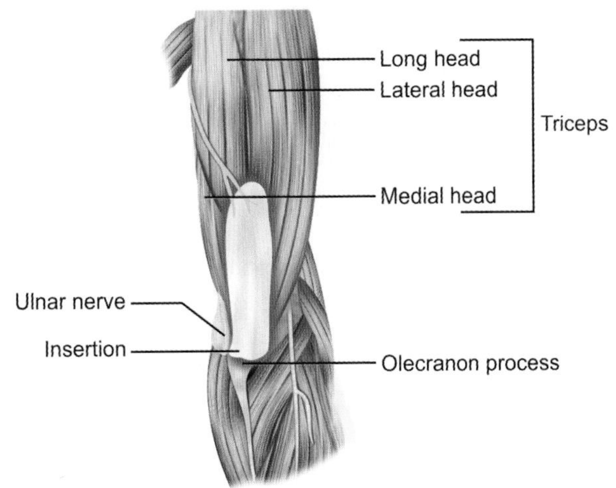

FIGURE 34 Superficial dissection of back of arm

extension of the forearm against resistance and see the tightening of the muscle. It is an extensor of the forearm at the elbow joint.

Dissection: Cut through the triceps muscle along the lateral border of the long head of triceps, between the long and lateral heads till you reach the lateral intermuscular septum. The cut passes through the spiral groove. Note the radial nerve and the profunda brachii artery. Trace this groove superiorly and note that the groove is continuous with the lower triangular space.

DEEP DISSECTION OF BACK OF ARM (Fig. 35)

The ***lower triangular space*** is bounded by teres major—superiorly long head of triceps medially, shaft of the humerus laterally. The radial nerve and profunda brachii artery pass through this. The ***radial nerve***—is a thick mixed nerve. This is a nerve of supply to the extensor compartment of the arm and forearm. It is motor to all these muscles as well as sensory to the skin over this region. See it in the spiral groove passing from medial to lateral side. Identify its muscular branches—the ***branches entering into the long head medial and lateral head of triceps, the nerve to anconeus,*** a long branch that runs down to supply the anconeus muscle. It gives off the ***posterior cutaneous nerve of forearm.*** This runs down along with the nerve to the anconeus and then becomes superficial. The ***profunda brachii artery*** gives branches to accompany the nerves. The ***lateral collateral artery*** arises from the profunda brachii artery near the lateral intermuscular septum and divides into an ***anterior and posterior lateral descending artery.*** Trace them down to lateral epicondyle. Look for its small ***nutrient artery*** which enters into the humerus in the spiral groove. Trace the ***radial nerve*** into the anterior compartment of arm. This reaches the anterior compartment above the lateral intermuscular septum, runs between the brachioradialis, extensor carpi radialis longus and the brachialis. Reidentify the muscular branches to all the three muscles.

Radial nerve is commonly injured in the spiral groove. Triceps muscle escapes total damage as the branches supplying long and lateral head are given off before the nerve enters spiral groove.

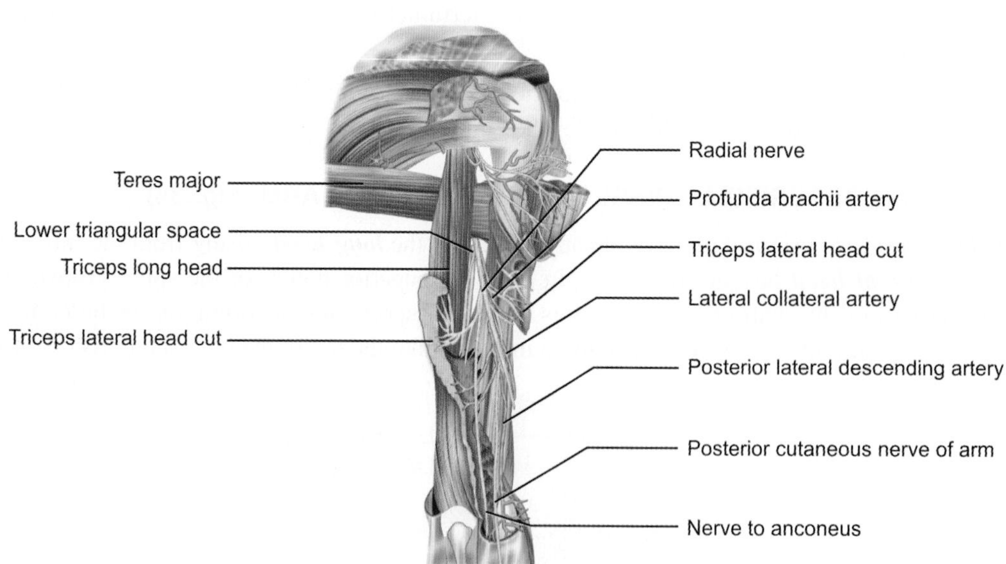

FIGURE 35 Deep dissection–back of arm

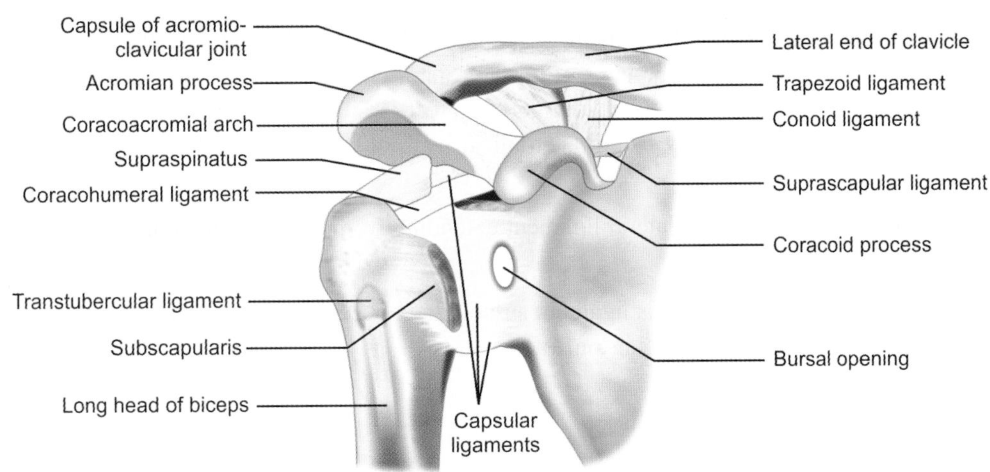

FIGURE 36 Pectoral girdle and shoulder joint

PECTORAL GIRDLE AND SHOULDER JOINT (Fig. 36)

The upper limb is a part for prehension and it has to pass the heavy weights that we carry, through the trunk to the ground. To perform these functions the shoulder joint is built with maximum freedom of movement, at the same time well protected by bones and musculature. The pectoral girdle helps in the movements of upper limb by suspending it by musculature except for the sternoclavicular joint. It is convenient to study the structural parts as acromioclavicular joint, coracoacromial arch, coracoclavicular ligaments, rotator cuff and the shoulder joint.

Acromioclavicular joint: This is a plane synovial joint. Identify the lateral end of the clavicle and the medial part of the acromian process on the dissected part. Identify these articulating surfaces on the dry bones. These are small plane articulating surfaces. *Note the capsule attached to the bones external to the articular surfaces. Slit the superior part of the capsule of the joint and see the interior. You will see a fibrocartilaginous articular disc.* This divides the joint into two compartments and permits two different movements in the compartments.

Coracoacromial arch: This is like a secondary socket for the shoulder joint. It is protective in nature, particularly in hyperabduction. ***See this arch extending from the anterior angle of the acromian process to the tip of the coracoid process***. ***Coracoclavicular ligament***—is a powerful ligament extending between the clavicle and the coracoid process. It helps in weight transmission from the upper limb to the trunk. *Try to see this ligament. It has two parts, the conoid part – is triangular in shape, the apex is attached to the root of the coracoid process and the base is attached to the conoid tubercle on the inferior surface of clavicle, the* ***trapezoid ligament****—a flat ligament extends from the rough edge on the medial border of the coracoid process to the oblique line on the inferior surface of the clavicle.* Identify these features on a dry bone.

Rotator cuff: You have seen all the muscles around the shoulder joint. *Reidentify them. Turn the part posteriorly and identify the insertion of* ***supraspinatus*** *passing under the coracoacromial arch to the supraglenoid tubercle. Identify the* ***infraspinatus*** *and* ***teres minor*** *below the supraspinatus extending on to the greater tubercle. Turn the part ventrally and note the* ***subscapularis*** *extending from the subscapular fossa to the lesser tubercle of the humerus. Pull the insertion of all these muscles and note that they are merging with the capsule.* Note the subscapular, supraspinous bursae under cover of the respective muscles. These stabilize the humerus on the scapula, particularly during rotatory movements.

SHOULDER JOINT

Shoulder joint is a polyaxial ball and socket joint. See the bony surfaces on dry bone. The scapular articulation is a pear shaped surface on the superolateral angle of the scapula. The humeral head is a hemispherical articulation. As you can see the surfaces are noncongruous.

Dissection: Detach the coracoacromial ligament near the coracoid process and saw through the acromian at the junction with the spine and remove the piece. Pull the rotator cuff muscles to their insertion into the greater and lesser tubercles. You can see the thin capsule. Note that it is attached proximally to the periphery of the articulating scapular surface and distally to the anatomical neck of the humerus.

Coracohumeral ligament: Identify this collateral ligament extending from the tip of the coracoid process to the greater tubercle of the humerus.

Transverse ligament of the humerus: See this ligament stretching between the greater and lesser tubercles of humerus. Note the long head of the biceps tendon coming out of it.

INTERIOR OF THE JOINT (Fig. 37)

Dissection: Open the joint cavity by a vertical cut through the posterior aspect of the capsule. Pull the head of the humerus laterally and see the interior.

Long head of the biceps: See this tendon extending from the supraglenoid tubercle of the scapula. Feel the stickiness of the synovial fluid. You can make out that the tendon as such is covered by the synovial membrane. It is because the tendon is outside the synovial membrane, though it is intracapsular.

Glenohumeral ligaments: Note these thickenings of the anterior wall of the capsule. The superior one extends from the root of the coracoid process to the lesser tubercle, the middle and inferior glenohumeral ligaments extend in the lower part of the capsule. The subscapular bursa lies between the superior and middle glenohumeral ligaments.

Labrum glenoidale: This is a triangular thickening on the periphery of the glenoid fossa. The base of it is attached to the bone and the apex projects free into the joint. This deepens the concavity of the glenoid fossa.

Synovial membrane: Note the sticky inner synovial membrane. It lines the innerside of the capsule and gets reflected off from here to the nonarticulating surfaces of the bone within the joint cavity.

Bursae around the joint: As number muscles cross the joint very closely, many a bursae intervene between them and the joint. Of them the ***subscapular,*** under cover of the subscapularis muscle and the ***infraspinatus*** under cover of the infraspinatus muscle are constant and communicate with the joint. There is a big subacromial bursa under cover of the ***deltoid*** and the ***coracoacromial arch.*** This bursa, though constant does not communicate with the joint cavity.

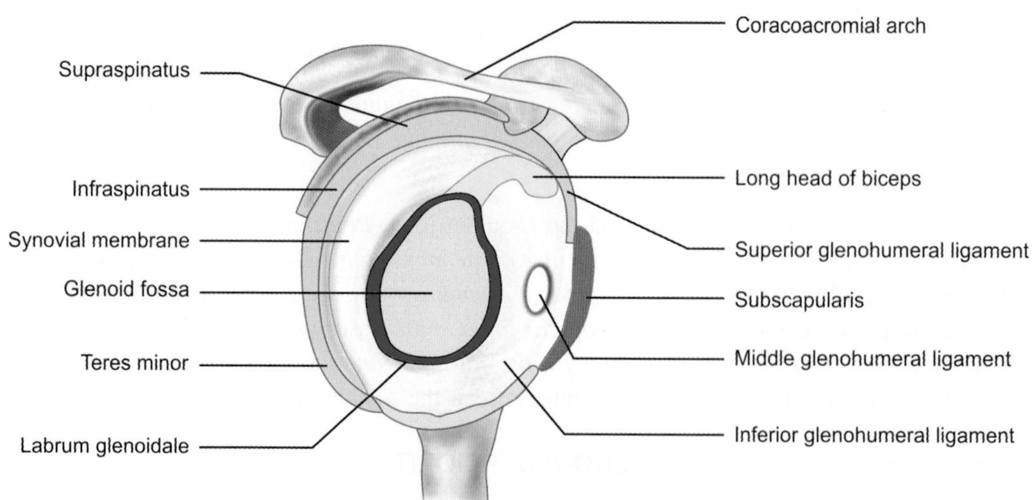

FIGURE 37 Interior of shoulder joint

MOVEMENTS

The ***pectoral girdle*** acts like the limbs of a pincer in attaching the upper limb to the trunk, with the clavicle in front and the scapula behind the thoracic cage. The scapula lies over the curvature of the chest wall and slides over it. The position of the shoulder joint is at the midaxillary line. The sternoclavicular and acromioclavicular joints form the joints of the pectoral girdle. Even though they are plane synovial joints, due to the intervention of the articular disc, movements around two axes are feasible at these joints. Elevation and depression around an anteroposterior axis and protraction and retraction around a shifting axis is feasible.

Elevation (shrugging) is produced by upper fibres of trapezius and depression is produced by the subclavius and pectoralis minor muscles. Protraction (boxing) of the scapula is produced by the serratus anterior muscle and retraction is produced by the middle fibres of trapezius and rhomboidei.

The ***shoulder joint*** being a polyaxial ball and socket type of joint, movement is possible in all possible planes. Observe the position of glenoid fossa of the scapula and the head of the humerus in an articulated skeleton. The ***flexion and extension*** takes place in a plane parallel to the glenoid fossa around a transverse axis passing through the center of the glenoid fossa. The coracobrachialis, short head of biceps and the anterior fibres of deltoid which cross the joint anteriorly cause flexion. The extension is produced by the posterior fibres of deltoid and the latissimus dorsi, which cross the joint posteriorly. The ***abduction and adduction*** are performed perpendicular to the glenoid fossa around an anteroposterior axis parallel to the glenoid fossa. The abduction is initiated by the supraspinatus and continued by the middle fibres of deltoid. These cross the joint superiorly. The adduction is a movement towards gravity. Latissimus dorsi, pectoralis major and teres major come into action when it is performed against resistance. In normal adduction, sustained relaxation of the abductors help in bringing about this action. Rotation of the humerus is an action that takes place around a vertical plane passing through the center of the humerus. Perform the ***medial and lateral rotation*** with a flexed forearm holding the humerus in your hand. Circumduction is a combination of all the movements. Here you make a cone with the apex near the glenoid fossa.

Scapular rotation: Except for the internal rotation of the humerus, all other movements at the shoulder joint are accompanied by the scapular rotation. For the scapular rotation the axis passes through the center of the scapula. Rotation of the scapula can be likened to the rotation of a wheel. The trapezius, serratus anterior and the scapular fibres of the latissimus dorsi pull in different direction and rotate the scapula.

FRONT OF THE FOREARM AND HAND

The forearm and hand is specialized to perform intricate movements. The hand has small intrinsic muscles to monitor the movements of the fingers. The muscles of forearm are long powerful muscles that add to the range of movement at the fingers. The pronation and supination is the rotator movement between the forearm bones. This gives a special ease to the movement of the hand.

SKELETON (Fig. 38)

Skeleton of the forearm is formed by the radius and ulna. Go to an articulated skeleton and identify the bones and their features.

Ulna: This is the medial bone of the forearm. The upper end is beak shaped and presents two processes. They are posterior ***olecranon process*** and anterior ***coronoid process.*** They clasp the trochlea of the humerus. Move the ulna over the humerus and see the sliding of the bone. Note that during extreme flexion and extension they fit into the coronoid fossa and olecranon fossa of the humerus. See the roughened depression on the anterior aspect of the coronoid fossa. This is for the insertion of the brachialis muscle. The shaft is triangular in nature. The lateral border is sharp and is called the ***interosseous border.*** The lower end presents a circular ***head*** and a projecting ***styloid process.***

Radius: See the rounded ***head*** at the upper end of radius. The upper surface of the head articulates with the capitulum of the humerus whereas the circumference of the head articulates with the notch on the ulna. Identify the ***neck*** below

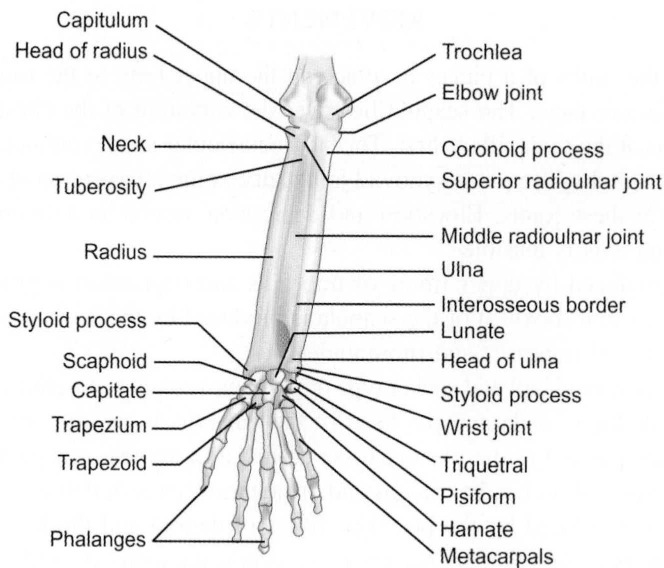

FIGURE 38 Skeleton—forearm and hand

the head. Note the ***radial tuberosity*** facing the medial side. This gives attachment to the biceps brachii muscle. The shaft of the radius is triangular with the medial sharp ***interosseous margin.*** The lateral margin shows a convexity. The distal end of the radius is more expanded. The part projects down to form the ***styloid process*** of the radius. The solid process of the radius is much lower than the styloid process of the ulna. The two interosseous borders are united by interosseous membrane. This is a fibrous joint. Both the upper and lower ends form a pivot joint.

Hand: ***Eight carpals, five metacarpals and fourteen phalanges*** form the skeleton of the hand. The carpals are arranged two rows—a proximal and a distal row. Identify the proximal row from lateral to medial—they are the ***scaphoid, lunate, triquetral*** and ***pisiform.*** The distal row is made up of ***trapezium, trapezoid, capitate and hamate*** bones. Note that carpals form a shallow concavity in the palmar surface. The pillars are formed by the pisiform and hook of hamate on the medial side and the tubercle of the scaphoid and the tubercle of trapezium on the lateral side. The concavity is converted into a tunnel by the attachment of the flexor retinaculum and lodges all the tendons entering into the palm. See the ***metacarpals.*** They are numbered from lateral to medial, first to fifth. Note that the first metacarpal is placed perpendicular to the remaining metacarpals. The metacarpals have a base, a triangular shaft and a rounded head. The metacarpals articulate with the base of the first phalange. The thumb has two phalanges whereas the remaining fingers have three phalanges each. Each phalange has a base, shaft and a head.

Joints of the hand: The distal end of the radius and articular disc of the ulna articulates with the proximal row of carpal bones. It forms the ellipsoidal ***wrist joint.*** It is a biaxial joint. Flexion extension, abduction and adduction takes place at this joint. All the ***intercarpal joints*** are plane synovial joints. Try to move the thumb and see. Note that the thumb has a free range of movement. It can produce flexion, extension, abduction, adduction, opposition and circumduction. All these movements are possible as the ***carpometacarpal*** and ***metacarpophalangeal*** joints are involved in unison in the movement of thumb. The ***metacarpophalangeal*** joints are biaxial ellipsoidal joints. Note that the midline passes through the center of the middle finger. Perform the flexion, extension, abduction and adduction of the other fingers here in relation to the middle finger. The ***interphalangeal*** joints are uniaxial condylar joints. Flexion and extension takes place here.

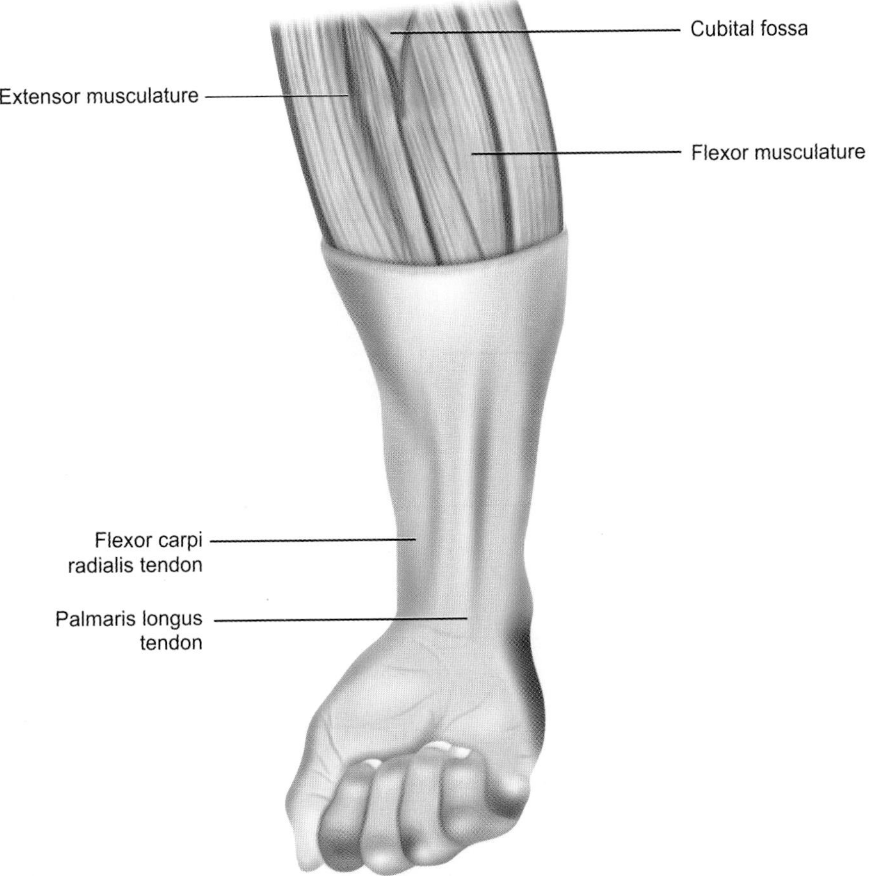

FIGURE 39 Surface anatomy—forearm and hand

SURFACE ANATOMY (Fig. 39)

Note that the ***flexor musculature*** forms a medial bulge and the ***extensor muscles*** form a lateral bulge near the proximal end of forearm. The depression between the two is the ***cubital fossa.*** Distally feel the ***radius and ulna*** and their ***styloid processes*** and note that the radial styloid process is more distal than the ulnar styloid process. Feel the ***pulsations of the radial artery*** at the distal end of radius. Make a tight fist and feel tendons near the wrist. Identify the flexor carpi ulnaris, palmaris longus and flexor carpi radialis.

Note that the skin over the front of the forearm is thin and the skin of the hand shows flexor creases. Note also that the flexor creases do not correspond to the joints. The study of the flexor creases and the dermal ridges on the palm and fingers is called dermatoglyphics.

Dermatoglyphics: Special methods are used to take the finger and palm prints. The patterns are genetically controlled and are formed in the uterine life and they are permanent. This is commonly used in forensic department to identify individuals. Some of the congenital disorders also show particular specific patterns. For example, the simian crease is a common pattern in Down's syndrome's people.

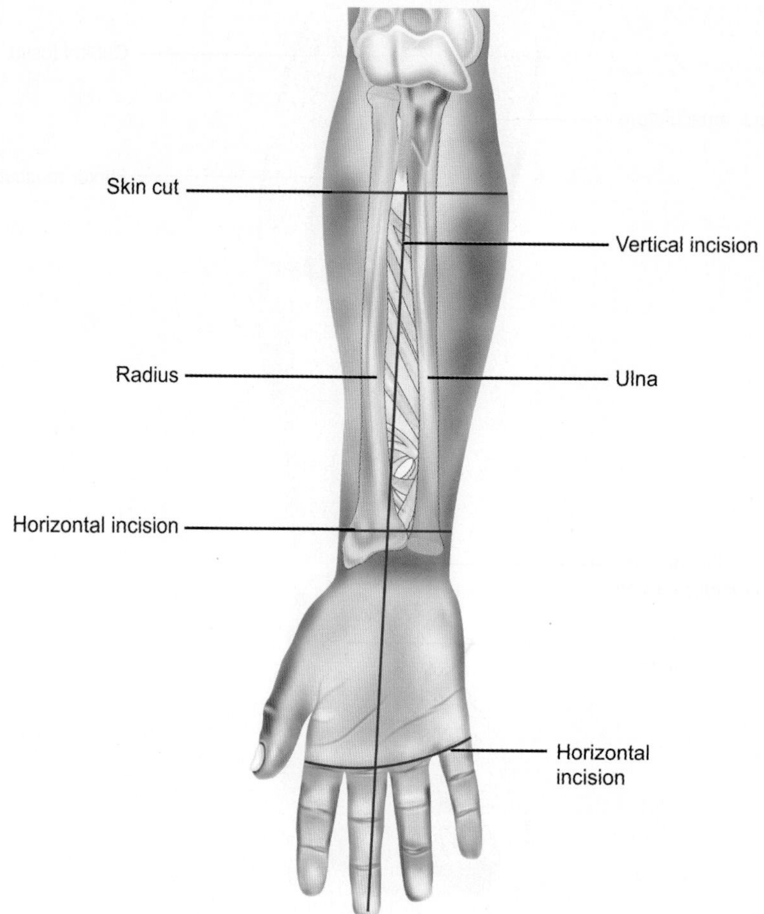

FIGURE 40 Skin incision—forearm and hand

SKIN INCISION (Fig. 40)

Dissection: Make a vertical incision from the middle of the forearm to the tip of the middle finger. Make a horizontal incision along the wrist. Make a horizontal incision along the bases of the phalanges. Reflect all the six flaps of the skin. The forearm skin is a thin skin and can be easily separated from the underlying superficial fascia. The skin over the palm and fingers is very thick and is adherent to the underlying deep fascia by thick connective tissue, the interstices of the connective tissue is filled with fat. This is protective in nature.

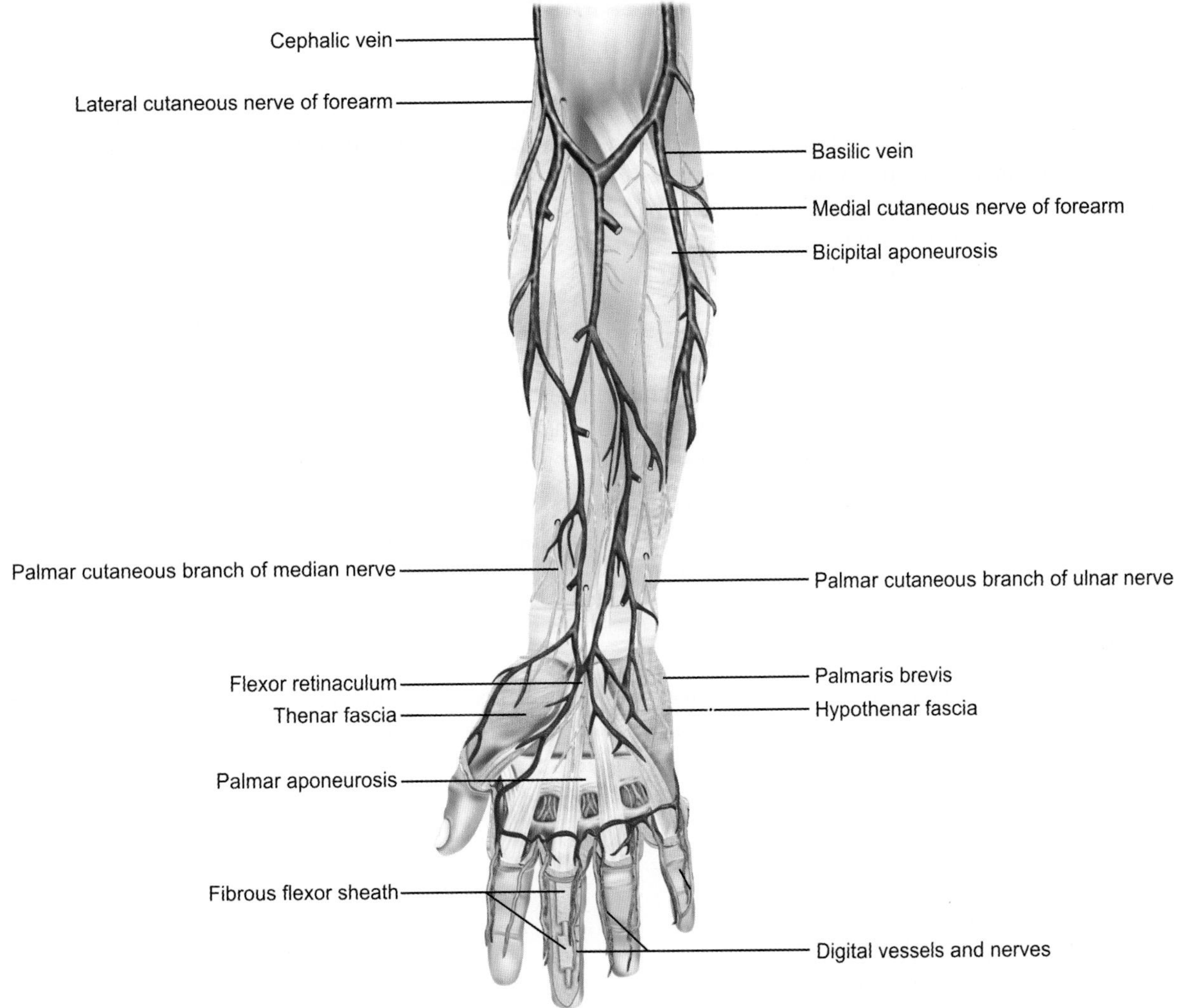

FIGURE 41 Cutaneous structures—forearm and hand

CUTANEOUS VESSELS AND NERVES (Fig. 41)

The cutaneous arteries are too fine to be identified. The cutaneous veins are irregular in position. The ***basilic and cephalic veins*** were already identified in the cubital fossa. See their continuations into the forearm and hand. Dissect the ***lateral cutaneous nerve*** into the forearm along the lateral border and the ***medial cutaneous nerve*** along the medial border of the forearm. The lateral cutaneous nerve is a continuation of the musculocutaneous nerve and the medial cutaneous nerve is an independent nerve from the medial cord of brachial plexus.

The palm of the hand is supplied by the ***palmar cutaneous branch of the ulnar nerve and median nerve.*** They pierce the deep fascia a little proximal to the wrist and supply the hand. Trace these branches.

Palmaris brevis is subcutaneous muscle. Identify this muscle on the medial side of hand. It extends from the palmar aponeurosis and flexor retinaculum to the side of the skin. It is supplied by the superficial branch of the ulnar nerve. When it contracts it pulls the skin towards the center, thus helps in deepening the cup of the hand **(Fig. 41)**.

Dissection: Cut the palmaris brevis muscle near the flexor retinaculum and reflect it. See the ulnar artery and nerve. Trace it distally.

The digital skin is supplied by the ***palmar digital branches of the arteries and nerves.*** They run along the sides of the digits. Identify these branches distal to the palmar aponeurosis between the webs of the fingers. Trace them to the side of the fingers up to the pulp.

DEEP FASCIA

Dissection: Remove the cutaneous nerves and identify the deep fascia. The deep fascia shows modifications. Identify and study it.

It is a thick white glistening sheet of connective tissue in the forearm. The ***bicipital aponeurosis*** gets inserted into its medial side of the upper end (this was already studied). The fascia is thickened to form ***flexor retinaculum*** near the wrist. This gives origin to the muscles. In the central part of the palm it is thickened and forms the ***palmar aponeurosis***. On the thenar and hypothenar eminence it is thinner. In the fingers the deep fascia is modified to form a protective covering for the tendons called the ***fibrous flexor sheaths.***

MUSCLES OF THE FOREARM

The forearm muscles are arranged in three layers, a superficial layer arising from the humerus, an intermediate flexor digitorum superficialis (considered as a superficial group by many authors) and a deep group arising from the shaft of radius and ulna. The median nerve and ulnar nerve share the supply. The radial and ulnar arteries share the arterial supply.

Dissection: Make a midline vertical incision through the deep fascia of the forearm. Reflect the fascia from the forearm. While reflecting, note that it has given origin to the muscles. Identify the origin of the superficial group of musculature (the insertions can be identified in a deeper dissection).

Superficial Layer (Fig. 42)

Origin of the superficial flexor muscles of the forearm. Identify this muscle mass arising from the medial epicondyle and the deep fascia. The muscles have a common muscular origin and become tendinous near the middle of the forearm. It is easy to identify them near their tendons. Identify the muscles from lateral to medial.

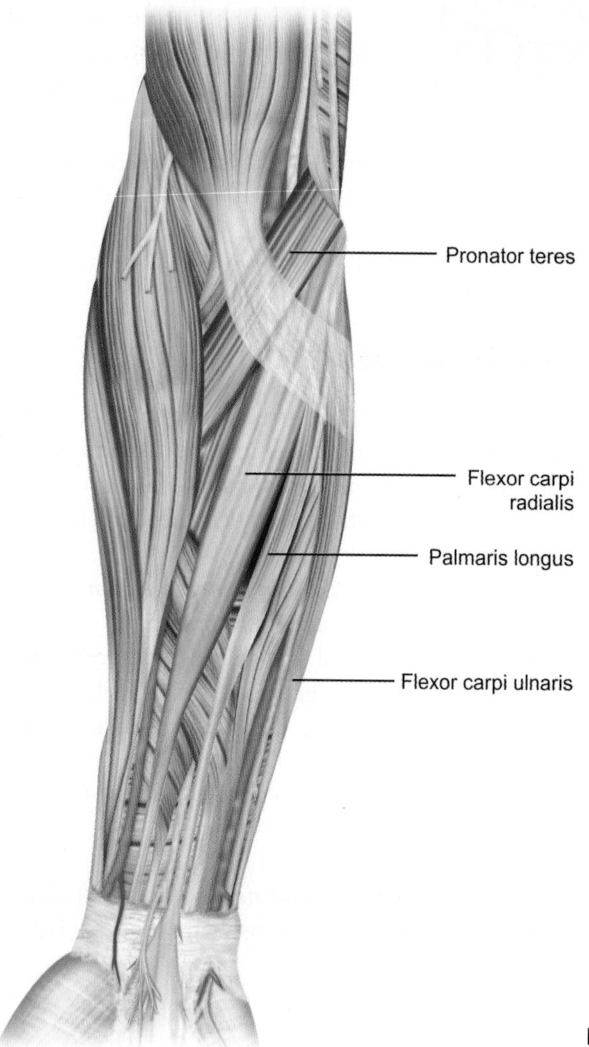

FIGURE 42 Superficial flexor muscles of forearm

The **pronator teres**: This is the most lateral muscle in the group. Reidentify the origin and note that it has two origins, the superficial slip from the medial epicondyle and the supracondylar ridge and the deep head from the coronoid process of the ulna. Note the median nerve passing between the two heads. Push the brachioradialis laterally and see the insertion of the pronatoteres into the convexity of the radius. This is a pronator of the forearm.

Flexor carpi radialis: This is the next muscle. Pick this muscle and trace it to its insertion. You can see it dipping deep to the thenar eminence. It is inserted into the base of the second and third metacarpal bone. Looking at the direction of its fibres it is clear that it is a flexor and an abductor of the hand.

Palmaris longus: Identify this muscle and note that it has a long tendon which becomes continuous with the palmar aponeurosis. Many a times this muscle may be absent. It is flexor of the hand.

This tendon is used for tendon grafting.

Flexor carpi ulnaris: This is the most medial of the muscles. Trace it down to the hand. Note that it dips deep to the hypothenar muscles and get inserted into the base of the fifth metatarsal bone.

Nerve supply: All the above muscles are supplied by the median nerve on their undersurface.

Dissection: Detach the superficial head of the pronator teres and pull it laterally. Cut the tendons of flexor carpi radialis and palmaris longus and flexor carpi ulnaris one inch proximal to the wrist joint. Lift and pull them medially. Note the branches of the median nerve entering into their undersurface. Study the flexor digitorum superficialis.

INTERMEDIATE LAYER (Fig. 43)

Flexor digitorum sperficialis. This muscle lies deep to the previous group of musculature. It has an origin from the medial epicondyle in common with the other superficial group of musculature. Note that this muscle stretches between the ulna and radius with a fibrous tunnel between the two. The radial head arises from a curved line on the lateral border of the radius. Note the median nerve and ulnar artery passing deep to the fibrous tunnel. Trace the muscle distally and identify its tendons. They arrange themselves in two rows. The tendons for middle and ring finger lie anterior to the tendons for the index and little finger.

Brachioradialis: This muscle belongs to the extensor compartment of the forearm. It arises from the lateral supracondylar line of the humerus. Note that this muscle forms the bulk on the lateral side of the forearm. It overlaps many a structures of the forearm. So it is better to study this muscle now. Note that it becomes tendinous in the middle of the forearm Trace it to its insertion to the styloid process of the radius.

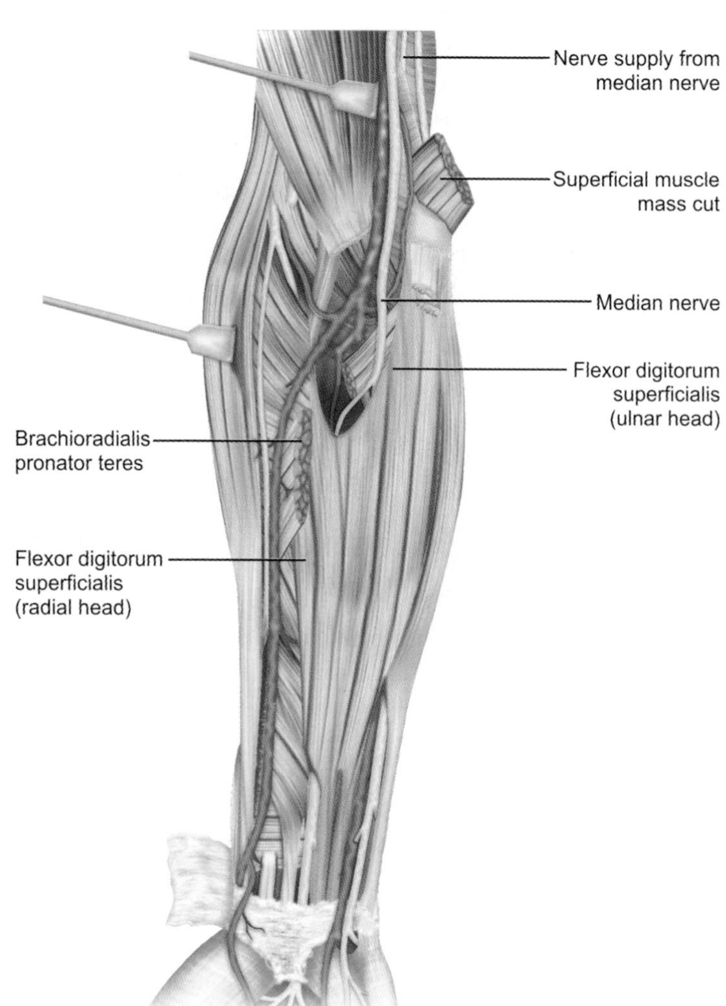

FIGURE 43 Flexor digitorum superficialis

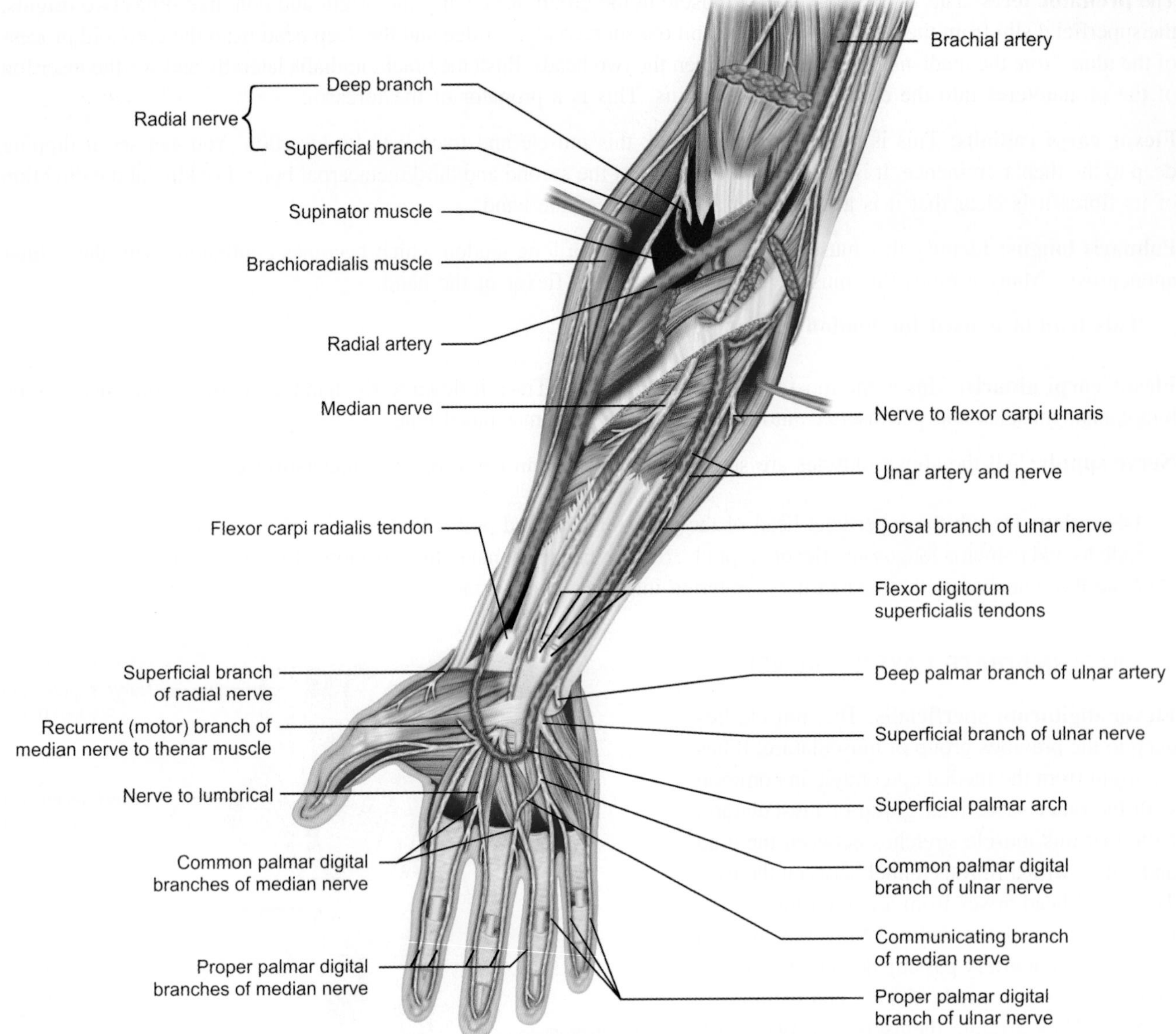

FIGURE 44 Neurovascular bundle of forearm and hand

SUPERFICIAL NEUROVASCULAR BUNDLE OF FOREARM AND HAND (Fig. 44)

Neurovascular bundle: The ulnar, median and radial nerves are seen in the forearm. The musculature of the forearm is supplied by the median nerve and ulnar nerve. The radial nerve passes through the forearm. The brachial artery and its two divisions, the radial and ulnar arteries are located here and give contribution. The venae comitantis accompany the arteries.

Dissection: Cut the flexor digitorum superficialis near its origin and near the wrist and remove the muscle. Pull the brachioradialis muscle laterally to see the deeper structures.

The ulnar nerve: Locate this nerve deep to the flexor carpi ulnaris. Trace its supply to the ***flexor carpi ulnaris.*** Trace it down further into the distal part of the forearm. See that it lies between the flexor carpi ulnaris and the flexor digitorum profundus. Note that it lies medial to the ulnar artery. Note its ***cutaneous*** branches. The dorsal branch is given off near the middle of the forearm. This deviates to the posterior aspect to supply the back of the forearm. See the ***palmar cutaneous branch*** which is given near the distal end. It supplies the skin of the palm (already identified).

Median nerve: Locate this nerve medial to the biceps brachii tendon. Trace its ***muscular branches*** into the pronator teres, flexor carpi radials, palmaris longus flexor digitorum superficialis and to elbow joint while it lies over brachialis muscle. Trace it to the fibrous tunnel deep to the flexor digitorum superficialis. It runs down between the flexor digitorum superficialis and profundus up to the wrist.

Radial nerve: This nerve lies under cover of the brachioradialis. Identify this nerve. Here it lies between the brachioradialis and extensor carpi radialis longus. See its nerve of supply to extensor carpi radialis longus. Note the radial nerve dividing into two branches. Trace its superficial, thin branch, superficial to the pronator teres. This deviates to the posterior aspect of the forearm near the middle of the forearm. This is a ***cutaneous branch.*** Trace the deep thick muscular branch into the supinator muscle. This is a nerve of the posterior compartment.

Brachial artery: Identify the brachial artery medial to the tendon of biceps brachii. See its two branches the ***radial and ulnar artery*** at the level of the neck of the radius.

Ulnar artery: This is the main artery of supply to the forearm and is a bigger branch. Note that it lies on the brachialis at its origin. Push the flexor muscles and identify the artery lying deep to the muscles. Trace it to the distal end of the forearm. Note that it runs between the flexor carpi ulnaris and the flexor digitorum superficialis. Identify the ulnar nerve on its medial side. Trace its lateral branches.

Radial artery: Trace the radial artery from its origin to the wrist and note that it lies on the pronator teres insertion, flexor digitorum superficialis and flexor pollicis longus. The radial artery pulsations are felt here. Trace the radial recurrent artery arising near the origin of the radial artery. Trace it up. It anastomoses with the radial collateral artery of the profunda brachii artery.

DEEP DISSECTION OF FOREARM (Fig. 45)

The floor of the cubital fossa is seen in the upper part of forearm. It is a slopping gutter shaped depression. Study the floor and contents of the cubital fossa.

Floor: This is formed by the ***insertion of brachialis*** muscle. Note that it is fleshy almost up to the insertion. It is inserted into the tubercle on the coronoid process of ulna. Note this area on the ulna. Appreciate its action as a flexor of the forearm. Note the tendon of biceps reaching the radial tuberosity. Pull it and realize that is separated from the anterior aspect by a bursa. Pull it, and see the possible rotatory action on the radius.

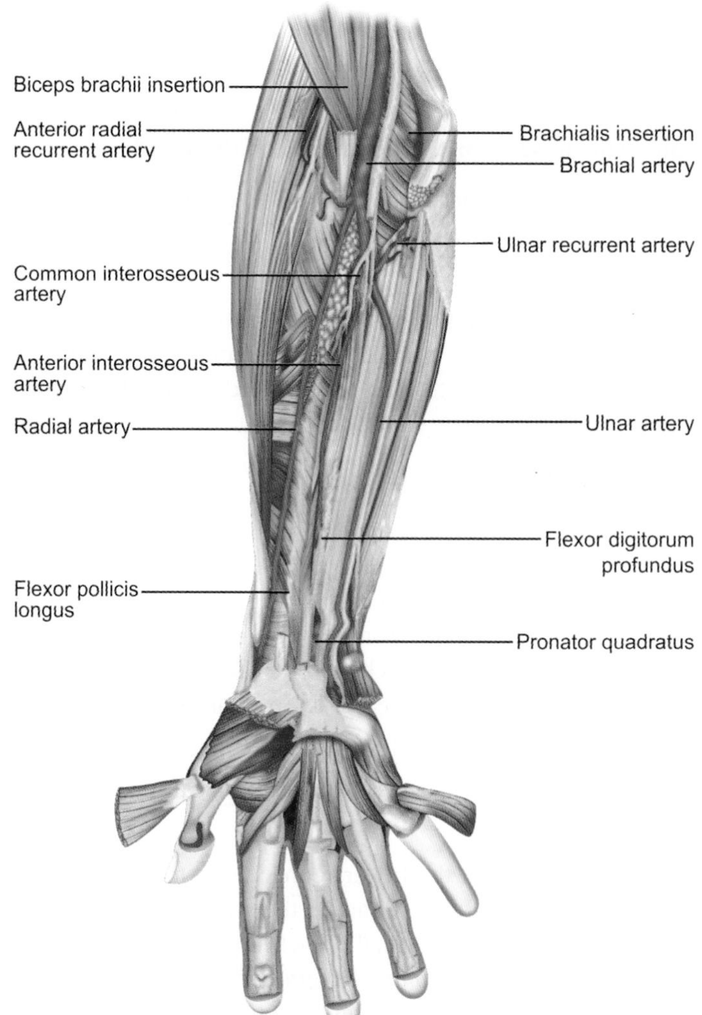

FIGURE 45 Deep dissection of forearm

Arteries of Forearm

Dissection: Trace the brachial artery to its division at the neck of the radius into ***radial*** and ***ulnar*** artery. From the ulnar artery trace the ***anterior ulnar recurrent artery*** proximal to the pronator teres muscle, in front of the medial epicondyle. The ***posterior ulnar recurrent artery***—trace it deep to the superficial group of muscles to the posterior aspect of the medial epicondyle. Pull the artery medially and trace its ***common interosseous branch***. See its division into an anterior and posterior interosseous branch, which passes in front and behind the interosseous membrane. Trace the ***anterior interosseous artery*** in front of the interosseous membrane between the flexor digitorum longus and pollicis longus. Identify the muscular branches into the superficial and deep group of muscles. Trace the ***radial recurrent***, from the radial artery to the anterior aspect of the lateral epicondyle (these above blood vessels are very thin, may be difficult to trace them, but it is essential to study the collateral circulation from a standard textbook).

Collateral circulation around the elbow: It is an arterial anastomosis between the arteries of the arm and forearm. They are located around the sides of the elbow. During flexion at elbow joint the major vessels get pressed. At this time the collateral circulation opens up and keeps up the continuity of blood flow.

Deep group of musculature: The muscles of this group arise from the radius and ulna. They consist of flexor digitorum profundus, flexor pollicis longus and pronator quadratus. The anterior interosseous artery and nerve constitute the neurovascular bundle of this group.

Dissection: Detach the flexor digitorum superficialis from its origin totally.

Flexor digitorum profundus: Locate this medial muscle below the coronoid process from the upper third of the anterior and medial aspects of the ulna and the interosseous membrane. Put your fingers medially and feel it up to the posterior border of ulna. Trace it down up to the wrist, where it gives rise to four tendons.

Flexor pollicis longus: Locate this lateral muscle arising from the anterior aspect of the radius and interosseous membrane between the origins of the flexor digitorum superficialis and the pronator quadratus. Trace it down to the wrist, where you can see its tendon.

The insertions of these muscles into the fingers and will be seen in the dissection of the hand.

Pronator quadratus: Locate this transversely placed muscle at the distal end of the forearm. It extends between the distal one-fourth of the anterior ends of radius and ulna. As the radius moves over the ulna the ulnar attachment is considered as the origin and the radial attachment is considered as the insertion.

Nerve and blood supply: Locate the anterior interosseous nerve and artery between the flexor digitorum profundus and the flexor pollicis longus and deep to the pronator quadratus. The nerve is a branch of the median nerve and ends in the anterior aspect of the forearm by supplying the wrist and carpal joints. The artery pierces the interosseous membrane and reaches the back of the forearm. They supply the muscles and joints.

SUPERFICIAL STRUCTURES OF THE HAND (Figs 41 and 44)

Palmar aponeurosis is the thick triangular central part of the palm. Proximally is the apex and it is continuous with the palmaris longus muscle. Its distal part is expanded and forms the base. Distally this divides into four slips for the medial four fingers. Each slip divides into two, encloses the digital tendons in their center. The slips dip deep and get attached to the deep transverse metacarpal ligaments. Medial and lateral septa arise from the sides dip deep. The medial septum gets attached to the third metacarpal bone whereas the lateral septum is attached to the fifth metacarpal bone. The fascia covering the thenar and hypothenar eminence is thinner compared to the central palmar aponeurosis.

Dissection: Cut the palmar aponeurosis near it apex and along the sides. Cut it near the distal slips and remove it totally. As you are detaching the palmar aponeurosis identify its medial and lateral septa, note its distal attachment to the deep transverse metacarpal ligaments.

Superficial palmar arch: It is an arterial arch. Identify the ulnar artery on the flexor retinaculum, trace it forward into the palm. Note that the arch is completed by branch from the radial artery. It can be the radialis indices or the princeps pollicis branch of the radial artery. Trace its distal branches. The most medial branch is the digital branch. It supplies the medial side of the little finger. The next three branches are ***common palmar digital branches.*** On reaching the webs of the fingers they divide into two proper digital arteries to supply the adjacent sides of the fingers.

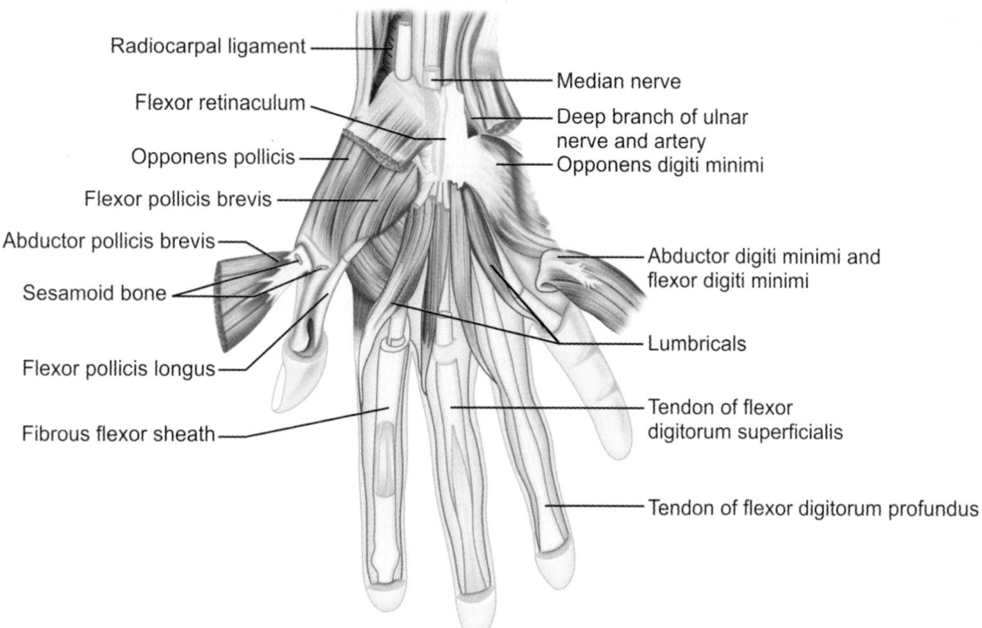

FIGURE 46 Superficial musculature of hand

Ulnar nerve: Identify the nerve medial to the ulnar artery in the distal part of the forearm, between the flexor carpi ulnaris and the palmaris longus. Trace its ***deep muscular branch*** given off from its medial side. This supplies the muscles of the hypothenar eminence. The deep branch leaves this area between the flexor and abductor digiti minimi. Trace the superficial ***cutaneous branch*** further forwards. Trace its branches to the medial side of little finger, lateral side of little finger, medial side of ring finger and a communicating branch to the median nerve.

Median nerve: Identify the median nerve distal to the flexor retinaculum (near the flexor retinaculum it lies deep to it in the carpal tunnel) and deep to the superficial palmar artery. It is a mixed nerve. Trace its branches into the ***muscles of the thenar eminence.*** Trace its ***cutaneous branches*** to either side of the thumb, either side of the index finger, either side of the middle finger and the lateral side of the ring finger. See its ***communicating branch*** with the ulnar nerve. Try to see the ***first and second lumbricals*** and the nerve supply into these muscles.

MUSCULATURE (Fig. 46)

Flexor retinaculum: Identify this thick fascia located near the wrist. Identify its medial attachment to the pisiform and hook of hamate. See its lateral attachment to the tubercle of scaphoid and tubercle of trapezium. Note that all the tendons of the musculature pass deep to it. Note the hand has got a central depression and a thenar eminence on the lateral side and the hypothenar eminence on the medial side. The thenar and hypothenar eminence is formed by the musculature of the thumb and little finger. The central area is occupied by the long tendons of the fingers (**Fig. 46**).

THENAR EMINENCE

It is formed by the ***abductor pollicis brevis, flexor pollicis brevis*** and opponens pollicis. They all have a common origin from the flexor retinaculum, scaphoid and trapezium. It is easy to identify them when traced to their insertions. The abductor is a lateral muscle. Trace it to the lateral side of the base of the first phalanx. The flexor is the medial muscle. Note that it divides into two parts. The medial part joins with the adductor (a deeper muscle) to be inserted into the base of the medial side of the first phalanx. Its lateral part joins the abductor pollicis brevis at its insertion.

Dissection: Cut the abductor pollicis brevis near its origin. Reflect to its insertion; while doing so, look for the nerve supply into the three muscles from the median nerve. Note that there are sesamoid bones located in the tendons of abductor and flexor pollicis. They are two in number, grooving the distal end of the head of the metacarpal bone.

Opponens pollicis: This is a deeper muscle. It is inserted into the anterior border of the first metacarpal bone. This muscle is a rotator of the metacarpal over the hamate. It turns the thumb, so as to reach the opposite side of the palm or other fingers.

Hypothenar eminence: It is made up of abductor digiti minimi, flexor digiti minimi and opponens digiti minimi. All the three muscles arise from the flexor retinaculum, pisiform bone and hook of hamate. The abductor and flexor form the superficial layer and the opponens forms the deep layer. Note that the abductor and flexor are closely united and they both insert into the medial side of base of the proximal phalanx.

Dissection: Cut the abductor and flexor digiti minimi near their origin and reflect them towards their insertion. While reflecting trace their nerve supply from the deep branch of the ulnar nerve.

Opponens digiti minimi: See this deeper muscle. It is inserted into the anterior border of the fifth metacarpal bone. It rotates the fifth metacarpal bone, thus helping the little finger to reach the opposite side of the palm and the thumb.

Long Tendons in the Palm

The tendons of flexor pollicis longus, flexor digitorum superficialis and profundus pass through the carpal tunnel, center of the palm and through the fibrous flexor sheaths of the fingers to reach their insertions on to the phalanges.

Dissection: Cut the superficial palmar arch, superficial branch of the ulnar nerve and the median nerve up to the metacarpophalangeal joints.

Carpal tunnel: It is a fibro-osseous tunnel formed by the carpal bones and the flexor retinaculum, the long flexor tendons of the hand pass through this. The flexor tendons are enclosed in ***synovial sheaths***. The synovial sheaths are bags of synovial fluid which have a parietal and a visceral layer. The parietal layer lines the boundaries and the visceral layer covers the tendons. The synovial fluid lies between the parietal and visceral layers.

The tendons insinuate themselves from the lateral aspect. They protect the tendons from getting rubbed in the osseofibrous carpal tunnel. The superficial and deep flexors of the fingers occupy one synovial sheath called ***ulnar bursa*** whereas the flexor pollicis longus occupies a separate synovial sheath called ***radial bursa.*** This is continuous up to the base of the distal phalanx. Generally the ulnar and radial bursae communicate proximally in the wrist region. The radial and ulnar bursae begin proximal to the wrist to the middle of the hand.

Dissection: Cut open the flexor retinaculum by a longitudinal cut. When you open the flexor retinaculum you are opening the fibrous part of the fibro-osseous tunnel and the parietal layer of the synovial sheaths. Feel the stickiness. It is due to the synovial fluid. Trace them into the palm.

The flexor pollicis longus: Identify this lateral tendon under the flexor retinaculum. Trace this to its insertion into the base of the distal phalanx of the thumb. This is enclosed in an independent synovial sheath. This is a thin sheet, which can be identified by making a fine slit into the sheath. This is called radial bursa. The radial bursa and ulnar bursa communicate generally proximal to the flexor retinaculum.

Identify the tendons of the flexor digitorum superficialis; they lie in two rows, the tendon of the index and little finger lie deep to the tendon of middle and ring finger. Deep to this note the four tendons of the flexor digitorum profundus. Trace them forward into the hand. The tendons spread out and the flexor digitorum superficialis tendons lie superficial to the flexor digitorum profundus tendons. Note that the synovial sheaths continue up to the middle of the hand. Slit open the synovial sheaths and note that two tendons are arranged for each finger, one from flexor digitorum superficialis and another flexor digitorum profundus.

Dissection: Pull the tendons of flexor digitorum superficialis and cut them transversely near the carpometacarpal joints and remove the proximal part of the muscle. See the tendons of the flexor digitorum profundus and the lumbrical muscles arising from them.

Lumbricals: These are small muscles arising from the lateral side of the flexor digitorum profundus tendons. Trace them forwards to the digital web where they move to the posterior aspect of the fingers. Nerve supply: The ulnar nerve supplies the medial two lumbricals, and the median nerve supplies the lateral two lumbricals. The ulnar nerve reaches the muscles on their deep surface whereas the median nerve reaches them on their superficial surface (you have already seen the supply to lateral two lumbricals, the nerve supply to medial two lumbricals you will see while reflecting the flexor digitorum profundus tendons). Note that these muscles cross the metacarpophalangeal joints anteriorly and laterally and cross the interphalangeal joints dorsally. These are flexors of fingers at metacarpophalangeal joints and extensors of the fingers at the interphalangeal joints.

Tendons in the fingers: The fibrous flexor sheaths, the phalanges and the interphalangeal joints form a continuous osseofibrous tunnel for the long tendons of the fingers. They are enclosed in common synovial sheaths.

Fibrous flexor sheaths: This is a modification of the deep fascia over the fingers. It extends from the heads of the metacarpal bones to the base of the distal phalanx. This protects the digital tendons. The muscles controlling the movements at the digits are tendinous when they reach the fingers. The tendons cross the metacarpophalangeal joints, the interphalangeal joints, and the phalanges to reach their insertions. To protect these tendons from rubbing, these are kept in osseofibrous tunnels. The fibrous flexor sheaths have transverse fibres over the phalanges and oblique fibres over the joints. This permits free movement over the joints. Posteriorly the sheaths are attached to the phalanges and palmar ligaments of the metacarpophalangeal and interphalangeal joints.

Dissection: Slit the fibrous flexor sheaths and trace the flexor digitorum superficialis and flexor digitorum profundus into the fingers. When you cut open the fibrous flexor sheaths you can feel the sticky synovial fluid.

The ***flexor digitorum superficialis*** flattens opposite the base of the proximal phalanx, divides into two slips, clasps the tendon of flexor digitorum profundus, gets inserted into the base of the second phalanx.

The ***flexor digitorum profundus*** tendon continues into the fingers, passes through the loop created by the flexor digitorum superficialis, and gets inserted into the base of the distal phalanx. Pull both the tendons forward and identify the long and short vincula. The vincula carry blood vessels and nerves to the tendons.

Movement: The flexor digitorum profundus initiates flexion at the distal interphalangeal joint, whereas the flexor digitorum superficialis initiates flexion at the proximal interphalangeal joint. Continued action of both the muscles causes flexion at the metacarpophalangeal, carpometacarpal and wrist joints. Pull the tendons of the muscles and see the movement performed by them.

PALMAR SPACES (Fig. 47)

Dissection: Catch the long tendons at the wrist level, lift them up and note the connective tissue septum extending from the deeper aspect of the lateral end of the tendons to the third metacarpal bone. This is lateral septum of the palmar aponeurosis.

Midpalmar space: It is the potential space seen between the long flexor tendons of the 3rd, 4th, 5th fingers and the fascia covering the interossei of 3rd and 4th intermetacarpal space.

Thenar space: It is the potential space between the long flexor tendons of the second finger and adductor pollicis **(Fig. 47).**

Proximally the spaces extend up to the distal palmar crease and distally they extend up to the proximal transverse palmar crease. Infection can accumulate in these spaces and may need surgical intervention to drain them.

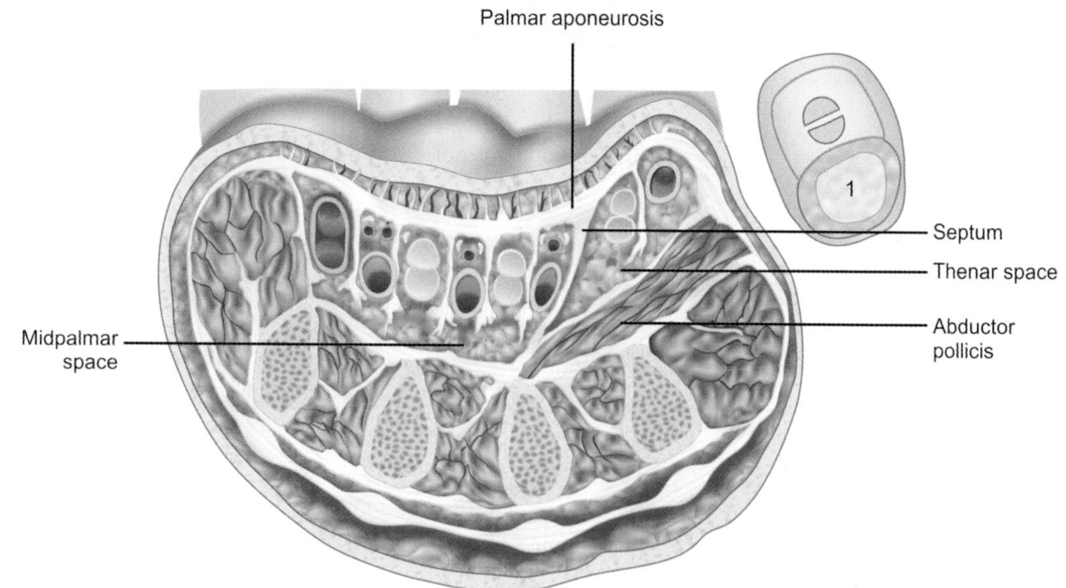

FIGURE 47 Palmar spaces—section through palm

Dissection: Cut the flexor digitorum profundus tendons and flexor pollicis longus tendon near the wrist and pull them up to the first phalange. While pulling the tendons note the nerve supply to the lateral two lumbricals from the ulnar nerve. Remove the connective tissue over the adductor pollicis and study the muscle.

Intrinsic Muscles of Hand (Fig. 48)

The adductor pollicis, palmar interossei and the dorsal interossei constitute the intrinsic muscles of the hand. The deep palmar arch and deep branch of the ulnar nerve form the neurovascular bundle.

Adductor pollicis muscle (Fig. 48). Identify this transversely placed muscle. Note its two origins. The transverse head takes origin from the third metacarpal bone. The oblique head arises from the second and third metacarpals and the adjoining carpal bones. See that they unite together and get inserted into the medial side of the base of the proximal phalanx. It is an adductor of the thumb.

Dissection: Cut the adductor muscle near its origins and reflect it towards the insertion. Clean the neurovascular bundle.

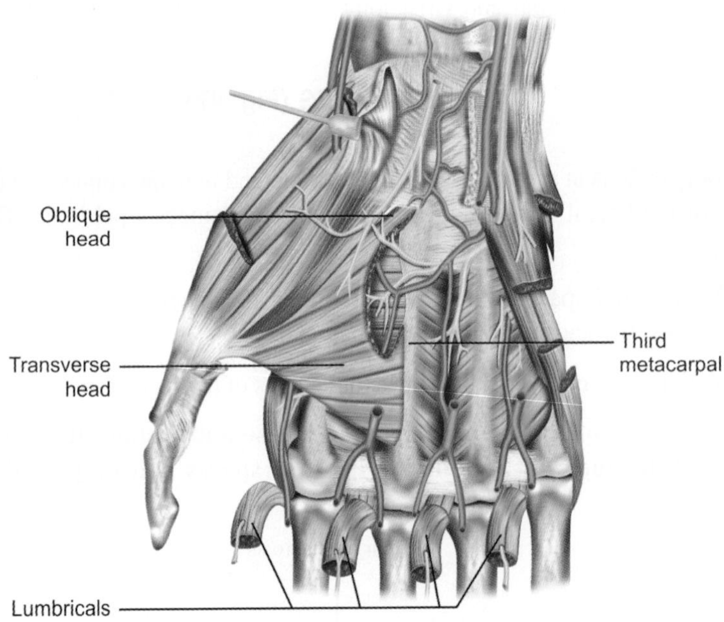

FIGURE 48 Adductor pollicis

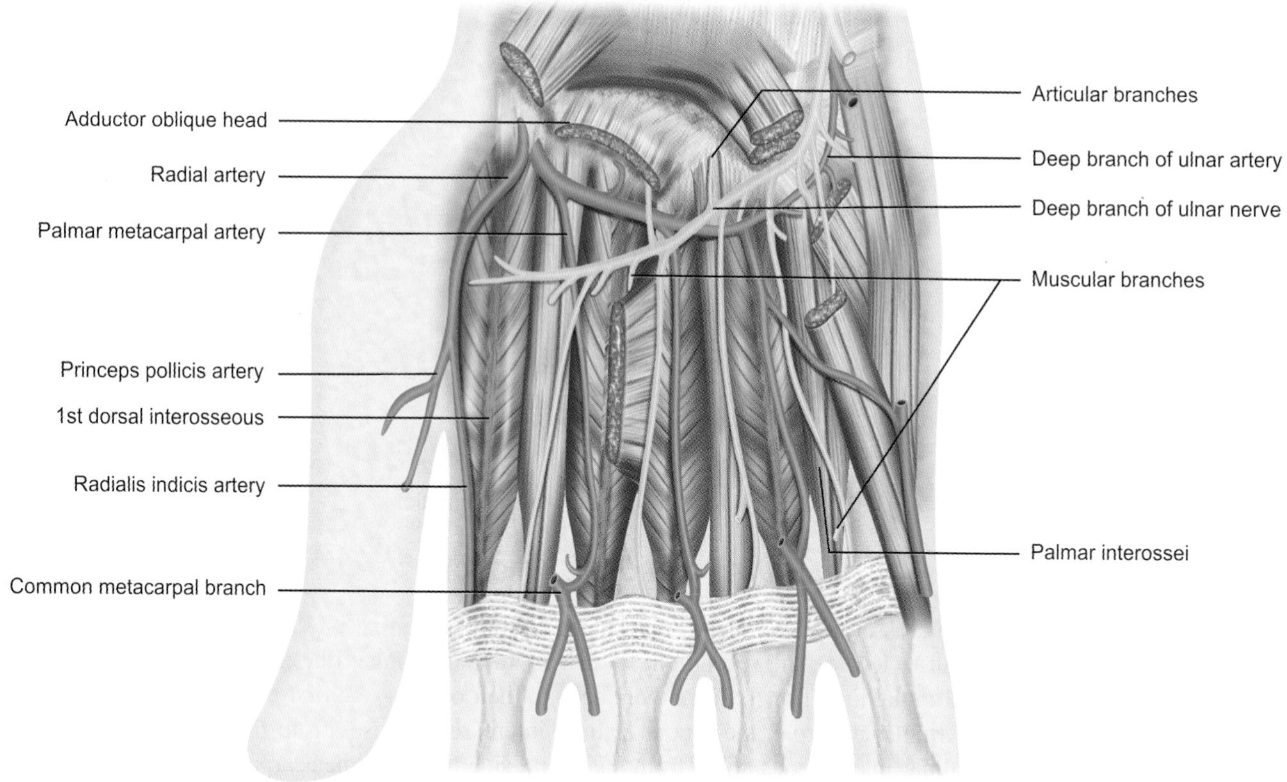

FIGURE 49 Neurovascular bundle

DEEP NEUROVASCULAR BUNDLE (Fig. 49)

The deep branch of the ulnar nerve and the deep palmar arch forms the neurovascular bundle here. It supplies all the deep muscles and the joints.

Deep Palmar Arch

Identify this. Note that it is firmed by the ***deep branch of the ulnar artery and the radial artery.*** Locate the radial artery entering the palm between the two heads of the first dorsal interosseous. The arch lies on the bases of the midcarpal bones. Trace the three ***palmar metacarpal arteries*** given off from its convexity. They traverse in the medial three interosseous space and join the distal ends of the common metacarpal arteries. They supply the muscles and metacarpals in these spaces.

Princeps pollicis artery: Trace this artery. It is a branch of the radial artery. This traverses in the thumb, divides into two palmar digital branches near the head of metacarpal bone, passes on either side of the flexor pollicis longus tendon and supplies the sides of the digits.

Radialis indices artery: This is a branch of the radial artery. Try to identify this artery over the first dorsal interosseous, and trace it along the lateral side of the index finger, where it is called as the lateral palmar digital artery of the index finger.

The Deep Branch of the Ulnar Nerve

Locate this nerve within the concavity of the deep palmar arterial arch. Trace it from the level of hook of hamate to the first dorsal interosseous. Trace its branches to all palmar interossei, all dorsal interossei, adductor pollicis and medial two lumbricals. It gives articular branches to the carpal joints and the metacarpophalangeal joints.

Dissection: Clean the connective tissue over the intermetacarpal space and identify the palmar and dorsal interossei muscles.

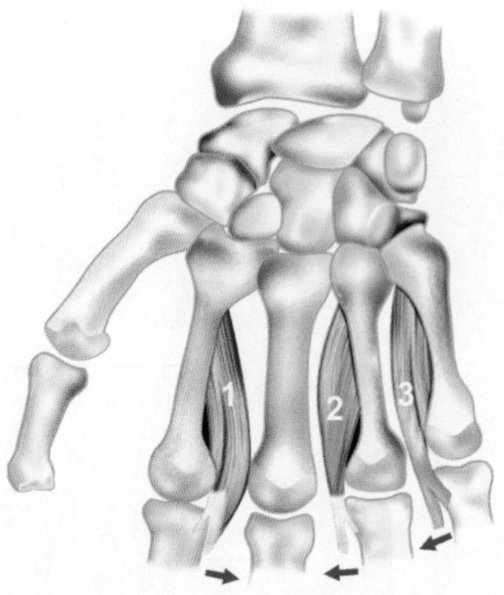

FIGURE 50 Palmar interossei—diagrammatic

PALMAR INTEROSSEI (Fig. 50)

Locate the tendons of palmar interossei near the metacarpophalangeal joint—the first one lateral to the thumb (this is a very small muscle and difficult to locate), the second one medial to the index finger, the third one lateral to the ring finger and the fourth one lateral to the little finger. Trace them back to their origin – the first palmar interosseous arises from the medial aspect of the first metacarpal, the second palmar interosseous arises from the medial aspect of the second metacarpal, the third palmar interosseous arises from the lateral side of fourth metacarpal and the fourth palmar interosseous arises from the lateral side of the fifth metacarpal bone. They are all adductors of the phalanges at the metacarpophalangeal joint. The axis for adduction is an anteroposterior axis passing through the head of the metacarpal bone.

DORSAL INTEROSSEI (Fig. 51)

These are four in number. Identify the tendons of the dorsal interossei—the first one lateral to the index; the second one is lateral to the middle finger; the third one medial to the middle finger and the fourth one medial to the ring finger. Trace them back to their origins. These are bipennate muscles. The first dorsal interosseous arises from the adjoining sides of the first and second metacarpal bones, the second one arises from the adjoining sides of the second and third metacarpal bones, the third one arises from the adjoining sides of the third and fourth metacarpal bones and forth interosseous arises from the adjoining sides of the fourth and fifth metacarpal bones. These are abductors of the fingers at the metacarpophalangeal joint. The axis for this movement passes through the heads of the metacarpal bones. The abduction and adduction takes place around the central line passing through the center of the middle finger.

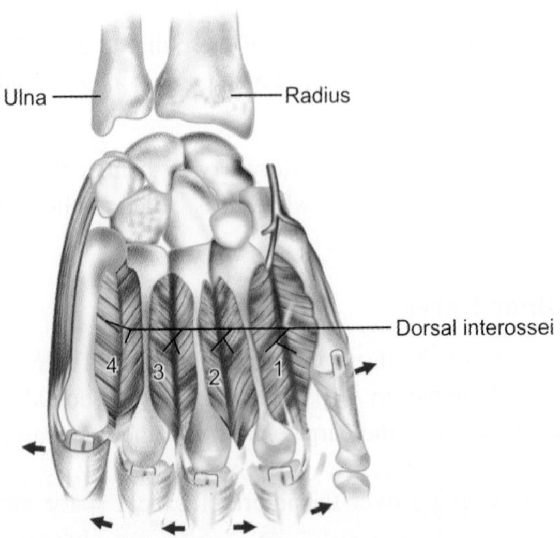

FIGURE 51 Dorsal interossei—diagrammatic

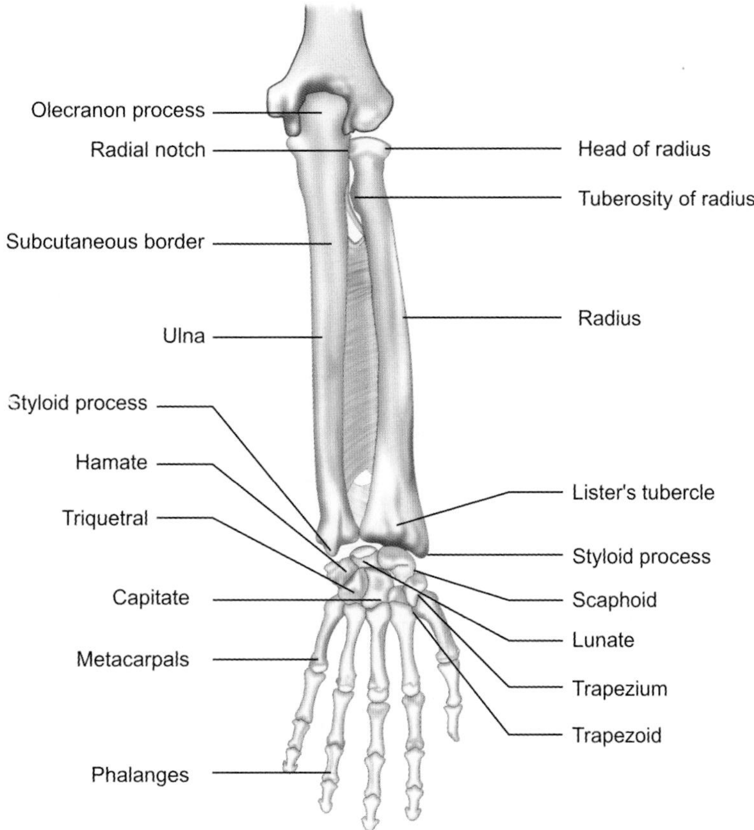

FIGURE 52 Skeleton of the back of the forearm and hand

BACK OF THE FOREARM AND HAND

The back of the forearm lodges the extensors of the forearm, wrist and the hand and supinator of the forearm. The posterior interosseous nerve, the deep branch of the radial nerve is the nerve of supply. The posterior interosseous artery, a branch of the common interosseous artery is the artery of supply.

SKELETON (Fig. 52)

Go to an articulated skeleton and see the posterior aspects of the bones of the forearm and hand.

Ulna: See the projecting ***olecranon process*** of the ulna. Identify its smooth and rough surfaces. The rough surface gives attachment to the triceps muscle and smooth surface lodges the bursa. Note that the triangular surface on the back of the olecranon process continues as the ***subcutaneous border*** of the ulna. See the ***styloid process*** of the ulna. It projects from the back of the ulna.

Radius: Note that the radius has the rounded head at the upper end and articulates with the radial notch of the ulna. The shaft of the radius bends outwards and presents a sharp medial border and a convex lateral border. Note that the lower end expands. Identify the lateral projecting styloid process and the dorsally placed Lister's tubercle.

Hand skeleton: Identify the ***scaphoid, lunate*** and ***triquetral*** from lateral medial in the proximal row of carpals; the ***trapezium, trapezoid, capitate and hamate*** from lateral to medial in the distal row of carpals. Note that they are wider on the dorsal aspect than on the ventral aspect. Identify the five metacarpals, note their bases, shaft and heads. Note that the shafts are wider on the dorsal aspect. See the ***phalanges,*** two to the thumb and three each to the remaining fingers. See their proximal bases, the shafts and the distal heads. Note that the dorsal surfaces of the phalanges are wider than the ventral surfaces.

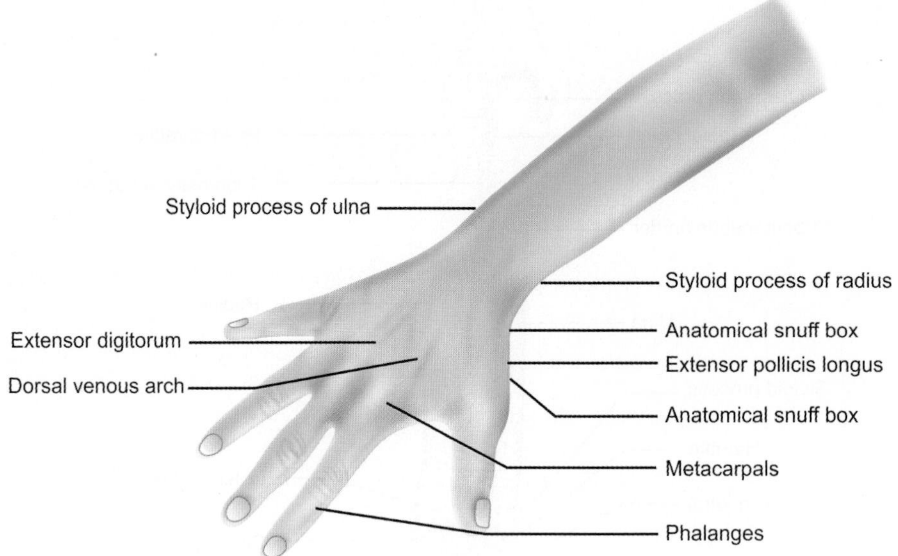

FIGURE 53 Surface anatomy—back of forearm and hand

SURFACE ANATOMY (Fig. 53)

Feel the subcutaneous border of the ulna throughout the extent of the back of the forearm. See that the extensors form the lateral bulge on the upper aspect of the forearm. At the distal end feel the distal ends of radius and the ulna. Note that they are the styloid processes of the radius and the ulna and the distal end of the radius is at a distal position compared to the ulnar styloid process.

In an extended hand identify the ***dorsal venous arch*** and the prominent extensor tendons. On the medial four fingers you can identify the tendons of the ***extensor digitorum.*** Extend the thumb and note the prominent tendons here. Medially it is formed by the ***extensor pollicis longus*** and laterally by the ***abductor pollicis longus*** and ***extensor pollicis brevis.*** This area is called ***anatomical snuff box.*** Put your finger in the area between the two and feel the pulsations of the radial artery. In the floor of the anatomical snuff box you can feel the styloid process of ulna and the trapezium and the base of the first metacarpal bone. On the dorsum of the hand you can feel all the *carpals,* ***metacarpals and phalanges.*** Make a fist and note the ***knuckles.*** They are formed by the heads of metacarpals and phalanges. Note that the metacarpophalangeal joints and interphalangeal joints are arranged along an arc. So when the fingers are extended they are separated and when they are flexed they come together, meet the hand at the same horizontal line.

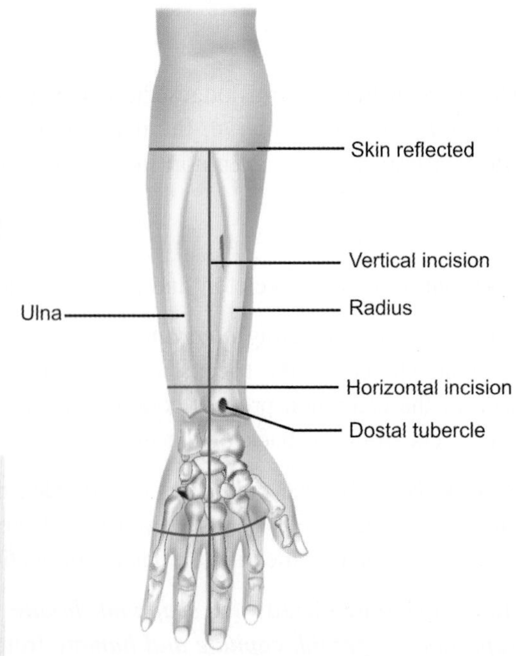

FIGURE 54 Skin incision—back of forearm and hand

SKIN INCISIONS (Fig. 54)

Dissection: Make a vertical incision in the midline from the olecranon process to the middle of the middle finger. Make a horizontal incision near the wrist, another horizontal incision along the knuckles and remove the skin from the back of the forearm and hand and over as many fingers as you feel like. Here the skin is ***thicker but easily separates from the deep fascia as the superficial fascia is loose.***

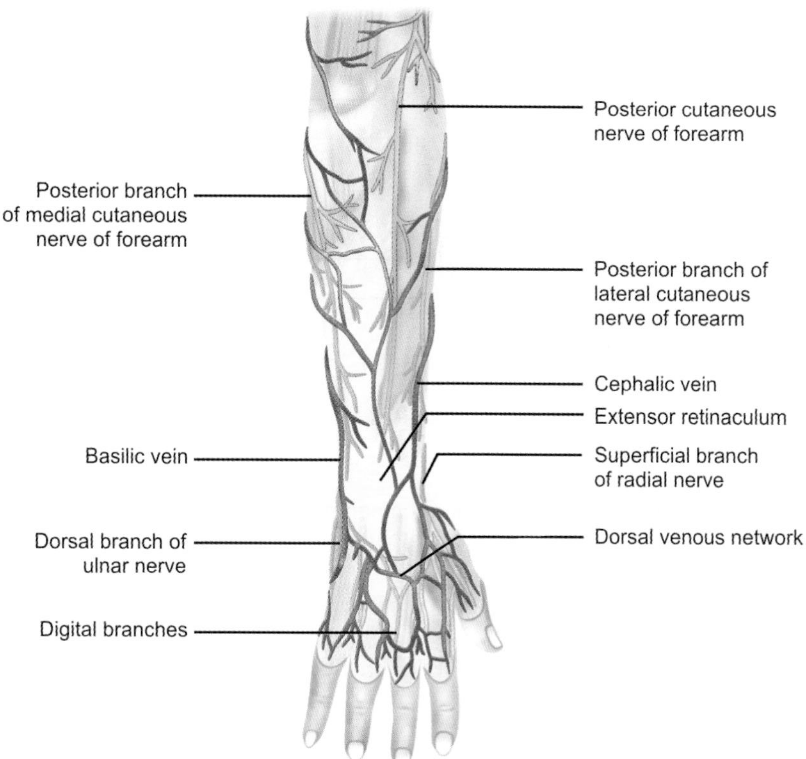

FIGURE 55 Superficial fascia—back of forearm and hand

SUPERFICIAL FASCIA (Fig. 55)

Venous system: Identify the irregular ***dorsal venous arch*** on the back of the hand. It is formed proximal to the knuckles. See the ***dorsal digital veins*** draining into it. Note that the dorsal venous arch continues as the *basilic vein* medially and as ***cephalic vein*** laterally. You have already seen their continuation on the anterior aspect.

Cutaneous nerves: Identify the ***posterior branch*** of the ***medial cutaneous nerve of the forearm*** accompanying the basilic vein; the ***lateral cutaneous nerve of the forearm,*** a continuation of the musculocutaneous nerve accompanying the cephalic vein and the ***posterior cutaneous nerve of the forearm,*** a branch of the radial nerve lying in the midline. On the hand trace the ***dorsal branch of the ulnar nerve*** supplying medial one and a half fingers and the dorsum of the hand. Note that the lateral three and a half fingers and the lateral side of the dorsum are supplied by the ***superficial branch of the radial nerve***.

Dissection: Remove the cutaneous structures and clean the deep fascia.

Deep fascia: Identify the deep fascia. Note that the fibres over the back of the forearm and the back of the hand run vertically and near the wrist they are supported by horizontal fibres. This is called the ***extensor retinaculum.*** Trace its attachment laterally to the anterior border of the lower end of the radius and medially it is attached to the styloid process of ulna, triquetral and pisiform bones. Pull it and note that it sends in vertical septa to reach the longitudinal ridges on the posterior surface of the lower end of the radius and forms six osteofibrous tunnels. The extensor tendons of the back of the hand pass through these. These tendons are covered by synovial sheaths. The synovial sheaths protect the tendons from getting rubbed away due to movement.

Dissection: Put a vertical incision along the middle of the back of the forearm from the elbow to the middle finger. Make a horizontal incision proximal to the extensor retinaculum, and remove the deep fascia from the back of the forearm, from the dorsum and from the back of the fingers. Retain the extensor retinaculum. Note that the deep fascia gives attachment to the musculature near their origin.

MUSCLES OF THE POSTERIOR COMPARTMENT OF FOREARM

Muscles of the posterior compartment of forearm are—extensors of the forearm, supinator of the forearm and extensors of the hand and fingers at wrist, intercarpal, carpometacarpal, metacarpophalangeal and interphalangeal joints. They are arranged in two layers, a superficial and a deep layer.

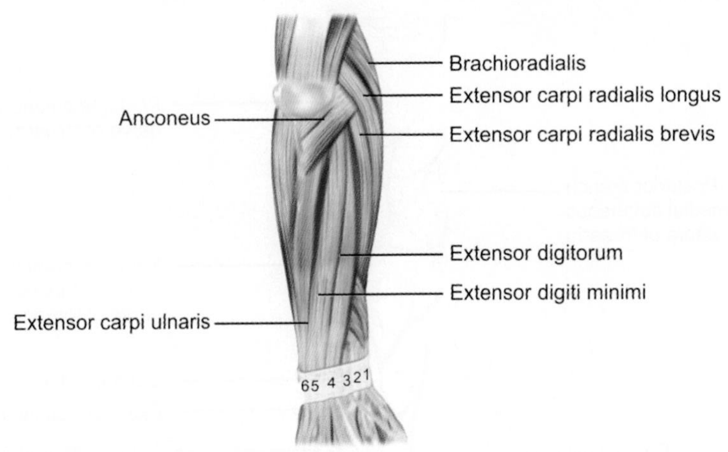

FIGURE 56 Muscles of posterior compartment of forearm superficial group

THE SUPERFICIAL GROUP OF MUSCULATURE (Fig. 56)

They arise by a common origin from the lateral epicondyle of the humerus. The origin of these muscles extends as high as the upper end of the lateral supracondylar line. Trace these muscles from lateral to medial. It is generally difficult to identify them individually at their origin. They become tendinous towards the distal part of the forearm where they can easily be identified.

Brachioradialis: This is better seen on the anterior side than on the posterior side. This is already identified in the anterior compartment. Try to see its origin on the lateral supracondylar line. Trace it down to the styloid process of the radius. It is a strong flexor in the mid prone position of the forearm. It also brings the forearm to the midprone position both from pure flexion and pure extension. Note its nerve supply from the radial nerve in the arm.

Extensor carpi radial longus: This is the next muscle. This also extends up to the supracondylar line of the humerus. Trace it down to the distal end. Note that it is under the second compartment of the extensor retinaculum along with the extensor carpi radialis brevis.

Extensor carpi radialis brevis: This muscle arises from the lateral epicondyle of the humerus. Trace it down to the extensor retinaculum. Note that this occupies the second compartment under extensor retinaculum.

Extensor digitorum: This is a thick muscle. It arises from the lateral epicondyle of the humerus. Trace it down to the extensor retinaculum and note that it splits into four tendons over the distal end of the forearm and pass deep to the fourth compartment of the extensor retinaculum.

Extensor digiti minimi: This muscle also arises from the lateral epicondyle of the humerus. It can be easily identified at the distal end of the forearm as it occupies a separate compartment under the extensor retinaculum, the fifth compartment.

Extensor carpi ulnaris: This is the next muscle taking origin from the lateral epicondyle. Trace it distally and note that it occupies the last compartment of the extensor retinaculum.

Anconeus: Identify this most medial muscle. Note that it extends from the posterior aspect of the lateral epicondyle to the lateral surface of the proximal third of ulna. It is an extensor and also acts as a pronator of the forearm.

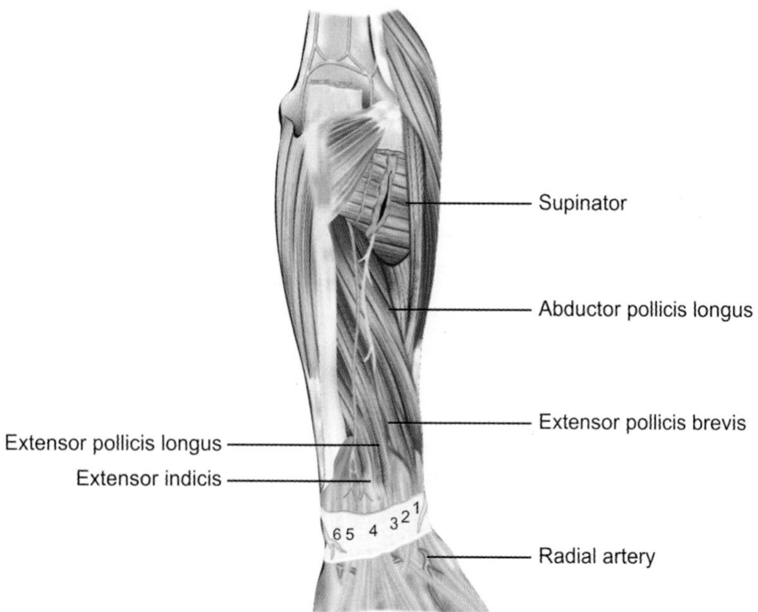

FIGURE 57 Muscles of posterior compartment of forearm—deep group

DEEP GROUP OF MUSCULATURE (Fig. 57)

Dissection: Cut the superficial group of muscles horizontally near their middle. Lift the proximal part superiorly and try to identify the deep group of musculature.

Supinator: This muscle extends between the radius and ulna. Identify its origin from the lateral part of the ulna below the radial notch and also from the fibrous capsule of the elbow and superior radioulnar joints. See how its wraps around the upper one third of the radius. See the posterior interosseous nerve piercing through it. It is a supinator of the forearm.

Abductor pollicis longus: This is the most lateral of the deep muscles. Identify this muscle. Note that it arises from both the radius ulna and the interosseous membrane. Trace it out distally and note that it occupies the first compartment of the extensor retinaculum.

Extensor pollicis brevis: Identify this muscle immediately beneath the abductor pollicis longus. Note that this muscle arises from the radius and accompanies the abductor pollicis longus into the first compartment of the extensor retinaculum. Both these muscles cross the radial carpal tendons which occupy the second compartment.

Extensor pollicis longus: Identify this muscle arising from the ulna. Trace this tendon down to the third compartment in the extensor retinaculum.

Extensor indicis: Identify this muscle distal to the extensor pollicis longus. It arises from the distal part of ulna. Trace it down and note that it passes deep to the extensor digitorum tendons into the extensor retinaculum. It lies in the fourth compartment along with the digitorum tendons.

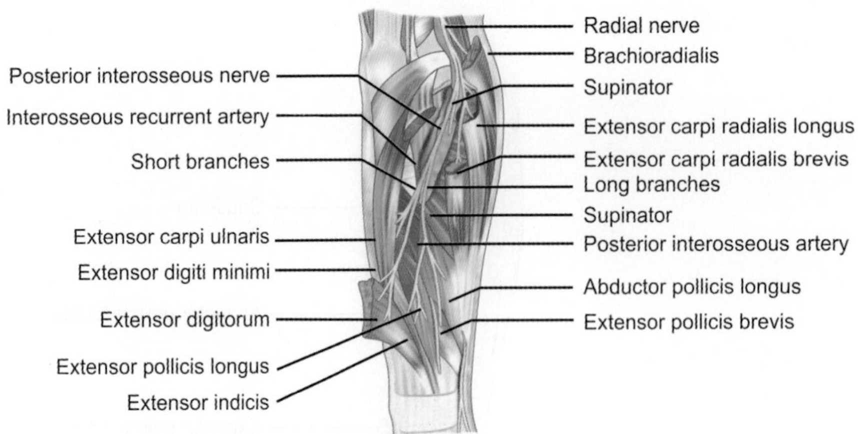

FIGURE 58 Neurovascular bundle of back of forearm

NEUROVASCULAR BUNDLE (Fig. 58)

The posterior interosseous nerve and the posterior interosseous artery form the neurovascular bundle of the back of the forearm.

Dissection: Reidentify the ***radial nerve*** in the lower part of the arm as it enters the front of the arm. Cut the muscles arising from the lateral epicondyle of the humerus and identify the nerves entering into the brachioradialis, extensor carpi radialis longus, extensor carpi radialis brevis and supinator. Further note that the radial nerve divides into an anterior and a posterior branch. You have already seen the superficial branch of the radial nerve in the anterior aspect of the forearm. Now trace the deep branch, called the ***posterior interosseous nerve*** into the back of the forearm through the supinator muscle. Trace its short branches which enter the undersurface of the extensor digitorum, extensor digiti minimi and extensor carpi ulnaris. See the long branches which descend down laterally to supply the abductor pollicis longus and extensor pollicis brevis. Identify its medial branches of supply to extensor pollicis longus and extensor indicis. Trace the posterior interosseous nerve to its termination where it supplies the wrist joint, intercarpal and metacarpal joints. Many a times you can identify the posterior interosseous nerve ending as a pseudoganglion near the distal end of the interosseous membrane.

Posterior interosseous artery: This is the smaller terminal branch of the common interosseous artery. Identify this artery between the supinator and the abductor pollicis longus, as it enters the posterior aspect of the forearm. Here it accompanies the posterior interosseous nerve and supplies the musculature of the back of the forearm. Try to identify the ***interosseous recurrent artery*** deep to the musculature, posterior to the lateral epicondyle. At the distal end it anastomoses with the anterior interosseous artery, which reaches by piercing the interosseous membrane.

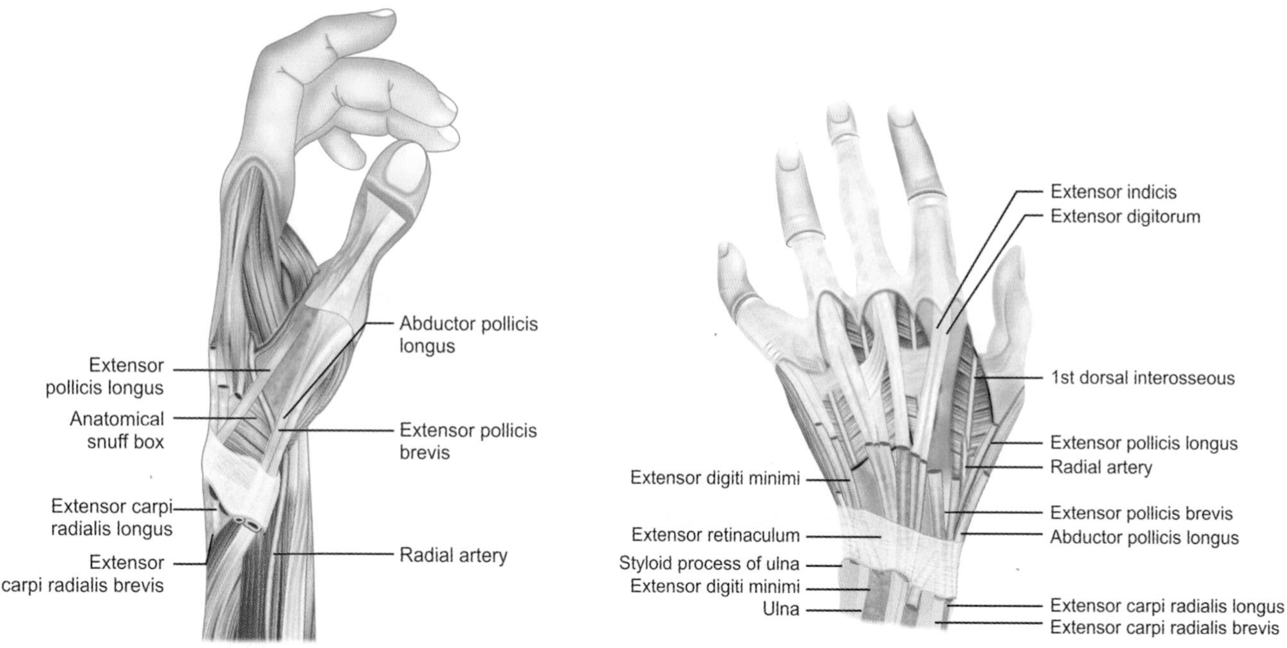

FIGURE 59 Tendons on the lateral side of hand

FIGURE 60 Tendons on the dorsum of the hand

TENDONS ON THE WRIST (Figs 59 and 60)

Dissection: Reidentify the tendons under cover of the extensor retinaculum. Note that they are all covered by the synovial sheaths. You may cut one or two compartments to identify these. Trace each tendon to its destination.

Abductor pollicis longus: This is the most lateral tendon in the most lateral compartment numbered as the first compartment. Identify this and trace it to its insertion into the base of the first metacarpal bone. Pull this muscle and see its abduction action on the thumb.

Extensor pollicis brevis: This is the second muscle of the first compartment. Trace its insertion into the base of the first phalanx of the thumb. Pull it and note its extension action on the thumb at the metacarpophalangeal joint.

Identify the second compartment with the extensor carpi radialis longus and brevis.

Trace the insertion of the ***extensor carpi radialis longus*** into the dorsum of the base of the second metacarpal. Trace the insertion of the ***extensor carpi radialis brevis*** into the dorsum of the base of the third metacarpal bone. Pull both the muscles and note their extension action on the wrist joint. They also act as the abductors of the hand at the wrist joint.

Extensor pollicis longus: This muscle occupies the third compartment. Trace it to its insertion into the dorsum of the base of the distal phalanx of the thumb. Pull the tendon and note the extension action of the muscle on the distal interphalangeal joint.

Extensor digitorum and extensor indicis: These muscles occupy the fourth compartment in the extensor retinaculum. Identify these two muscles and their tendons. Trace the tendons into the fingers. Note that the tendons are interconnected on the dorsum of the hand. Try to perform the extension action on individual fingers and note that it is not possible to perform a complete extension of the finger without involving the other fingers. This is due to the interconnections. You can easily perform the extension of the index finger and little finger as they have an extra muscle. Trace the insertion of the tendons into the fingers. Each extensor tendon is further supported by the interossei and lumbricals from the palmar aspect, and they form an expansion on the medial four fingers called the extensor expansion.

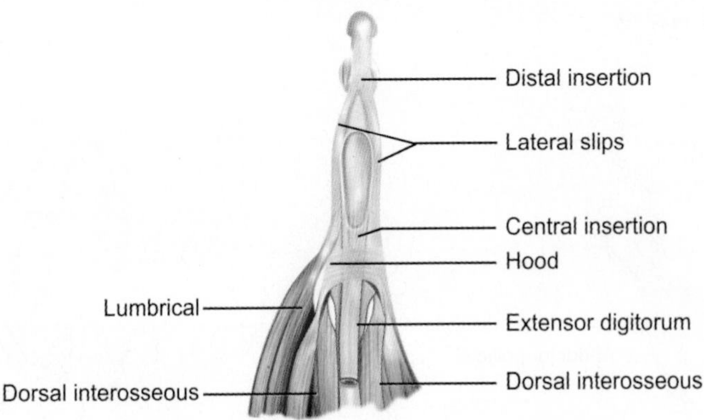

FIGURE 61 Extensor expansion over middle fingers

EXTENSOR EXPANSION (Fig. 61)

Clean extensor expansion on at least two of the fingers. It is a diamond shaped expansion formed proximal to the metcarpophalangeal joint. It crosses over the joint as its posterior part of the capsule. It is attached to the deep metatarsal ligaments on its sides. Note the tendons of the lumbrical and interosseous muscles join the extensor expansion after it crosses the metatarsophalangeal joint. The expansion divides into three parts near the proximal phalanx. The middle part gets inserted into the base of the second phalanx. The parts which are along the sides join together and get inserted into the base of the distal phalanx. The extensor expansion forms the dorsal aspect of the metatarsophalangeal and interphalangeal joints. Note that the extensor digitorum, lumbricals and the interossei are all extensors of the phalanges at the interphalangeal joints. Pull the muscles and confirm this. However, note that the lumbricals and interossei cross the metacarpophalangeal joint from front to the back. These are flexors at this joint.

Note that the extensor expansion of the middle finger is contributed by the extensor digitorum tendon, second lumbrical, second and third dorsal interossei. Note that the extensor expansion of the index finger is contributed by the extensor digitorum tendon, extensor indicis tendon, first lumbrical, first dorsal interosseous and second palmar interosseous.

Extensor digiti minimi: See this muscle in the fifth compartment under the extensor retinaculum. This is an extra extensor for the little finger. This joins the extensor expansion of the little finger.

Extensor carpi ulnaris: See this tendon in the sixth compartment of the extensor retinaculum. Trace its insertion into the base of the fifth metacarpal bone. Pull it and see that it is an extensor of the hand at the wrist joint. It is also a medial deviator or adductor of the hand at the wrist joint.

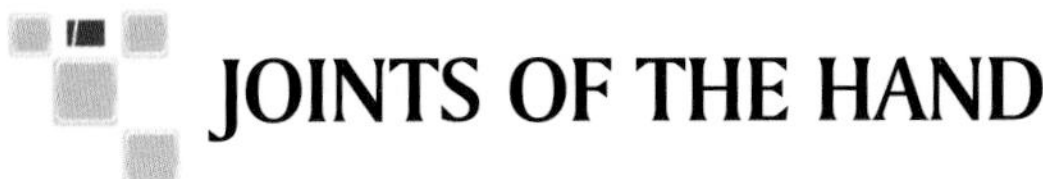

JOINTS OF THE HAND

ELBOW JOINT AND SUPERIOR RADIOULNAR JOINT (Fig. 62)

The **elbow** joint is a uniaxial hinge joint between the distal end of the humerus and proximal ends of radius and ulna. The superior radioulnar joint is a pivot joint between the ulna and radius.

Study the bones on an articulated skeleton. Proximal articulation of the elbow joint is formed by the ***trochlea*** and the ***capitulum*** of the humerus. The trochlea is a pulley shaped medial process and the capitulum is a half circle projection seen only on the anterior side. It also includes the ***radial*** and ***ulnar fossae*** anteriorly and the ***olecranon fossa*** posteriorly. They receive the corresponding processes during articulation. The distal articulation is formed medially by the ***olecranon process*** and the ***coronoid process*** of the ulna. These articulate with the trochlea. The lateral capitulum of the humerus articulates with the upper surface of the head of the radius.

In the superior radioulnar joint the radial notch of the ulna and the annular ligament forms the rim in which the head of the radius rotates.

Dissection: Identify the radial, median, ulnar and posterior interosseous nerve around the joint and trace their supply into the joint. Remove all the muscles and nerves around the elbow joint and study the capsule.

Capsule: Note that the elbow joint and the superior radioulnar joints have a common capsule and it includes the olecranon, radial and ulnar fossae. The capsule shows thin and oblique fibres both in the anterior and posterior aspects of the joint. See its proximal attachment on the humerus proximal to the fossae. Identify the distal attachment of the capsule into the margins of the olecranon process, coronoid process of the ulna and the annular ligament.

Radial collateral ligament: Identify this thick ligament on the lateral side extending from the distal end of the lateral epicondyle to the lateral and posterior parts of the annular ligament.

Ulnar collateral ligament: Identify this triangular ligament on the medial side of the joint extending from the distal end of the medial epicondyle to the edges of the olecranon and coronoid processes of the ulna. The thinner central part is attached to the oblique band that extends between the olecranon and coronoid process.

Dissection: Cut across the joint capsule from lateral to medial end. Extend the forearm fully and see the interior. This opens the elbow joint and the superior radioulnar joint.

Synovial membrane: Feel the stickiness of the synovial membrane on the inner side of the capsule and note that it is reflected from the capsule on to the nonarticulating surfaces of the bones. Identify the articulating surfaces of the bones within the joint cavity. Perform flexion and extension and see how the bones move during movement.

Superior radioulnar joint: See the articulating surfaces of this joint. See the glistening head of the radius. The annular ligament is collar shaped, holds the head of the radius snugly. It is attached to the anterior and posterior margins of the ulnar notch. Distally it is attached to the neck of the radius. Perform the movement pronation and supination on the part and see how it moves.

Nerve supply: Both the joints are supplied by the radial, posterior interosseous, ulnar and the median nerves.

Movement: Flexion and extension are the movements performed around a transverse axis at the elbow joint. The biceps, brachialis are prime movers to perform flexion and all the flexors arising from the medial epicondyle are agonists for flexion. Extension is performed by the triceps muscle, which crosses the joint posteriorly.

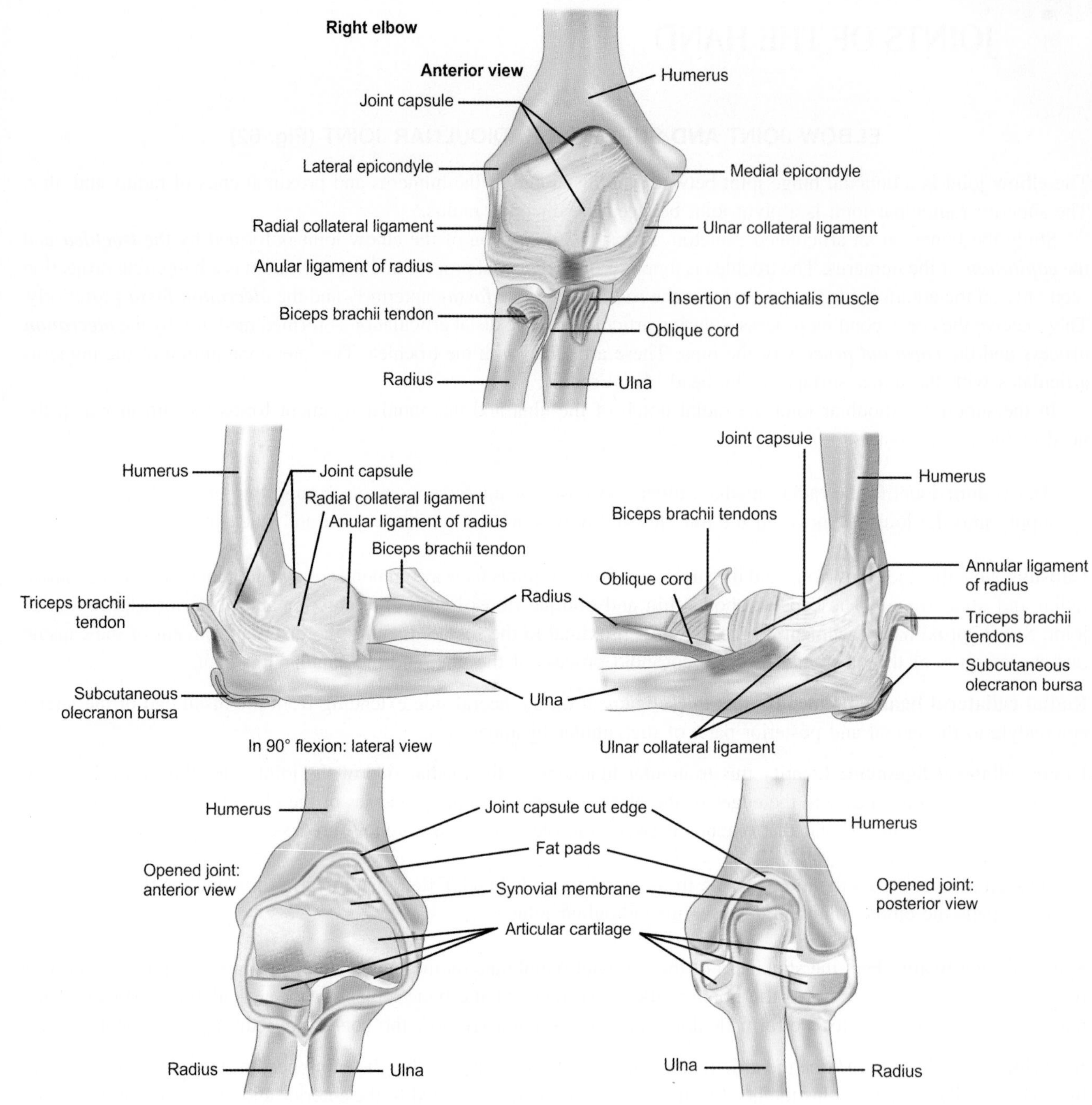

FIGURE 62 Elbow joint and superior radioulnar joint

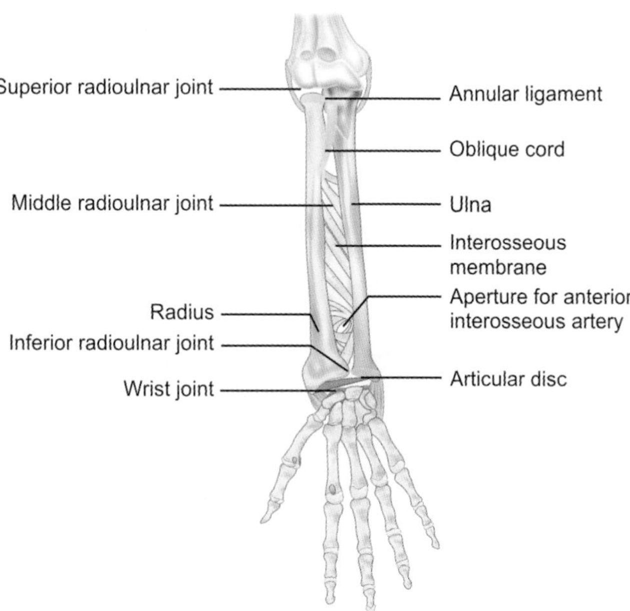

FIGURE 63 Radioulnar joints

RADIOULNAR JOINTS (Fig. 63)

Radioulnar joints are three in number: The superior radioulnar joint is a pivot joint, the middle radioulnar joint is a fibrous joint united by the interosseous membrane and quadrate ligament, the inferior radioulnar joint is a pivot joint.

Dissection: Remove all the muscles arising from the interosseous membrane both anteriorly and posteriorly.

SUPERIOR RADIOULNAR JOINT

It is already studied as it lies within the same joint capsule of the Joint.

Quadrate ligament/oblique cord: See this extending between the radial notch on the ulna to below the radial tuberosity of the radius.

MIDDLE RADIOULNAR JOINT

It is a fibrous joint formed by the ***interosseous ligament.*** Identify this connective tissue sheet extending from below the radial tuberosity to the ulna. It runs downward and medially from the interosseous border of radius to the interosseous border of ulna. This helps in directing the compressional force from the radius to the ulna.

INFERIOR RADIOULNAR JOINT

It is a pivot joint. It is an articulation between the distal end of the radius and the head of the ulna and the articular disc. The distal end of the radius has a broad distal surface and has a notched medial surface. The circumference of the head articulates with the distal radial notch. The distal end of the head of the ulna articulates with the intra-articular disc. This separates the ulna from articulating with the carpals.

Movement: This being a pivot joint permits rotation around a vertical axis. Rotate the hand and observe that the movement takes place in the distal radioulnar joint. Here the ulna remains stationery and the distal end of the radius along with the articular disc rotates over the head of the ulna. The hand is a passive accompanied of the radius. The movement is pronation and supination. Pronation is produced by the pronator teres and pronator quadratus whereas the supination is produced by the supinator. The brachioradialis acts as a pronator as well as a supinator to bring the hand to midprone position.

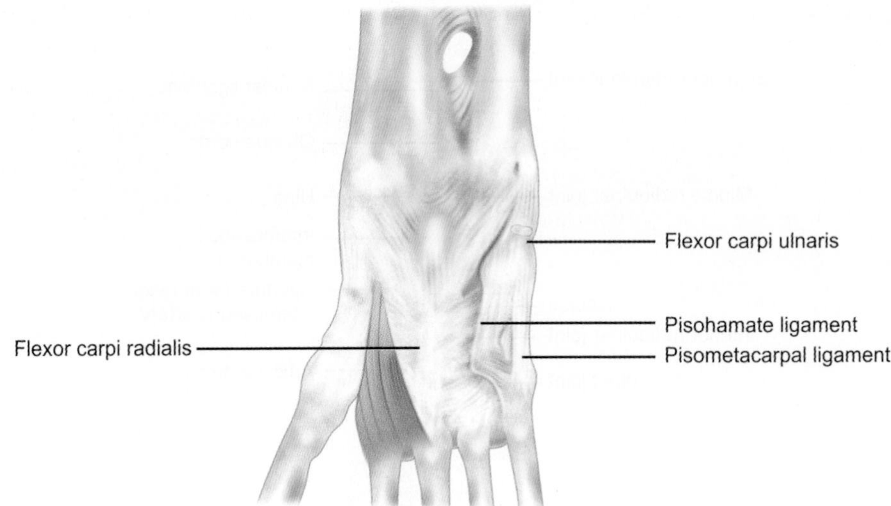

FIGURE 64 Wrist joint

WRIST JOINT (Fig. 64)

Skeleton: Study the bones on an articulated skeleton. The distal surface of radius shows two articulating surfaces. The lateral one is for the scaphoid and the medial one is for the lunate. The articular disc separates the ulna from articulating with the carpals. It is the articular disc which articulates with the triquetral to form the wrist joint.

Carpals: See the proximal row of carpal bones—they are scaphoid, lunate and triquetral from lateral to medial. The scaphoid and lunate articulate with the distal end of radius whereas the triquetral articulates with the articular disc.

Identify the insertion of ***flexor carpi ulnaris*** into the pisiform bone, further on as ***pisohamate*** ligament extending from the pisiform to the hook of the hamate, and ***pisometacarpal*** extending from the pisiform to the base of the fifth metacarpal bone Identify the ***flexor carpi radialis*** inserting into the bases of the second and third metacarpal bones.

Turn the wrist to the back and identify the insertions of ***extensor carpi radialis longus*** into the base of the second metacarpal and ***extensor carpiradialis brevis*** into the third metacarpal. See the insertion of ***extensor carpi ulnaris*** into the base of the fifth metacarpal bone.

Dissection: Remove the tendons from both the anterior as well as the posterior aspect.

The capsule is thin anteriorly and posteriorly. The fibres of the capsule run obliquely and medially. It extends from the distal margins of the radius and ulna to the proximal margins of the scaphoid, lunate and triquetral bones. It encloses the articular disc. See the lateral radial collateral ligament extending from the radial styloid process to the lateral side of the scaphoid bone. Identify the medial collateral ligament extending from the ulnar styloid process to the medial side of the triquetral bone. These are thicker and support the capsule. Open the joint cavity by a transverse incision extending from lateral to medial side and see the interior.

Articular disc: See this triangular fibrocartilaginous structure extending from the styloid process of the ulna to the medial margin of the distal end of the radius. Note that this separates the joint cavities of the inferior radioulnar joint from the wrist joint.

Nerve supply: These joints are supplied by the anterior and posterior interosseous nerves and the dorsal branch of the ulnar nerve.

Movement: In an opened joint observe that the wrist joint is obliquely placed, the lateral and dorsal margins of the radius extend farther distally compared to the ulnar styloid process. This being a biaxial ellipsoid joint permits flexion and extension around a transverse axis and abduction and adduction around an anteroposterior axis. Perform the movement on your hand. The extension and adduction has a greater range of movement here compared to the flexion and abduction. You can observe this fact by looking at the articular surfaces of the carpal bones. Their auricular surface extends far posteriorly. In resting position of the hand the scaphoid and part of the lunate articulate with the radius and the remaining part of the lunate lies on the articular disc, whereas the triquetrum is more on the medial part of the capsule. During adduction note that the carpal bones slide more laterally with the lunate articulating with the radius and the triquetrum coming on to the articular disc.

Flexion is produced by all the carpal and digital flexors—the flexor digitorum longus and profundus, flexor carpi radialis and ulnaris and palmaris longus. Extension is produced by all long extensors and carpal extensors – the extensor digitorum, extensor indicis, extensor digiti minimi, extensor carpi radialis longus and brevis and extensor carpi ulnaris. Note that it has far more extensors than flexors as it is a powerful movement and against gravity. Abduction is produced by the flexor carpi radials, extensor radialis longus and brevis. This movement in spite of having three muscle has a smaller range of movement as it has mechanical disadvantage due to the positioning of bones. The adduction is produced by the flexor carpi ulnaris and extensor carpi ulnaris. This has a greater range of movement. Test the movements by pulling the tendons.

JOINTS OF THE HAND

Intercarpal Joints

Skeleton: See an articulated hand and identify the following. The ***scaphoid*** is a boat shaped bone. It is the lateral bone of the proximal row. Proximally it articulates with the radius and distally with the trapezium and trapezoid. The ***lunate*** is the moon shaped middle bone. Proximally, it articulates with the radius and distally with the capitate and hamate. The ***triquetrum*** is the medial bone of the proximal row. Proximally it articulates with the articular disc and distally with the hamate. The ***pisiform*** bone is considered a bone of the proximal row and articulates on the ventral aspect of the triquetrum.

The second row of carpal bones are four in number. The most lateral bone is the ***trapezium,*** this articulates proximally with the scaphoid and distally with the first metacarpal bone. The ***trapezoid*** is the next bone, this proximally articulates with the scaphoid and distally with the second metacarpal bone. The central bone is the ***capitate.*** It has a rounded head and proximally it articulates with the lunate and scaphoid and distally with the third metacarpal bone. The medial most bone is the ***hamate*** which presents a hook on its ventral aspect. This articulates proximally with the lunate and triquetrum.

Intercarpal joints are the joints between the first row of carpal bones, the second row of carpal bones and also the joints between the carpal bones of the same row. All these joints are synovial and plane except for the joint between the capitate and lunate where a rotatory movement is possible due to the shape of the bones. The pisiform is a sesamoid bone in the tendon of the flexor carpi ulnaris.

Capsule: All joints are held together by capsule, dorsal, ventral and interosseous ligaments.

Carpometacarpal Joints

Carpometacarpal joints are also plane synovial joints. They are held together by the dorsal, ventral and interosseous ligaments.

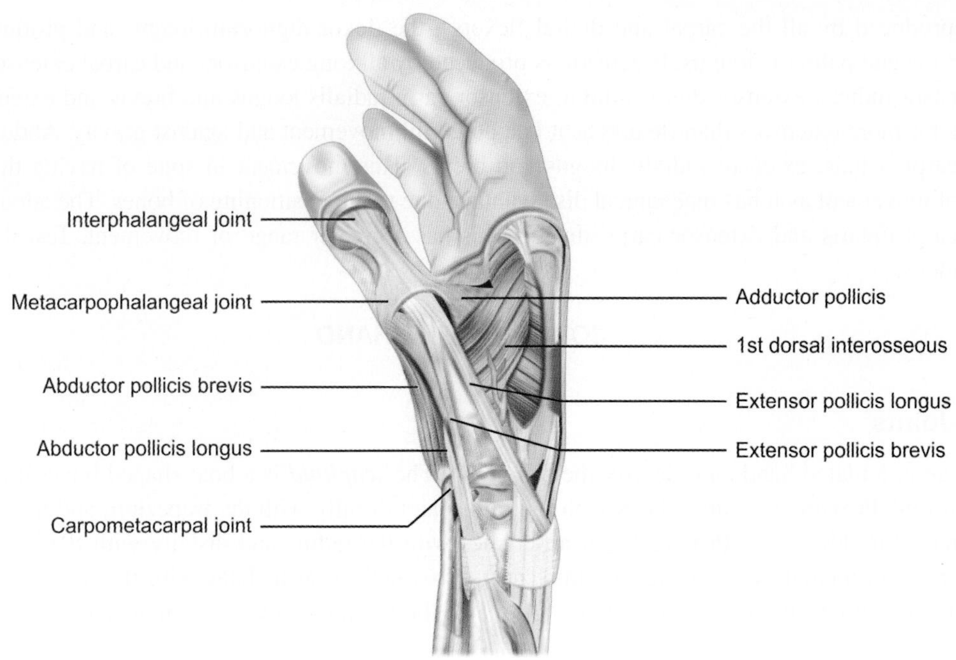

FIGURE 65 Joints of thumb

JOINTS OF THE THUMB (Fig. 65)

Joints of the thumb need special mention due to its importance in our hand.

These are three in number – the carpometacarpal joint, the metacarpophalangeal and the interphalangeal joint of the thumb. The thumb lies perpendicular to the other fingers. All the joints of the thumb move in unison to bring about an action in thumb.

THE CARPOMETACARPAL JOINT

The first metacarpal bone articulates with the trapezium of the distal row of carpal bones. It is a biaxial saddle joint. Identify them on a skeleton and see their articulating surfaces. They show a reciprocally fitting concavoconvex surfaces.

Capsule: This is attached to the periphery of the articulating surfaces. The capsule is loose fitting over the bones.

THE METACARPOPHALANGEAL JOINT

It is a condyloid joint. The rounded head of the metacarpal, articulates with the concave base of the first phalanx. The **capsule** of the joint is loose ventrally, forms the collateral ligaments laterally. The capsule is thin posteriorly.

THE INTERPHALANGEAL JOINT

Thumb has only two phalanges and so has only one interphalangeal joint. It is a uniaxial condylar joint. The base of the first phalanx has two knuckle shaped articulating surface. This articulates with the concave base of the second phalanx.

The **capsule** encloses the articulating surfaces and is supported by collateral ligaments.

Movements of thumb: Here flexion and extension takes place around an anteroposterior axis. ***Flexion*** is produced by the flexor pollicis longus at the interphalangeal joint and by the flexor pollicis brevis at the metacarpophalangeal and carpometacarpal joint. In flexion, the thumb moves parallel to the other fingers. ***Extension*** is produced by the extensor pollicis longus at the interphalangeal joint and by the extensor pollicis brevis at the metacarpophalangeal and carpometacarpal joint. In extension, the thumb moves parallel and away from the other fingers. Abduction and adduction takes place around a transverse axis. In this the thumb moves away from the other fingers and in adduction it moves towards the other fingers. The ***abduction*** is produced by the abductor pollicis longus and brevis. ***Adduction*** is produced by the adductor pollicis. ***Opposition*** is a rotatory movement where the metacarpal moves around a longitudinal axis. This brings about touching of the ventral surface of the thumb with the other fingers. This is an accessory movement.

Nerve supply: All the intercarpal and metacarpal joints are supplied by the posterior interosseous nerve and deep branches of ulnar nerve.

METACARPOPHALANGEAL AND INTERPHALANGEAL JOINTS OF THE MEDIAL FOUR FINGERS

The metacarpophalangeal joints are biaxial ellipsoidal joints. The heads of the metacarpal are oval in shape fitting into the concavity of the base of the first phalanx.

The **interphalangeal joints** are uniaxial condylar joints. They present two knuckle like projections on the heads which fit into the reciprocal concavities on the base of the phalanges.

Dissection: Clean the tendons and trace them to their insertions. Clean the capsule and collateral ligaments of the joints. Clean and identify the fibrous flexor sheaths on the ventral aspect and the extensor expansions on the dorsal aspects. Clean the deep transverse metacarpal ligaments extending between the necks of metacarpal bones.

The capsule is attached to the peripheries of the articulating surfaces of the bones. It is thickened on the anterior aspect and forms the palmar ligament and thickening on the lateral aspect forms the lateral collateral ligaments. Posteriorly the capsule is replaced by the extensor expansion.

Deep transverse metatarsal ligaments: These ligaments extend from the bases of the first phalanx and the necks of the metacarpal bones of one finger to the bases of the first phalanx and necks of the next finger.

Movements: Flexion and extension takes place around a transverse axis. Flexion at distal interphalangeal joint is brought by flexor digitorum profundus, flexion at proximal interphalangeal joint is initiated by flexor digitorum superficialis and flexion at metacarpophalangeal joint is brought by both flexor digitorum superficialis and profundus. Extension at the metacarpophalangeal joint is brought about by the extensor digitorum in all the fingers and supported by the extensor indicis in index finger and extensor digiti minimi in little finger. Extension at the interphalangeal joint is brought about by the interossei and lumbricals as well as the extensor digitorum tendons.

The midline for abduction and adduction is the line passing through the center of the middle finger. Movement away from the central line is abduction and towards the central line is the adduction. The movement takes place around an anteroposterior axis.

Abduction is brought about by the dorsal interossei and adduction is brought by palmar interossei. The middle finger has only abduction and coming back to the midline is by elastic recoil of the finger.

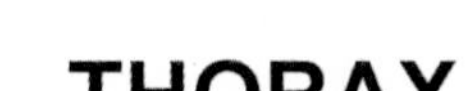

THORAX

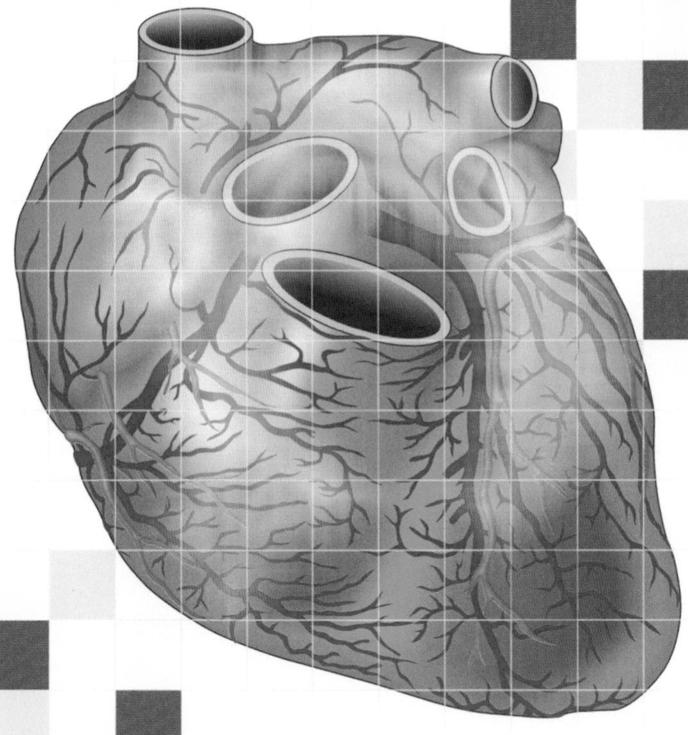

Introduction

Thoracic Wall
Pleural Cavity
Anterior Mediastinum
Middle Mediastinum
Superior Mediastinum
Posterior Mediastinum

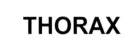

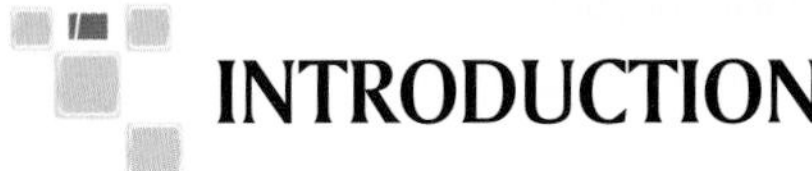

INTRODUCTION

Thorax is the upper part of the trunk. It lodges and protects the lungs and heart. The bones form the outer thoracic cage and the organs are located inside. For convenience of description and dissection, it can be divided into three parts: (i) the thoracic wall with the bony architecture and the muscles that move them, (ii) the pleural cavities—these lodge the lungs in the pleura (iii) the mediastinum—this lodges the heart and other structures passing through the thorax from the neck to the abdomen.

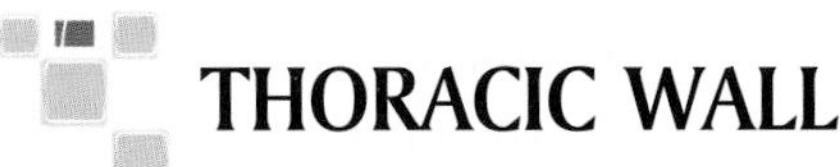

THORACIC WALL

THORACIC CAGE (Fig. 1)

Go to an articulated skeleton and identify the thoracic cage. It is truncated in shape. It is made up of 12 thoracic vertebrae intervertebral discs 12 pairs of ribs 2 costal cartilages and the sternum. It has a superior aperture called the inlet through which it communicates with the neck. It has an inferior aperture which is closed by the diaphragm and it separates it from the abdomen.

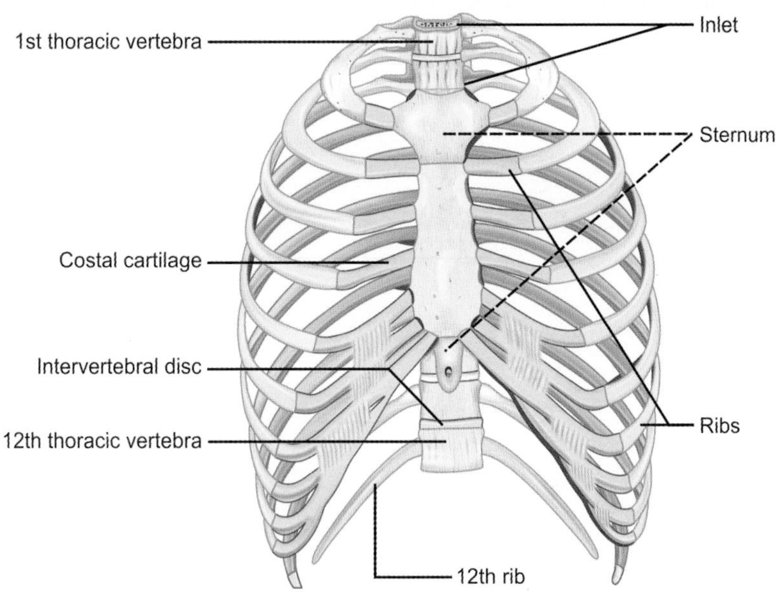

FIGURE 1 Bony architecture

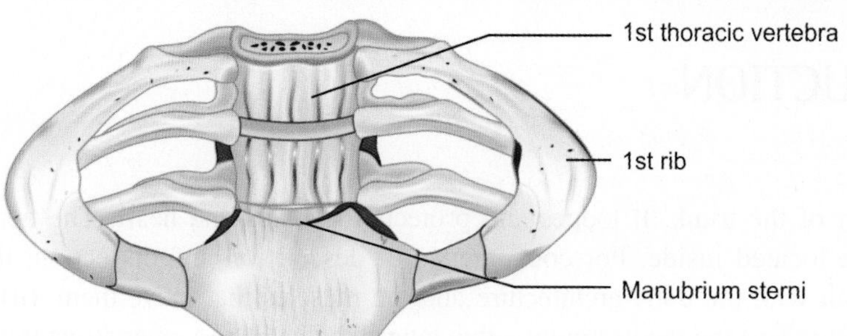

FIGURE 2 Inlet of thorax

INLET OF THORAX (Fig. 2)

The inlet is posteriorly formed by the ***first thoracic vertebra***. The medial border of ***first rib*** forms the lateral boundary. It presents a superior surface and an inferior surface with medial and lateral borders. The upper border of the ***manubrium sterni*** forms the anterior boundary. Note that the aperture is oblique and the upper border of the manubrium sterni corresponds to the lower border of the second thoracic vertebra.

OUTLET OF THORAX

It is formed by 12th thoracic vertebra, 12th rib, 12th to 7th costal cartilages (costal margin) and xiphisternum.

ANTERIOR BOUNDARY (Fig. 3)

Anteriorly it is formed by the ***sternum***. The sternum has three parts, an upper manubrium sterni, a middle body of sternum and a lower small xiphoid process. The manubrium and the body meet at manubriosternal angle or angle of Louie.

Take a separate sternum and observe the anterior surface. It is a rough surface, due to muscular attachements. Look at the smooth posterior surface. It is related to the pleura and pericardium. Identify its parts—the manubrium, body and the xiphoid process. Note the lateral articulating facets for the costal cartilages.

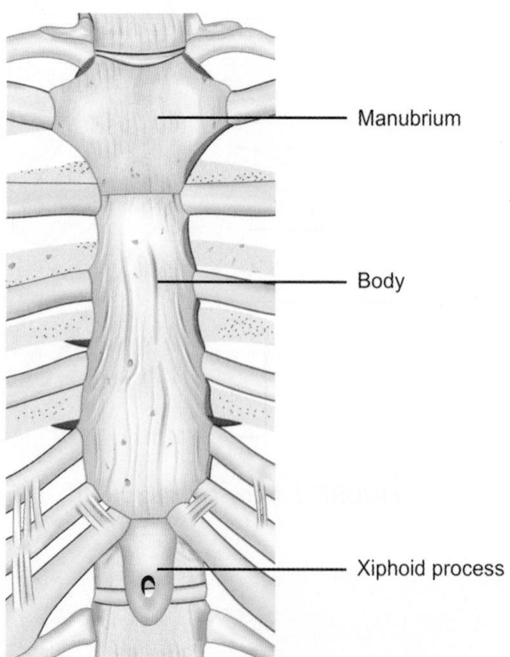

FIGURE 3 Anterior boundary – sternum

LATERAL BOUNDARY

Laterally, it is formed by ***12 pairs of ribs***. The 1st to 6th rib are called ***true ribs*** as they articulate anteriorly with the sternum.The 1st articulates with the manubrium of the sternum.The 2nd articulates with the manubrium and the body. The 3rd to 6th articulate with the body. The 7th articulates with the body and xiphisternum. The 8th to 12th are called ***false ribs*** as they do not reach the sternum anteriorly. The 8th to 10th ribs articulate with the costal cartilage above. The 11th and 12th ribs are called floating ribs as they are free at their anterior ends.

Take any typical rib and identify the features. Feel its thick upper border. It gives attachment to the muscles. Feel its sharp lower border. It gives attachment only to external oblique muscle. Identify its costal groove on the inner side near the lower border. It lodges the neurovascular bundle. See the head. It has two articulating surfaces and an intermediate ridge. The upper articulating surface articulates with vertebra above, the lower surface articulates with the corresponding vertebra and the intermediate ridge lies opposite to the intervertebral disc. Identify the posterior tubercle. This articulates with the transverse process and its nonarticular part gives attachment to the ligaments. Note the neck which lies between the head and the tubercle. Note sharp posterior angle and indistinguishable anterior angle (Fig. 4).

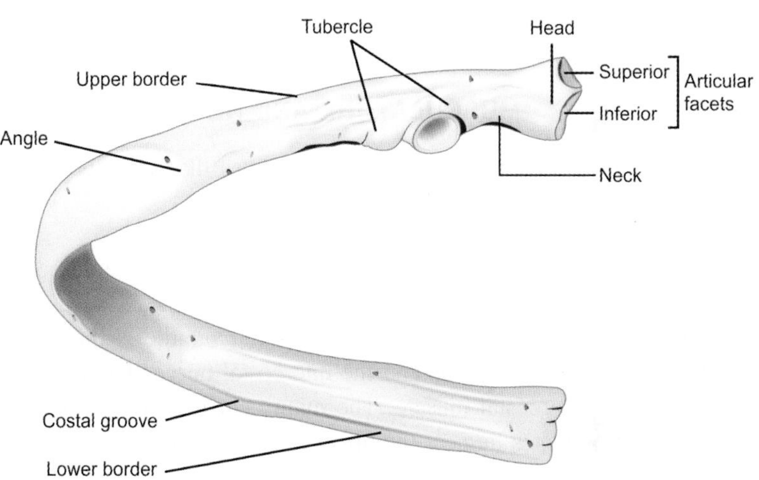

FIGURE 4 Typical rib

POSTERIOR BOUNDARY

Posteriorly the thoracic cage is formed by ***12 thoracic vertebrae.*** The ribs articulate with the vertebrae posteriorly. The first rib articulates with 1st vertebra. The 2nd rib articulates with the 1st and 2nd vertebra. Till 10th rib each rib articulates with its own corresponding vertebra and the vertebra above. The 11th and 12th ribs articulate with their own corresponding vertebrae.

Take any typical thoracic vertebra and identify the features. The vertebral body is the thick, anterior heart shaped part. It is the part which transmits weight of the body. The posterior part is the neural arch. It protects the spinal cord. Note the pedicle, lamina of the neural arch. Note the transverse process, the spine and the superior and inferior articular facets (Fig. 5).

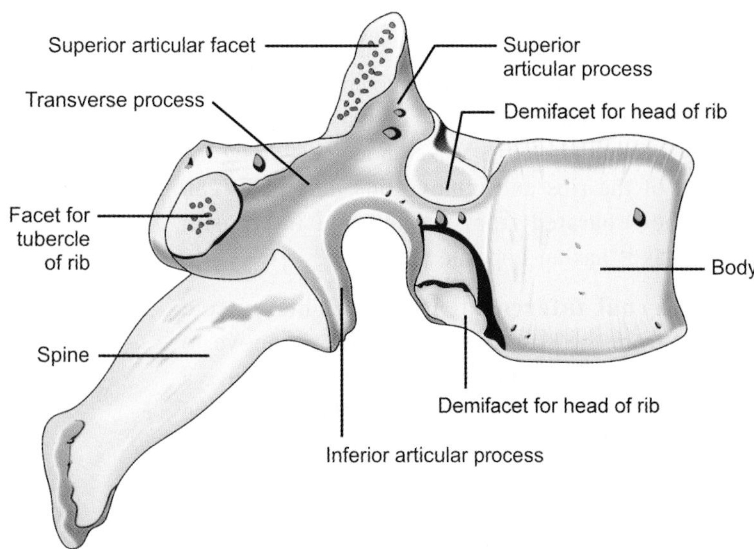

FIGURE 5 Typical thoracic vertebra—side view

SURFACE ANATOMY

On a living body anteriorly identify the suprasternal notch, sternum, sternal angle and xiphisternum.

Slip your fingers below the clavicle in midclavicular line. The depression that you feel is the first intercostals space and the rib that you feel is the second rib. Note that the second rib articulates with the sternal angle. Count the ribs from this point downwards. Feel the costal margin from the xiphisternum to the midaxillary line. The rib that you are feeling is the 10th rib. Posteriorly identify the vertebral spines. The 4th spine lies opposite to the spine of the scapula and the 7th spine lies opposite to the inferior angle of the scapula. To understand the location of the internal organs these surface landmarks are very much useful.

Draw and practice the projections of the heart, lungs and pleura on a cadaver.

JOINTS

In living, the thoracic cage is constantly expanding: To achieve this, the above said bones have to constantly move. The joints between the sternal parts are secondary cartilaginous joints. All the joints of the ribs with the vertebrae are plane synovial joints. The costochondral joints are primary cartilaginous joints. The sternocostal joints are plane synovial joints. This signifies that the movement feasible between the bones is minimal. These cartilages act like struts between the ribs and the sternum.

MUSCULATURE AND NEUROVASCULAR BUNDLE (Figs 6 and 7)

Dissection: Clean all the upper limb muscles like serratus anterior, pectoralis minor and pectoralis major from the thoracic cage.

The wall of the thorax is formed by the ribs and eleven intercostals spaces. The intercostals spaces are filled with three intercostal muscles and the neurovascular bundle. The muscles are external intercostal, internal intercostal and transversus thoracis muscle. The neurovascular bundle is the anterior and posterior intercostal arteries, the anterior and posterior intercostal veins and the intercostal nerve. The neurovascular bundle lies between the internal intercostal and innermost intercostal muscle. The main neurovascular bundle lies in the costal groove of the rib above, whereas the collateral branches lie near the upper border of the lower rib. All the intercostal spaces show the same architecture, so generally it is convenient to dissect middle spaces between the 3rd to 6th.

Dissection: Lift the body and let it lie on its sides supported by wooden blocks, try to observe the muscles from the posterior tubercle of the ribs to the sternum. Identify the anterior and lateral cutaneous branches of the intercostal nerves.

External Intercostal Muscle (Fig. 6)

This muscle extends from the lower margin of the upper rib to the upper margin of the rib below. The muscle is replaced by external intercostal membrane between the costal cartilages. The muscle fibres run downwards and forwards. Make an incision along the borders of the ribs and remove this muscle. It can easily be separated from the internal intercostal muscle, as it has an opposite slant.

The internal intercostal muscle: This muscle extends from the costal groove of the rib above to the upper margin of the rib below. The fibres have a posterior slant. It is muscular from the side of the sternum to the angle of the rib. Between the angle of the rib and the tubercle it is replaced by the internal intercostal membrane.

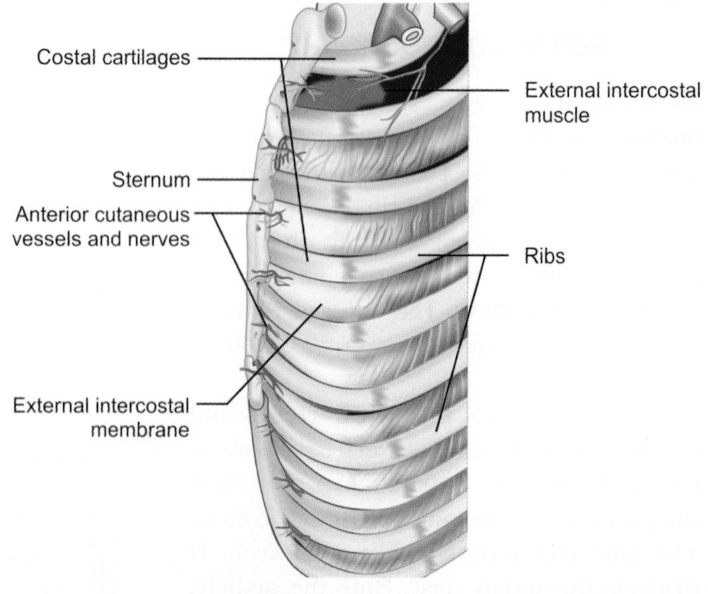

FIGURE 6 External intercostal muscle

The internal intercostal muscle and the neurovascular bundle will be seen in a later dissection, as it can be best viewed from the inner aspect.

The deepest layer of the muscles is split into three parts—***subcostalis*** is the posterior part. It covers two ribs near the angles. ***The intercostalis intimi*** is the middle part. It extends from the upper border of the costal groove of the rib above to the innermost aspect of the upper border of the rib below. The ***sternocostalis*** is the anterior part. It extends from the body of the sternum to the 2nd to 6th costal cartilages.

There are 11 pairs of ***intercostal nerves.*** They are mixed nerves. They supply the intercostal musculature and the skin of the trunk. It enters the intercostal space deep to the internal intercostal membrane and runs in the costal groove. It gives off the collateral branch at the angle of the rib. This runs in the upper border of the lower rib. The lateral cutaneous branch is given off beyond the angle of the rib and pierces the muscle near the middle of the space. The intercostal nerve supplies the intercostal muscles by fine branches as the nerve passes along the muscles.

This above description holds good for 3rd to 6th intercostal nerves. The first thoracic nerve joins with the eighth cervical nerve to form brachial plexus, the lateral cutaneous branch of the second forms the intercostobrachial nerve, the 7th onwards the intercostal nerves supply the musculature and the skin of the abdomen.

There are two arteries supplying each space. The ***posterior intercostal arteries*** are branches of the thoracic aorta. They enter the intercostal space along with the nerve. Each artery gives a collateral branch. This accompanies the nerve along the upper border of the lower rib. The veins drain into azygos system of veins. The ***anterior intercostal arteries*** are two in each space. They lie between the sternum and the transversus thoracis muscle. One passes along the upper border of the rib and the other along the lower border. In the upper six spaces these are branches of the internal thoracic artery and between 7th to 9th spaces they arise from musculophrenic artery. In the last two spaces there is no anterior intercostal artery. The anterior branches of the 2nd to 6th anterior intercostals arteries enlarge to supply mammary gland is the female. The veins accompany the arteries as the venae commitantis and drain into the corresponding bigger veins.

Dissection: Removal of anterolateral wall of the thoracic cage.

Use a circular small saw for this dissection. Cut through the manubrium sternum horizontally between the articulation of the 1st and 2nd rib. Cut through the body horizontally above the xiphisternum. Cut through the cage anterior to the angle of the ribs, and through the intercostal muscles from 2nd rib to the 6th rib, on both sides. Carefully separate the rib cage and take it out. While doing this you should have separated this at the endothoracic fascia which lies immediately deeper to this. Try to leave it behind. The endothoracic fascia is the loose areolar tissue inner to the thoracic cage which separates it from the pleura. Turn the detached part of the cage onto the inner surface and identify the following **(Fig. 7)**.

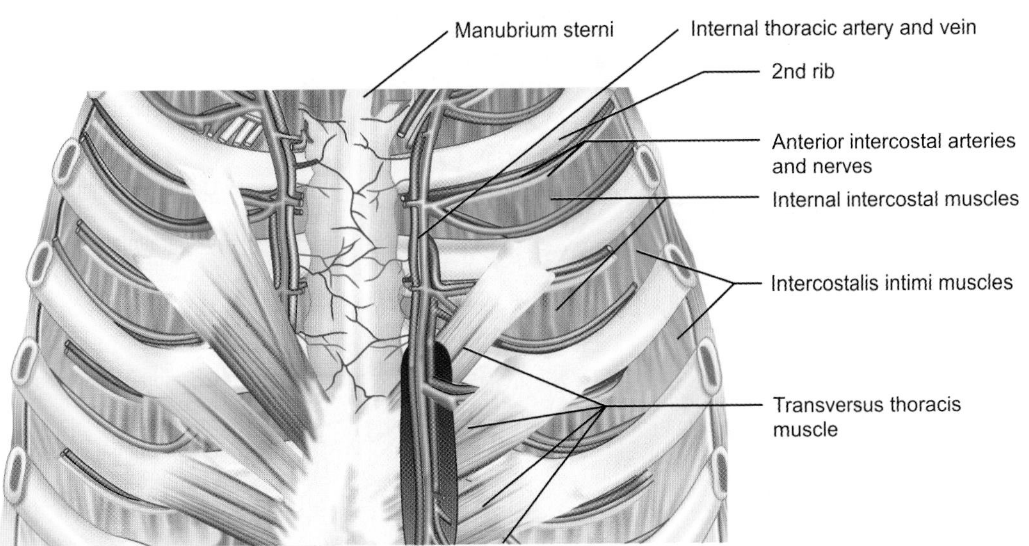

FIGURE 7 Anterior wall of thoracic cage viewed from inside

Transversus thoracis: It has 4 slips of origin from the body of the sternum and will get inserted into the 2nd to 6th costal cartilages and ribs.

Internal thoracic artery and vein run along the lateral border of the sternum. This is a branch of the subclavian artery. Pull the artery and locate two anterior intercostals arteries given off in each intercostals space.

The internal intercostal muscle lies nearer to the anterior part of the space.

The intercostalis intimi: Remove this thin muscle. This lies in the middle part of the space. Its direction of fibres is same as the internal intercostal muscle.

Dissection: Cut and remove the intercostalis intimi muscle and see the neurovascular bundle within the costal groove, and also along the upper border of the lower rib, at least in two to three spaces.

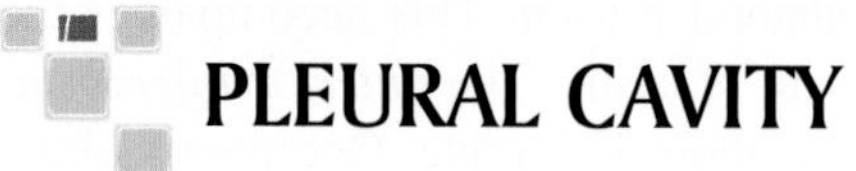

PLEURAL CAVITY

The thoracic cavity has got a central mediastinum where the heart and the other organs which traverse through the thorax lie. It has two lateral pleural cavities for the lungs and pleura.

PLEURA (Fig. 8)

Pleura: The pleura is the outer serous sac which envelops the lung. It has an outer parietal layer which lines the wall and an inner serous layer which covers the lung. Between the two layers lies the pleural cavity. This is filled with serous fluid, which lubricates the surfaces. For convenience of description the parietal layer is described as mediastinal, costal, diaphragmatic and cervical pleura, according to the areas it is related to. The visceral pleura is adherent to the lung tissue. The parietal layer and visceral layer are continuous with each other near the root/hilum of the lung. The parietal pleura is supplied by intercostal nerves and phrenic nerve. So it is sensitive to general sensations, where as the visceral pleura is supplied by the pulmonary plexus of nerves. This is a part of the autonomic nervous system. It also supplies the lung parenchyma, so is not sensitive to external stimuli.

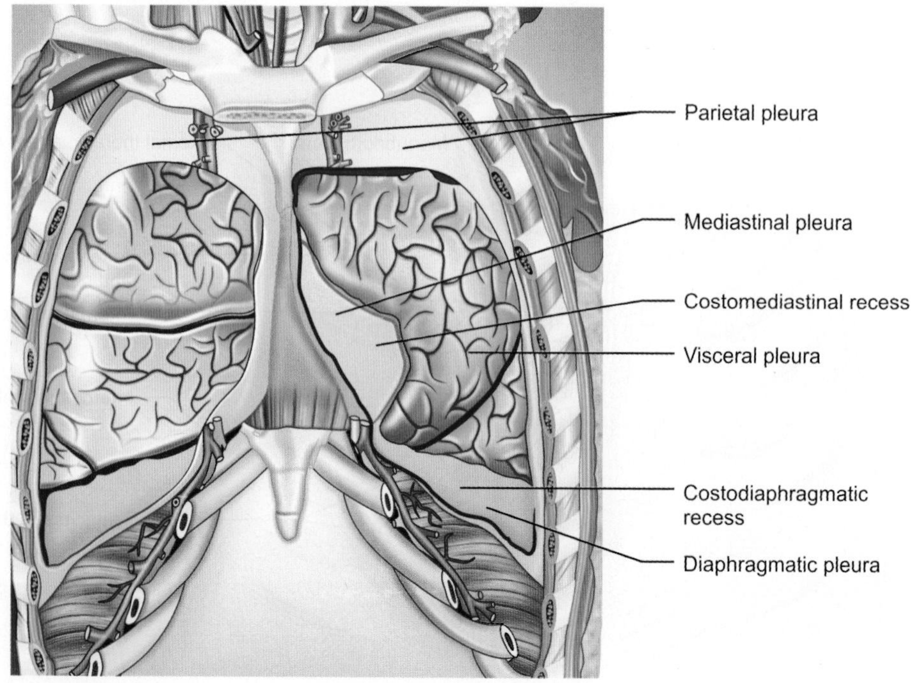

FIGURE 8 Pleura

Dissection: When the thoracic wall was removed it was removed at the endothoracic fasica. This is the connective tissue separating the thoracic wall and the pleural sacs. The thin sheet that is seen covering the lung is the parietal layer of pleura. The parietal pleura is the layer which lines the parieties. This is named according to the parts that it is related to. Note that the costal pleura is related to the ribs. Put your fingers below the lung and feel the diaphragm. The part of the parietal pleura sticking to the diaphragm is the diaphragmatic pleura. Put your fingers over the apex of the lung push it up—the resistance encountered is because of the supra pleural membrane which covers the apex. The part of the pleura which covers this area is called the cervical pleura. Put your fingers medially and feel the mediastinal pleura. Invariably the parietal pleura is adherent with the endothoracic fascia and is ruptured. Cut the anterior part of the parietal pleura and visualize the visceral pleura.

Pleural recess: It is the part of the pleural cavity normally not occupied by the lung except in deep inspiration. It is generally described as two recesses, the costomediastinal and costodiaphragmatic.

The surface projection of lung and pleura has to be studied on a cadaver by drawing with a chalk piece.

Dissection: Feel the root of the lung along the mediastinal surface of lung and clasp it. Pull the lung laterally and cut through the root of the lung and separate the lungs. Wash the lungs well with water and clean the pleural cavities with cotton and under take study of the lung. While studying the lungs constantly put them back into the body and understand the position and relations of the lungs.

LUNGS

The lungs are respiratory organs where exchange of gases takes place. It is made up of spongy parenchyma and is heavily supplied by blood vessels. It appears pink in young children and it appears slate gray in adults due to the deposition of carbon particles. They weigh approximately 500 to 600 grams and float when immersed in water due to the presence of air, where as the fetal lung sinks in water due to lack of air. Each lung is somewhat half a cone in shape and presents a base, apex, costal surface and the mediastinal surface.

RIGHT LUNG (Fig. 9)

Hold the right lung with the base in your right palm with the anterior border facing anteromedially. Identify the following features and relations.

The right lung is divided into three lobes, the ***superior, middle*** and ***inferior*** lobes by two fissures.

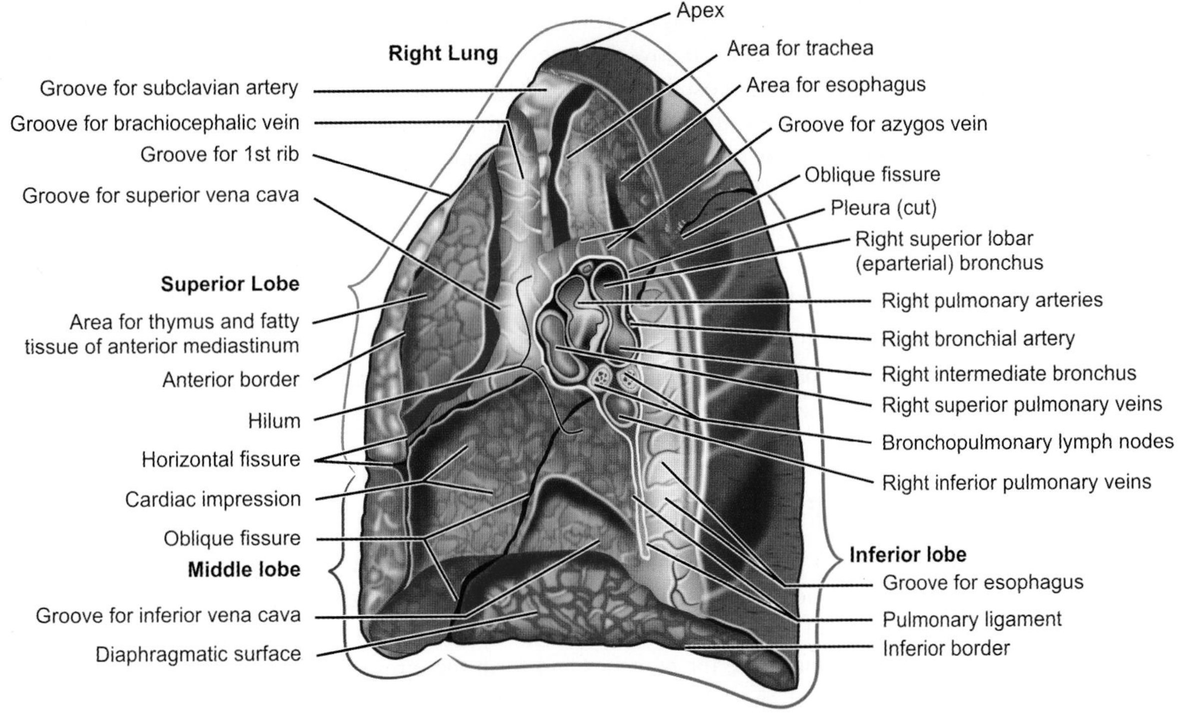

FIGURE 9 Right lung

Oblique fissure: Put your fingers in this and trace it to the hilum. Note that it cuts the inferior border anteriorly and separates the inferior lobe from the superior and middle lobes. ***Horizontal fissure*** runs from the oblique fissure to the anterior border and to the hilus of the lung. This separates the superior lobe from the middle lobe.

BORDERS AND SURFACES

Anterior border: It is the sharp margin which separates the costal surface from the mediastinal surface. This projects into the costomediastinal recess in deep inspiration. ***Inferior border*** is another sharp margin which separates the costal surface from the diaphragmatic surface. This projects into the costodiaphragmatic recess in deep inspiration. ***Costal surface*** is the most extensive lateral surface. It is related to the ribs and intercostal spaces. It shows depressions corresponding to the ribs. ***Apex*** is the projecting upper part. Look for the impression of the 1st rib. The part of the lung above this is the apex. This projects 1 to 2 cm above the middle 3rd of the clavicle and 3 to 5 cm above the sloping anterior part of the 1st rib. This part of the lung is related to the structures of the neck but in separated from them by the supra pleural membrane. Look for the indentation caused by the subclavian artery on the summit of the lung behind the indentation of the 1st rib.

Medial surface can be divided into three parts, the flat mediastinal surface and the rounded vertebral part and the root through which the lung communicates.

The ***mediastinal surface*** is hardened around the soft mediastinal structures which form identifiable impressions on this surface. The ***cardiac impression*** is the area in front of the hilus. It is much depressed as it is related to heart. The ***right atrium,*** the right ventricle and the ***infundibulum*** of the heart are related here. The ***superior vena caval*** impression can be well-identified in continuation with the cardiac impression. The ***trachea*** and ***esophagus*** form well identifiable impressions behind the vena caval impression. The azygos vein forms an impression above and behind the hilum. The ***inferior vena caval*** impression can be identified in front of the pulmonary ligament.

The ***vertebral part*** is related to the vertebrae, intervertebral discs and the structures lying on them. They are the sympathetic chain, thoracic nerves and vessels. These generally do not raise any elevations.

Hilus is the root of the lung, the area through which the lung communicates. Identify the cut margin of the pleura. This is the point where the serous layer and parietal layer of the pleura become continuous. The narrow lower part is called the pulmonary ligament. It has the bronchi, pulmonary artery, veins, lymphatics and plexus of nerves. ***Pulmonary veins*** carry oxygenated blood from the lungs to the heart. They are two in number. Being veins these have thin walls. Superior pulmonary vein is the most anterior structure within the hilus. The inferior pulmonary vein occupies the pulmonary ligament. ***Pulmonary artery*** presents thick wall and is behind the vein. Depending upon the cut at the hilus it may show up as a single branch, or could be two branches. This carries impure blood from the heart to the lung. ***Bronchus*** can easily be identified by feeling the cartilage present within the wall. On the right side the bronchus normally divides into 1st division before entering into the lung, so it is seen as two branches, one is generally behind and above the artery called eparterial bronchus. The other below the artery called hyparterial bronchus. ***Bronchial artery*** is a small artery, is a branch of the first right intercostal artery, lies posterior to the bronchus. This supplies the bronchial tree and parenchyma of lung. ***Lymph nodes*** are the black rounded to oval cut parts of the lymph nodes. They are pulmonary lymph nodes. ***Pulmonary plexus of nerves*** belong to the autonomic nervous system. They accompany the blood vessels and the bronchial tree.

Between the pleura and pericardium the ***phrenic nerve*** and the ***pericardiacophrenic artery*** passes down to reach the diaphragm.

(There can be adhesions in a cadaver, but in the living the superior middle and inferior lobes can easily be separated).

Diaphragmatic surface forms the base of the lung. Note that the diaphragm is bulging into the thorax due to the abdominal organs. To suit to this, the base is very much depressed but the circular inferior margin project down into the gap between the diaphragm and the thoracic cage. On the right side the diaphragm separates the lung from the right lobe of the liver.

Bronchopulmonary Segments (Fig. 10)

The trachea divides into right and left primary bronchi to reach each lung. The primary bronchus of the right lung divides into three lobar bronchi. Each lobar bronchus further divides into segmental tertiary bronchi. The part of the lung tissue connected to each segmental tertiary bronchus is called the bronchopulmonary segment. The superior lobar bronchus divides into apical, anterior and posterior branches and form the corresponding bronchopulmonary segments. The middle lobar bronchus forms medial and lateral bronchopulmonary segments. The inferior lobar bronchus forms apical, anterior, posterior, medial and lateral basal bronchopulmonary segments. Each bronchopulmonary segment is

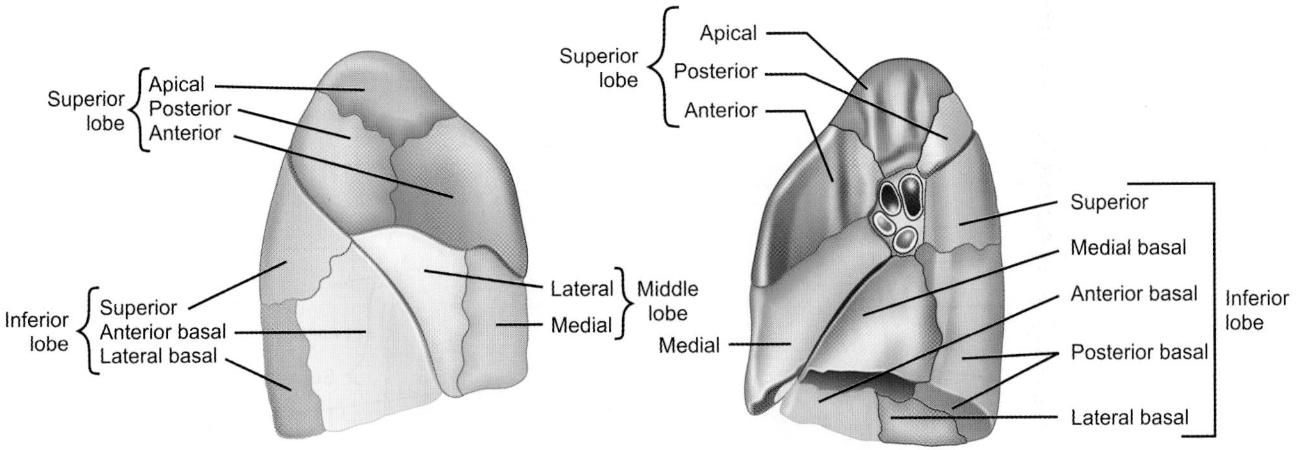

FIGURE 10 Right lung—bronchopulmonary segments

pyramidal in shape with the base facing outward and the apex facing towards the hilus. Each bronchus is accompanied by the pulmonary artery whereas the vein lies within the connective tissue between the segments.

LEFT LUNG (Fig. 11)

Hold the left lung with the base in your left palm and the anterior border facing medially and try to identify the following features. The left lung is divided into two lobes by the ***oblique fissure.*** It cuts through the lung form the hilus and through the inferior border of the lung.

The left is longer and narrower than the right lung. It weighs little less than the right lung. The ***anterior border*** presents the ***cardiac notch*** the indentation caused by the left tilt of the heart. The inferior border is shaper and longer separates the diaphragmatic surface from the costal surface. It enters the costodiaphragmatic recess during deep inspiration. ***Costal surface*** is the most extensive lateral surface and shows the depression caused by the ribs**.** ***Apex*** of the left lung shows the indentation for the left subclavian artery at its summit.

The medial surface presents a vertebral part, mediastinal surface and a hilus.

Hilum is the area where the lung communicates with the others. The parietal and visceral layers of the pleura are reflected here and you can see the cut surface. Identify the ***Superior pulmonary vein*** which is the most anterior structure. The ***inferior pulmonary vein*** is seen in the pulmonary ligament. The veins show thin wall and show a collapsed appearance. Note the left pulmonary artery. It has a thick wall and is the most superior structure in the hilus. Note the thick cartilaginous left principle bronchus which lies below the pulmonary artery and behind the pulmonary vein**.** See the ***bronchial arteries,*** which are two in number. They arise from the thoracic aorta, and are seen sticking to the bronchus posterior and superior to it. Note the dark black rounded ***lymph nodes*** cut in the hilus. The ***Pulmonary plexus of nerves*** is a part of autonomic nervous system accompanying the bronchus and the blood vessels.

Mediastinal surface: In front of the hilum note the deep cardiac impression formed by the heart. It is related to the left ventricle below and infundibulum of right ventricle above. Above and arching around the hilus, it is related to the ***ascending aorta, the arch of the aorta and the descending aorta,*** which continues down to form an impression along the posterior border of the hilus. The part above the aorta is related to ***the thymus, left common carotid artery and left subclavian artery*** in that order from front to the back.

The left phrenic nerve and pericardiacophrenic vessels lie between the pleura and the pericardium.

The ***vertebral surface*** is the rounded posterior part of the medial surface of the lung. It is related to the ***thoracic vertebrae, intervertebral discs, sympathetic chain; the segmental inter costal vessels*** and nerves.

Diaphragmatic surface is separated from the stomach**,** *Spleen and the left lobe of the liver* by the diaphragm.

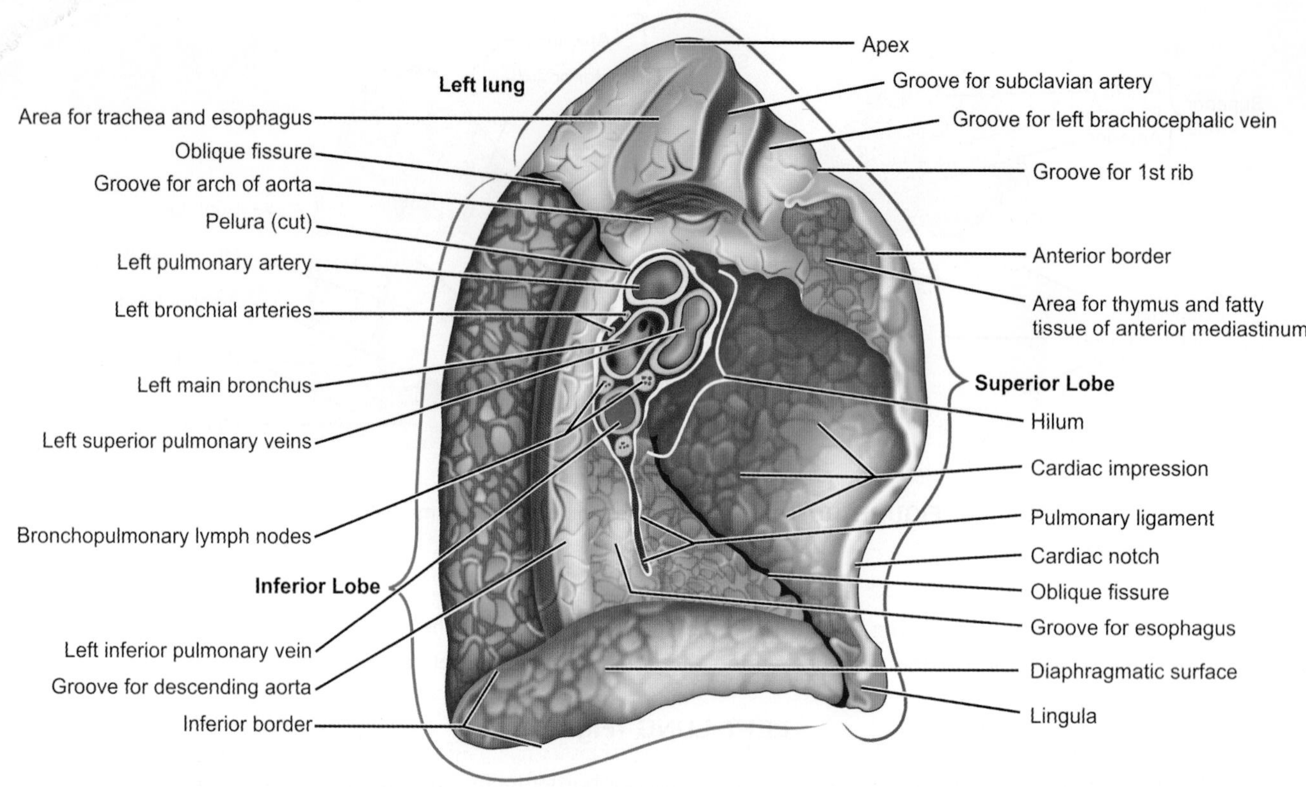

FIGURE 11 Left lung

Bronchopulmonary Segments (Figs 12 and 13)

The superior lobar bronchus divides into five branches: apical, posterior, anterior (many a times the apical and posterior can have a common stem), superior and inferior lingular segment each forming the bronchopulmonary segments of the same name. The inferior lobar bronchus gives off the superior and divides into medial, lateral, anterior and posterior lobar branches and caters to the bronhopulmonary segments of the same name. Many a books describe the anterior and medial basal segments as a combined anteromedial segment.

Dissection: Start at the bronchus near the hilum of the right lung and trace it into the lung pinching off the lung tissue as you go deeper. Trace, up to its next division which are the tertiary or segmental bronchi. Identify that the superior lobar bronchus divides into apical, anterior and posterior branches and form the corresponding bronchopulmonary segments. The middle lobar bronchus forms medial and lateral bronchopulmonary segments. The inferior lobar bronchus forms apical, anterior, posterior, medial and lateral basal bronchopulmonary segments.

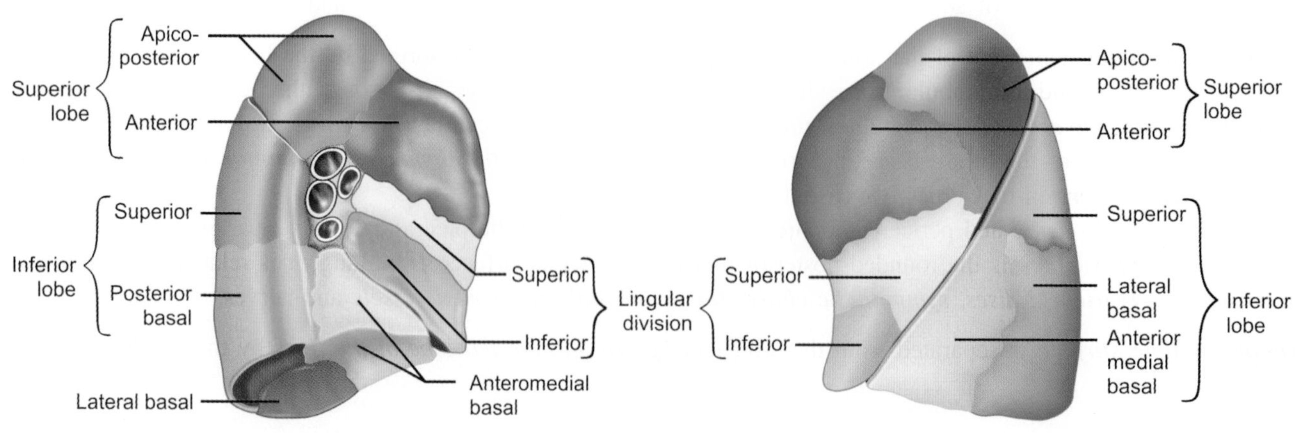

FIGURE 12 Left lung—bronchopulmonary segments

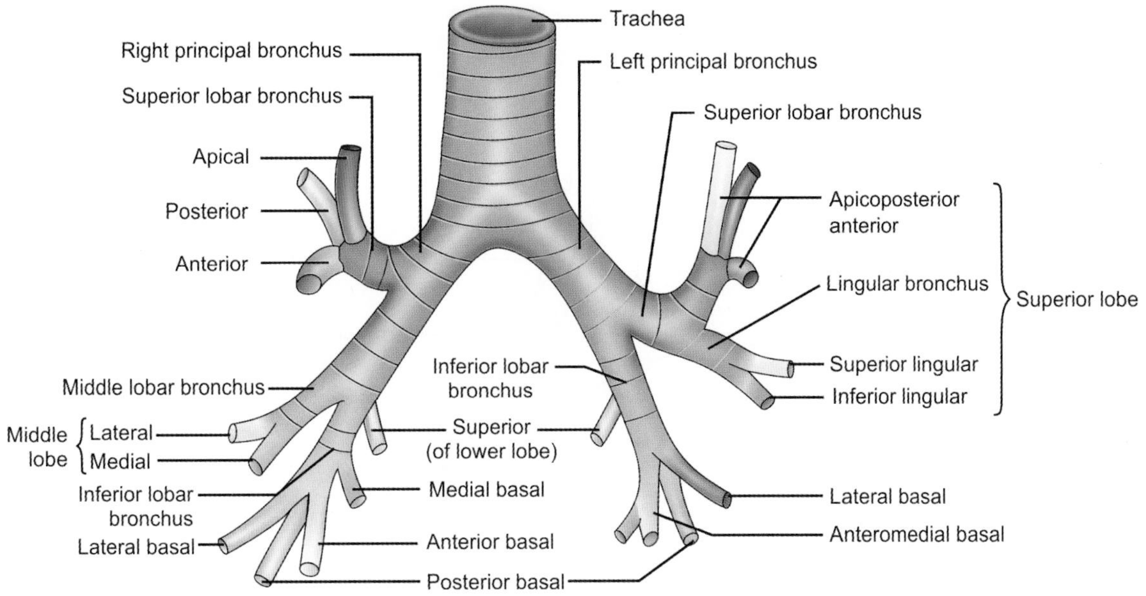

FIGURE 13 Bronchi

In the left lung the superior lobar bronchus gives rise to five branches: apical, posterior, anterior, superior lingular and inferior lingular branches. The lower lobar bronchus gives off the superior, medial basal, lateral basal, anterior basal and posterior basal branches. Partial removal of lung tissue is very common nowadays and knowledge of the variations in this field is very essential.

DIVISIONS OF MEDIASTINUM (Fig. 14)

The intact central part of the thorax is the mediastinum. It lodges all the structures that pass to neck and to abdomen. For convenience of description it is divided into a superior mediastinum and an inferior mediastinum by passing an imaginary line from the level of the manubriosternal joint to the lower border of the 4th vertebra.

The superior mediastinum lodges the blood vessels to and from the heart, the trachea and the esophagus. The inferior mediastinum is further divided into three parts, due to the presence of the heart. The part which lodges the heart is called the middle mediastinum, the part anterior to the heart is the anterior mediastinum and the part behind the heart is the posterior mediastinum.

Let us study in detail the structures in the mediastinum as they reveal in the mediastinum.

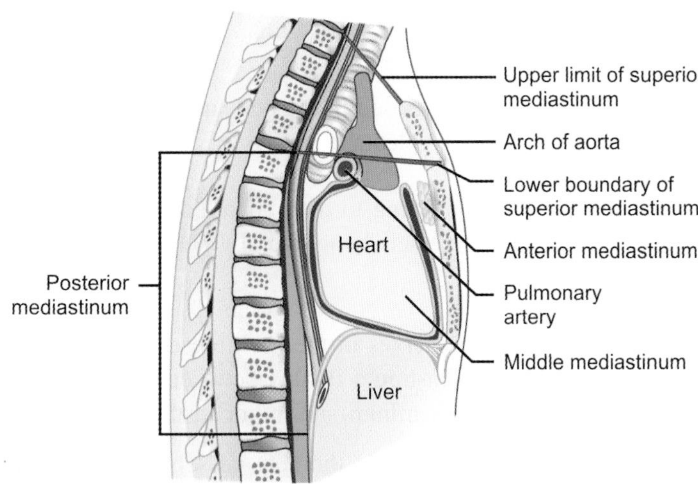

FIGURE 14 Divisions of mediastinum

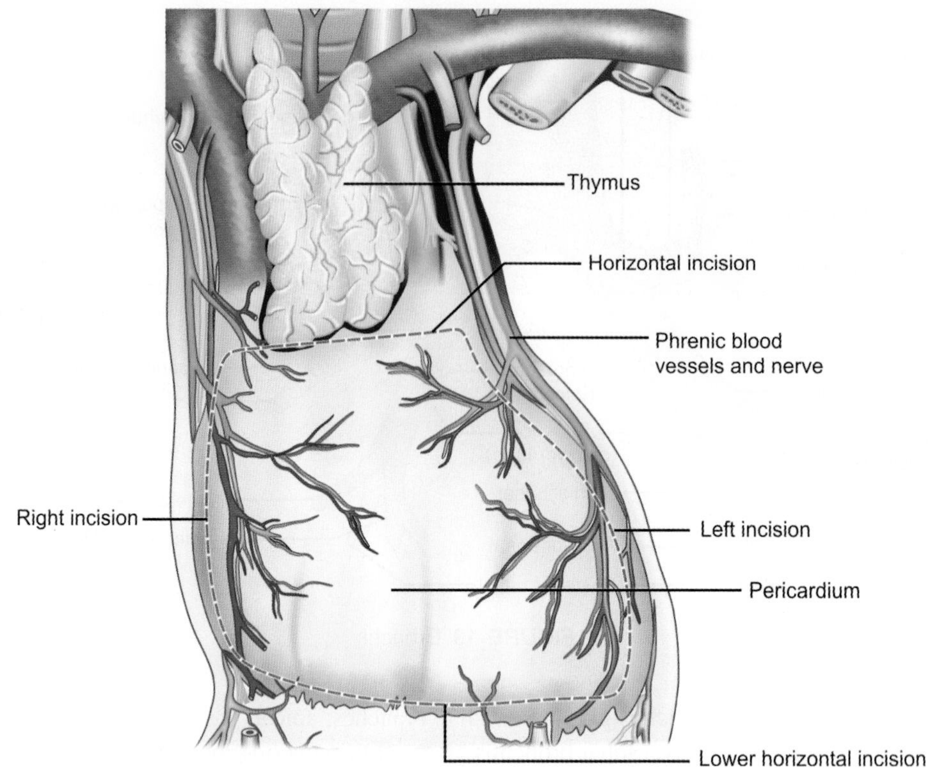

FIGURE 15 Pericardium and dissection lines

ANTERIOR MEDIASTINUM

This is a narrow space that lies in front of the heart up to the thoracic wall. It shows the remnants of the thymus in the adult/old people. In the young and in fetus thymus is a big gland occupying the anterior mediastinum.

MIDDLE MEDIASTINUM

The middle mediastinum is occupied by the heart enclosed in the pericardium. The phrenic nerve and the pericardiaco phrenic vessels lie between the pericardium and the pleura.

Dissection: Clean the thymus and the pleura sticking to the pericardium both anteriorly and laterally. Identify the phrenic nerve and the pericardiacophrenic vessels lying laterally between the pericardium and pleura. Trace them superiorly as far as you can.

Phrenic nerve (C3, 4, 5) arises from the cervical nerves in the neck, descends down into the superior mediastinum, along with the blood vessels. In the middle mediastinum it runs between the pleura and pericardium to reach the diaphragm. It is sensory to mediastinal pleura, pericardium and motor to the diaphragm.

Pericardiacophrenic vessels are branches of the internal thoracic vessels. These are given off in the neck region. They descend down along with the phrenic nerve and supply the mediastinal pleura, pericardium and the diaphragm.

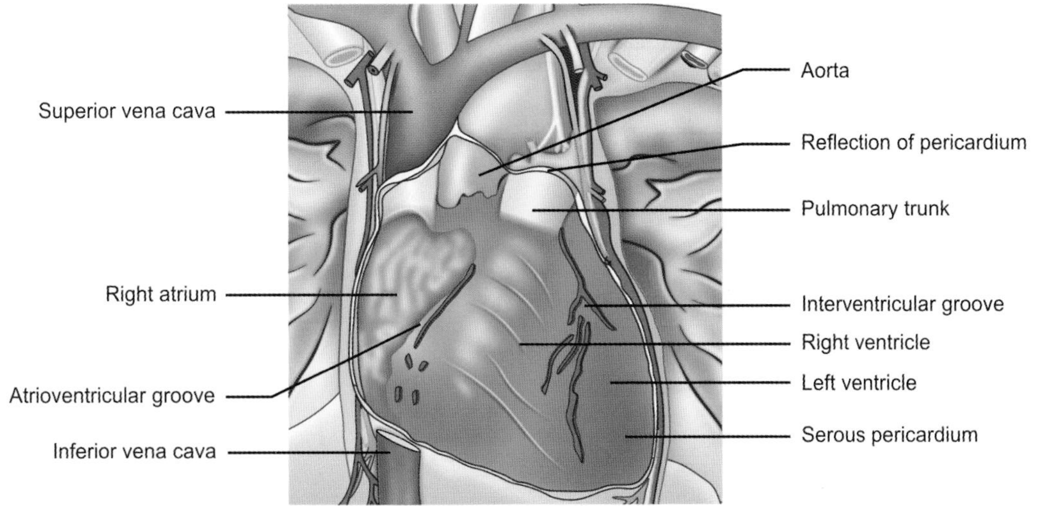

FIGURE 16 Heart in situ

PERICARDIUM (Fig. 15)

The heart is located within the fibrous pericardium, a thick connective tissue covering. The serous pericardium is a thin sac which encloses the heart and lies between the fibrous pericardium and the heart. The serous pericardium presents a parietal layer lining the fibrous pericardium and a visceral layer covering the heart. They get reflected at the root of the heart, where the blood vessels enter or leave the heart. The pericardial cavity between the two layers is filled with pericardial fluid. This helps in the smooth movement of the heart within the pericardium.

Dissection: Make a window in the pericardium as is shown in the diagram. A horizontal incision across the root of the heart. A right incision connecting the superior and inferior vena cavae. A lower horizontal incision near the diaphragm. A left incision along the left side of the heart.

Reflect the flap. Note that you are in the pericardial cavity. The fibrous pericardium has both fibrous pericardium and the parietal layer of the serous pericardium. The heart has the visceral layer of the serous pericardium. Run your fingers on all sides of the heart. Note the point of reflection of parietal layer and visceral layer of serous pericardium around the entry of blood vessels.

Heart in Situ (Fig. 16)

Try to identify the heart *in situ*. See the area of reflection of the parietal layer of pericardium with the serous layer of the pericardium. The heart is covered by serous layer of pericardium. Identify the superior and inferior vena cava. Note the right atrium between the two vena cavae. Note the right and left ventricles. They occupy most of the anterior surface of the heart. Note the atrioventricular and interventricular grooves. Make out that these areas are occupied by the blood vessels and are supported by the fat. Note the pulmonary trunk arising from the right ventricle and the aorta from the left ventricle.

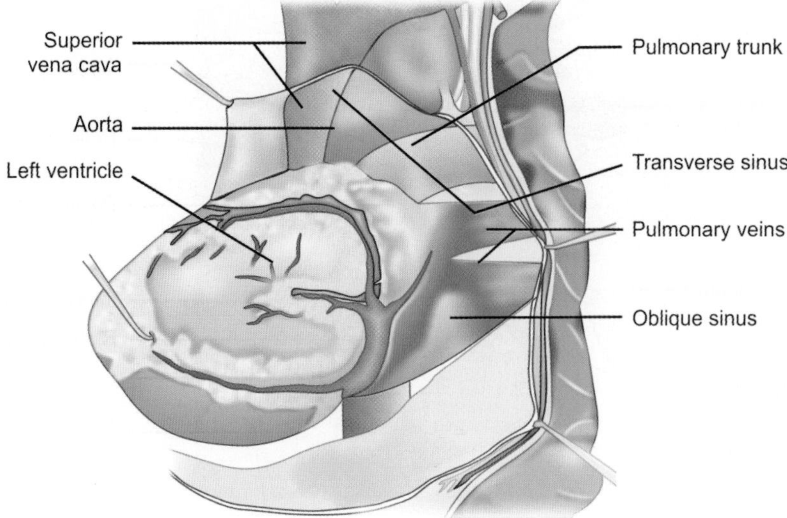

FIGURE 17 Sinuses of pericardium

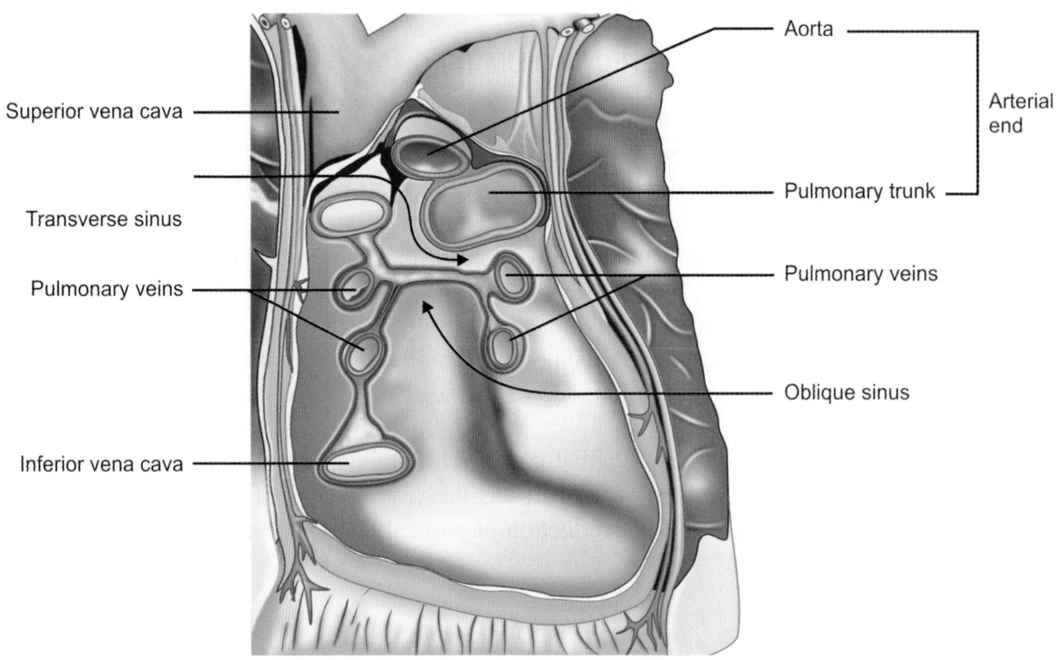

FIGURE 18 Sinus of pericardium after removing the heart

SINUSES OF PERICARDIUM (Figs 17 and 18)

Oblique sinus: Put your fingers from the left side of the heart to the back of the heart. You encounter resistance on all sides. This is due to the entry of pulmonary veins and inferior vena cava into the heart. The space in which your fingers lie is called the oblique sinus. It is the posterior extension of the pericardial cavity. Pull the heart forwards and to the right, to visualize it better.

Transverse sinus: Put your finger in front of the superior vena cava and behind the aorta and pulmonary trunk. It is a gap between the arterial and venous end of the heart and is called the transverse sinus.

Dissection: Identify the inferior vena cava piercing the diaphragm and entering into the right atrium. Cut it near the diaphragm. Identify the superior vena cava, ascending aorta and pulmonary trunk from right to left at the upper end and cut them across. Turn the heart to the right and cut through the pulmonary veins entering into the heart on the posterior aspect. Take the heart out of the body and study the details of the heart. Note the posterior part of the pericardium and the blood vessels opening into it.

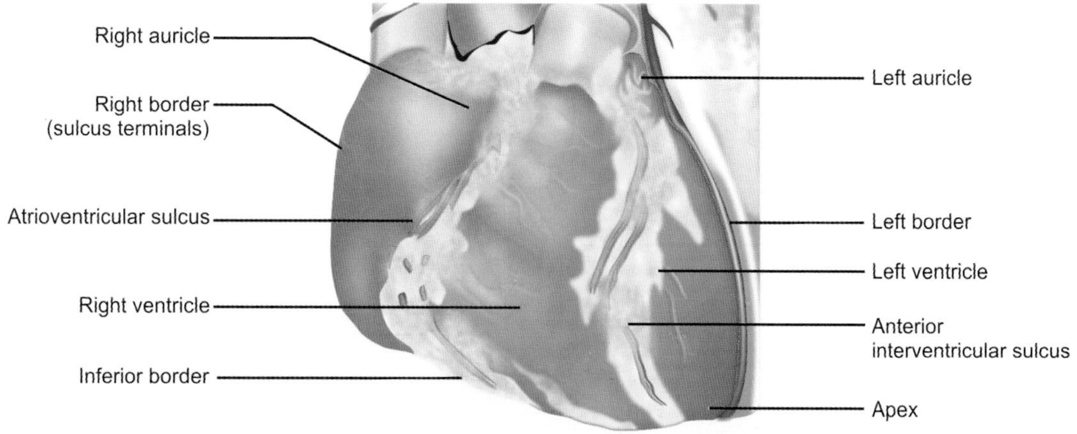

FIGURE 19 Heart—external features anterior surface/sternocostal surface

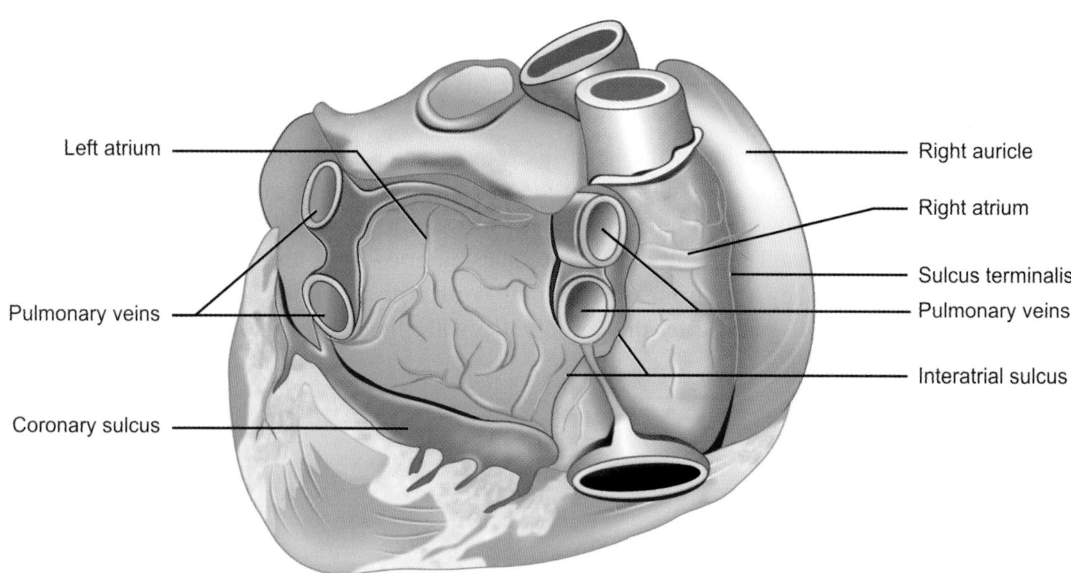

FIGURE 20 Heart—external features base/posterior surface

HEART

EXTERNAL FEATURES (Figs 19 to 21)

Put the heart, with the diaphragmatic surface in your right palm with the apex in line with the middle finger. This is as it lies in your body. Keep turning the heart as you identify each part.

The ***right border*** extending from the superior vena cava to the inferior vena cava, can easily be identified because of the sharp depression called sulcus terminalis. The ***left border*** is a rounded border extending from right auricle to the apex. Note the ***inferior border*** extending from the inferior vena cava to the apex of the heart. It is a sharp margin. The ***anterior surface/sternocostal surface*** is formed by the ***right and left auricles; right and left ventricles.*** The two ventricles are separated by ***anterior interventricular sulcus. Base or posterior surface*** is formed by the right and left atria. Two atria are separated by a shallow ***interatrial sulcus.*** The 4 pulmonary veins enter the left atrium and superior and inferior vena cava open into the right atrium. The ***coronary sulcus*** separates the posterior surface from the diaphragmatic surface. The diaphragmatic surface is the undersurface of the heart formed by the right and left ventricles. They are separated by ***posterior interventricular sulcus.*** The atria and ventricles are separated by a 'C' shaped ***atrioventricular sulcus/coronary sulcus.***

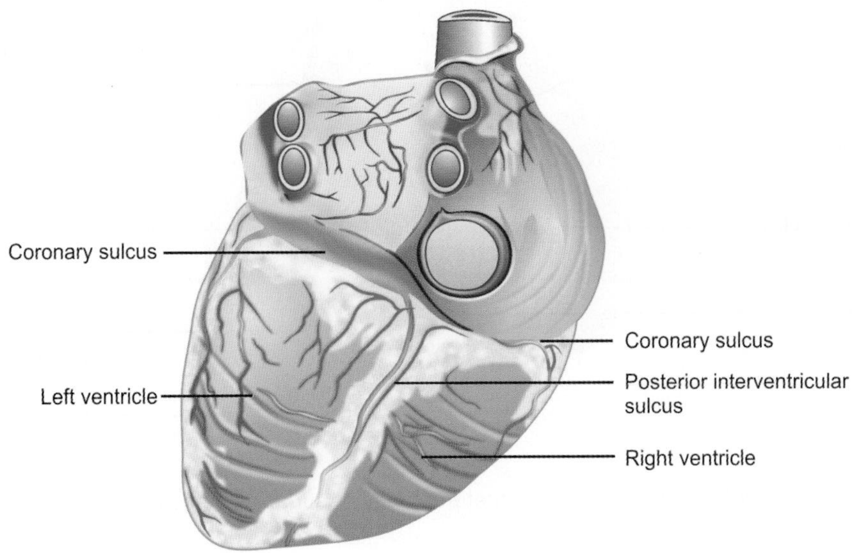

FIGURE 21 Heart—external features: diaphragmatic surface

BLOOD SUPPLY OF THE HEART (Figs 22 and 23)

Dissection: The major arteries and veins of the heart lie in the grooves between the chambers. There is a good amount of fat accompanying the blood vessels. Clean the visceral pericardium and the thin epicardium sticking to the pericardium. This is the adventitial covering of the heart. In a cadaver it is inseparable from the serous pericardium. Identify the vessels. The right and left coronary arteries share the supply of the heart. They are the first branches of the aorta. They arise from the ascending aorta. The ascending aorta exhibits three dilatations, one anterior two posterior and is guarded by the aortic valve with three cusps. Note these structures by seeing through the cut end of the aorta.

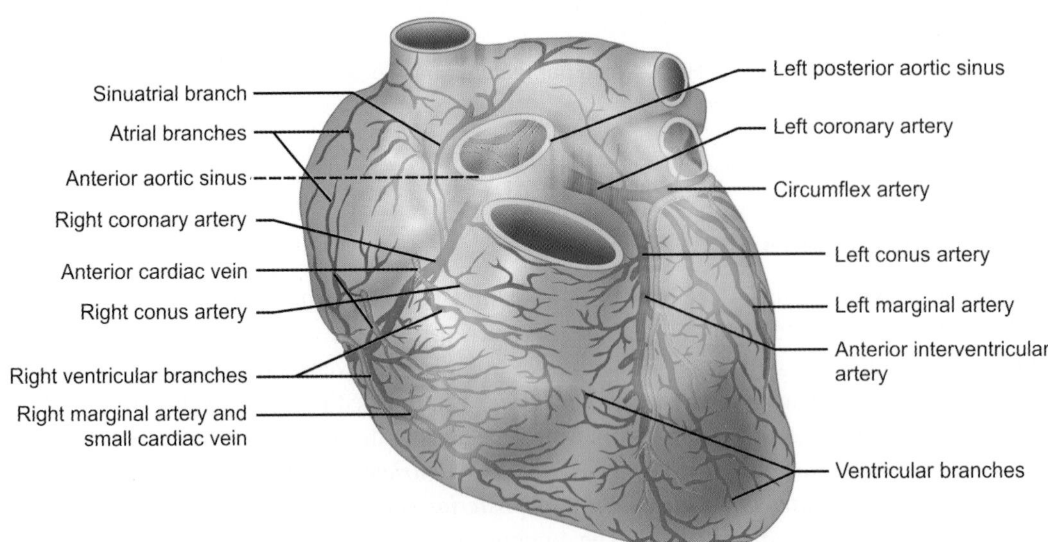

FIGURE 22 Heart—blood supply: anterior aspect

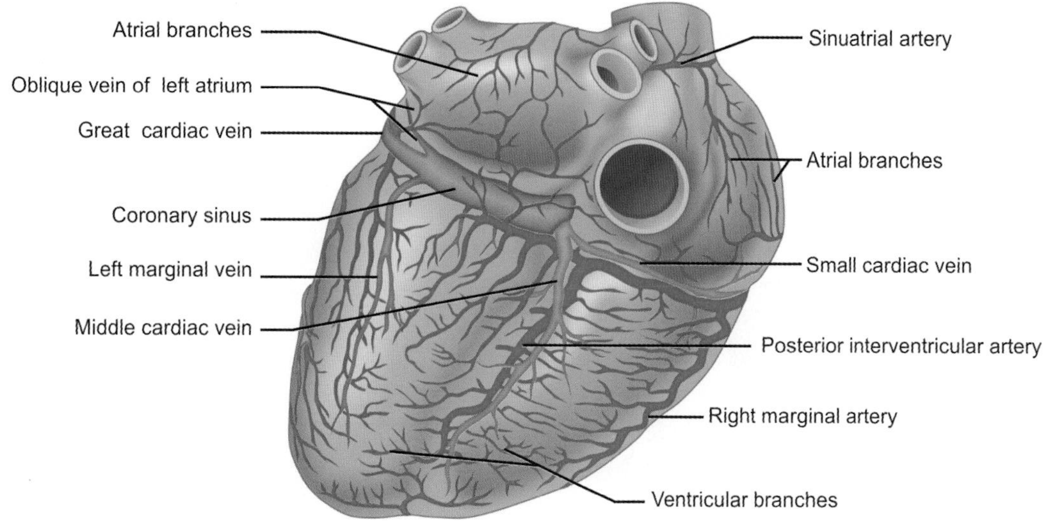

FIGURE 23 Heart—blood supply: posterior aspect

Coronary sulcus is a 'C' shaped groove separating the atria from the ventricles. Anteriorly it is overlapped by the ascending aorta and pulmonary trunk. Posteriorly it lodges the coronary sinus.

The right coronary artery: Locate the origin of this artery from the anterior aortic sinus by passing a probe through the opening of the artery. Separate the right auricle and trace the artery in the right anterior part of the coronary sulcus up to the lower end of the atrium. Trace the ***sinoatrial artery*** and the ***atrial branches*** from the right side of the artery. Trace them as far as you can. The sinuatrial nodal artery is the artery of importance here as it supplies the SA node. From the left side of the artery, trace the ***conus artery*** and ***right ventricular branches*** along the wall of the right ventricle. These arteries supply the infudibulum and the anterior wall of the right ventricle. Biggest of the ventricular branch is called the ***marginal artery*** and it runs along the inferior border.

Dissection: Turn the heart to the base and continue tracing the right coronary artery in the atrioventricular sulcus, till it anastomses with the left coronary. Trace the big **posterior interventricular branch** into the posterior interventricular groove on the diaphragmatic surface of the heart. This artery anastomoses with the anterior interventricular branch around the apex. Trace the **atrial, ventricular branches** given off from the right coronary. Trace the right and left ventricular branches that are given off from the posterior interventricular artery.

Left coronary artery: Trace the left coronary artery from the left posterior aortic sinus. Lift the left auricle; trace the artery between the auricle and the infundibulum. Note that this artery has a very short stem. It gives off the ***left conus artery.*** Trace the left conus artery to the infundibulum.This anastomoses with the right conus artery, given off from the right coronary artery. The left coronary artery divides into two branches. They are the ***anterior interventricular branch*** which runs in the anterior interventricular groove and the ***circumflex branch*** which runs in the atrioventricular sulcus. Trace the circumflex branch till it anastomoses with the right coronary artery. From the anterior interventricular artery trace its ***right and left ventricular branches.*** From the circumflex branch trace the big ***left marginal branch,*** other ventricular and the ***left atrial branches*** into the corresponding walls.

Note: That the branches of distribution are highly variable in different subjects.

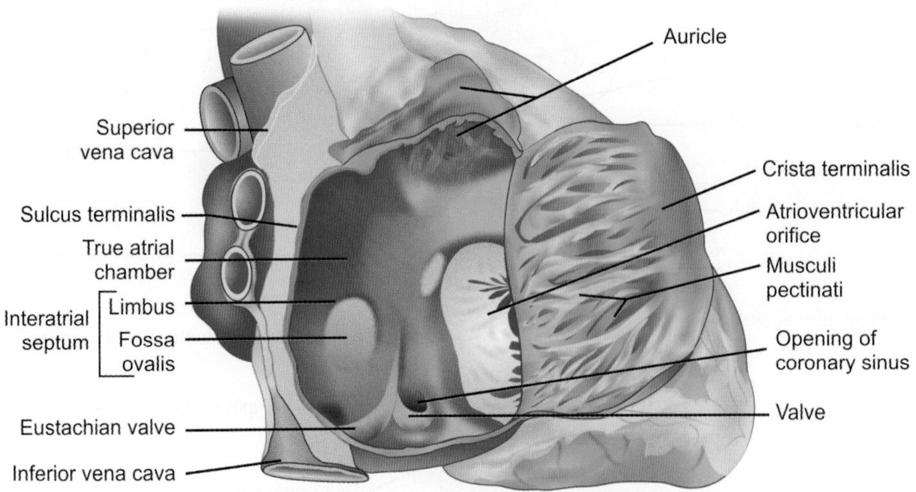

FIGURE 24 Heart—right atrium

VEINS OF THE HEART

The ***coronary sinus*** is the venous channel which returns the blood from the heart into the right atrium. It traverses from left to right, and is located in the atrioventricular sulcus in the posterior border of the heart. Note that all its tributaries accompany the arteries. ***Great cardiac vein*** lies in the anterior interventricular groove and its continuation forms the beginning of coronary sinus. Left ventricular branches drain into the coronary sinus at its left end. ***Middle cardiac vein*** runs in the posterior interventricular sulcus. ***Oblique vein of left atrium*** is a small tributary. It is seen on the wall of left atrium. Anterior cardiac vein drains the right ventricle into the right atrium. ***Small cardiac vein*** accompanies the right marginal vein along the inferior border of the heart turns on the right side of the heart to drain into right end of the coronary sinus.

Venae cardis minimi are small veins which drain directly into all the chambers of the heart.

CHAMBERS OF THE HEART

The heart is made up of two atria and two ventricles. The atria lie superiorly and posteriorly whereas the ventricles lie anteriorly and inferiorly. The atria are the receiving ends, and the vessels that enter into the atria are veins. The ventricles send blood out, through the arteries. The right side of the heart has the impure blood and the left side of the heart has pure blood. Study each chamber in detail.

RIGHT ATRIUM (Fig. 24)

The ***right atrium*** receives the deoxygenated blood from the whole body and pushes it down to the right ventricle. It forms the right margin, anterior and posterior surfaces of the heart. ***Sulcus terminalis*** is the depression extending from the superior vena cava to inferior vena cava along the right margin. Feel and identify this. ***The right auricle*** is ear shaped part from the sulcus terminalis on to the anterior surface. ***Cut through the auricle behind and parallel to the sulcus terminalis. Open the atrial chamber.*** Note that the auricular part shows muscle fibres radiating from the ***crista terminalis*** the projection in the atrial chamber corresponding to the sulcus terminalis on the exterior. These are called ***musculi pectinati,*** as they resemble the arrangement of feathers. Note that the remaining part of the right atrium is smooth and it is the ***true atrial chamber.***

The interatrial septum: This extends obliquely, from back to the front. This separates the right atrium from left atrium. Due to the obliquity of the septum the right atrium lies in front of the left atrium. Note that it presents two parts—the elevated inverted U shaped ***limbus*** and central depressed ***fossa ovalis.***

(Study their embryology and the associated defects).

Identify the Vessels Entering into the Right Atrium

The ***superior vena cava*** opens into the chamber superiorly. It drains the blood from the head and neck, upper limb and thorax. It is devoid of valves as it drains towards gravity. The ***inferior vena cava*** opens at inferior angle. It is guarded by the eustachian valve, which directs the blood towards the left atrium in the fetal life. It is continuous with the anterior limb of limbus. The ***coronary sinus*** opens into the right atrium, to the left of inferior vena caval opening and between it and the interventricular orifice. It is guarded by Thabecian valve.

Atrioventricular orifice: It is located more anteriorly. Put your fingers and feel the atrioventricular valve and the right ventricular chamber.

RIGHT VENTRICLE (Fig. 25)

The right ventricle receives the blood from the right atrium and pumps it to the lungs for purification. It occupies the sternocostal surface and diaphragmatic surface of the heart.

Dissection: Cut and reflect the anterior wall as per the incision shown in the diagram.

Note that the wall of the ventricle is far thicker in comparison to the atrium. This is due to its thick musculature. The musculature raises elevations within the interior and these are called ***trabeculae corneae*** and ***papillary muscles.*** The papillary muscles projecting into the interior are connected to the atrioventricular valve by chordae tendineae. Identify the papillary muscles and note the following—The anterior papillary muscle is larger and is attached from the anterior wall to the anterior and posterior cusps of the atrioventricular valve. The posterior papillary muscle extends from the inferior wall to the posterior and septal cusps of the atrioventricular valve. The septal papillary muscles are 3 to 4 small muscles attached from the interventricular septum to the septal and anterior cusp of the atrioventricular valve. These muscles contract during the ventricular systole, pull the cusps of the atrioventricular valve together, thus closing it tightly. ***Infundibulum*** is the smooth anterosuperior part of the ventricle. It continues up to form the pulmonary trunk. Here it is guarded by pulmonary valve. Identify the ***interventricular septum.*** Note that it has two parts. The upper membranous part separates the right atrium and the right ventricle from the left ventricle. The lower muscular part, separates the two ventricles, but it bulges into the right ventricle. So in a cross-section the right ventricle appears more or less C shaped. The trabecula in the interventricular wall raises a longitudinal elevation called ***septomarginal trabecula/ moderator band.*** Note that it ends into the anterior papillary muscle. It carries the conducting system of the heart to the right ventricle. It is called the atrioventricular bundle.

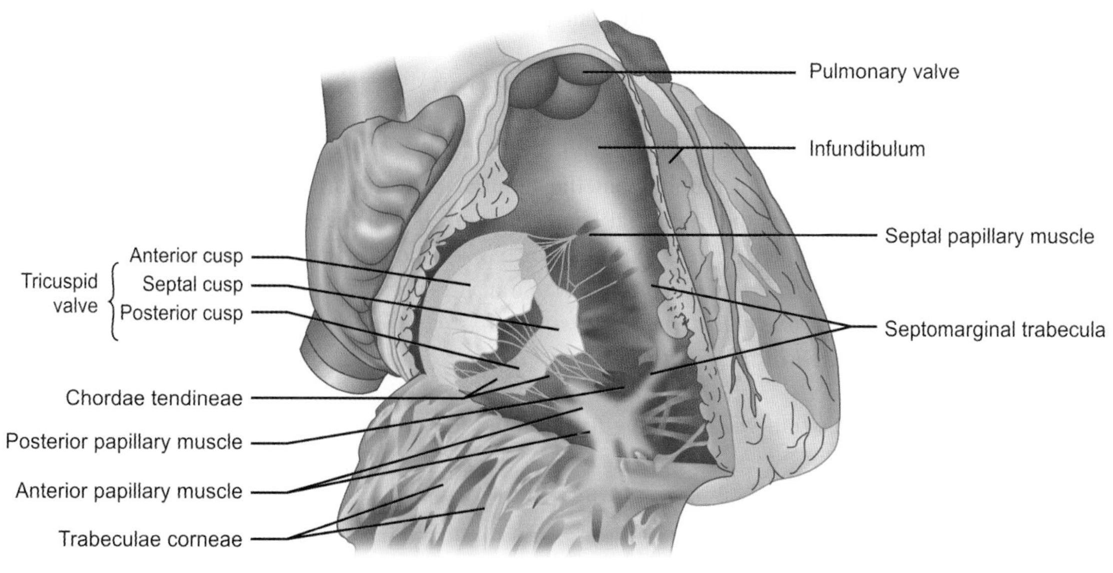

FIGURE 25 Heart—right ventricle

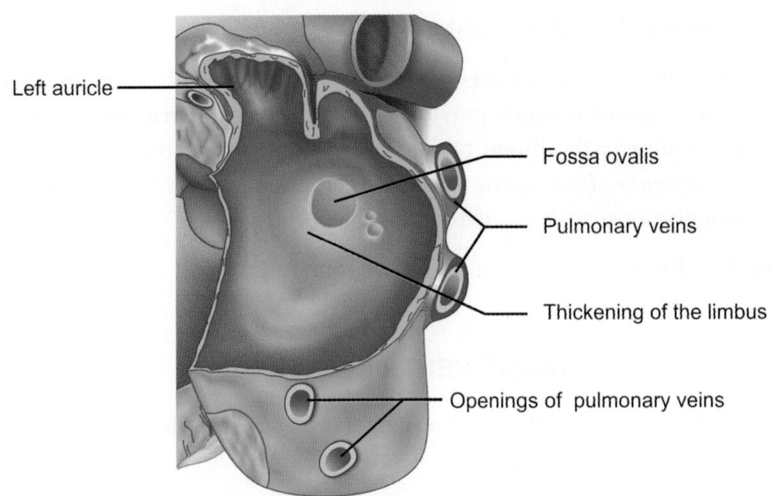

FIGURE 26 Heart—left atrium

Right atrioventricular orifice: It is the communication between the right atrium and the right ventricle. It is around 2.5 cm in diameter. The ***atrioventricular or tricuspid valve*** guards this orifice. It presents three cusps named according to their attachment to the walls of the ventricle. They are the ***anterior, posterior and septal cusps.*** They are anchored to the orifice by a fibrous ring. These cusps are irregular in shape and the septal is smaller than the other two. They present a smooth part towards the atrial surface due to the constant passage of the blood from atrium to the ventricle. The ventricular surface presents a rough surface due to the attachment of the ***chordae tendineae*** of the papillary muscles.

Pulmonary orifice: Note that at the upper end of the ***infundibulum*** where it continues into the pulmonary trunk in presents a orifice guarded by a valve the pulmonary valve. Pulmonary valve presents three semilunar cusps, the anterior, right and left. ***Make a vertical slit through the pulmonary trunk and examine the cusps.*** They are attached to the wall by means of a fibrous ring. The free margins of the cusps show a fibrous thickening and its center presents a thick nodule. The total cusp is thin and is called ***lunule.*** During the ventricular systole the blood is pushed into the pulmonary trunk through the gap between the cusps by the contracting ventricular musculature. During ventricular diastole the blood in the pulmonary trunk fills the cusps thus approximating them. They are tightly held together as the nodules approximate each other. They prevent the blood from going back into the ventricle.

LEFT ATRIUM (Fig. 26)

Left atrium: Turn the heart to the back and identify that the base of the heart is formed primarily by the left atrium. The left atrium receives the blood from the lungs by four pulmonary veins. It pumps the blood to the left ventricle.

Dissection: Cut through the left atrium in a ∩ shaped manner passing through the auricle and the true atrial part. Reflect it downwards to view the interior.

Pulmonary veins are generally four in number but the number can be variable. Note that the part between the pulmonary veins appears smooth. This is the true atrial chamber. ***Auricle***—of the left atrium is a small projection to the left of the atrium and projects to the anterior sternocostal surface of the heart. It presents rough surface due to muscular projections called musculi pectinati. ***Interatrial septum***—note that it is located inferiorly and to the right of the cavity.

See this against light and note the thick limbus fossa ovalis and the thin fossa ovalis within the curve of the limbus. (These are already explained in the right atrium.)

Atrioventricular orifice: Note this thin wide opening towards the left, put your fingers in it and feel the left ventricle which is in front of it.

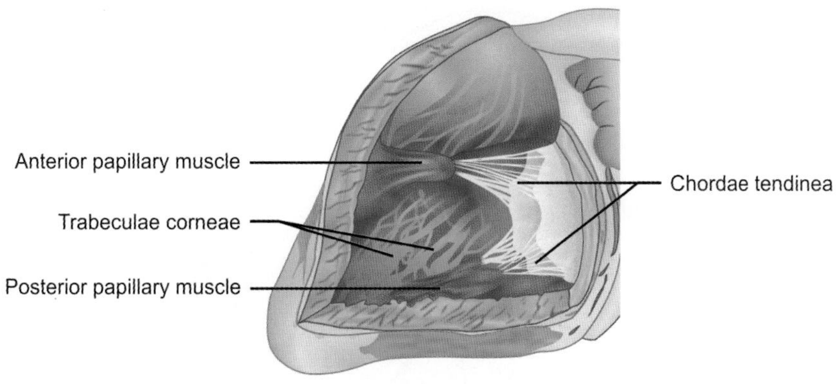

FIGURE 27 Heart—left ventricle

LEFT VENTRICLE (Fig. 27)

Left ventricle: This receives the oxygenated blood from the left atrium and pumps it to the whole body through the aorta.

Dissection: Turn the heart to its left side. Identify the left ventricle. Make a L shaped cut as shown in the diagram and open the chamber.

Note that this has the thickest wall of all the four chambers. Identify the well elevated ***trabeculae corneae*** and papillary muscles. The ***papillary muscles are two*** in number, the anterior and the posterior. The chordae tendineae of the both the muscles attach to both the cusps of the atrioventricular valve.

Atrioventricular valve: The atrioventricular valve has two cusps—the anterior and the posterior. The atrial surface of the cusps present a smooth appearance and the ventricular surface is rough due to the attachment of the chordae tendineae of the papillary muscles.

Aortic vestibule: Cut the anterior papillary muscle from the wall, pull it down and look for the aortic vestibule. Put your fingers in, and feel the smooth part the aortic sinus. Note that your fingers are just behind the infundibulum of the right ventricle. Put your fingers in the ventricles and feel the thin membranous part of the interventricular septum. The aortic vestibule continues into the ascending aorta.

Aortic valve: It is located at the junction of the aortic vestibule and the ascending aorta. It has three cusps. Like the pulmonary valve the aortic valve also attaches itself into the peripheral fibrous ring, presents nodules in the center of the free margin and a central lunules.

Ascending aorta: It runs from the aortic vestibule upwards forwards and to the right of pulmonary trunk and presents three aortic sinuses. These are one anterior and two posterior aortic sinuses.

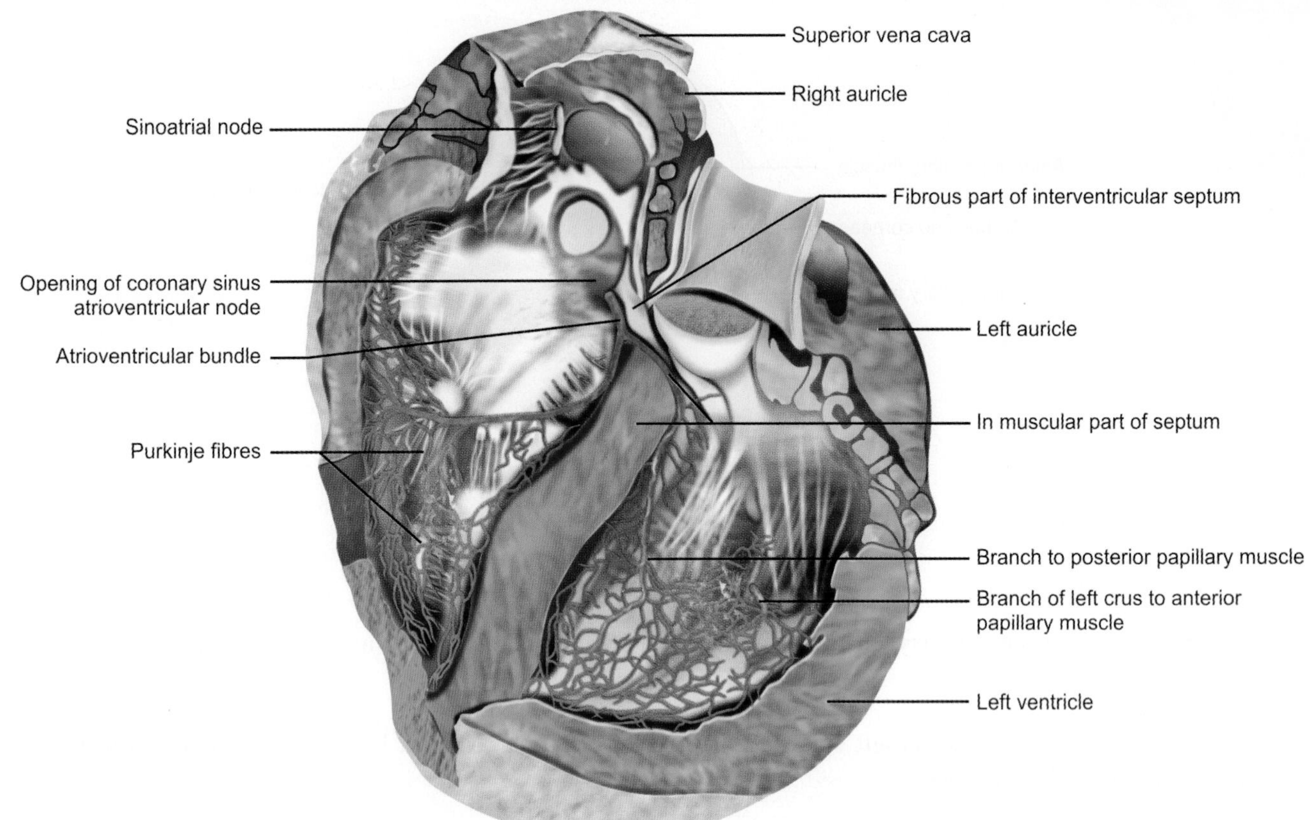

FIGURE 28 Conducting system of the heart

CONDUCTING SYSTEM (Fig. 28)

The conducting system of the heart is the intrinsic modified musculature of the heart. It initiates and conducts the impulse to different chamber of the heart. The ***sinoatrial node*** is located near the upper end of the crista terminalis. It is called the pacemaker and initiates the impulse and passes it onto the atrial chambers. The ***atrioventricular node*** lies in the interatrial septum above the opening of coronary sinus. This picks up the impulse from the atrial musculature and passes it onto both the ventricles through the ***atrioventricular bundle***. The right branch of the atrioventricular bundle raises the elevation—septomarginal band in the interventricular septum facing the right ventricle. ***Purkinje fibres*** are the fine branches that reach the musculature. The atrioventricular node, atrioventricular bundle, the right and left branches and purkinje fibres, pass on the impulse to the ventricles. These fibres are too fine to be visualized in the dissection. Try to identify the location of the parts of punkinje system on the heart.

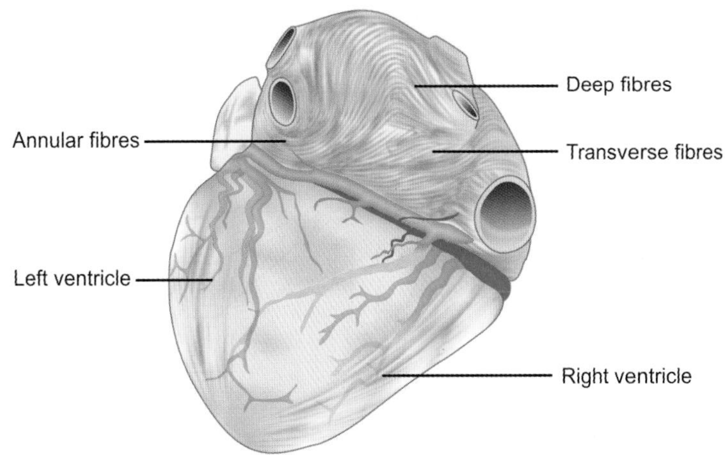

FIGURE 29 Myocardium

MYOCARDIUM (Fig. 29)

The musculature of the heart constitutes the main bulk of the heart.

Dissection: Peel the pericardium and try to see the musculature.

The **atrial muscle** presents three parts:

1. Superficial fibres run transversely and cover both the atria.
2. Deep fibres run in the form of an S from the right atrium to the left atrium.
3. The deepest annular fibres are prominent near the orifices and are continuous with the musculature of the vessels.

The ***ventricular fibres*** begin at the atrioventricular orifice whorl near the apex go deeper to reach the papillary muscles. The deeper fibres form a loop with the center in the interventricular septum. They also reach the papillary musculature.

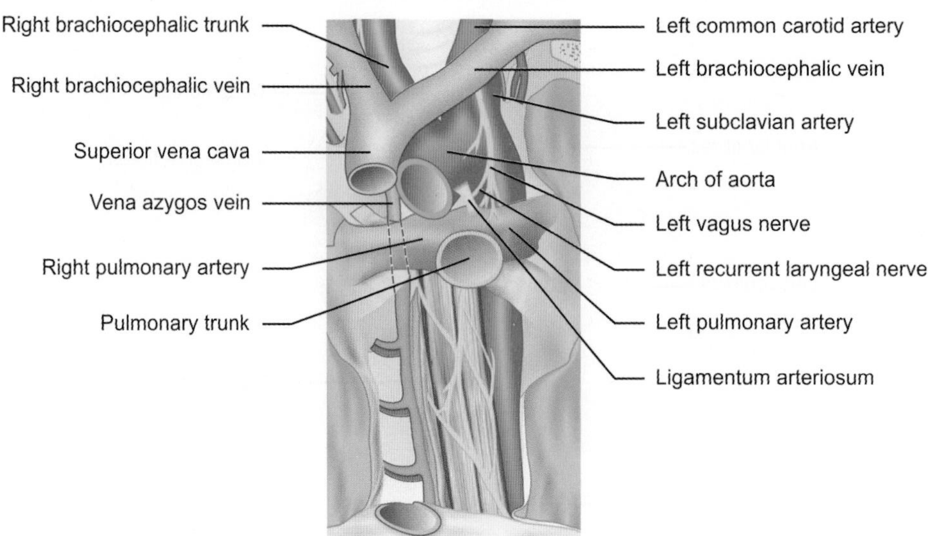

FIGURE 30 Superior mediastinum

SUPERIOR MEDIASTINUM (Figs 30 and 31)

The superior mediastinum lodges the superior vena cava and its tributaries, the aorta and its branches, lymphatics, the vagus and phrenic nerves, the sympathetic chain and its branches, trachea and esophagus.

Dissection: Clean the remnants of the pericardium and see the following structures.

Superior vena cava and associated veins: The superior vena cava drains the upper half of the body. This is the most anterior of the structures the superior mediastinum and is located on the right side.

Vena azygos: This vein opens into the posterior aspect of the superior vena cava at the level of the second rib. Locate this vessel. Note, its arch over the hilum of the right lung. Trace it down into the posterior mediastinum. It drains blood from the intercostal spaces. It lies in front of thoracic vertebrae.

Right and left brachiocephalic veins: Note these two vessels which join on the right side to form the superior vena cava. The right brachiocephalic vein is short and looks like a continuation of superior vena cava. The left brachiocephalic vein crosses from the left to the right at the level of the 1st thoracic vertebra.

AORTA AND ITS BRANCHES

Ascending aorta: This was already noted in the heart. It arises from the left ventricle at the level of 2nd costal cartilage. The ***arch of aorta*** is the continuation of the ascending aorta. Note this thick vessel to the left of the superior vena cava. The arch of the aorta begins and ends at the level of the second costal cartilage with an arch superiorly and to the left. It can be divided into three parts for convenience of description. Note its three branches—***brachiocephalic trunk*** the first and biggest branch. It arises behind the center of the manubrium sterni and moves to the ***right of the trachea*** to the right sternoclavicular joint**.** The ***left common carotid artery*** is the next branch. It moves to the left side of the trachea to the left sternoclavicular joint. The ***left subclavian artery*** is the most posterior of the branches. It ascends upwards and laterally to reach the left rib. The ***descending aorta*** is a posterior mediastinal structure.

Pulmonary trunk: Identify this artery below the aorta. It arises from the right ventricle and divides into two branches—the right and left pulmonary arteries. The pulmonary trunk and pulmonary arteries lie within the curvature of the arch the aorta. They enter the lungs at the hilum. These vessels lie in front of the trachea. Put a probe into this vessel and see the cut parts of the pulmonary trunk and right and left pulmonary arteries.

The ligamentum arteriosum: Pull the pulmonary trunk downwards and note this connection between the left pulmonary artery and the left part of the arch of the aorta. It is a functional vessel in the embryological state but in the adult anatomy it is a fibrosed structure.

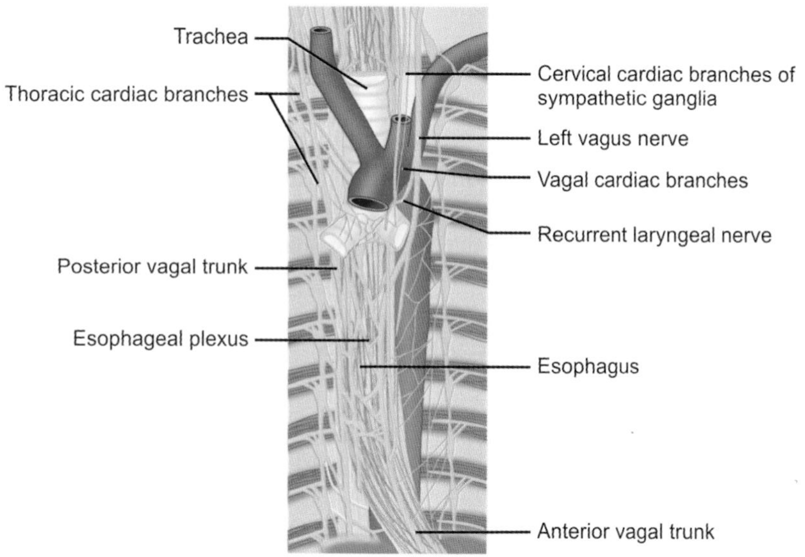

FIGURE 31 Cardiac plexus, trachea, and esophagus

Left vagus nerve: The left vagus crosses the left common carotid and arch of the aorta and goes behind the left pulmonary vein to reach the hilus of the lung and to the left side of the esophagus to form pulmonary and esophageal plexus.

Left recurrent laryngeal nerve: Note this thick branch of the vagus that is given off at the arch of the aorta. It winds round the ligamentum arteriosum goes posteriorly to lie between the trachea and esophagus.

Dissection: Cut the brachiocephalic veins near the inlet. Cut the azygos vein near its termination into the superior vena cava. Remove the superior vena cava and brachiocephalic veins. Remove the pulmonary trunk and the right and left pulmonary arteries.

THE TRACHEA

The lower part of the trachea is seen here deep to the aorta. It is a midline structure. It divides into right and left bronchi at the level of the 4th thoracic vertebra. Note these cut ends which were a part of the hilus of the lung. Note the C shaped tracheal and bronchial cartilages. Note that the right bronchus is in line with the trachea whereas the left bronchus shows a left deviation and relatively narrower.

THE CARDIAC PLEXUS

It is a plexus of nerves located between the trachea and arch of the aorta. Locate this nerve plexus position. It is a plexus of autonomic nervous system contributed by sympathetic trunk and vagus. The sympathetic branches come from the cervical ganglia and upper four thoracic ganglia. The vagus gives branches at the cervical level as well as thoracic level. The recurrent laryngeal branch of vagus also gives direct cardiac branches to the plexus. It is normally described as superficial part in front of the trachea and the deep part at the lowest part of trachea. The plexuses lie with the trachea behind and pulmonary trunk and arch of aorta in front.

POSTERIOR MEDIASTINUM (Figs 32 and 33)

All the structures that lie between the vertebral column and the heart constitute the posterior mediastinal structures. They are the esophagus, the thoracic aorta with its branches, the azygos system of veins, the thoracic duct and the associated lymphatic system, the segmental thoracic nerves, the sympathetic chain and its branches and the prevertebral muscles.

ESOPHAGUS

Dissection: Trace the blood vessels reaching esophagus from the thoracic aorta. Trace the right and left vagus nerves supplying the esophagus. They form a plexus deep to the adventitia.

It is around 25 cm long. It extends from the pharynx in the neck to the stomach in the abdomen. In the thorax it passes through the superior and posterior mediastinum. Note the position of the esophagus. It is the deepest structure in the superior mediastinum. Trace the esophagus throughout the extent. Note that in its course it lies deep to the aorta, lies behind the trachea in the superior mediastinum and heart in the posterior mediastinum. It lies in front of the thoracic vertebrae throughout its extent. Note that it reaches the midline at the 4th thoracic vertebra and continues in that position until 6th thoracic vertebra. Later it deviates to the left and more anteriorly. It passes through the muscular part of the diaphragm at the level of 10th thoracic vertebra, 3 cm to the left of the midline.

Dissections: Reidentify all the structures related to the esophagus. Anteriorly from above downwards trachea, right principal bronchus, right pulmonary artery, left atrium are related to it. Cut and remove the trachea, bronchi, pulmonary arteries, pulmonary trunk and clear the nerve plexusses. The esophageal plexus of nerves closely accompany the esophagus throughout its extent. It is an autonomic plexus of nerves contributed by sympathetic trunk and vagus. Peel the adventitia on the esophagus and identify the esophageal plexus of nerves. Note that the right vagus nerve goes to the back to form the posterior vagal trunk and the left vagus nerve turns forward to form the anterior vagal trunk. Cut the esophagus near the inlet of thorax superiorly and inferiorly nearer to the left crus of the diaphragm. Take it out and study its interior.

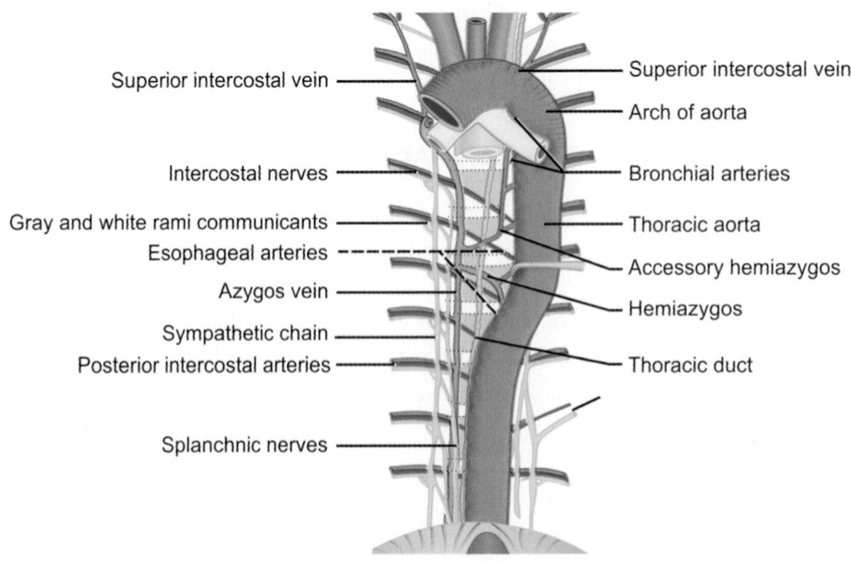

FIGURE 32 Posterior mediastinal structures

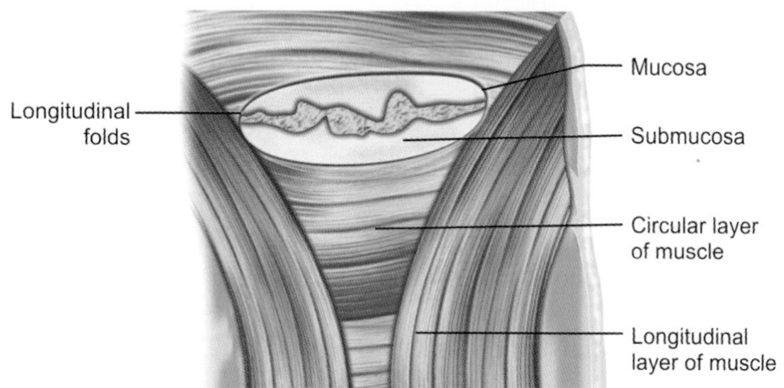

FIGURE 33 Esophagus structure

Structure of Esophagus

It is a part of the gastrointestinal (GI) tract. It exhibits the typical features of the GI tract. It is made up of four layers. ***Slit the esophagus longitudinally to see the layers.*** The outer thin connective tissue covering is the adventitia. Peel it. Note the thick muscular layer. It shows an outer longitudinal and an inner circular layer. See the inner folded mucosa. Pull the inner mucosa, and appreciate the submucosa which lies between the mucosa and the muscular layer. The submucosa is a loose layer.

THORACIC AORTA

It is the part of the aorta below the level of the 4th thoracic vertebra to the level of 12th thoracic vertebra. At this level it passes through the diaphragm. Note that it is the most posterior structure in the thorax and it lies to the right and behind the esophagus.

Pull the artery laterally and try to identify the following branches.

Two left ***bronchial*** arteries.

Several ***esophageal*** branches.

Nine pairs of ***posterior intercostals*** arteries and one pair of subcostal artery. Trace them from the back of aorta to the intercostal spaces. Note that the right side arteries cross the thoracic vertebrae to reach the right intercostals spaces. Note that the first two intercostal arteries come from highest intercostal artery a branch of the costocervical trunk which comes down from neck region.

AZYGOS SYSTEM OF VEINS

Azygos system of veins drains the venous blood from the thorax.

Tributaries from esophagus and trachea are minute and drain directly into the azygos veins. The intercostal veins accompany the posterior intercostal arteries.

Dissection: Clean the spaces near the vertebrae and look for their drainage.

The first or highest intercostal vein drains directly into the corresponding brachiocephalic veins. Generally the second and third unite to form the superior intercostal vein. On the right side it enters the azygos vein, on the left side it drains into the left brachiocephalic vein. All the remaining right posterior intercostals veins drain into the azygos vein directly. The posterior intercostal veins of the left side drain into the azygos veins through the hemiazygos veins. The veins from the 4th to 8th intercostals spaces join to form a common trunk, ***the accessory hemiazygos vein,*** whereas the 9th to 12th intercostal veins join to form ***the hemiazygos vein.*** Both accessory and the hemiazygos veins cross the thoracic vertebrae to join the azygos vein.

The azygos vein on the right and hemiazygos on the left pierces the diaphragm to reach the abdomen and join the renal or inferior vena cava. The azygos vein is a direct connection between the superior and inferior vena cavae.

THORACIC DUCT

Thoracic duct is the biggest lymphatic channel of the body. It drains lymph from the lower limbs, pelvis, abdomen and lower part of thorax. It begins in the abdomen as cysterna chili.

Dissection: Locate this vessel between the aorta and the azygos vein.

It is very thin, presents a beaded appearance due to the droplets of fat which enter this. Trace this vessel up and note that at the 4th thoracic vertebra it deviates to the left. In the superior mediastinum note that it lies between the esophagus and the pleura.

Right lymphatic duct: It is a small thin vessel. This drains the upper right side of the thorax. Its further course is in the neck region.

The lymph that it drains pass through the regional nodes. They are described as the parasternal intercostals, phrenic, posterior mediastinal, tracheobronchial, bronchopulmonary and anterior mediastinal nodes.

INTERCOSTAL NERVES AND SYMPATHETIC CHAIN

Dissection: Clean the sympathetic chain. Clean the intercostals nerves. Identify the gray and white rami communicantis passing between them. Clean the splanchnic nerves arising from the sympathetic chain.

Locate this thick chain on the lateral side of the thoracic vertebrae. It presents segmental ganglionic enlargements with the intermitant connecting chain. Relocate the intercostal nerves between the thoracic vertebrae and the internal intercostal muscle**.** ***Gray and white rami communicantes*** are the connecting branches between the sympathetic ganglia and the intercostal nerves. Identify these small branches from the lateral side of the chain to the intercostal nerves. The white rami communicantes carries the preganglionic fibres and the gray ramus carries the postganglionic fibres.

Splanchnic nerves: Locate these nerves arising from the medial side of the chain. The branches from 5th to 9th thoracic ganglia join to form the greater splanchnic nerve. The branches from the 10th and 11th from the lesser splanchnic nerve. The branch form the 12th thoracic ganglia continues as the least splanchnic nerve. All pierce the diaphragm and reach the abdomen. The ***ventral branches*** are small branches and arise from the ventral aspect and reach the cardiac, oesophageal and pulmonary plexuses.

PREVERTEBRAL MUSCULATURE (Fig. 34)

Subcostal muscle: This is a segmental thin muscle present near the lower ribs. They arise from the lower border near the angle of a rib. They cross a rib and get attached to the upper border of a second or third rib below. It is a part of the innermost layer of muscles here, and is in line with the innermost intercostal muscle. Identify this muscle.

Internal intercostal membrane: It is seen as a thin sheet and is a continuation of the interal intercostal muscle. It extends from the neck of the rib to the costotransverse ligament. It is deeper to the subcostal muscle. Identify this in few of the spaces and note that the neurovascular bundle lies between this and the subcostal muscle.

Longus colli: This is a part of the ventral muscle mass which extends from the neck region. Try to locate it on the anterior aspect of the upper thoracic vertebrae.

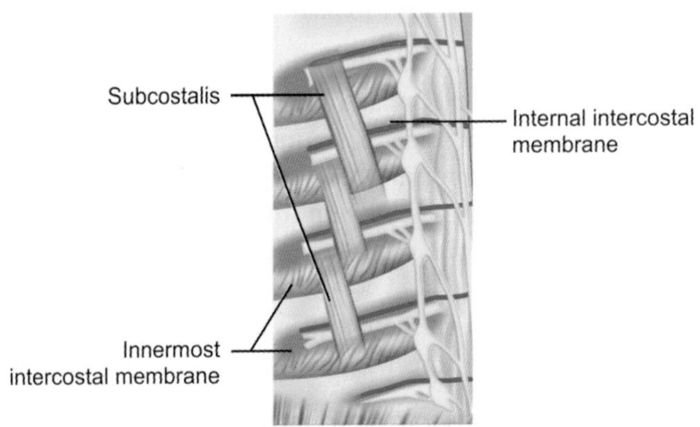

FIGURE 34 Subcostalis muscle

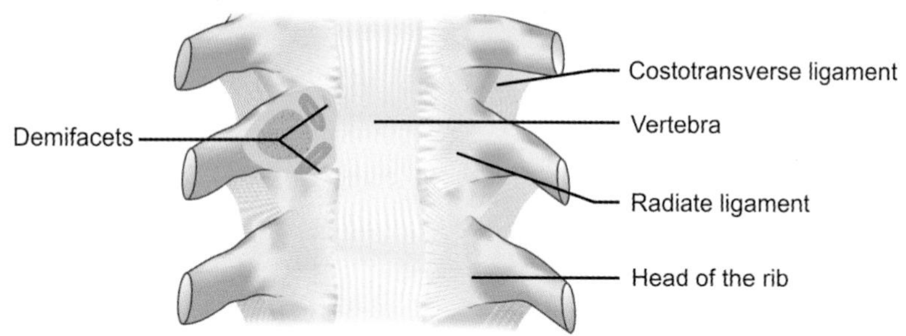

FIGURE 35 Costovertebral joint

COSTOVERTEBRAL JOINTS (Fig. 35)

Dissection: Try to clean at least one or two joints to get an idea about the arrangement of the articulation and the ligaments.

Costovertebral joints: Each rib articulates with the vertebra at three places. The tubercle of the rib articulates with the costal surface on the transverse process of the vertebra. The head of the rib has two demifacets in a typical rib. The upper demifacet articulates with the body of the vertebra above whereas the lower facet articulates with the corresponding body. All the three articulations are plane synovial joints. These are enclosed in a radiate capsular ligament. The costotransverse ligaments connect the nonarticular part of the neck of the rib to the transverse process. The intervertebral disc is connected to the head of the rib by the intra-articular ligament.

CHAPTER 4

ABDOMEN

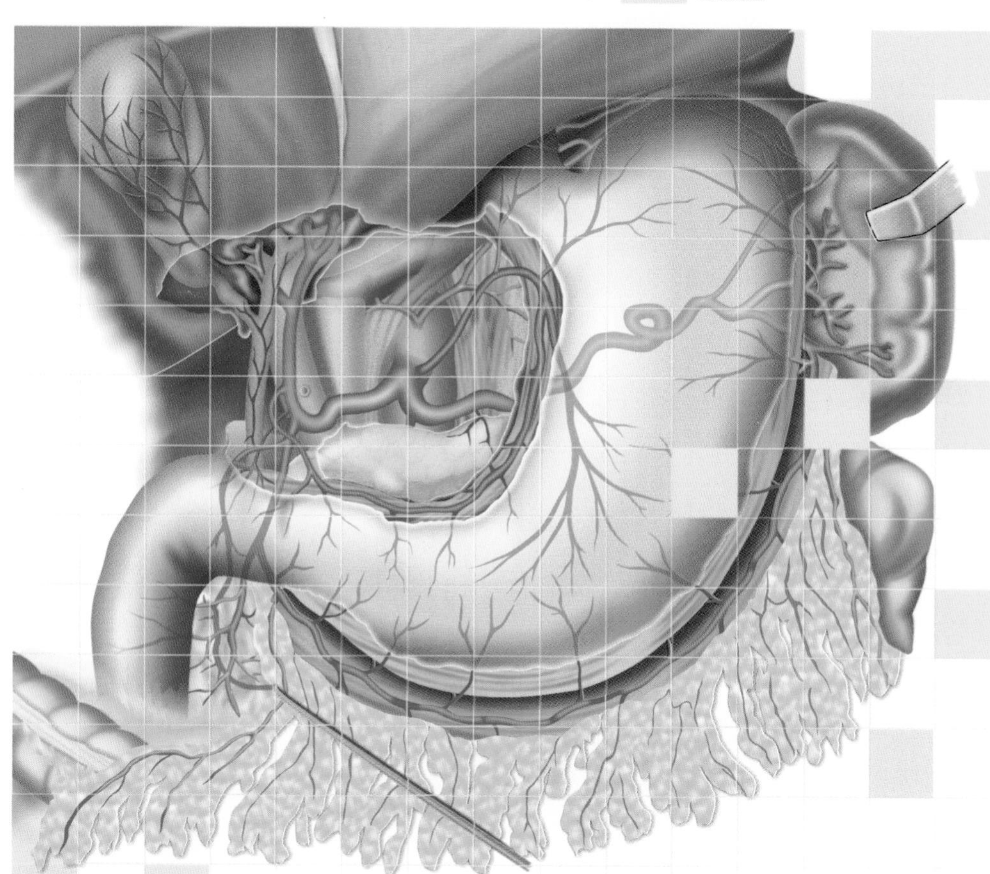

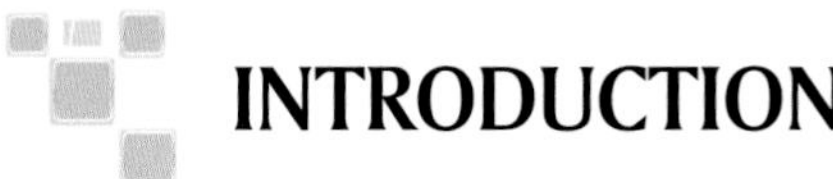

INTRODUCTION

The abdomen is the lower, most extensive part of the trunk. It is divided into ***abdomen proper, pelvis and perineum.*** It is partly supported by bones. The lower thoracic cage protects the abdomen superiorly, the bony pelvis protects it inferiorly and lumbar vertebrae protect it posteriorly. The remaining anterolateral wall is formed by musculature. This helps in the expansion of the abdominal contents. The abdominal cavity is separated from the thoracic cavity by the dome shaped diaphragm. The abdominal cavity is continuous with the pelvic cavity at the inlet of the pelvis. The pelvic cavity is separated from the perineum by the pelvic diaphragm. The abdomen is filled with viscera. They are parts of the gastrointestinal tract, urinary system, genital system, endocrine gland suprarenal and lymphoid organ spleen, and their neurovascular bundle. As there are too many organs in the abdomen, to understand their position in the body, the abdomen is divided into regions by imaginary lines. Loin is the posterior aspect of the abdomen and is occupied by the postvertebral muscles.

SURFACE ANATOMY (Fig. 1)

Bony boundaries: Try to identify the bony boundaries on the living and on the skeleton. Superiorly feel the ***xiphisternum*** in the midline. Anterolaterally feel the ***costal margin*** (formed by costal cartilages of 7th rib to 10th rib), lower end of the costal margin is formed by 10th rib. Inferiorly feel the ***pubic symphysis*** in the midline**.** It is the secondary cartilaginous joint formed between the two pubic bones. Run your fingers along the ***pubic crest.*** It is a part of pubic bone and the ***pubic tubercle*** is the lateral end of crest. Laterally identify the ***anterior superior iliac spine,*** the most anterior projection of the iliac crest, and the ***iliac crest,*** the upper surface of the iliac bone **(Fig. 1).**

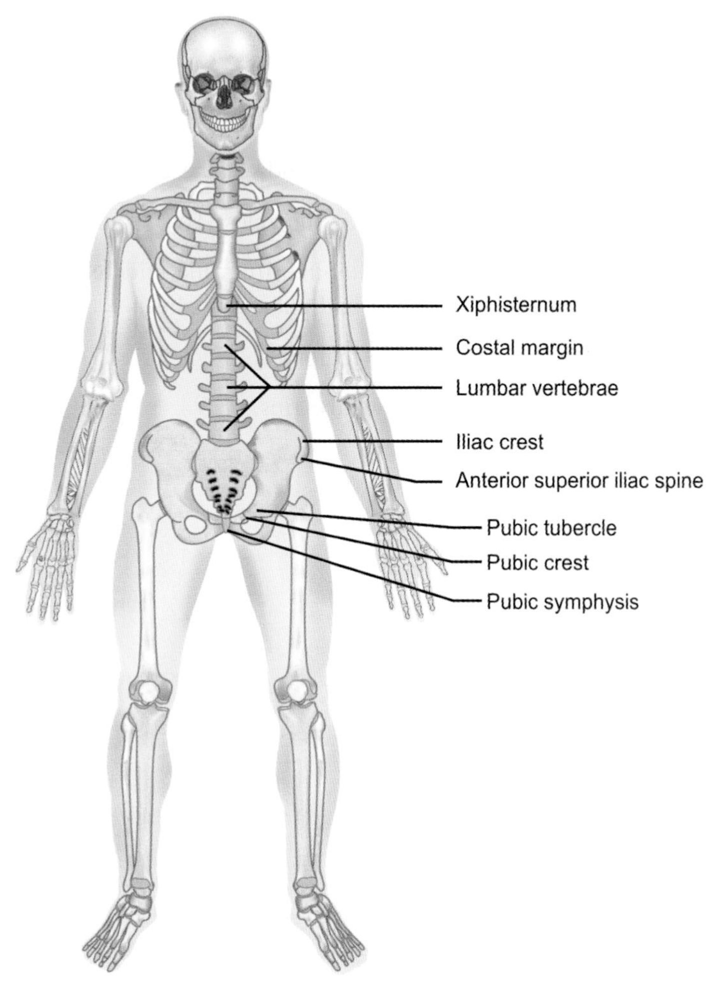

FIGURE 1 Surface anatomy

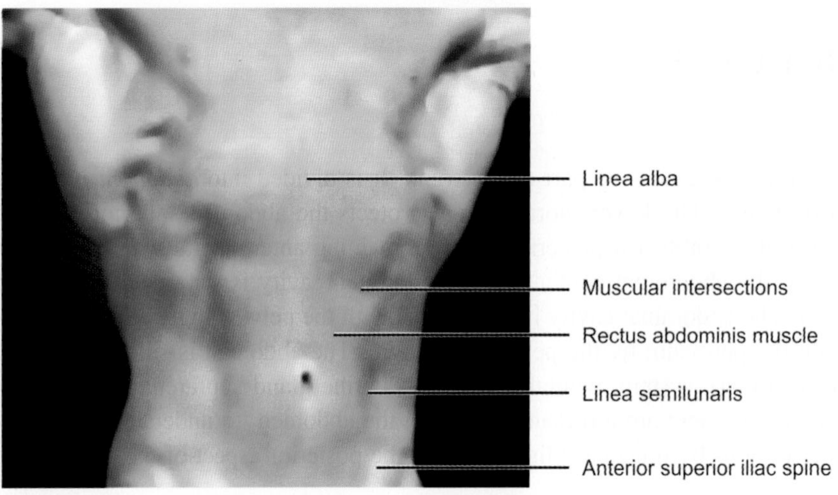

FIGURE 2 Surface anatomy—muscle elevations

Surface anatomy (Fig. 2): In a muscular person we can see a midline depression that extends from xiphisternum to pubic symphysis. This is due to a midline tendinous raphae called ***linea alba***. ***Linea semilunaris*** extends from 9th costal cartilage to the pubic tubercle. This is the depression to the side of the rectus abdominis muscle. ***Intersections*** of rectus abdominis muscle can also be visible as transverse lines.

REGIONS OF ABDOMEN (Fig. 3)

Draw the following lines on the cadaver:

Transpyloric plane: This is a horizontal line cutting across the tip of 9th costal cartilage. This will cut the first lumbar vertebra.

Subcostal plane: This line passes below the 10th rib. This would cut the upper border of third lumbar vertebra.

Transtubercular plane: It is a line connecting the two iliac tubercles. This would cut the lower border of L5.

Midinguinal or midclavicular line/vertical line: Draw this line from the middle of the clavicle to the midinguinal point (point midway between anterior superior iliac spine and pubic symphysis).

The above lines are used to divide the abdomen into nine regions.

Right and left hypochondriac regions lie under cover of the ribs.

Epigastric region lies below the xiphisternum.

Right and left lumbar regions lie below the hypochondriac regions.

Umbilical region is in the midline around the umbilicus.

Right and left inguinal regions lie in relation to iliac fossa.

Hypogastric region lies above the pubic symphysis.

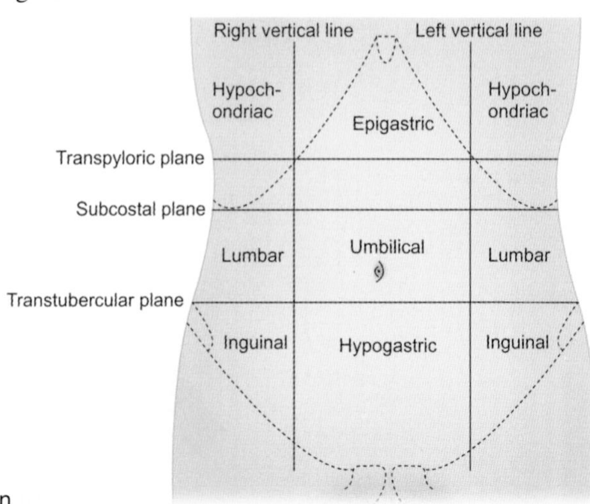

FIGURE 3 Regions of abdomen

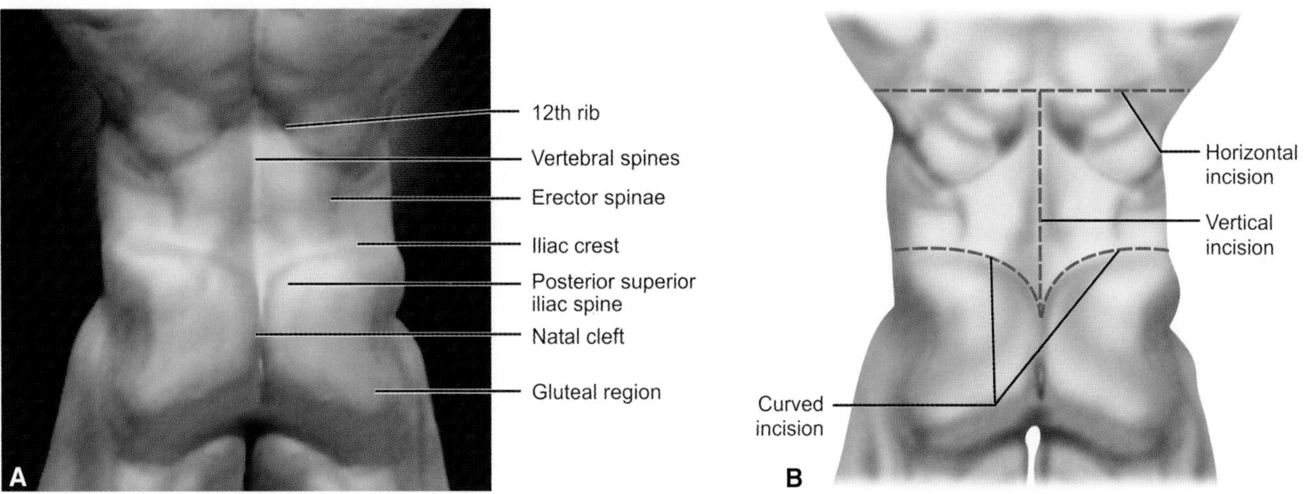

FIGURES 4A AND B (A) Surface anatomy—posterior aspects and (B) Skin incisions

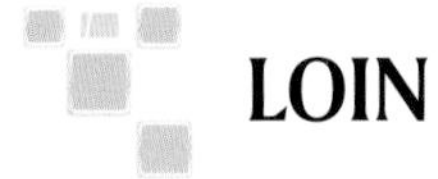

LOIN

Loin is the area lateral to the lumbar vertebrae. It is occupied by three layers of muscle and the fascia separating them. The most superficial layer here is the latissimus dorsi, belonging to the upper limb. This gives a firm anchorage to the upper limb. Deep to this is the extensor muscle of the vertebral column—the erector spinae. The deepest layer is the quadratus lumborum, the lateral rotator of the lumbar region.

SURFACE ANATOMY (Fig. 4A)

Turn the body to a prone position and identify the following:

12th rib: Feel the tip of the 12th rib lateral to the erector spinae muscle.

Spines of vertebrae: Feel them from 12th thoracic to 2nd sacral in midline.

Iliac crest: Feel and trace it posteriorly.

Posterior superior iliac spine can be seen as a dimple on the posterior aspect **(Figs 4A and B)**.

Erector spinae: This is the postvertebral muscle and raises a vertical elevation.

Natal cleft: This is the depression between the two gluteal regions.

MUSCULATURE

Skin Incision (Fig. 4B)

Dissection: Make a horizontal incision at the level of 8th thoracic spine to the mid axillary line. Make a vertical incision in the midline from T8 spines to coccyx. Make a curved incision from the posterior superior iliac spine along the iliac crest to the mid axillary line. Reflect the skin laterally to the midaxillary line.

The posterior cutaneous nerves and posterior branches of the lateral cutaneous nerves supply this area. Both these branches are too tiny to be located.

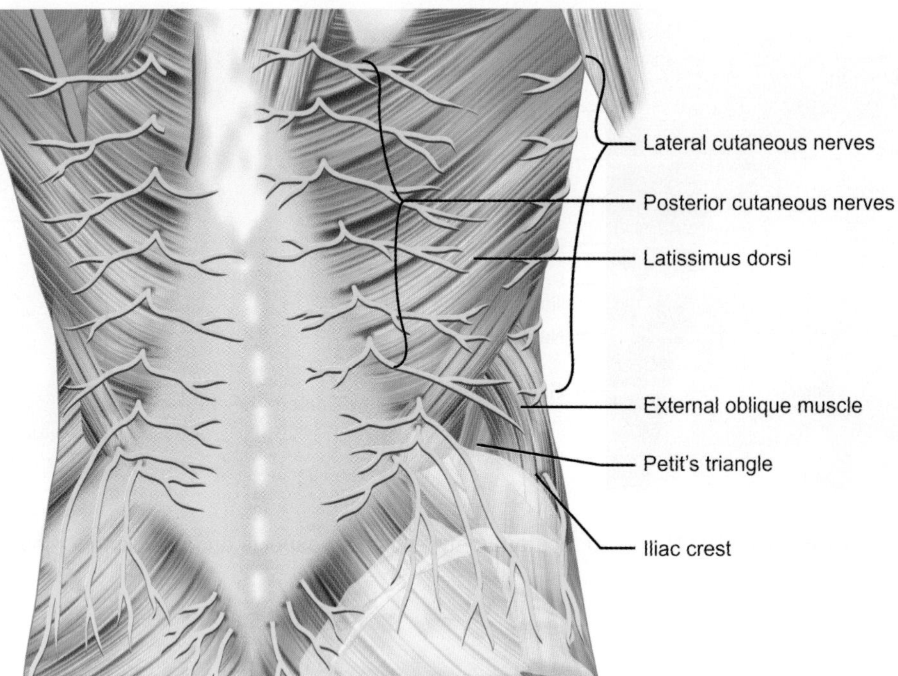

FIGURE 5 Loin—Latissimus dorsi

Latissimus dorsi (Fig. 5): Study its origin from the lower thoracic, lumbar and sacral spines, supraspinous ligaments and outer lip of posterior part of iliac crest.

Lumbar/petit's triangle: This is a muscular triangle in this region. Look for the posterior border of the external oblique muscle, this forms the anterior boundary. The inferior border is formed by the iliac crest. The medial border is formed by lateral border of latissimus dorsi.

Dissection: Cut the latissimus dorsi by the side of the spines and remove it. (It is already cut in the upper limb dissection).

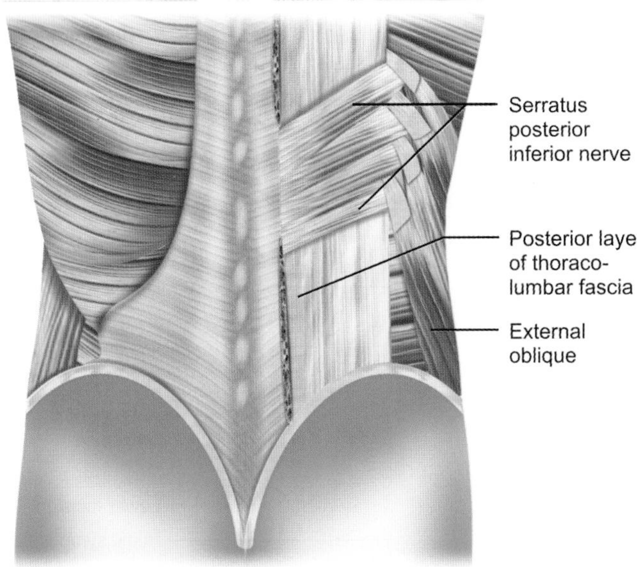

FIGURE 6 Loin—serratus posterior inferior

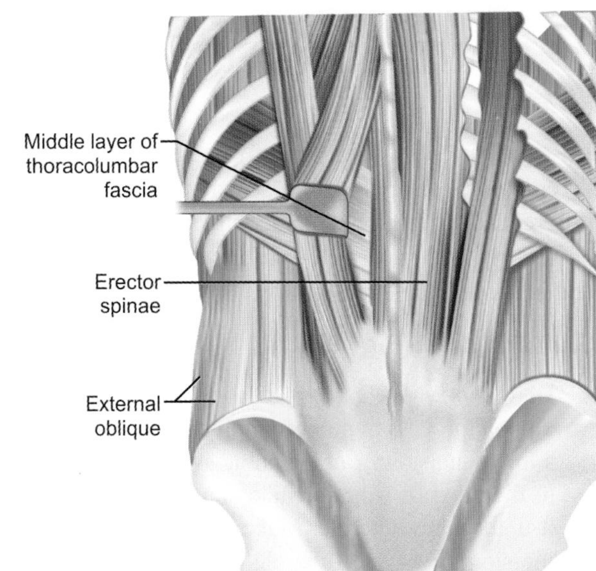

FIGURE 7 Erector spinae muscle

Serratus posterior inferior (Fig. 6): It has 4 slips. They extend from spines to the posterior angles of the lower 4 ribs. Identify them.

Dissection: Detach and remove the serratus posterior inferior.

Thoracolumbar fascia: It has three layers of fascia and envelops two muscles. The erector spinae is enclosed between the posterior and middle layer and the quadratus lumborum muscle is enclosed between the middle and anterior layer. All the three layers unite laterally and give attachment to the anterolateral musculature of the abdomen.

Posterior layer of thoracolumbar fascia: Identify this thick layer deep to the latissimus dorsi and serratus posterior inferior.

Dissection: Cut through the posterior layer of thoracolumbar fascia by a vertical incision parallel to the spines. clean the fascia and study the erector spinae muscle.

Erector spinae muscle (Fig. 7): It is the extensor muscle of the vertebral column. It extends from the sacrum to the occiput. The muscle extends between the spines and posterior angles of the ribs. It is divided into three layers horizontally and three layers superficial to deep. This muscle is best developed in the neck region. This will be studied in detail there.

Middle layer of thoracolumbar fascia: Pull the erector spinae muscle laterally and see the deeper, middle layer of thoracolumbar fascia.

The posterior and middle layer of thoracolumbar fascia unite laterally. This further unites with anterior layer of thoracolumbar facia which will be seen later.

Study the Morris parallelogram. This is the projection of the kidney posteriorly. This is very much essential to approach the kidney posteriorly for surgical procedures. Study the attachments of the fasciae and the muscles on the lumbar vertebrae.

ANTEROLATERAL ABDOMINAL WALL

It is made up of three layers of muscles. The direction of fibres of these muscles is different. They reach the thoracolumbar fascia posteriorly, ribs superiorly, midline anteriorly and inguinal ligament inferiorly.

Skin Incision (Fig. 8)

Dissection: Mak]e a vertical incision from xiphoid process to pubic symphysis. Make a lower incision from the pubic symphysis to the anterior superior iliac spine extend it upto pubic tubercle. Make a horizontal incision from one tubercle to the other. Horizontal incision above xiphisternum. Reflect and remove the skin totally in four flaps.

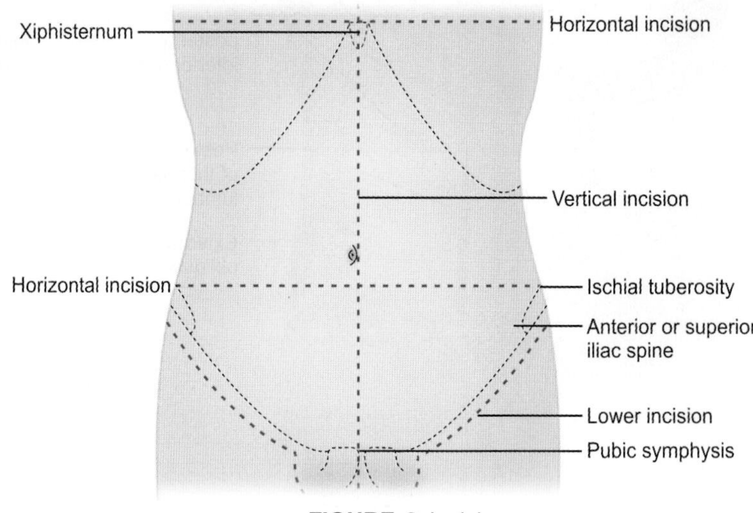

FIGURE 8 Incisions

Superficial Fascia (Fig. 9)

It is made up of two layers—a superficial fatty layer called fascia of Camper and a deep membranous layer called, fascia of Scarpa. The amount of fat is variable in different individuals. The lower part of the abdomen is filled with more fat. Cutaneous veins are seen here.

Dissection: Cut through the superficial fatty layer and reflect it. As you reflect you will note on its undersurface there is a thick sheet of connective tissue. This is the membranous, Scarpa's fascia. Inferiorly it is attached to the deep fascia of thigh below the inguinal ligament.

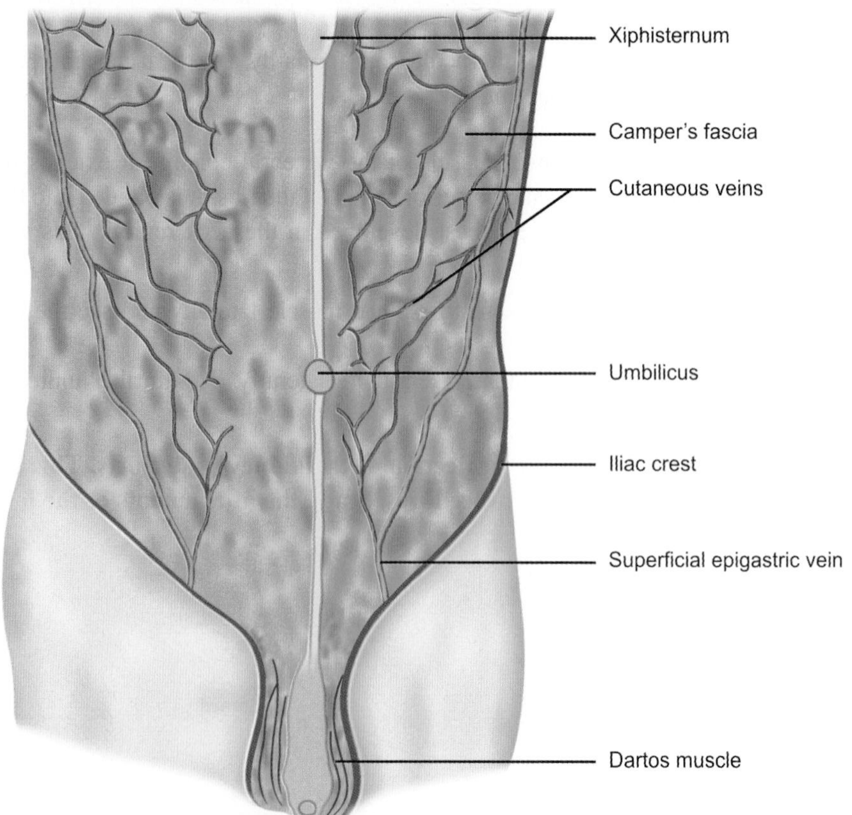

FIGURE 9 Superficial fascia–anterior abdominal wall and scrotum

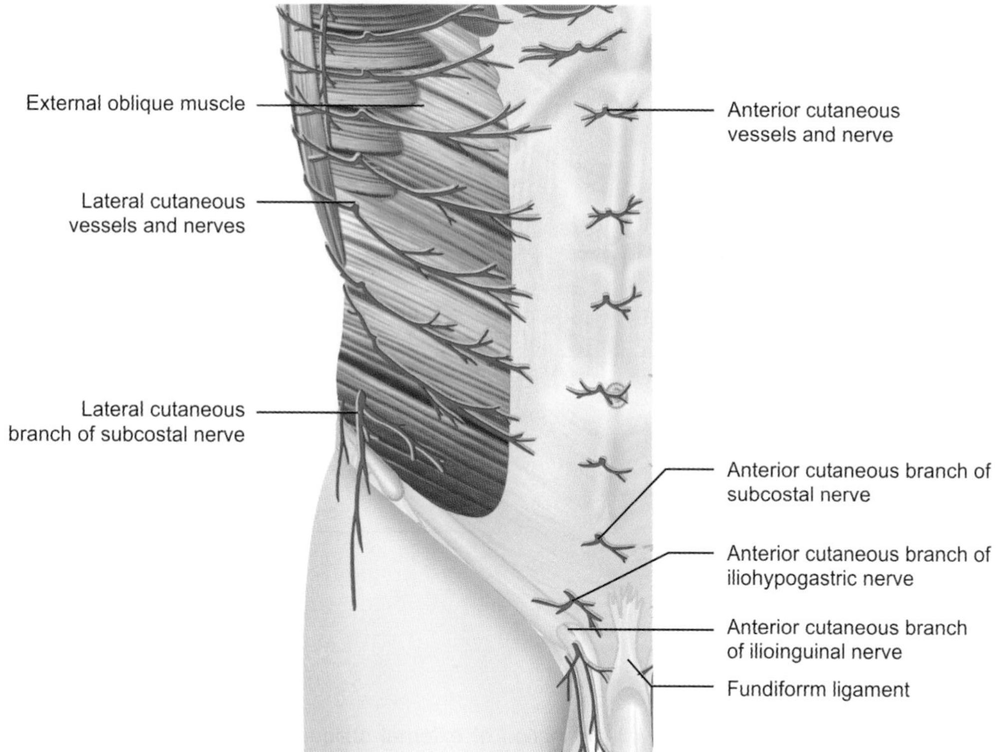

FIGURE 10 Anterior abdominal wall—cutaneous vessels and nerves

CUTANEOUS STRUCTURES (Fig. 10)

Anterior cutaneous vessels and nerves: These are small fine branches lateral to the midline. These are branches of intercostal vessels and nerves. The 12th thoracic branches reach the pubic region. Anterior cutaneous branches of iliohypogastric and ilioinguinal reach abdominal wall lateral to the linea semilunaris.

Lateral cutaneous branches of intercostals, subcostal and iliohypogastric reach the skin along the midaxillary line and supply the skin.

Fundiform ligament is the thick connective tissue sheet which connects the top of penis to the anterior abdominal wall.

Deep fascia: There is no deep fascia in the anterior abdominal wall. The function of the deep fascia is to hold the underlying structures tightly in position. In abdomen as most of the organs need to expand there cannot be a deep fascia.

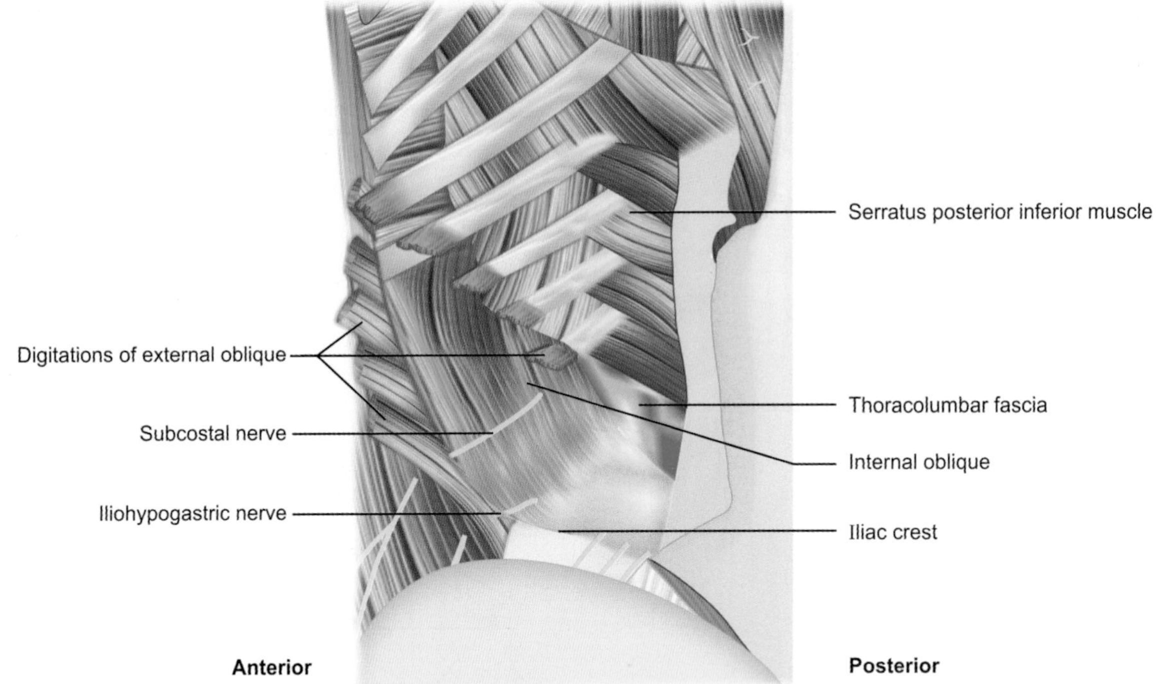

FIGURE 11 Anterior abdominal wall—reflection of external oblique muscle posterior side view

MUSCLES OF ABDOMEN

External oblique muscle: It is the most superficial of the muscle. It arises from the lower eight ribs near their anterior angles. The fibres run downward and forward to reach the linea semilunaris, where they become aponeurotic. Inferiorly the muscle is ligamentous and is called the inguinal ligament. It extends between the anterior superior iliac spine to the pubic tubercles.

Dissection (Fig. 11): Turn the body to sides and note that the fibres arising from the 11th and 12th rib run vertically downward to reach the anterior 2/3rd of the outerlip of the iliac crest. Detach the muscle from the ribs near its origin, and from the iliac crest. Cut across the muscle from the anterior superior iliac spine to the linea semilunaris and turn the muscle medially to the linea semilunaris.

Iliohypogastric nerve: Note this nerve while reflecting the external oblique. It pierces the internal oblique and passes through the external oblique to become cutaneous. Note the ***subcostal*** nerve piercing through the muscle.

Internal oblique (Fig. 12): It is the muscle seen deeper to the external oblique. Note the direction of the fibres. They run downwards and posteriorly. The muscle extends from lower borders of the lower six ribs from the thoracolumbar fascia, anterior 2/3rd of the middle lip of iliac crest and the lateral 2/3rd of the inguinal ligament.

Dissection: Turn the body to the side. Cut the internal oblique in front of the thoracolumbar fascia and detach the muscle from ribs and iliac crest. Cut the muscle across the anterior superior iliac spine to the linea semilunaris in line with the external oblique muscle. While reflecting the muscle note the neurovascular bundle which lies deep to it between internal oblique and transversus abdominis muscle.

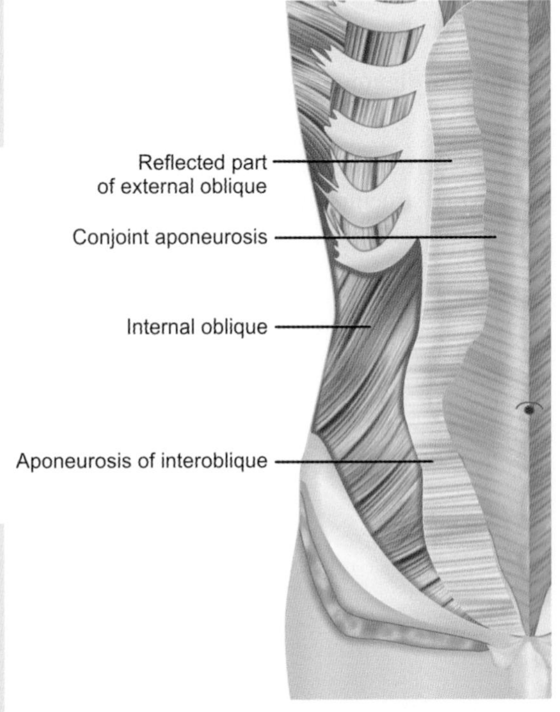

FIGURE 12 Anterior abdominal wall—Internal oblique muscle

Transversus abdominis muscle (Fig. 13): Note the transversely running fibres of this muscle. It extends from the inner aspect of the lower six ribs, thoracolumbar fascia and anterior 2/3rd of the inner lip of the iliac crest and the lateral 1/3rd of the inguinal ligament. Trace these fibres medially to the linea semilunaris.

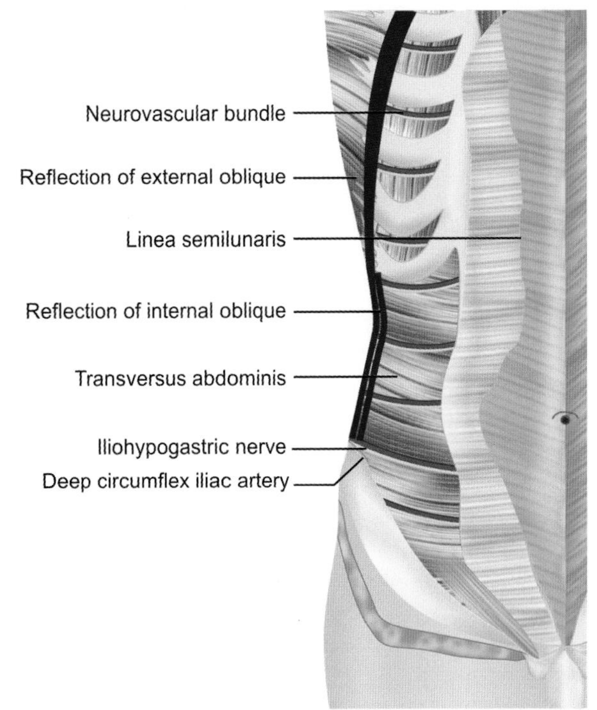

FIGURE 13 Anterior abdominal wall—transversus abdominis

RECTUS SHEATH

Rectus abdominis muscle is present between the linea semilunaris and linea alba and is enclosed in the rectus sheath.

Linea semilunaris is the curved lateral margin of rectus sheath. Note all the three muscles, the external oblique, internal oblique and transversus abdominis have united here and the neurovascular bundle passes through it.

Linea alba is the midline white glistening structure extending from the xiphisternum to the pubic symphysis. This is a raphae of six muscles—the anterolateral muscles of both right and left side.

Anterior layer of rectus sheath is formed by aponeurosis of external oblique and anterior layer of internal oblique muscle.

Dissection: Cut vertically through the rectus sheath next to linea alba. Separate the rectus muscle from its anterior wall. Note that the rectus abdominis is adherent to the anterior wall by three intersections between xiphisternum and umbilicus. Cut through them.
Push your fingers to the laterally towards the lineal semilunaris and note that the internal oblique has split into two layers—one merging anteriorly with the external oblique muscle and the deeper layer going posteriorly and merging with the transversus abdominis.

Rectus abdominis muscle (Fig. 14): It arises by two slips from the pubic symphysis and pubic crest, ascends up, to be inserted into 5th, 6th and 7th costal cartilages along a horizontal line. Not that this muscle shows three tendinous intersections between the umbilicus and xiphisternum, denoting the segmental origin.

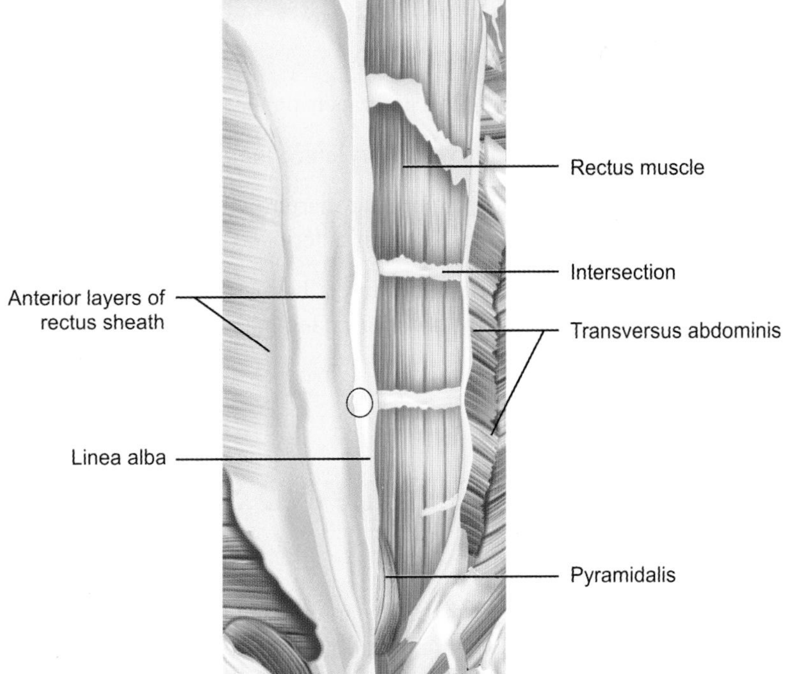

FIGURE 14 Anterior abdominal wall—rectus muscle

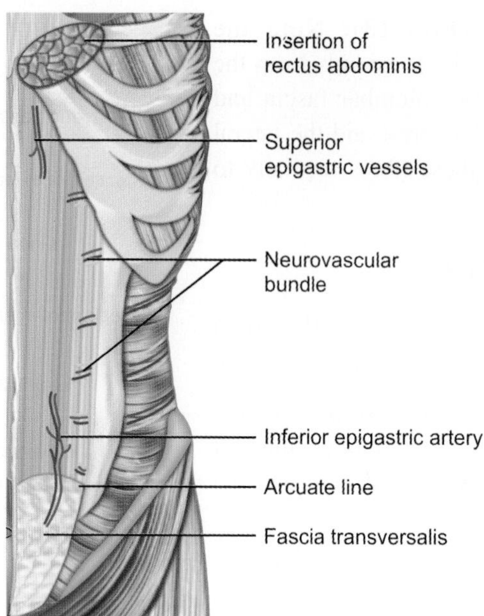

FIGURE 15 Anterior abdominal wall—rectus sheath

Pyramidalis: It is a small muscle present in the lower part, superficial to rectus muscle. It arises from the pubic crest and is inserted into the linea alba.

Dissection: Cut through the rectus muscle transversely near the umbilicus. Lift it superiorly and inferiorly and identify the structures deep to the muscle **(Fig. 15).**

Superior epigastric artery: This runs down from the space lateral to the xiphisternum. It is one of the terminal branches of the internal thoracic artery.

Inferior epigastric artery: This is branch of the external iliac and enters the rectus sheath from below.

Intercostals vessels and nerves: They enter the rectus sheath along the linea semilunaris.

Arcuate line: Note the sharp semilunar margin within the posterior wall between the umbilicus and pubic symphysis. At this level all the three muscles turn anterior to the rectus muscle thus leaving a sharp posterior margin.

Fascia transversalis: Note this thin fascia below the arcuate line. This is similar to the endothoracic fascia of thorax. It lines the inner aspect of the anterior abdominal wall.

INGUINAL CANAL AND SCROTUM

Inguinal region is the area where the anterior and posterior walls of the abdomen meet. The testis which develops anterior to the posterior abdominal wall on either side of the vertebral column migrates downwards and anteriorly to reach the ***scrotum*** located in front of the pubic bones, below the anterior abdominal wall. While doing so it passes through the anterior abdominal wall musculature and superficial fascia, thus getting covered by them. The passage through which the testis passes is called ***inguinal canal***. In the adult anatomy the male gonad, the ***testis*** and the ***epididymis*** lies in the scrotum. The ***ductus deference*** continues from the epididymis and passes through the inguinal canal with its neurovascular bundle. It is called ***spermatic cord***.

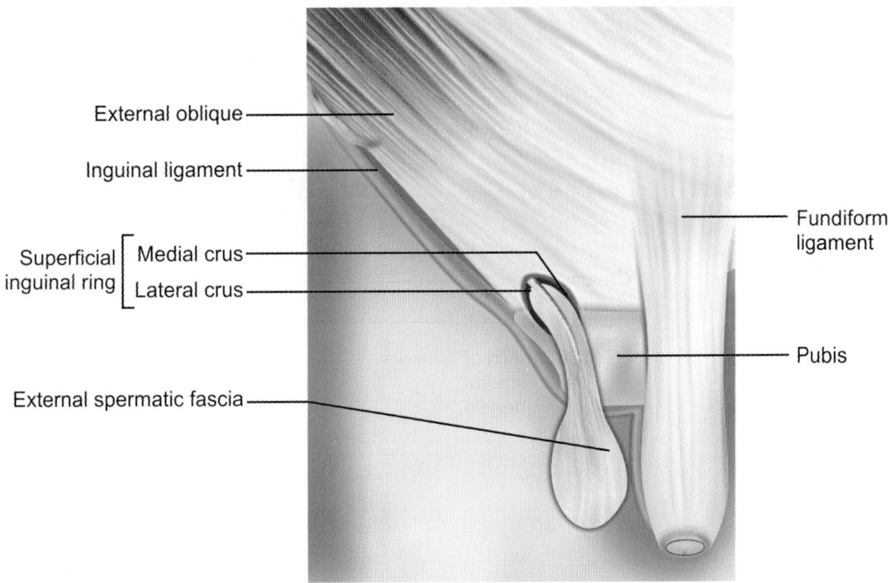

FIGURE 16 Inguinal canal and scrotum—external oblique muscle

SCROTUM

Dissection: Feel the scrotum. Put a midline incision on each half of the scrotal sac. Reflect the skin to either side. The skin here is very thin and should be reflected carefully. Deep to the skin the fatty layer of the superficial fascia is replaced here by dartos muscle. The muscle fibres can be identified because of the coloration. Clean and identify the scrotal vessels and nerves, the cutaneous nerves of this region.

Dartos muscle: It is the subcutaneous muscle present within the superficial fascia. It is attached to the skin and causes the wrinkles of the scrotal skin. It helps in controlling the temperature for the testis.

Scrotal vessels and nerves: The two parallel vessels and nerves can be easily identified on the anterior aspect within the superficial fascia. These are branches of the pudendal nerve and vessels.

Membranous layer of superficial fascia: lies deep to the dartos muscle and is a thick fascia.

External oblique (Fig. 16): *Locate the lower unreflected part of the external oblique muscle. Push your fingers downward deep to the external oblique muscle toward the superficial inguinal ring and feel the thick sheet covering your fingers. This is the* ***external spermatic fascia****. It is a continuation of the external oblique aponeurosis into the scrotum.*

Superficial inguinal ring: It is the thick margin within the external oblique aponeurosis from where the external spermatic fascia continues. It shows two thick margins—the lateral and medial walls called crura. The lateral crus is attached to the pubic tubercle and the medial crus to the pubic symphysis.

Intercrural fibres are aponeurotic fibres crossing across the superficial inguinal ring, can be seen clearly against light.

Dissection: Reflect the cut external oblique aponeurosis downward to the inguinal ligament. It can easily be separated from the internal oblique aponeurosis. As you reflect it, the deeply lying internal oblique muscle, its continuation the cremaster muscle, ilioinguinal nerves and genital branch of genitofemoral nerves can be identified **(Fig. 17).**

Iliohypogastric nerve (L1) traverses between the internal oblique and external oblique muscles to supply both the muscles.

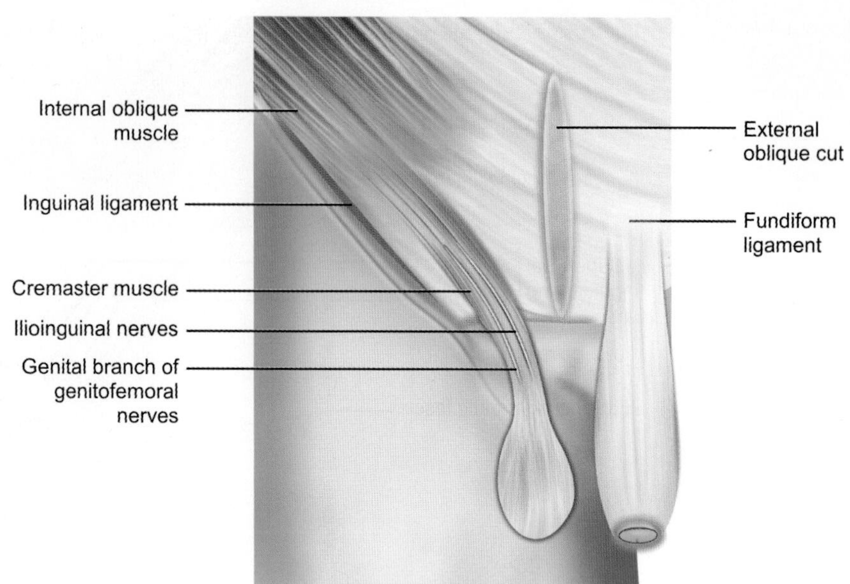

FIGURE 17 Inguinal canal and scrotum—internal oblique muscle

Ilioinguinal nerve (L1) is below the iliohypogastric nerve, traverses between the internal and external oblique muscles parallel to the inguinal ligament, passes through the superficial inguinal ring to reach the skin of the thigh.

Internal oblique muscle arises from the lateral 2/3rd of the inguinal ligament. ***Identify its fleshy fibres. Trace the internal oblique fibres continuing over the spermatic cord. Trace these fibres through the superficial inguinal ring into the scrotum.*** Note that these fibres loop around the testis and reach the pubic tubercle medially. This muscle is the *cremaster muscle*. It is supplied by the cremasteric nerve, a branch of the genitofemoral nerve which will be seen later, in the posterior abdominal wall dissection. The lateral fibres of the internal oblique traverse above the spermatic cord, arch over it to reach the pubic crest medially. Here it joins with the aponeurosis of the transverse abdominis and get inserted into the pubic tubercle as ***conjoint tendon***.

Dissection: Detach the internal oblique muscle from the inguinal ligament and reflect it medially towards the linea semilunaris. See the transverse abdominis muscle and the neurovascular bundle. Separate the cremasteric muscle fibres and see the deeply placed internal spermatic fascia **(Fig. 18).**

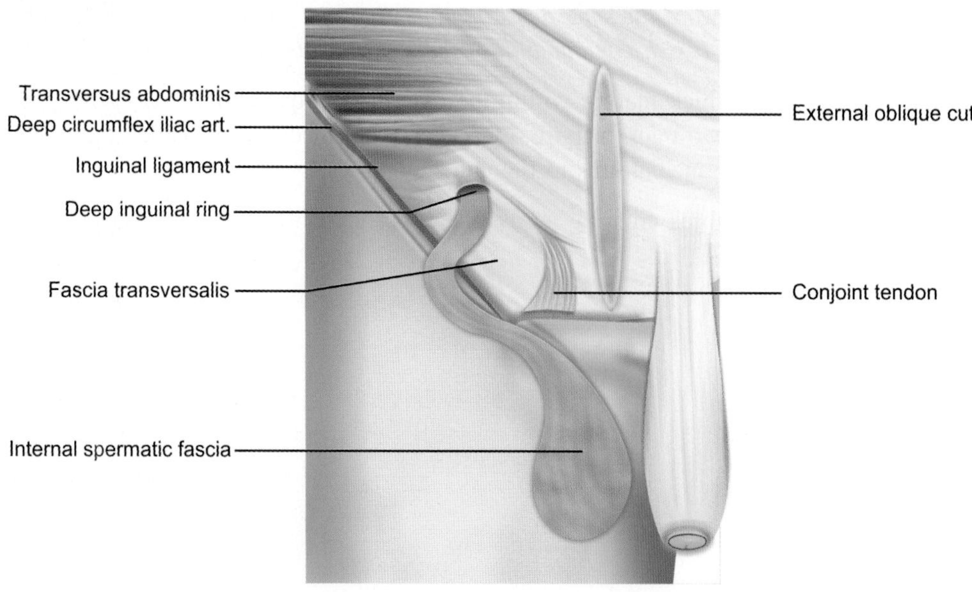

FIGURE 18 Inguinal canal and scrotum—deep structures

Transversus abdominis lies deep to the internal oblique muscle. It takes origin from the lateral 1/3rd of the inguinal ligament. Note that it is lateral to the deep inguinal ring. The fibres arch over the spermatic cord to join the tendon of internal oblique to form ***conjoint tendon.*** Run your fingers along the conjoint tendon and see its insertion into the pubic crest behind the superficial inguinal ring.

Deep circumflex iliac artery is the artery of supply to this region. It runs in a curve along the iliac crest, gives an ascending branch. They travel between the internal oblique and transversus abdominis muscle to supply this region.

Deep inguinal ring: Feel the spermatic cord passing deep into the abdomen below the transversus abdominis muscle. It passes through a slit in the connective tissue sheath deep to the transversus abdominis muscle. This sheath is the ***fascia transversalis*** and the slit is the ***deep inguinal ring***. It is 1 cm above the inguinal ligament at midinguinal point. Midinguinal point is the point midway between anterior superior iliac spine and pubic symphysis.

Lacunar ligament: Put your finger lateral to the pubic tubercle and press it to the back, towards the bone. The structure you feel is lacunar ligament. This is an extra insertion of the external oblique muscle. It extends between the inguinal ligament and the superior ramus of the pubis.

INGUINAL CANAL BOUNDARIES (Fig. 19)

Identify all the boundaries and appreciate the canal formation.

Extent: It extends from deep inguinal ring to superficial inguinal ring.

Anterior wall is formed by the skin, the superficial fascia, and is supported by the external oblique and internal oblique muscles in its lateral 1/3rd.

Floor is formed by the upturned part of the inguinal ligament and is medially supported by the lacunar ligament.

Posterior wall is formed by the fascia trasversalis, extraperitoneal tissue and peritoneum, and is medially supported by conjoint tendon.

Roof is formed by the arching fibres of internal oblique and transversus abdominis muscle.

INGUINAL HERNIA: Study the boundaries, contents, coverings and etiology of the inguinal hernia.

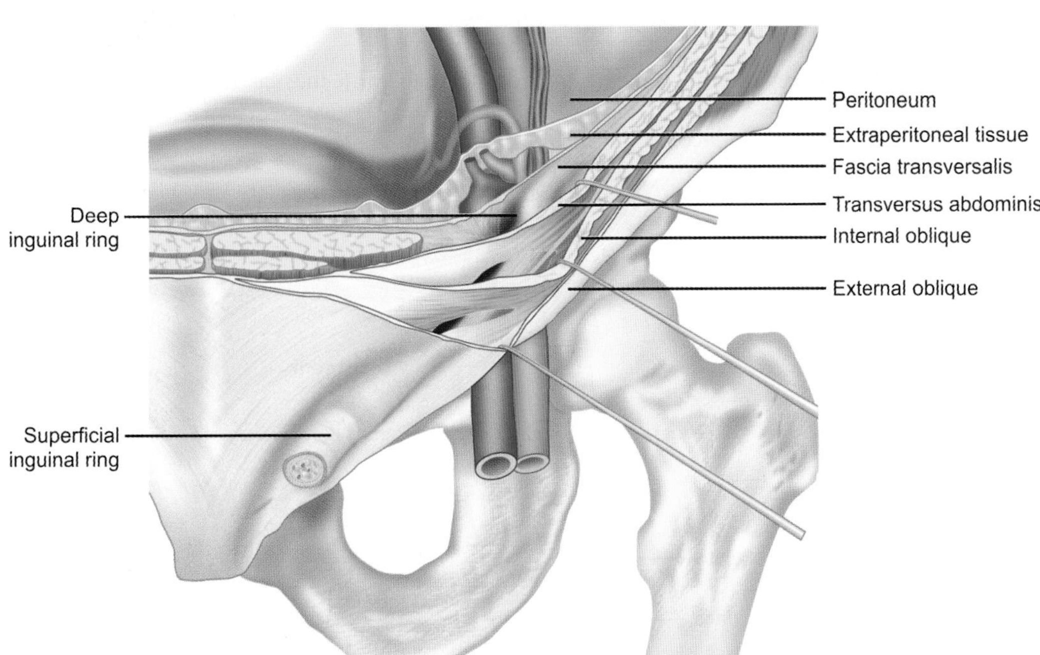

FIGURE 19 Inguinal canal—diagrammatic representation

SPERMATIC CORD AND COVERINGS

Extent: Spermatic cord extends from the deep inguinal ring to the top of the testis. It is 4 cm long.

Coverings from superficial to deep.

External spermatic fascia is derived from the external oblique muscle at superficial inguinal ring. ***Cremasteric muscle and fascia*** is derived from the medial part of origin of internal oblique form the inguinal ligament. ***Internal spermatic fascia*** extends from fascia transversalis at the deep inguinal ring.

CONTENTS OF SPERMATIC CORD (Fig. 20)

Dissection: Here note that in a cadaver all the layers covering the testis are adherent and they are inseparable from the parietal layer of the processes vaginalis. Make a slit from upper pole to the lower pole along the anterior border of this. The cavity that is seen, is the cavity of processus vaginalis between the parietal and visceral layers of processus vaginalis. The visceral layer is adherent to the tunica albuginea. Note that the parietal and visceral layers are continuous with each other posteriorly leaving epididymis and vas deferens to lie outside the processus vaginalis.

Cut the spermatic cord midway between the deep and superficial inguinal rings. Lift it up from the anterior abdominal wall and the scrotum along with the testis. The testis that is removed is with the tunica albuginea and the visceral layer of the processus vaginalis. Put it into a bowl of water, separate the covering of spermatic cord and study the following:

Vas deferens is the thick tube. It can be easily felt as a cord like structure.

Pampiniform plexus is the plexus of veins draining the testis.

Artery to the vas is a branch of the superior vesical artery. It is a small branch seen very close to the vas deferens.

Artery to the testis is a big artery, and it is a branch of the abdominal aorta. It can be easily identified because of its lumen.

Cremasteric branch is a small branch of the inferior epigastric artery and supplies the cremasteric muscle.

Remains of processus vaginalis, sympathetic plexus of nerves and genital branch of genitofemoral nerve, though tiny to distinguish are present there.

Dissection: Trace the structures of the spermatic cord down to the posterior aspect of the testis and appreciate the following:

Epididymis lies along the posterior border of the testis and lateral to the vas deferens. Identify the bulging head on the superior pole, body and tail along the posterior border.

Vas deferens is the tail of the epididymis takes a turn on itself to form the vas deferens. It lies medial to the epididymis.

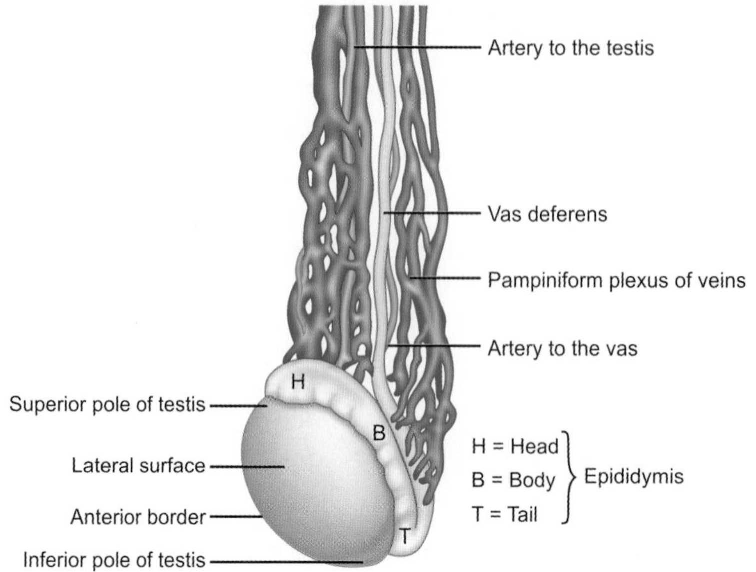

FIGURE 20 Contents of spermatic cord and testis

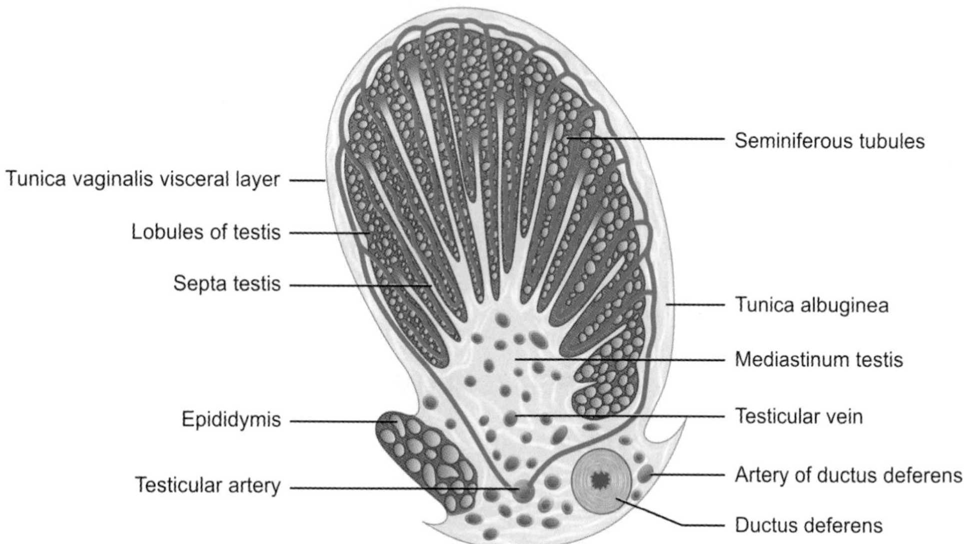

FIGURE 21 Transverse section of testis

TESTIS

Tunica vaginalis is the extended peritoneal covering of the testis. The parietal layer is thick and is adherent with the internal spermatic fascia. The visceral layer is thin and is adherent with the covering of the testis, the tunica albuginea. The two layers are continuous at the posterior aspect of the testis.

Testis: It is the male sex organ, suspended by the spermatic cord and manufactures sperms. ***Superior pole*** is rounded and the spermatic cord is attached here. ***Anterior border*** is convex, connecting the superior and inferior poles. ***Inferior pole*** is rounded**. *Posterior border* is straight**.

Side identification: Medial position of the vas deferens is a point of identification of the side of testis. Hang the testis by spermatic cord, feel the vas deferens and epididymis and confirm the side.

Interior of Testis (Fig. 21)

Dissection: Cut the testis transversely and identify ***tunica albuginea***. It is the thick outer covering of testis. White septa pass from the tunica albuginea to the interior of testis. It divides the testis into 200 compartments. The compartments lodge the seminiferous tubules.

Mediastinum testis is the posterior part of the testis where all the seminiferous tubules come together and form a mesh work.

Head of the epididymis is formed by the 15/20 efferent ductules which start from the upper part of mediastinum testis. They are highly coiled and form the bulk of the head. One single duct arises from the ductules and coils and forms the body and tail of epididymis.

Vas deferens begins at the lower end of the tail of the epididymis and ascends up as a straight duct.

Epididymis and vas deferens carry the sperms.

ABDOMINOPELVIC CAVITY

Abdominopelvic cavity lodges the major part of gastrointestinal tract along with its associated glands, urogenital system, spleen, suprarenal and the associated neurovascular bundle. As there are many organs, knowledge of the disposition of viscera within the abdominal cavity is very much essential. The recent diagnostic methods like ultrasonography, CT and MRI scans produce sectional views of the abdomen. It is advisable to study the sections available in the department. The abdomen appears kidney shaped in a transverse section and J shaped in a sagittal section.

PERITONEUM

The peritoneum like the pericardium and the pleura is a closed sac, filled with peritoneal fluid. All abdominal viscera lie inside the abdominal cavity but outside the peritoneal sac. The peritoneum lines the walls of the abdomen gets reflected on to the organs from the posterior abdominal wall. The part of the peritoneum which lines the walls is called the parietal peritoneum and the part which covers the organs is called the visceral peritoneum. In the abdomen as there are too many organs the visceral peritoneum presents varying lengths as it passes from one organ to the other organ. So the visceral peritoneum is named by different names like ligaments when it is small, omentum when it is connected to the stomach, mesentery when it is connected to the small intestine, mesocolon when it is connected to the large intestine.

The peritoneal cavity is the space between the parietal and visceral peritoneum and it is only a capillary space in the living. The peritoneal cavity is filled by peritoneal fluid, manufactured by the peritoneum. The fluid avoids friction between the organs and helps in their free movement. The peritoneal cavity is a closed space in the males, whereas in females as the uterine tube opens into the pelvic cavity, the peritoneal cavity is continuous to the exterior through the uterus and vagina. The peritoneal sac is divided into two parts, the greater and lesser sacs. The lesser sac is the part behind the stomach, lesser and greater omenta, whereas the remaining part is called the greater sac. The greater and lesser sacs communicate with each other through the epiploic foramen.

Study the longitudinal as well as horizontal sections of the abdomen kept in the museum. Study the CT/MRI scans of abdomen to get an orientation of the disposition of the abdominal viscera.

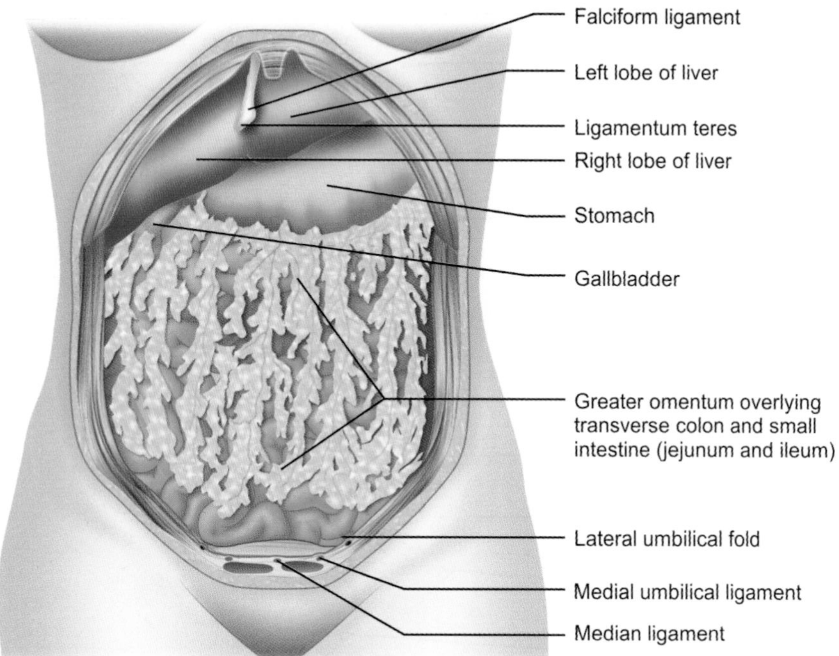

FIGURE 22 Abdominal cavity

Dissection: Open the abdomen by a cruciate incision. Put the longitudinal incision to the left of the midline. This should extend from the xiphisternum to the pubic symphysis. The transverse incision should extend laterally from the umbilicus. Reflect the wall as four flaps. Now you are within the peritoneal cavity. The parietal layer sticks to the wall and the visceral layer sticks to the viscera.

In the cadaver the thin connective tissue layers adhere and it is difficult to separate them. Transversalis fascia is the connective tissue layer deep to the anterior abdominal wall musculature. The transversalis fascia is separated from the parietal layer of peritoneum by the extraperitoneal connective tissue. It is laden with fat in a well-fed individual. Transversalis fascia the extraperitoneal connective tissue and the parietal peritoneum, all look like a single sheet. Peel the peritoneal layer from the inner side and see the structures within the extraperitoneal connective tissue.

ANTERIOR LIGAMENTS (Fig. 22)

Median umbilical ligament: Identify this ligament extending from the apex of the bladder to the umbilicus. It is the remnant of the allantoic diverticulum. The proximal part gives rise to urinary bladder and the distal part gets obliterated and is called urachus.

Medial umbilical ligament: Note this fibrosed structure lateral to the urachus extending from the superior vesical artery. This is the obliterated part of the umbilical artery. This was functional during fetal life.

The lateral umbilical fold: Note this peritoneal fold over the inferior epigastric artery.

Falciform ligament and ligamentum teres: Trace the falciform ligament from the umbilicus to the inferior border of the liver. It is two layered, and its size increase as it reaches the liver. Feel it and note that its free margin has a thick round structure. Separate the two layers of falciform ligament and identify the round ligament of liver/ligamentum teres. This is the obliterated left umbilical artery. This extends from placenta to the left branch of the portal vein in the fetal life. It carries the oxygenated blood to the fetus.

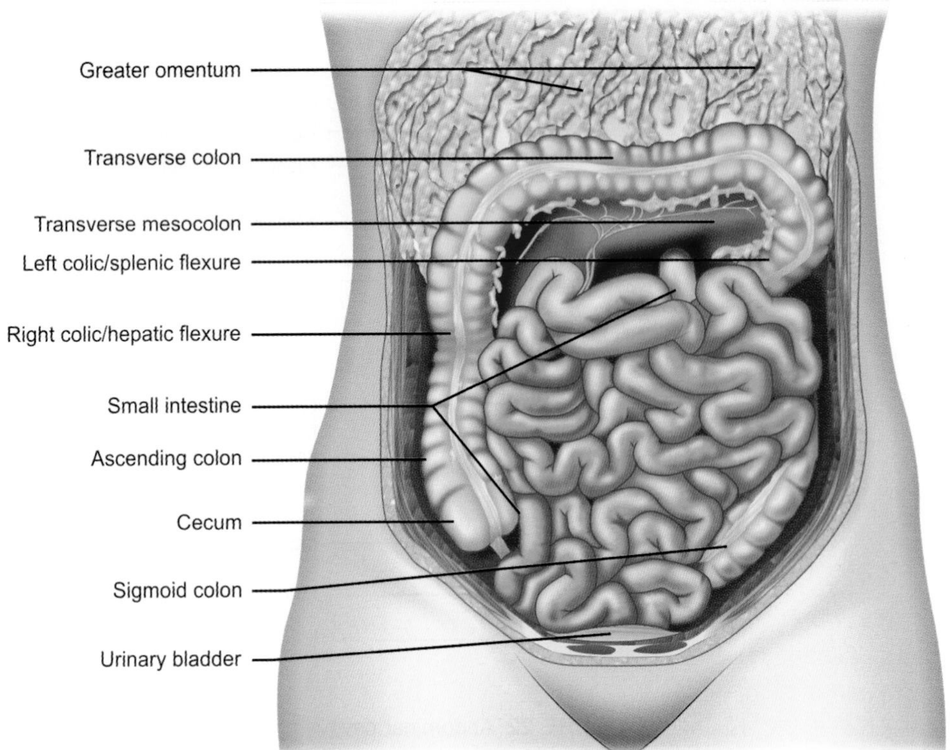

FIGURE 23 Infracolic compartment

ARRANGEMENT OF VISCERA

The viscera in the abdomen are tightly arranged within the available space. They show an anteroposterior disposition as well as a superoinferior disposition. The vertical disposition can be divided into a supracolic and an infracolic compartment by the position of the transverse colon. The stomach, liver and spleen belong to supracolic compartment. The small intestine lies in the infracolic compartment.

Try to identify the viscera and understand their relative position in the abdomen.

Greater omentum: This is the most superficial structure seen here overlapping all other structures, It can be loose or condensed. This is the peritoneum extending from the greater curvature of stomach. It is filled with fat.

Stomach: Pull the greater omentum downward and identify the stomach. Note that it is under cover of the left ribs. You can see the major part of the stomach extending across the abdomen.

Liver: Push your fingers under cover of the right costal margin and feel the bulky liver. Note that it crosses from right side to the left side and extends from anterior wall to the posterior wall. It is light brown in color.

Spleen: Put your hand deep to the diaphragm on the left side and feel deep in. You can clasp the spleen in your hands to the left of the stomach.

Infracolic compartment (Fig. 23): Lift the greater omentum and reflect it superiorly. Note that the deeper part of the greater omentum is attached to the transverse colon. Note the centrally located jejunal and ileal part of the ***small intestine***. It is almost 5 to 6 meters long. It is highly coiled tube.

Mesentery: Push the mesentery to one side and note this peritoneal covering attaching the small intestine to the posterior abdominal wall.

Large intestine: The large intestine lies peripheral to the small intestine. Identify its parts from the right to the left. The *cecum* occupies the right iliac fossa, the ***appendix*** descending from the posterior aspect of the cecum, the ***ascending colon*** lies in the right paracolic gutter, the ***hepatic flexure*** is related to the liver, the ***transverse colon*** extends from right to left, the ***splenic flexure*** is related to spleen, the ***descending colon*** lies in the left paracolic gutter, and the ***sigmoid colon*** crosses into the pelvis. The ascending and descending colons are held to the posterior abdominal wall by the peritoneum. The transverse colon is suspended by the ***transverse mesocolon*** to the posterior abdominal wall.

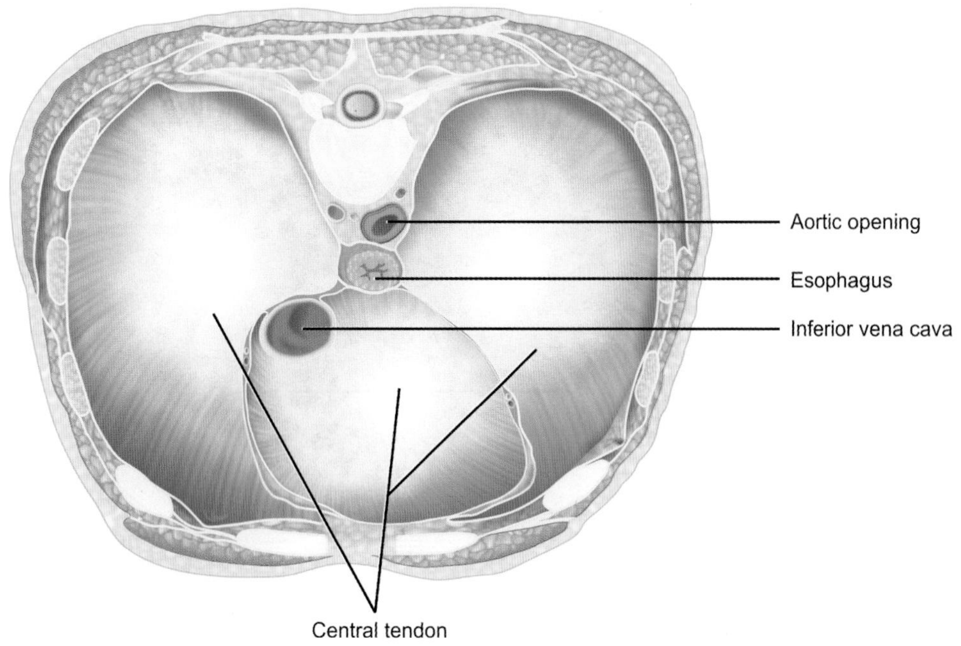

FIGURE 24 Diaphragm—superior aspect

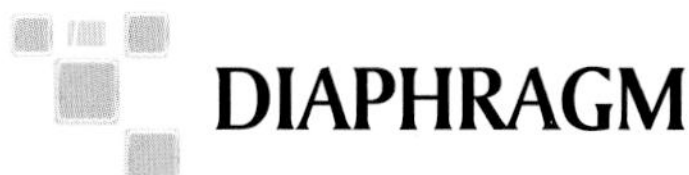

DIAPHRAGM

The diaphragm **(Fig. 24)** is the partition between the thorax and the abdomen. This muscle takes origin from the inner aspect of the costal cartilages of the lower six ribs, xiphisternum and from the anterior aspect of the lumbar vertebrae. It also arises from the upper end of the fascia over the psoas major and quadratus lumborum muscle. The muscle moves from the periphery to the center to get inserted into the triangular central tendon. As the neurovascular bundle and the esophagus pass from the thorax to the abdomen, there are number of orifices within the diaphragm to let them go.

At this stage, try to identify the diaphragm from the thoracic aspect. Note the inferior vena caval opening within the central tendon of the diaphragm. As it passes through the thick central tendon, it is all the time kept open.

The other details will be studied at a later stage.

Dissection: Look for the xiphisternal and costal cartilage origin of diaphragm at this stage. Detach the muscle from these places. Cut the ribs vertically in line with other ribs and remove the lower part of the thoracic cage. This gives more freedom to observe the abdominal viscera.

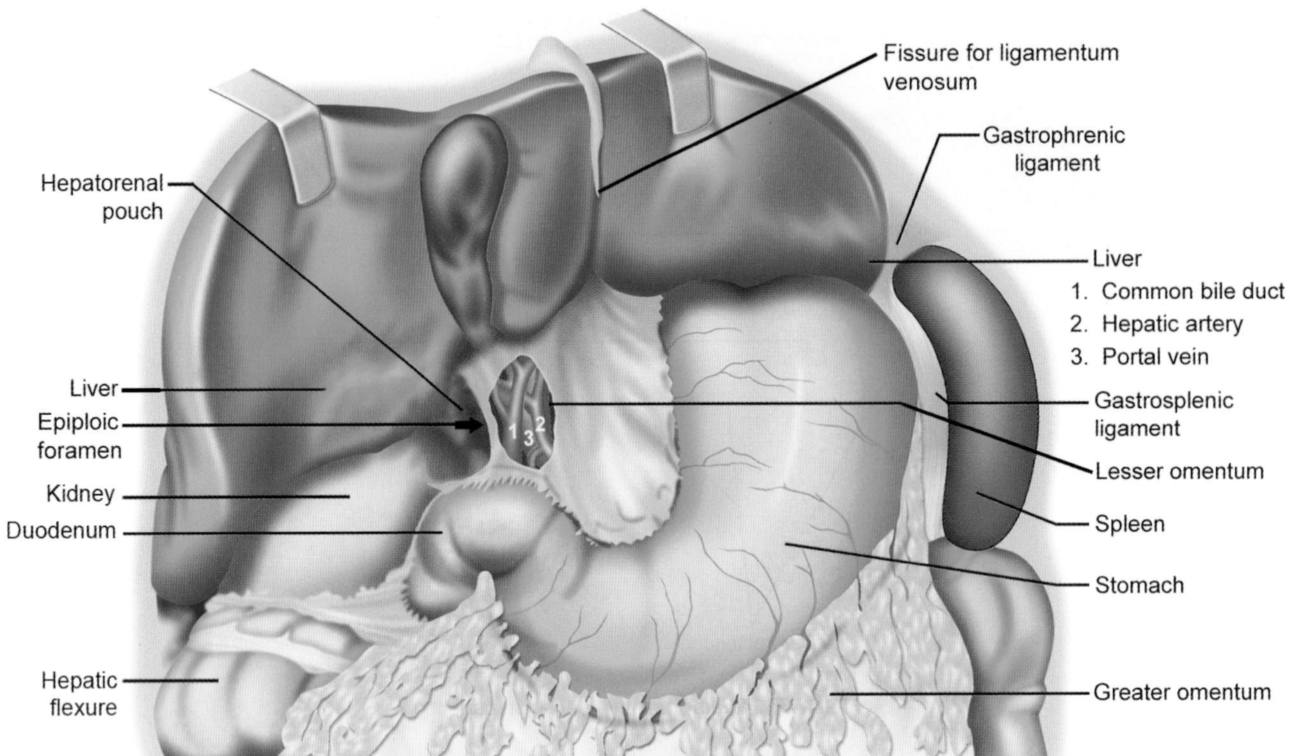

FIGURE 25 Lesser sac

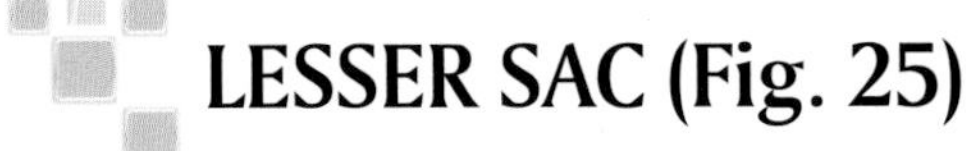

LESSER SAC (Fig. 25)

Hepatorenal pouch of Morrison: This is the space bounded anteriorly by the right lobe of liver and posteriorly by the kidney, duodenum and hepatic flexure of colon. This is one of the important spaces used for peritoneal fluid drainage.

Lesser sac: It is the cul de sac of the peritoneal cavity tucked behind the stomach and its omenta. It communicates with the greater sac through the ***epiploic foramen***. The ***anterior wall*** of the lesser sac is formed by the lesser omentum, the stomach and the anterior two layers of the greater omentum. The ***superior boundary*** is formed by the lesser omentum getting reflected above the caudate lobe of liver. The ***inferior boundary*** is formed by the lower end of the greater omentum, laterally limited by the spleen, the ***posterior boundary*** is formed by the posterior two layers of the greater omentum and the stomach bed—the diaphragm, suprarenal, kidney, splenic artery, spleen, pancreas, transverse mesocolon and transverse colon.

Epiploic foramen: This is the communication from the greater sac to the lesser sac. Put your fingers as shown in the figure and observe the foramen. Press your fingers and feel the boundaries. Superiorly it is limited by the ***caudate lobe of liver***. Inferiorly it is limited by the ***first part of the duodenum***. Posteriorly it is formed by the *inferior* ***vena cava***. Anteriorly it is formed by the free margin of the ***lesser omentum.***

Dissection: Peel the anterior layer of the free margin of the lesser omentum and identify the structures.

Common bile duct: This is the duct which carries the bile from the liver to the duodenum. It lies anteriorly and to the right. It is formed by the union of common hepatic duct from the liver and the cystic duct from the gallbladder.

Hepatic artery: This is the artery of supply to the gallbladder and liver. It lies to the left of the common hepatic duct.

Portal vein: This lies in a deeper plane. It carries nutritive blood from the gastrointestinal tract to the liver.

Lesser omentum: This is the part of the peritoneum extending between the liver and the stomach. Proximally, on the liver it is attached around the porta hepatis, to the left of this extends into the fissure for ligamentum venosum (In fetal life the ductus venosus connects the left branch of the portal vein to the inferior vena cava). Distally it is attached to the lesser curvature of the stomach and the first part of duodenum.

Gastrophrenic ligament: Identify this ligament extending from the upper end of the greater curvature of the stomach to the diaphragm.

Gastrosplenic ligament: Pull the spleen slightly and clasp the part between the spleen and the stomach. This is the gastrosplenic ligament and it feels thick as it has the short gastric vessels in it.

 Greater omentum: Trace this curtain type structure from the level of spleen to the first part of duodenum.

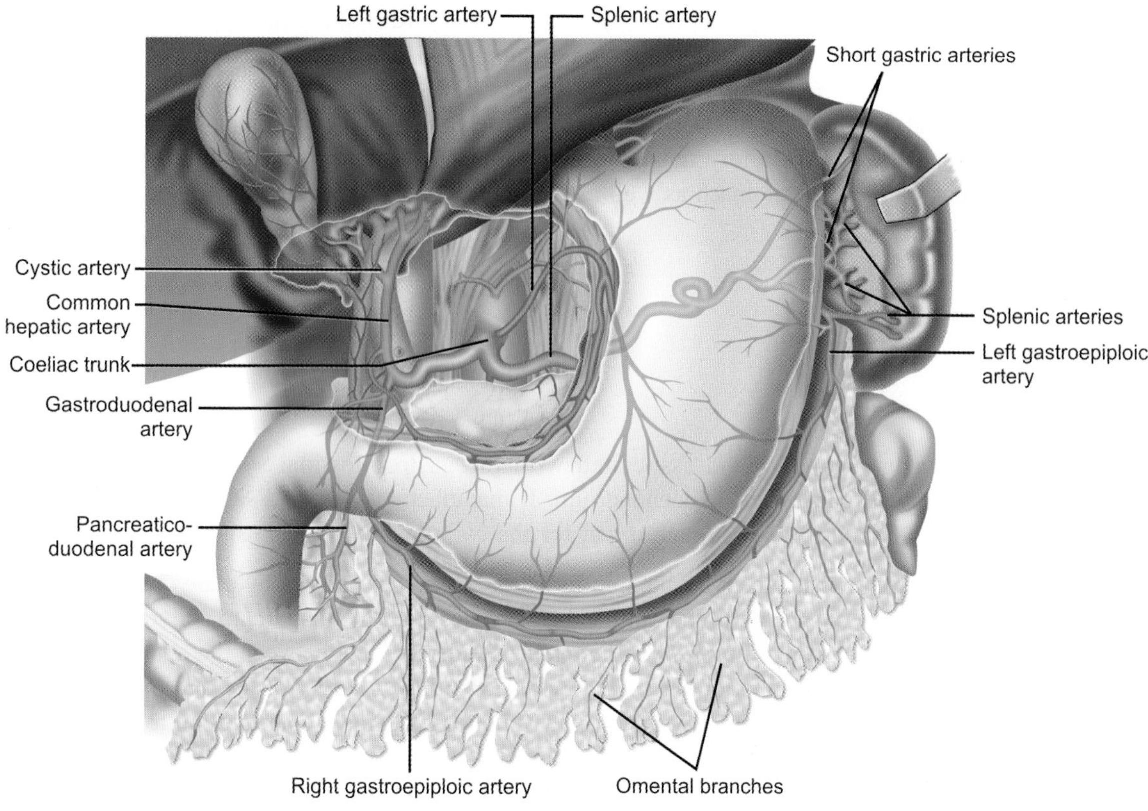

FIGURE 26 Coeliac trunk

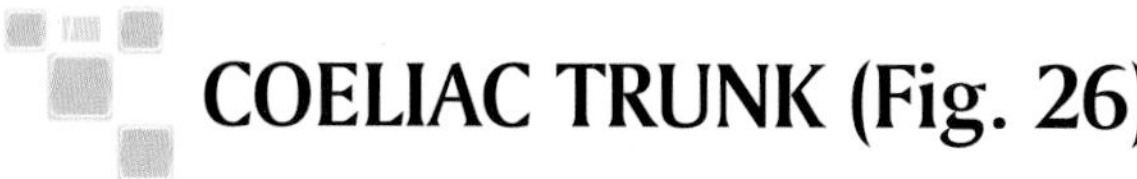

COELIAC TRUNK (Fig. 26)

This is the artery of supply to the foregut. This is the first ventral branch of the abdominal aorta. It is given off at the level of T12 vertebra. As soon as it is given off it divides into three branches—the left gastric, the common hepatic and the splenic artery.

Dissection: The blood vessels lie between the two layers of the peritoneum as near as possible to the organ. Peel the peritoneal layers near the greater and lesser curvature of the stomach, free margin of the lesser omentum and identify the arteries, veins, lymphatics and the nerves accompanying them.

Left gastric artery: Identify this artery along the upper part of the lesser cuvature of the stomach. Trace it down to the coeliac artery. It supplies the stomach on either side along the lesser curvature.

Common hepatic artery: Trace this artery arising from the coeliac trunk. It runs to the right and divides into two branches. Generally it gives off the right gastric artery. ***Right gastric artery***—trace it along the left side of the lesser curvature of the stomach. Trace it to the origin of the artery. It may arise either from the common hepatic artery or hepatic artery proper. It supplies the stomach along the lesser curvature. The branch which ascends up is the hepatic artery proper. It runs in the free margin of the lesser omentum. Trace its fine ***cystic branch*** which runs to the right to supply the gallbladder. The hepatic artery proper divides into two branches and enters the hilus of the liver. ***Gastroduodenal artery***—This branch descends downward behind the first part of the duodenum to reach the greater curvature of the stomach. ***Duodenal branches—superior duodenal, anterior and posterior pancreaticoduodenal branches*** arise from the gastroduodenal artery. The ***right gastroepiploic artery*** is given off from the gastroduodenal artery near the right end of the greater curvature of the stomach. It supplies both the greater curvature of the stomach and the greater omentum.

Splenic artery: Trace this artery from the celiac trunk. It is a big artery, runs along the upper border of the pancreas in a tortuous course. It gives number of *pancreatic branches* to supply the pancreas. It divides into number of branches and enters the hilum of the spleen. ***Short gastric arteries*** arise from the splenic artery. They traverse the gastrosplenic ligament and supply the fundic part of the stomach. The ***left gastroepiploic artery*** is another artery given off from the splenic artery near its termination. This artery runs along the greater curvature of the stomach. It gives number of branches to the greater curvature of the stomach as well as the greater omentum. These are called ***omental branches.***

LIVER

The liver is the largest wedge-shaped gland associated with the gastrointestinal system. It occupies the right hypochondrium, epigastrium and part of left hypochondrium. It manufactures bile and sends it to the second part of the duodenum through the bile duct. It is a storage organ for the carbohydrates and fats.

Ligaments of liver (Fig. 27): Note that except for the inferior surface all other parts of liver are covered by diaphragm. In the midclavicular line the liver extends up to the 5th intercostal space. Pull the diaphragm and identify the ligaments extending between the liver and diaphragm. ***Falciform ligament:*** Reidentify this between the anterior abdominal wall and the liver, from the umbilicus to the anterior surface of liver. At the lower border of the liver note the ***ligamentum teres*** round ligament. This diverges and goes deep, whereas the falciform ligament continues on to the anterior surface of the liver. Put your hands on either side of the falciform ligament and trace it up. Trace the left layer of the falciform ligament. Note that it continues and forms the ***left triangular ligament.*** Trace the right layer of the falciform ligament. It continues as the anterior layer of the ***coronary ligament*** on the superior surface. Run your fingers towards the right side and note that the coronary ligament ends as the ***right triangular ligament.*** This continues posteriorly to form the inferior layer of the coronary ligament. The two layers of the coronary ligament are widely separated. The gap between the two layers is called the bare area of liver.

Dissection: Cut the ligamentum teres, the falciform ligament, left triangular ligament, anterior and posterior layers of coronary ligaments, and the right triangular ligament. On the inferior surface cut the structures in the free border of the lesser omentum nearer to the porta hepatis. Cut the inferior vena cava from the diaphragm and also near the caudate lobe. This totally releases the liver from the abdomen. Take it out of the abdomen and study the organ.

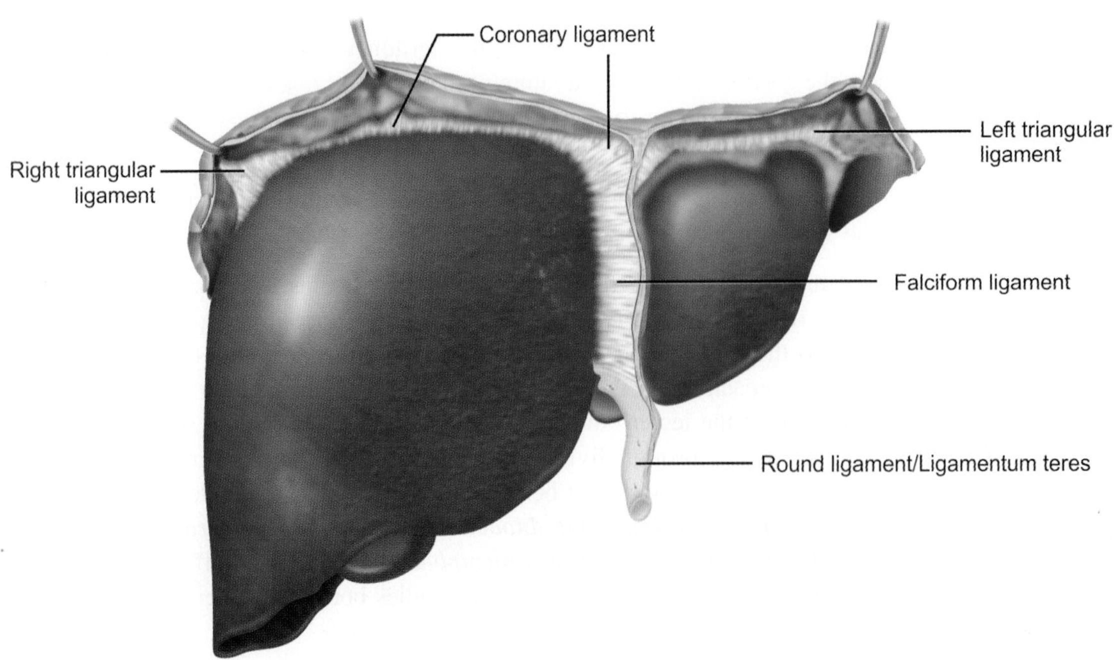

FIGURE 27 Liver ligaments

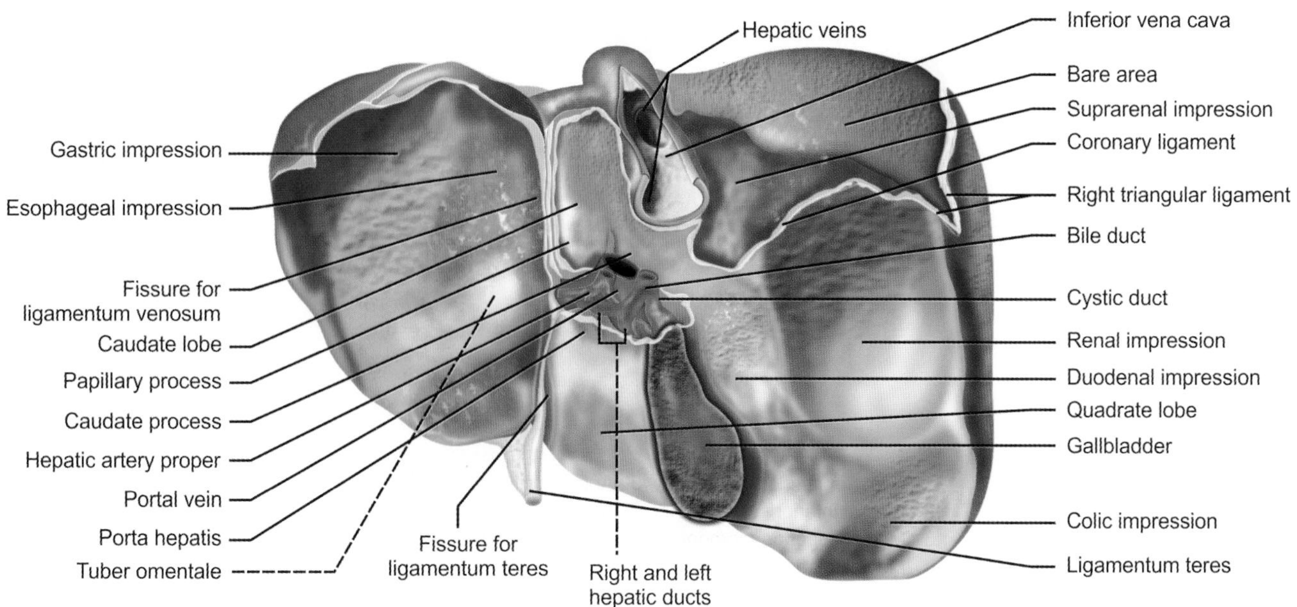

FIGURE 28 Posterior and visceral surface of liver

Anatomical position (Fig. 28): Hold the liver in your right hand, with the anterior surface facing forwards, the right surface facing the right side, the superior surface facing above, the inferior surface facing down and the posterior vertebral surface facing back. The sharp inferior border should run obliquely from left to the right. Note that the anterior surface, superior surface and right surface merge with each other and mould itself to the space available under the thoracic cage. The sharp inferior border separates the anterior surface from the visceral surface.

Relations*:** The ***anterior surface and ***right surface*** are related to the lower six ribs and intercostal spaces separated by the diaphragm. The ***superior surface*** and ***right surface*** are related to the lungs and the heart, separated by the diaphragm. The ***posterior vertebral surface*** is related to the vertebrae, intervertebral dksc, esophagus and inferior vena cava. The ***inferior surface*** is otherwise called as the visceral surface. The organs located below the liver cause impressions on its inferior surface in the cadaver. The impressions can easily be identified. They are from left to right—the gastric impression, duodenal impression, colic impression, renal and suprarenal impressions. The same structures should be identified on the body and their relations should be confirmed.

Lobes of liver: Anatomically the liver is divided into ***right* and *left lobes*** by the attachment of the falciform ligament anteriorly and ligamentum teres and venosum posteriorly. The left lobe is much smaller compared to the right lobe. ***Tuber omentale***—is the most prominent part on the left lobe and this is related to the lesser omentum. ***Fissure for ligamentum teres***—trace it from the inferior border to the porta hepatis. This is a fibrosed structure in the adult anatomy. But in the fetal life it is the left umbilical vein. It carries oxygenated blood from the mother to the portal vein. ***Fissure for ligamentum venosum***—trace this extending from the porta hepatis to the inferior vena cava. Look at the two layers of the lesser omentum. Within the depths of the fissure, the ***ligamentum venosum*** is located. Again this is fibrosed in the adult anatomy. In the fetal life blood passes from the portal vein to the inferior vena cava, by passing the liver. It is called the ductus venosus and carries the oxygenated blood to the developing fetus. Identify the ***caudate lobe***—it lies between the groove for inferior vena cava and the fissure for the ligamentum venosum**.** ***Caudate process:*** See this small extension from the caudate lobe. It joins the right lobe between the porta hepatis and the inferior vena cava. ***Papillary process*** is another extension of the caudate lobe parallel and to the right of the caudate process. The ***quadrate lobe*** lies between the fissure for the ligamentum teres and the gallbladder. These two are parts of the right lobe of liver anatomically.

Bare areas of liver: The space between the superior and the inferior layer of the coronary ligament is closely related to the diaphragm, suprarenal and the kidney, without the intervention of the peritoneum. This is called the bare area of the liver. Similarly, the gallbladder and the inferior vena cava are also directly connected to the liver by connective tissue without a peritoneal separation. These are also considered as bare areas.

Porta hepatis: This is the entry point for the blood vessels and nerves. Note that the ***right* and *left hepatic ducts*** leave the liver. These are the most anterior structures here. Trace it down and see the union of these ducts forming the

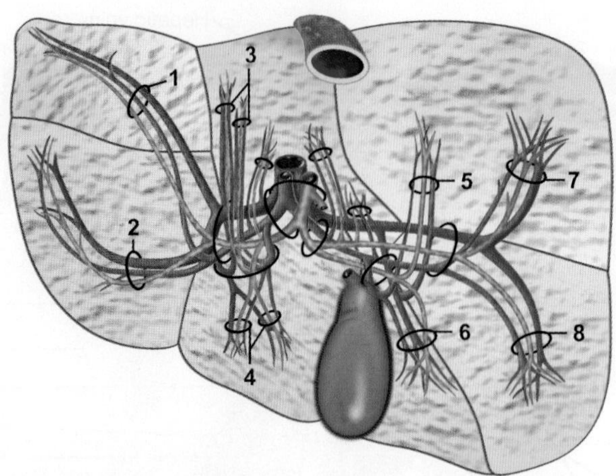

1. Superior inferior segment
2. Lateral inferior segment
3. Medial superior segment
4. Medial inferior segment
5. Anterior superior segment
6. Anterior inferior segment
7. Posterior superior segment
8. Posterior inferior segment

FIGURE 29 Segmentation of liver

common hepatic duct. Trace the cystic duct arising from the gallbladder joining the bile duct. Beyond this point it is called ***common bile duct. Portal vein*** is the most deep structure within the porta hepatis. Right and left branches of the hepatic artery enter through the porta hepatis. There are nerves and lymphatics accompanying these structures.

Inferior vena cava: See that inferior vena cava makes a deep impression on the posterior surface of liver. Slit it open and note that it receives the hepatic veins, generally two in number.

Segments of Liver (Fig. 29)

The liver is divided into eight functional segments. These are made use, while doing liver surgery. The structures in the porta hepatis follow the same pathway in dividing the liver into subdivisions. Liver can be put into a solution of hydrogen peroxide for few hours and can be dissected. Keep removing the liver tissue following the structures in the porta hepatis. This would enable you to identify the eight lobes of liver.

GALLBLADDER (Fig. 30)

Identify the gallbladder under cover of the liver. It concentrates the bile secreted by the liver. It stores the bile till it is to be released into the duodenum.

Parts: The part which projects beyond the inferior border of the liver, is related to the 9th costal cartilage. It is called the ***fundus.*** The part succeeding this and related to the liver is called the ***body.*** The right wall of the gallbladder shows a slight enlargement. It is called the infundibulum or the Hartmann's pouch. Then suddenly it narrows down and is called the *neck.* The neck follows as the ***cystic duct.***

Slit open the gallbladder from cystic duct to the fundus. You will see that the fundus and body are smooth and the neck and cystic duct shows raised mucous membrane. It is called spiral valve in the cystic duct.

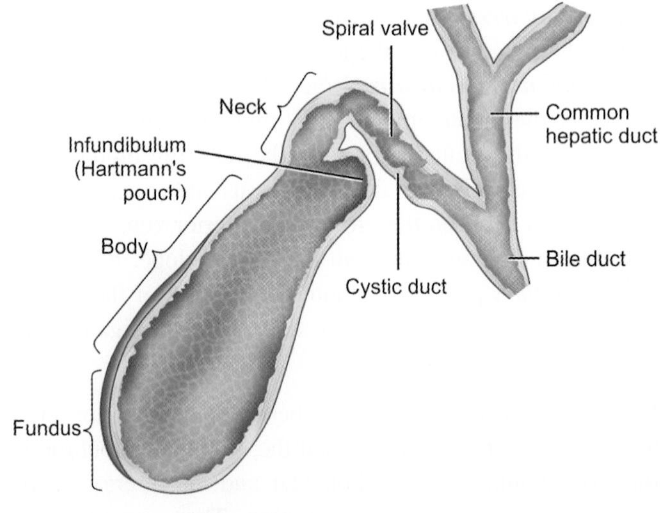

FIGURE 30 Gallbladder

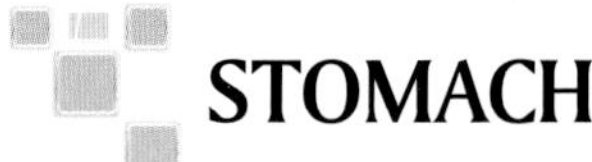

STOMACH

Stomach is the most dilated part of the gastrointestinal tract. It lies in the upper left part of the abdominal cavity. It occupies the left hypochondrium, umbilical region to the epigastrium. Its shape is variable. It presents from a J shape to a steer horn shape.

Peritoneal connections: Reidentify the *lesser omentum, gastrophrenic ligament, gastrosplenic ligament,* and *greater omentum.*

Dissection: Take two pairs of thick twine thread. Tie two strings near the cardiac end and two near the pyloric end. Cut the stomach between the two strings at both the ends. Cut it along the greater curvature, cutting through all the ligaments and remove the stomach out of the body.

Anatomical position: Put the stomach on the table exactly as you had seen it in the cadaver. The surface that faces you is the anterior surface and the surface that lies on the table is the posterior surface.

Parts of Stomach (Fig. 31)

See the ***cardiac end*** of stomach. This is where the esophagus meets the stomach. The point where the esophagus joins the greater curvature is called the ***cardiac notch.*** Draw an imaginary line from here horizontally. The part of the stomach which lies above this is called the ***fundus.*** Feel the margin from the esophagus along the right border. This is the ***lesser curvature.*** See the sharp constriction on the right end. It is the ***pyloric end*** of the stomach. Identify the sharp angle on the lesser curvature. It is called the ***incisura angularis.*** The part between the incisura and the pyloric end is the ***pylorus of the stomach.*** This is divided into two parts, the ***pyloric antrum*** **and** ***pyloric canal.*** These are better seen when the stomach is opened.

Relations: ***Anteriorly,*** the stomach is related to the left lobe of liver, the diaphragm and the anterior abdominal wall (these structures you have already seen). ***Posteriorly,*** the structures that are related to the stomach are called structures of stomach bed.

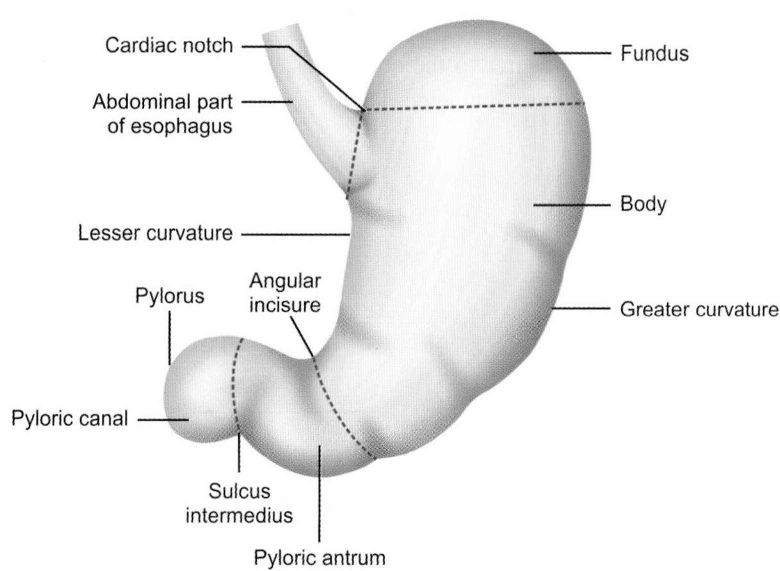

FIGURE 31 Parts of stomach

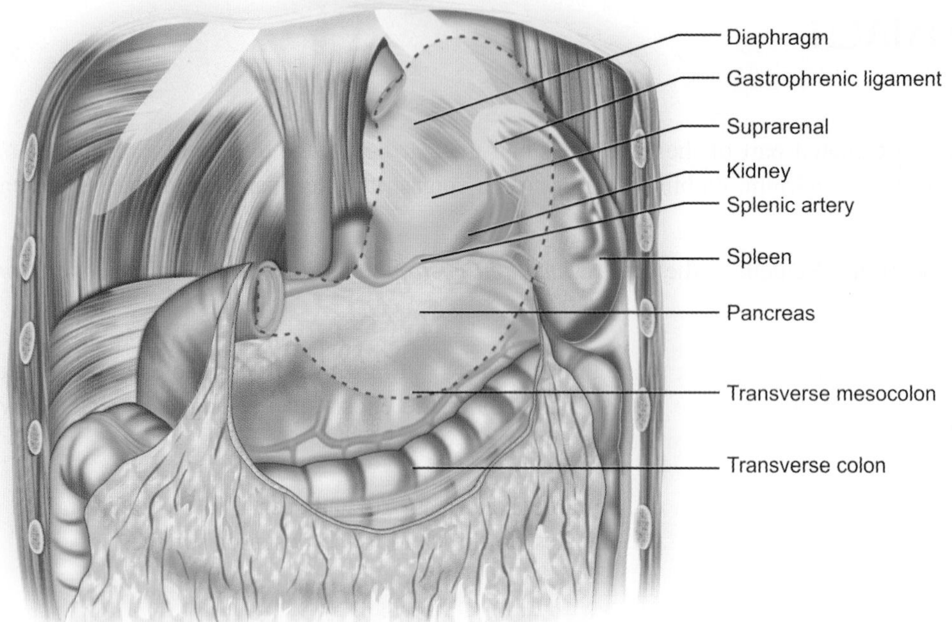

FIGURE 32 Stomach bed

Stomach Bed (Fig. 32)

It is formed by the diaphragm, left suprarenal, left kidney, spleen, splenic artery, pancreas, transverse mesocolon and transverse colon. (Identify all these structures on the cadaver).

Dissection: Peel the peritoneum from the outer surface of the stomach and try to observe the ***blood vessels*** along the curvatures of stomach (these were already studied). The stomach is supplied by the right and left gastric arteries, right and left gastroepiploic arteries and short gastric arteries. Clean and identify the vagus nerve. The nerve seen on the anterior aspect is the ***left vagus*** and the one seen on the posterior part is the ***right vagus***. Peel the peritoneum and the adventia on the stomach and see the musculature layer by layer.

Musculature (Fig. 33)

The longitudinal muscle is better developed nearer to the curvatures. See the circular muscle deep to the longitudinal muscle. This is best developed near the pyloric sphincter. The deepest is the oblique muscle fibres. On cleaning the circular fibres you will see the oblique fibres.

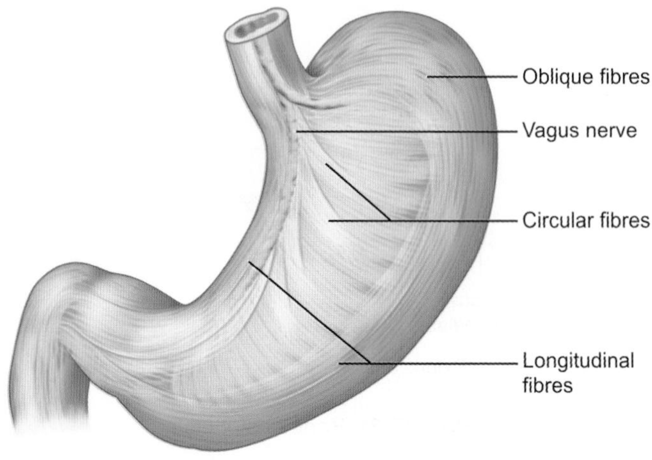

FIGURE 33 Musculature of stomach

Interior of Stomach (Fig. 34)

Slit open the stomach along its greater curvature. Get it washed well and observe the interior. The mucous membrane of the stomach is thrown into folds called rugae. The folds are longitudinal along the lesser curvature of the stomach. Move the mucous membrane and observe the loose ***submucosa.***

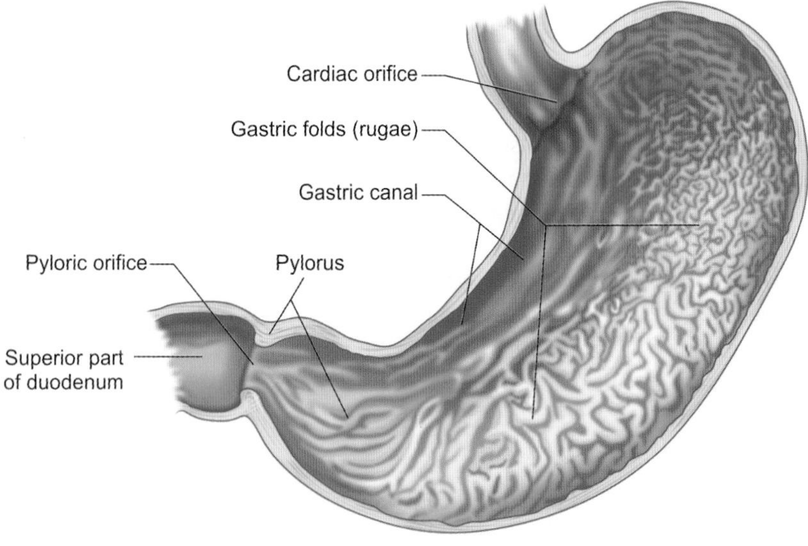

FIGURE 34 Stomach—inferior

SPLEEN

Spleen is the lymphoid organ located in the left hypochondrium, under cover of the diaphragm. Clasp the spleen in your hands and note that it is covered by peritoneum on all sides. Look at the hilum where the splenic vessels enter. Feel the ligaments extending from here. The gastrosplenic ligament is already identified and cut. Feel the lienorenal ligament extending from the spleen to the kidney below. Feel the tail of the pancreas in it.

Dissection: Pull the spleen laterally and cut the lienorenal ligament and remove the spleen from the body.

Anatomical position: Hold the spleen in your left hand. Put the hand in an oblique position.

External Features (Fig. 35)

Diaphragmatic surface is the smooth surface. Put it in your palm. ***Superior border*** is notched, generally, it is due to the fact that the organ develops as small splenic nodules. These fuse later in development. The ***posterior end*** is more medial in position. It is nearer to the 10th vertebral body. The ***anterior end*** is more lateral in position. It reaches the midaxillary line. The long axis of the spleen lies along the 10th rib. It is posteriorly related to the 9th, 10th and 11th ribs. It is separated from the ribs by the diaphragm. ***Visceral surface*** is irregular in shape. The hilum occupies the central position. The area between the hilum and the superior border is related to the stomach, called the ***gastric impression.*** The elevated border between the hilum and the posterior end is called the ***intermediate border.*** The area between the hilum and the ***inferior border*** is related to the kidney, called the ***renal impression.*** The anterior end is more flattened and is related to the splenic flexure of the colon, called ***colic impression.*** The ***hilum*** receives the splenic arteries, veins, lymphatics and the nerves.

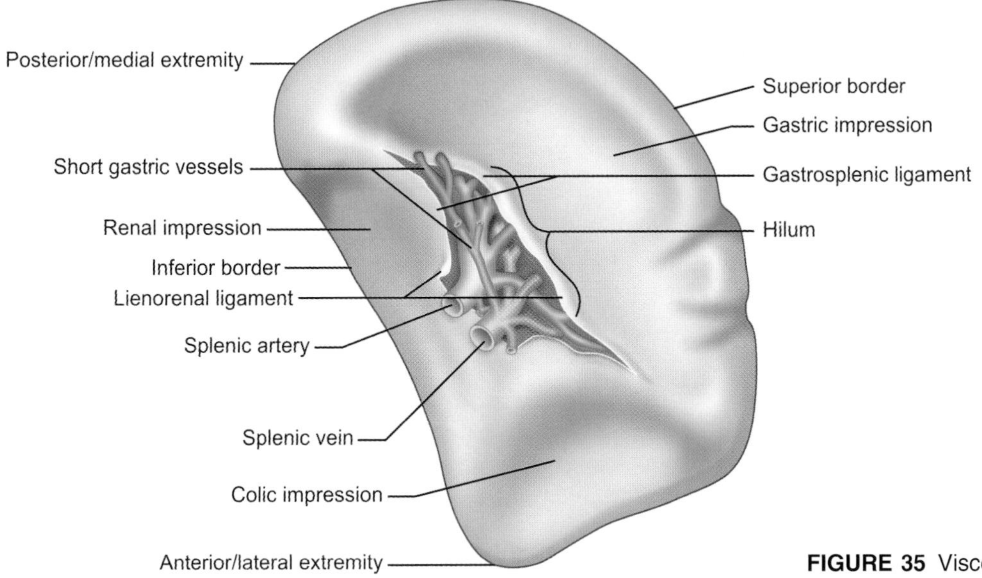

FIGURE 35 Visceral surface of spleen

JEJUNUM AND ILEUM

Small intestine follows the stomach. Duodenum, jejunum and ileum constitute the small intestine. The duodenum is a retroperitoneal organ. The jejunum and ileum lie in the infracolic compartment of the abdomen. They are attached to the abdominal wall by mesentery. Superior mesenteric vessels supply the small intestine.

Dissection: Lift the greater omentum, reflect it up along with the transverse colon. You will see the transverse mesocolon extending from the transverse colon to the posterior abdominal wall and small intestine with the mesentery, attached to the posterior abdominal wall. Turn the small intestine to the left side and visualize the mesentery in full. Clean right layer of the mesentery and see the neurovascular bundle.

Mesentery (Fig. 36)

It is the double layered peritoneal fold which encloses the jejunum and ileum of the small intestine in its free border. It attaches the gut to the posterior abdominal wall. Note that it extends from the duodenojejunal flexure to the ileocecal junction. It is around 15 cm long at its attached border. It is around 5.5 meters long at its free border. Note that the mesentery is highly folded due to the difference in length. The height from the attached margin to the free margin can be up to 15 to 20 cm. The superior mesenteric artery, vein, lymphatics, the nerve plexus and the fat are the contents of the mesentery.

Superior mesenteric artery: It is the artery of supply to the midgut. It arises from the abdominal aorta at the level of L1 vertebra. At its origin it lies behind the pancreas and supplies the lower part of pancreas and duodenum. Soon it enters the mesentery, passing over the uncinate process of the pancreas. In the mesentery it gives off branches from its left to supply the jejunum and ileum. Branches arising from the right side supply the large intestine up to the right 2/3rds of the transverse colon.

Jejunal and ileal branches: They are around 15 to 20 in number. Note that all these branches form arcades by dividing and anastomosing with each other. This helps to maintain the flow of blood to the organ. The arcades are fewer near the jejunal side, whereas they are three to four levels of arcades near the ileal end. The arteries arising from the last arcade nearer to the gut are straight branches called vasa recti. These are end arteries. As they reach the gut,

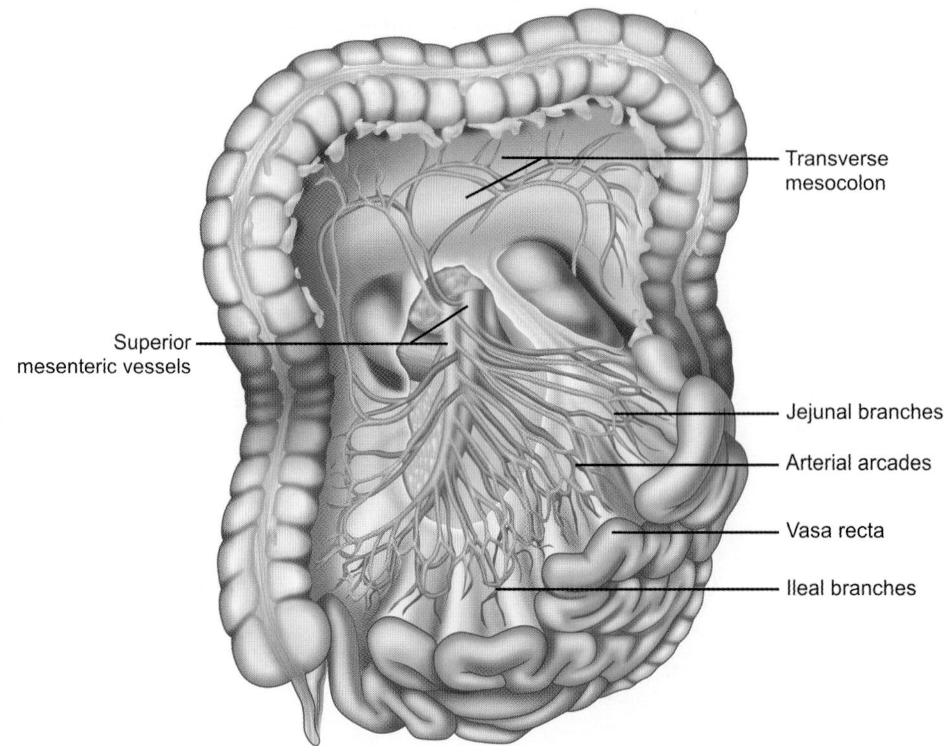

FIGURE 36 Small intestine

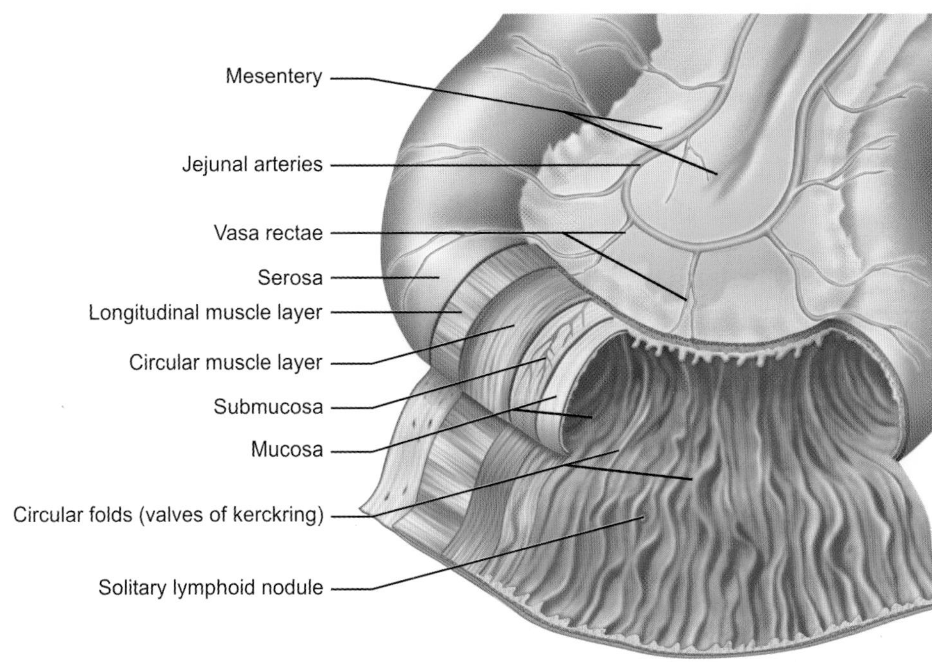

FIGURE 37 Jejunum—inferior

they enter the gut on to the right and to the left side alternatively. Note that in the jejunal side fat is far less compared to the ileal side of the mesentery. So seeing the mesentery against light is easier on the jejunal side as it has fewer arcades and less amount of fat. These are generally described as windows.

Dissection: Take two sets of twine thread, tie one set near the jejunal end and the other set near the ileal end of the gut. Cut the gut between the ties. Detach the jejunum and ileum by cutting near its attached border. Take the gut out of the body, remove the ties and get it washed well under tap water. Slit the gut along the mesenteric border of the gut and observe the interior.

Interior of Jejunum (Fig. 37)

The mucous membrane is folded horizontally, these are called *plicae circulares.* These folds are very near, and this makes the jejunal wall thick when felt by hand (feel it and see). Move the mucous membrane and see the submucosa. Peel the peritoneum from the surface and identify the outer longitudinal layer of musculature and the inner circular layer of musculature.

Interior of ileum (Fig. 38): Note that there are *plicae* within the ileum but they are far apart compared to the jejunum. Feel the ileal wall, it feels thinner compared to the jejunum. Look the ileum against light. You will see darkened 1 cm long areas along the antimesenteric border. These are the aggregated lymphoid follicles called the ***Peyer's patches***.

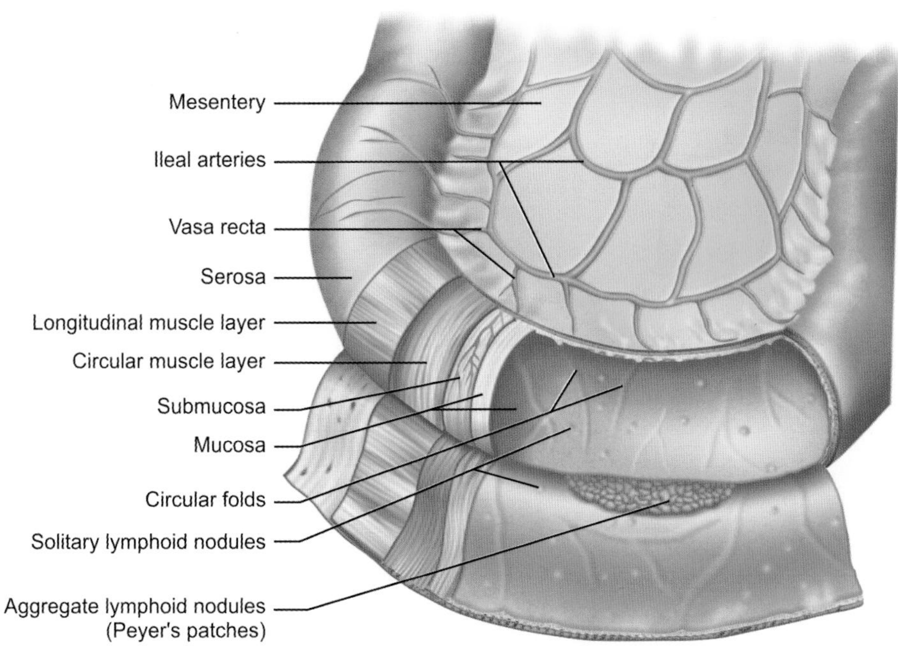

FIGURE 38 Ileum—inferior

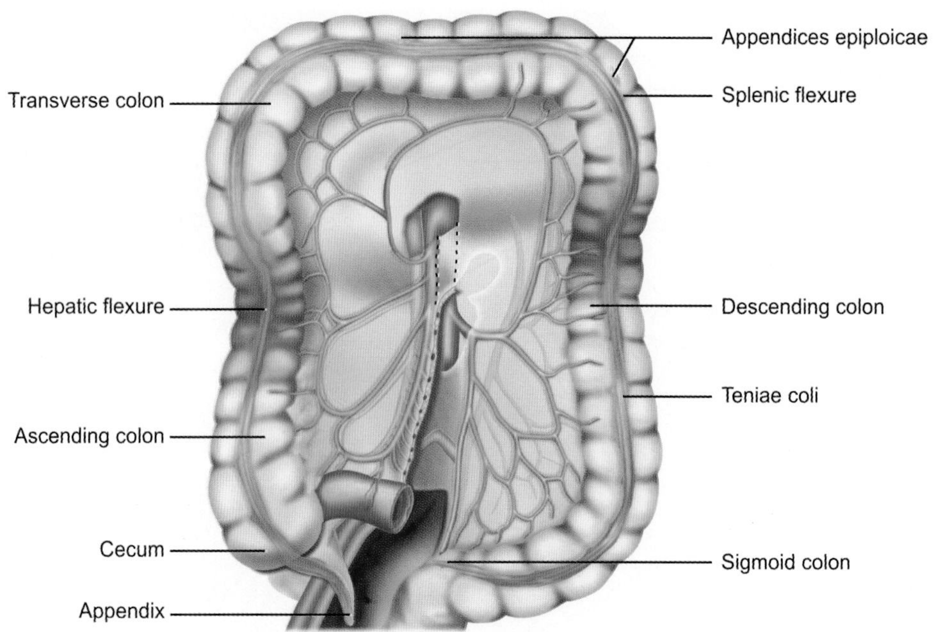

FIGURE 39 Large intestine–general features

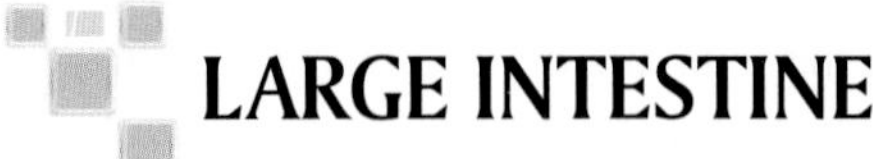

LARGE INTESTINE

Large Intestine (Fig. 39)

It is 1.5 meters long, made up of cecum, vermiform appendix, ascending colon, hepatic flexure, transverse colon, splenic flexure, descending colon, sigmoid colon, rectum and anal canal. Identify the parts on the body.

Large intestine can easily be distinguished from the small intestine, by its position and by its ***bigger caliber***. It also presents ***sacculations/haustrations,*** fatty sacs in its peritoneal covering called *appendices epiploicae*. The longitudinal musculature of the large intestine presents as three bands called ***taeniae coli***. On the ascending and descending colon they are one anterior and two posterior in position. Follow them through the whole large intestine and note that they cover the vermiform appendix and the rectum in full.

Peritoneal Attachments (Fig. 40)

Cecum and appendix: Note that the cecum is covered by peritoneum on all sides. Note the ***vascular fold*** extending from the front of the cecum to the mesentery. Put your finger into the gap between the two. It is called the ***superior***

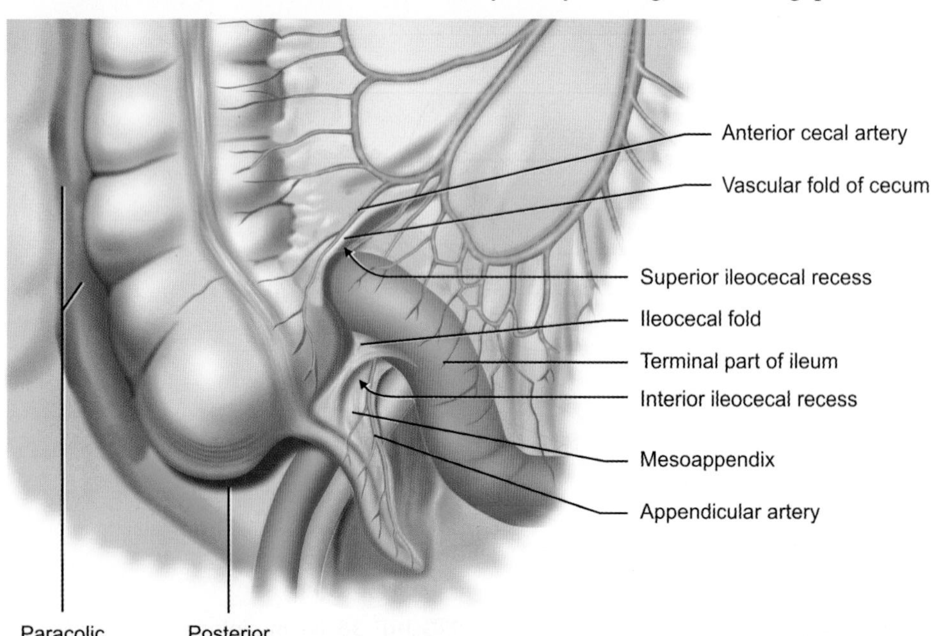

FIGURE 40 Cecum—peritoneal coverings

ileocecal recess. Note the ***ileocecal fold/Treves ligament*** from the anterior aspect of the lower part of the cecum to the ileum. Put your finger between this and the mesoappendix. It is called the ***inferior ileocecal recess.*** Put your fingers behind the cecum. You can make out that laterally it is limited by the lateral ligament, superiorly by reflection of the peritoneum. This is called the ***posterior cecal recess.*** Many a times you may find the appendix in this fossa.

Appendix: Identify this long narrow blind tube of the large intestine. It starts from the back of the cecum. Identify the ***mesoappendix*** from the posterior layer of the mesentery.

The ascending colon and descending colon are attached to the posterior abdominal wall by the peritoneum which covers them on their anterior aspect. The area on either side of the ascending and descending colon is called ***paracolic gutter.*** The ***transverse mesocolon*** extends from the transverse colon to the posterior abdominal wall along the duedenum head and body of pancreas. The sigmoid colon is attached to the pelvic wall by the ***sigmoid mesocolon.*** It presents two limbs, a lateral limb and a medial limb. The lateral limb is along the pelvic brim and the medial is vertical, extends from the division of the common iliac artery to the 3rd piece of sacrum. Touch and feel these limbs (Fig. 41).

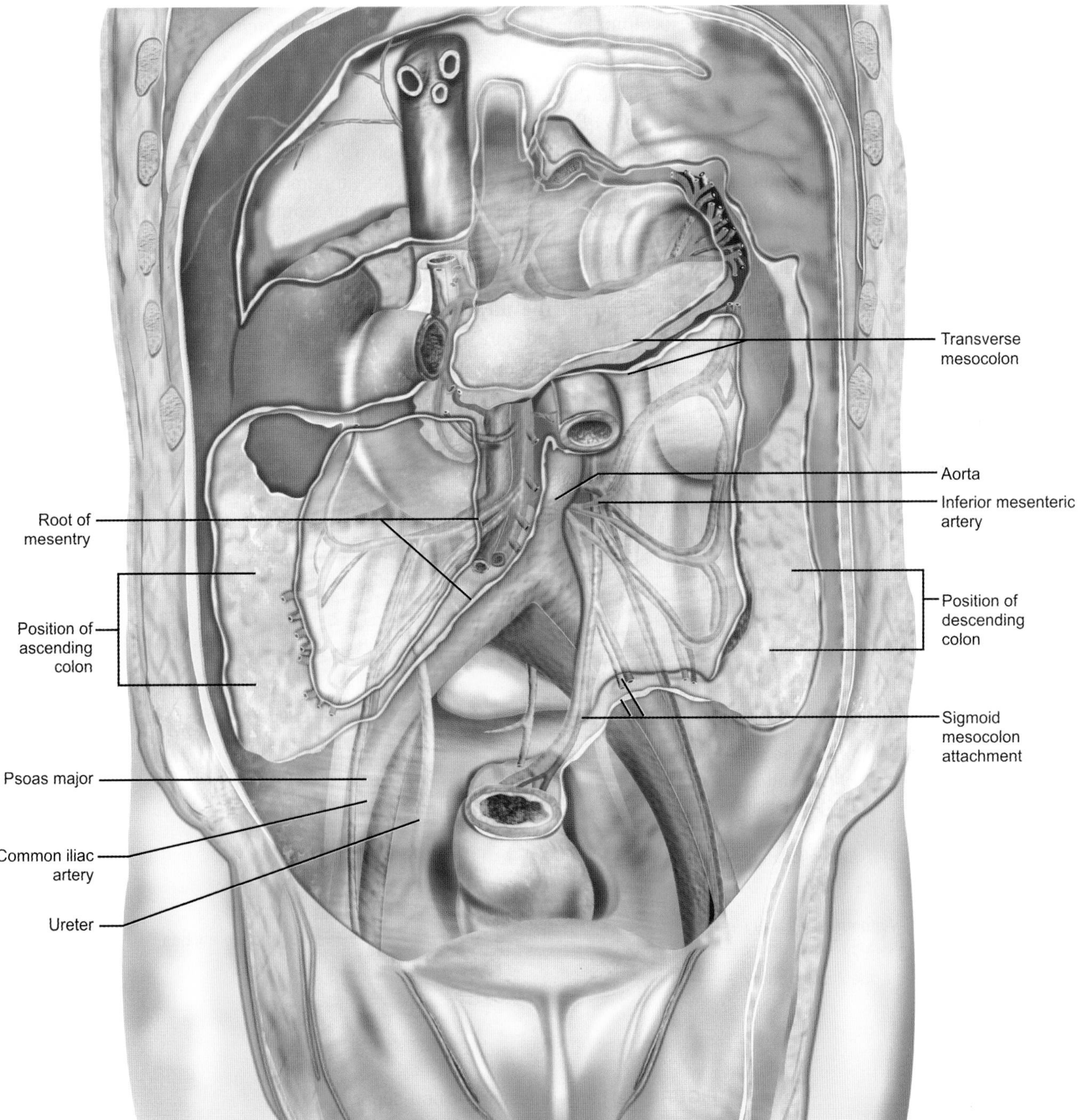

FIGURE 41 Peritoneal attachment of large intestine

Dissection: Clean the peritoneum, on the posterior abdominal wall, of the transverse mesocolon and of the sigmoid mesocolon to identify the blood vessels. The large intestine is supplied by the superior mesenteric as well as the inferior mesenteric artery. The branches from the superior mesenteric arise from the right side of the artery.

Blood Supply (Figs 41 and 42)

From superior mesenteric artery: The ***ileocolic*** is the lowest of the branches. Identify this and note that it divides into ascending and descending branch. The descending branch anastomoses with the terminal part of the superior mesenteric artery. Trace its ***ileal branches*** to the terminal part of the ileum, anterior and posterior ***cecal branches*** to the cecum, ***appendicular artery*** from the posterior caecal artery to the appendix, ***colic branches*** to the lower part of the ascending colon. The ***right colic artery*** is the next branch. On reaching the colon it divides into an ***ascending*** and a ***descending branch,*** they anastomose with the ileocolic and middle colic branches. It supplies the upper part of the ascending colon and the hepatic flexure. The ***middle colic*** artery arises from the upper part of the superior mesenteric artery. See its entry into the transverse mesocolon. This divides into ***right and left branches***. These anastomose with the middle colic and left colic branches.

Inferior mesenteric artery: This is the lower of the three ventral branches of the abdominal aorta. Identify its origin at the level of the 3rd lumbar vertebra. Trace the ***left colic branch*** arising from this. This divides into an ***ascending*** and a ***descending*** branch. These anastomose with the middle colic and first sigmoid branch. This supplies the left part of transverse colon, splenic flexure and descending colon. ***Sigmoid branches*** generally 2 to 3 in number anastomose with the left colic artery and supply the sigmoid colon. Note that all these arteries supplying the large intestine form a continuous artery called ***marginal artery of Drummond.*** The vasa recti arise from here to supply the large intestine. Further trace the inferior mesenteric artery into the pelvic region where it supplies the rectum as ***superior rectal artery.***

Relations of the superior mesenteric artery (root of the mesentery): Lift the superior mesenteric artery and see the structures that it crosses from left to right—the second part of duodenum, inferior vena cava, right psoas major, right ureter, and genitofemoral nerve. The superior mesenteric vein lies on its right side.

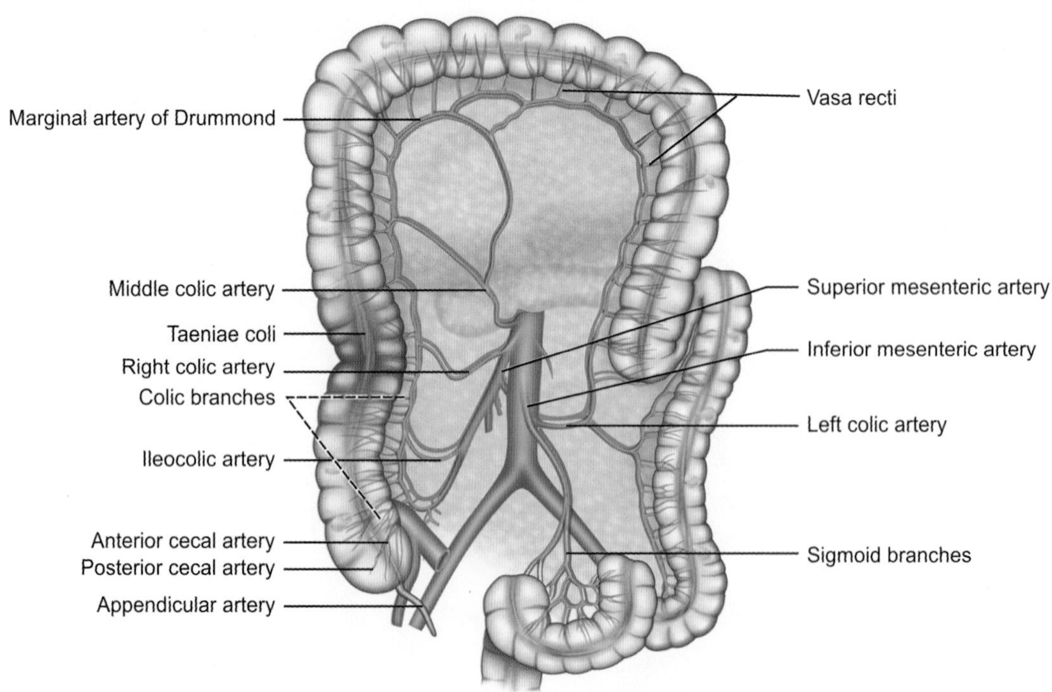

FIGURE 42 Large intestine—blood supply

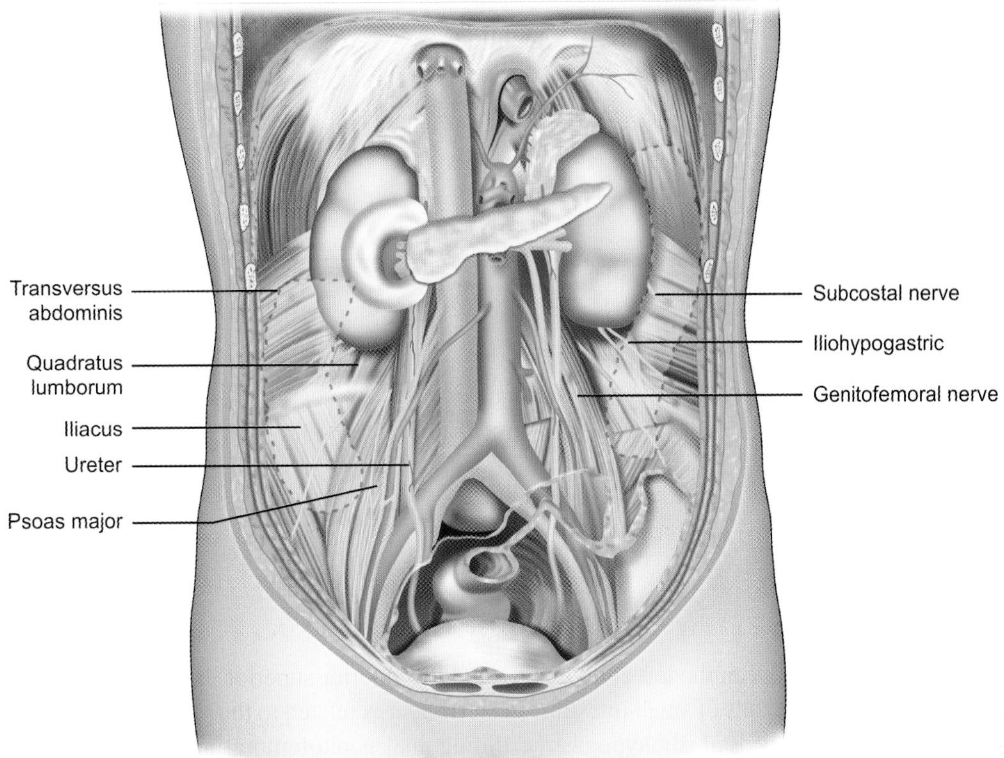

FIGURE 43 Large intestine—posterior relations

Relations of the inferior mesenteric artery: Identify it behind the horizontal part of the duodenum. Note its posterior relations as it passes to the left. It crosses the aorta, left sympathetic chain, left psoas major muscle, division of left common iliac artery. The inferior mesenteric vein lies to the left of the artery.

Dissection: Keep lifting and detaching the colon as you proceed to see the relations. Take two strings and tie the sigmoid colon near the pelvic brim. Cut it between the strings. Cut the superior mesenteric artery and vein below the duodenum and the inferior mesenteric artery and vein near the abdominal aorta. Remove the colon along with the blood vessels and study the posterior relations.

Posterior Relations of Large Intestine (Fig. 43)

Cecum: The cecum lies in the right iliac fossa. Anteriorly it is related to the anterior abdominal wall. Lift the cecum and note the structures that are posteriorly related. Here it lies on the iliacus and psoas major muscles, lateral cutaneous nerve of thigh femoral nerve, genitofemoral nerve, external iliac artery and posterior cecal artery.

Vermiform appendix: This is a vestigial lymphoid organ. Pull it and see that it is attached to the posteromedial wall of the cecum. The length and position of the appendix is variable. Its position is generally likened to the hands of the clock. It may present a 1 o' clock position (paracolic), 12 o'clock position (retrocecal), 2 o' clock position (ileal), 5 o'clock position (pelvic), 6 o' cock position (midinguinal). It is enclosed in the ***mesoappendix***. The mesoappendix varies in length, this may expose the artery. Peel the peritoneum and note that the ***Taeniae coli*** are continuous and cover the whole appendix. See the appendicular artery and vein in here.

Ascending colon: Anteriorly it is related to the anterior abdominal wall, coils of small intestine and part of greater omentum. Posteriorly it is related to the iliacus, transversus abdominis and quadratus lumborum muscle, right kidney, subcostal vessels and nerve, iliohypogastric vessels and nerve.

Hepatic flexure: Anteriorly it is related to the right lobe of liver. Posteriorly it is related to the right kidney and transversus abdominis muscle.

Transverse colon: It is variable in length. Anteriorly it is covered by the greater omentum. Posteriorly it is variable as it is freely mobile in the living.

Splenic flexure: Anteriorly it is related to stomach and left costal margin. Posteriorly it is related to spleen and stomach.

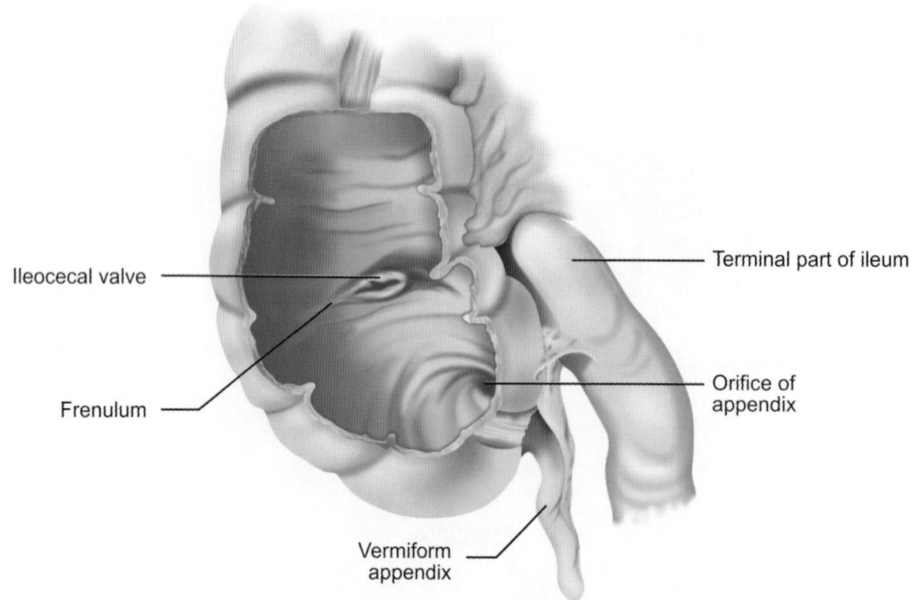

FIGURE 44 Cecum interior

Descending colon: The extent between the left colic flexure and the anterior superior iliac spine is called the descending colon. It is anteriorly related to the coils of small intestine. Posteriorly it is related to the psoas major, quadratus lumborum, transversus abdominis muscle, subcostal, iliohypogastric, ilioinguinal genitofemoral and femoral nerves.

Sigmoid colon: It is shaped like a S, crosses the pelvic brim to enter the pelvis.

Dissection: Slit the large intestine open, wash well and see the interior.

Interior of Cecum (Fig. 44)

Cut open cecum by removing a small part of the anterior wall and see the interior. **Ileocecal opening** is on the posteromedial wall. It is a transverse slit protected by two horizontal folds of mucous membrane. Mucosal extensions of the valve are called frenula.

Appendicular opening: Note this slit like opening below the cecal opening.

Interior of the large intestine (Fig. 45): *Open any part of the large intestine and see its interior.* It shows ***semilunar folds*** of the mucous membrane corresponding to the external constrictions. Move the mucosa and note that the ***submucosa*** is far thinner here, as it does not have glands here. Peel the external peritoneal layer and identify the musculature. Note the three bands of the ***longitudinal muscle*** layer and deeper continuous ***circular muscle*** layer.

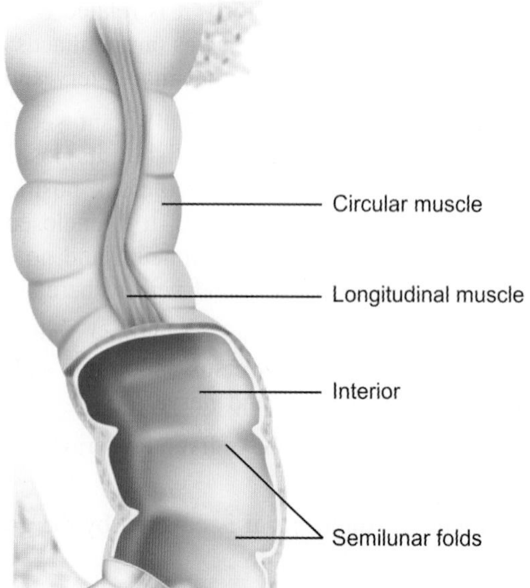

FIGURE 45 Large intestine—interior

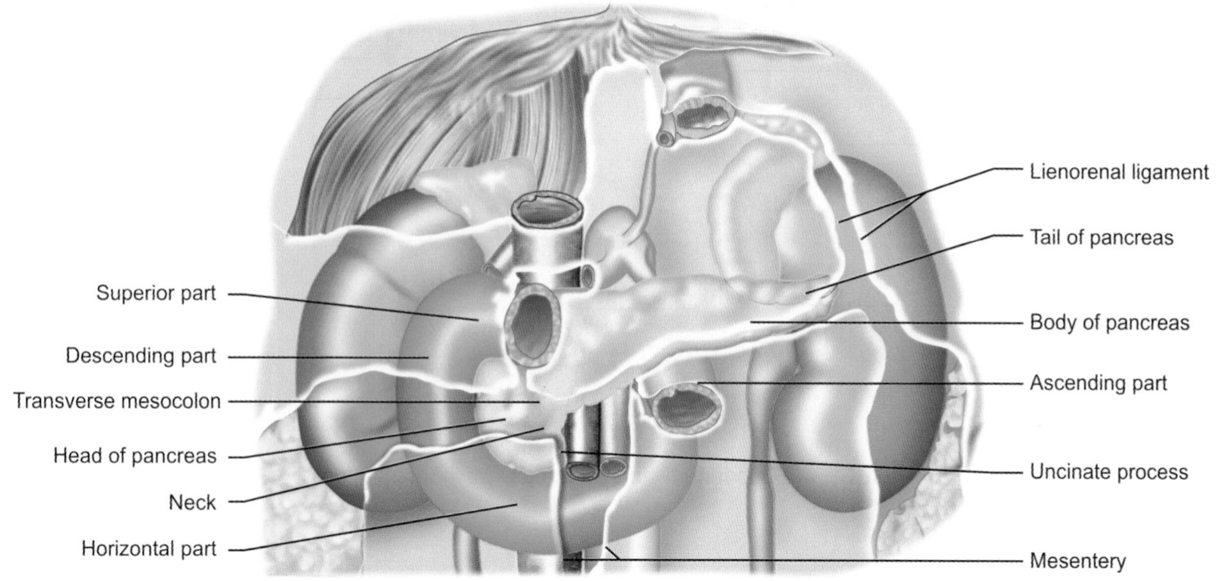

FIGURE 46 Duodenum and pancreas—parts and peritoneal coverings

DUODENUM AND PANCREAS (Fig. 46)

Duodenum is a retroperitoneal part of the gastrointestinal system. This is the first part of the small intestine. It extends between L1 to L3 vertebra. Identify this on the anterior aspect of the right kidney. It is a C shaped organ placed around the head of the pancreas. The pancreas is the gland associated with the digestive system. The duodenum and the pancreas together extend from the right kidney to the left kidney, across the posterior abdominal wall. Duodenum is generally described as having the superior, descending, horizontal and ascending parts. The pancreas is described as having the head, neck, body and tail.

Peritoneal coverings: Note that the first 2.5 cm at the beginning of the superior part is covered by the lesser omentum. The second part is crossed by the transverse mesocolon. The horizontal part is crossed by the beginning of the mesentery with the superior mesenteric vessels. The ascending part turns forward to join the jejunum.

The head of the pancreas snugly fits into the duodenum. It is crossed by the transverse mesocolon. The uncinate process of the head is crossed by the superior mesenteric vessels. The root of the transverse mesocolon is attached along the anterior border of the pancreas. The tail is covered by the lienorenal ligament of the peritoneum.

Duodenal Fossae (Fig. 47)

Pull the duodenum to the right and try to identify the fossae associated with this. Generally the peritoneum extending from the posterior aspect of the ascending part of the duodenum reaches the posterior abdominal wall in cresent shaped manner. These folds are limited on the left side by the inferior mesenteric vein. These are called superior, inferior and paraduodenal recesses. Sometimes you can pass a finger from the lateral side to the posterior aspect of the horizontal part of the duodenum. This is called the retroduodenal recess. These can be areas for internal hernias in the adult.

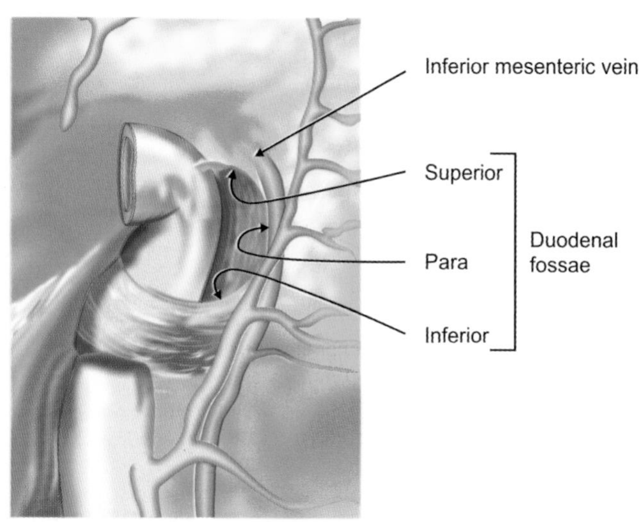

FIGURE 47 Duodenal fossae

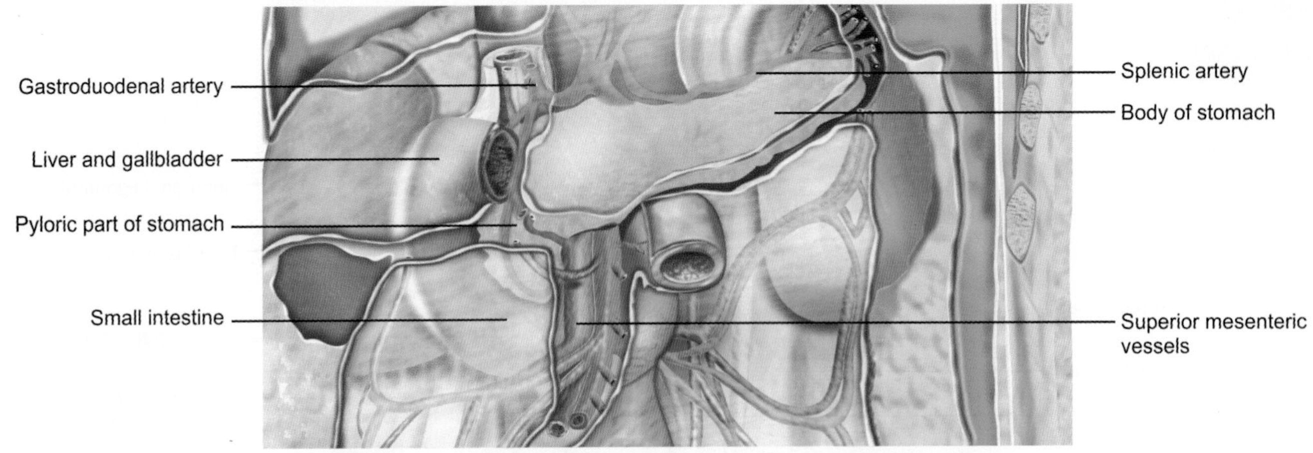

FIGURE 48 Duodenum and pancreas—anterior relations

Anterior Relations (Fig. 48)

The organs that were already removed form the anterior relations. Note that above the attachment of the transverse colon, the duodenum is related to the quadrate lobe of liver and the gallbladder. The remaining part of the duodenum is related to the small intestine except at the area where the superior mesenteric vessels cross it. The head, neck, body of the pancreas above the attachment of the transverse mesocolon, is related to the stomach. The head and neck are related to the pyloric part and the body is related to the body of the stomach. They are separated from the pancreas by the lesser sac of peritoneum. Below the attachment of the transverse mesocolon, it is related to the small intestine. The part of the pancreas which lies above the attachment of the transverse colon, is called the anterior surface and the part below is called the inferior surface. The superior border lies along the upper end of the anterior surface. The superior border is related to the beginning of the coeliac trunk, reidentify this. Note the elevation on the border here. It is called tuber omentale. The superior border along its total length is related to the splenic artery.

Dissection: Cut and remove the duodenum and pancreas enmass along with the superior mesenteric vessels, portal vein, the splenic artery, vein and inferior mesenteric vein. Carefully separate the organs from the deeper abdominal structures, and identify the portal vein and its tributaries.

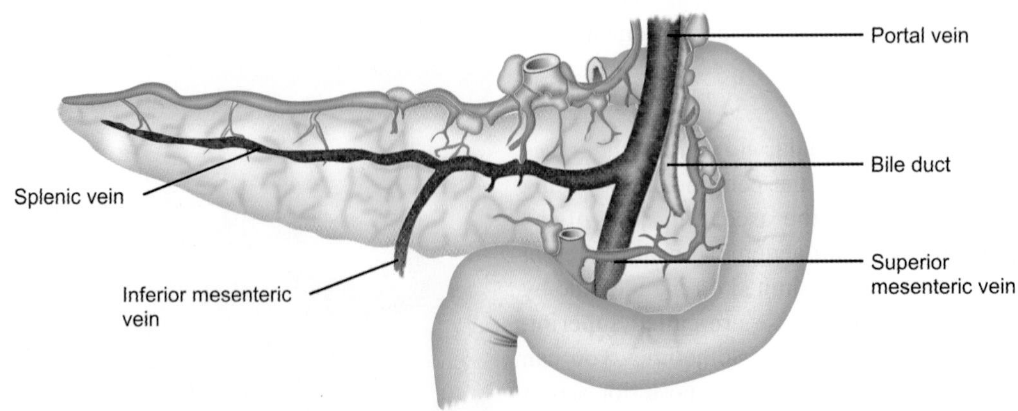

FIGURE 49 Portal vein and tributaries

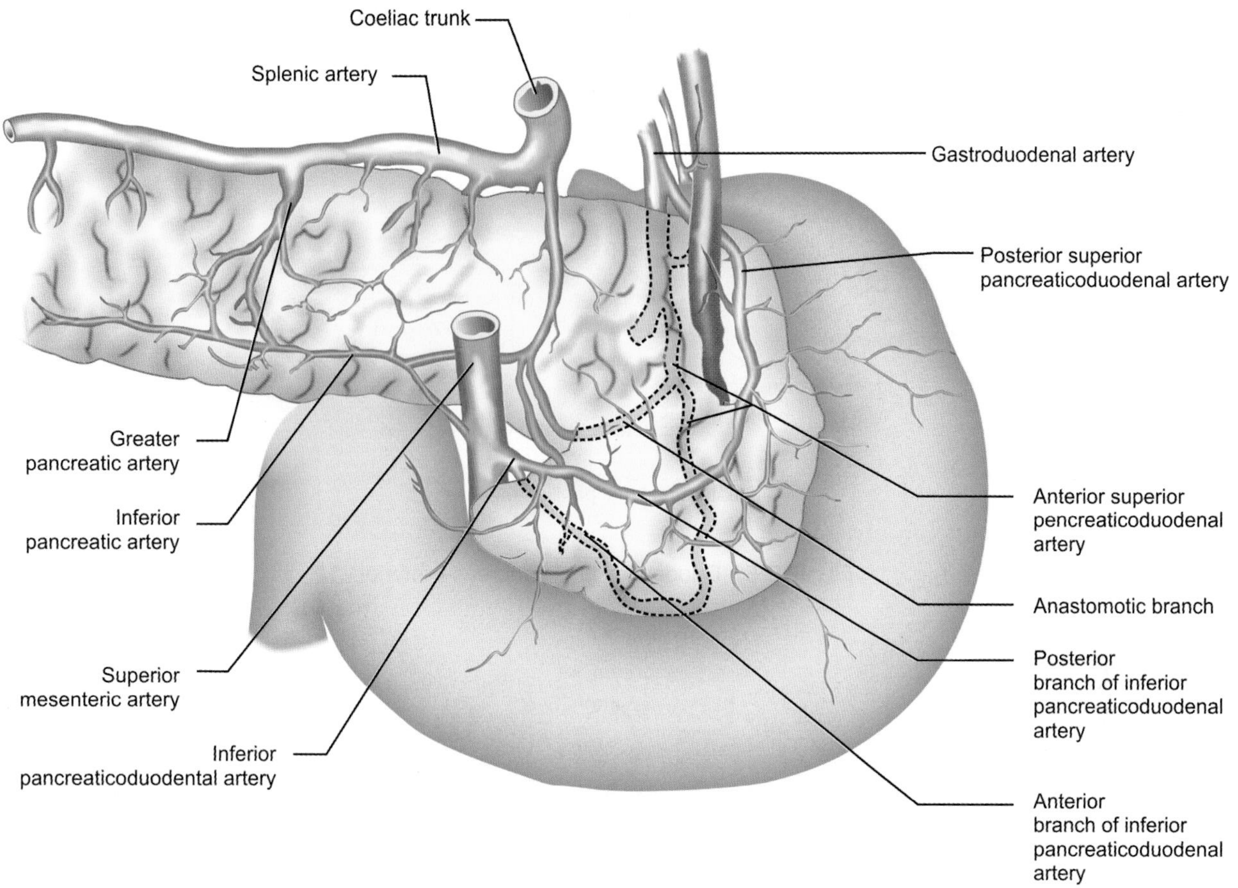

FIGURE 50 Duodenum and pancreas—posterior aspect—blood vessels

Portal Vein (Fig. 49)

The portal vein is the vein of drainage for the gastrointestinal tract. It brings the nutritive blood from the gastrointestinal tract to be stored in the liver. The inferior mesenteric vein which accompanies the artery drains blood from rectum, descending colon and transverse colon. This drains into the splenic vein. The superior mesenteric vein drains blood from the transverse colon, ascending colon, cecum and vermiform appendix. The splenic vein which drains the spleen also drains the pancreas and joins with the superior mesenteric vein behind the neck of the pancreas to form the portal vein. Trace these veins on the posterior aspect of the pancreas and trace it up into the lesser omentum.

Portal vein is an important topic. Study the vein from the textbook particularly the position of portosystemic anastomosis and its applied aspect.

Dissection: Remove the portal vein and it cleans the blood vessels supplying the duodenum and pancreas.

Blood Supply (Fig. 50)

Duodenum and head of the pancreas are supplied by the superior and inferior pancreaticoduodenal arteries. The ***superior pancreaticoduodenal artery*** is a branch of the gastroduodenal artery and ***inferior pancreaticoduodenal artery*** is a branch of the superior mesenteric artery. Identify their anterior and posterior branches in the gap between the pancreas and duodenum. Trace the branches of the ***splenic artery*** into the spleen. One of the splenic branches is big and is called ***major pancreatic artery***.

Dissection: Remove the blood vessels and dissect the bile duct, pancreatic ducts and the duodenal papillae.

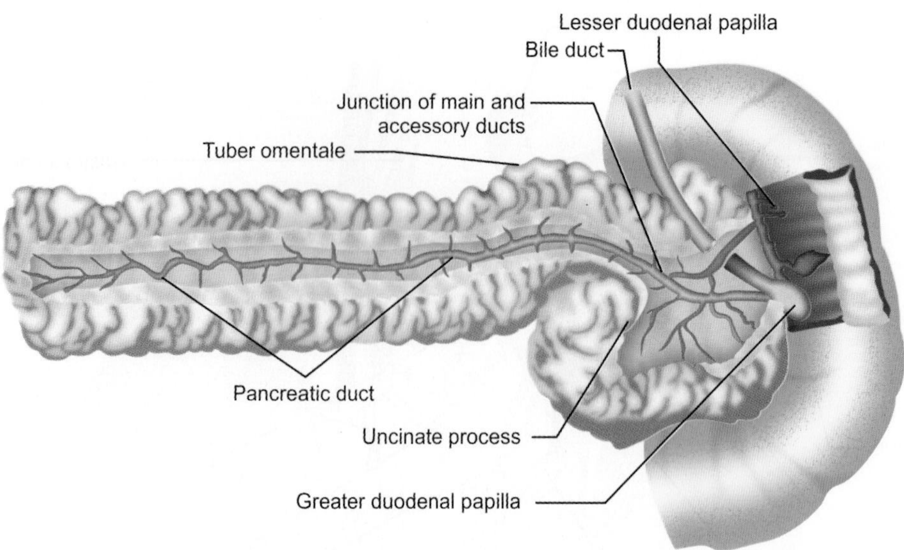

FIGURE 51 Duodenum and pancreas—interior

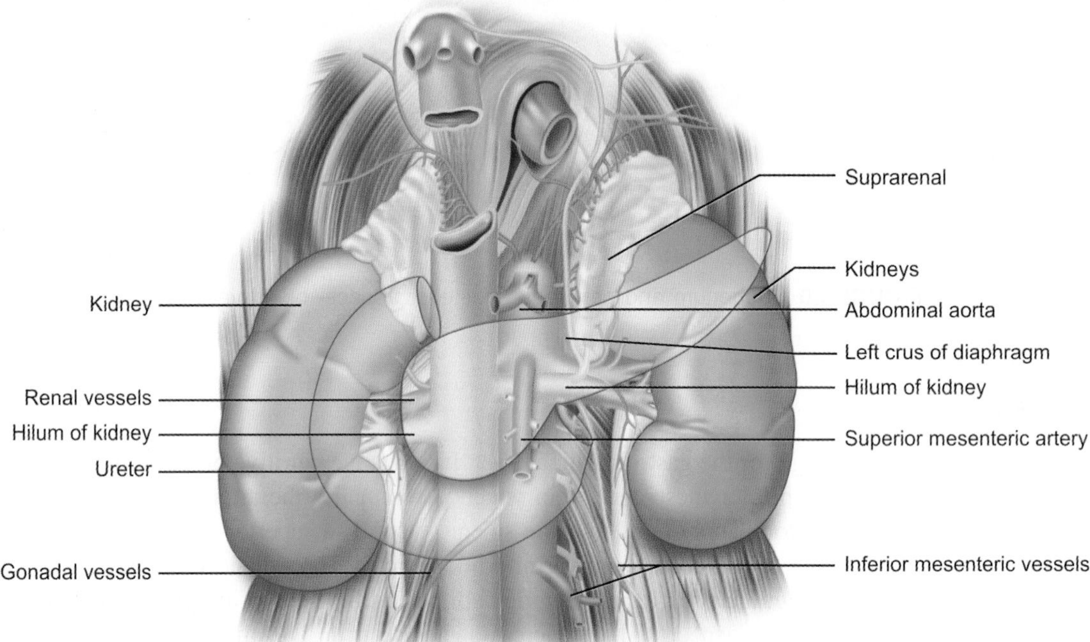

FIGURE 52 Duodenum and pancreas—posterior relations

Pancreatic Duct (Fig. 51)

Pancreas is a gland. It pours its secretion into the descending part of the duodenum along with the bile duct. Dissect through the pancreas and identify the Herringbone patterned pancreatic duct. Trace the bile duct in the groove between the duodenum and pancreas and see its union with the pancreatic duct. The combined part is called the hepatopancreatic ampulla of Vater, this passes through the thick wall of the duodenum to empty into it.

Interior of duodenum: Make a window dissection to identify the interior. Folds of the mucous membrane seen here are called the plicae circularis. Identify the two prominent papillae, the lower ***major duodenal papilla,*** formed by the union of the bile duct and the pancreatic duct, the ***minor duodenal papilla*** draining the head of the pancreas. You can see the submucosa clearly by removing the mucosa. It is studded with ***Brunner's gland.*** This is better seen under microscope. The muscle layer is outer circular and inner longitudinal layers.

Duodenum and Pancreas Posterior Relations (Fig. 52)

Identify the structures on the posterior abdominal wall, on which the duodenum and pancreas were resting. From right to left see the kidney, renal vessels entering the hilum of the kidney, abdominal aorta with its superior mesenteric artery, gonadal arteries and inferior mesenteric artery, left crus of diaphragm, left suprarenal and the left kidney.

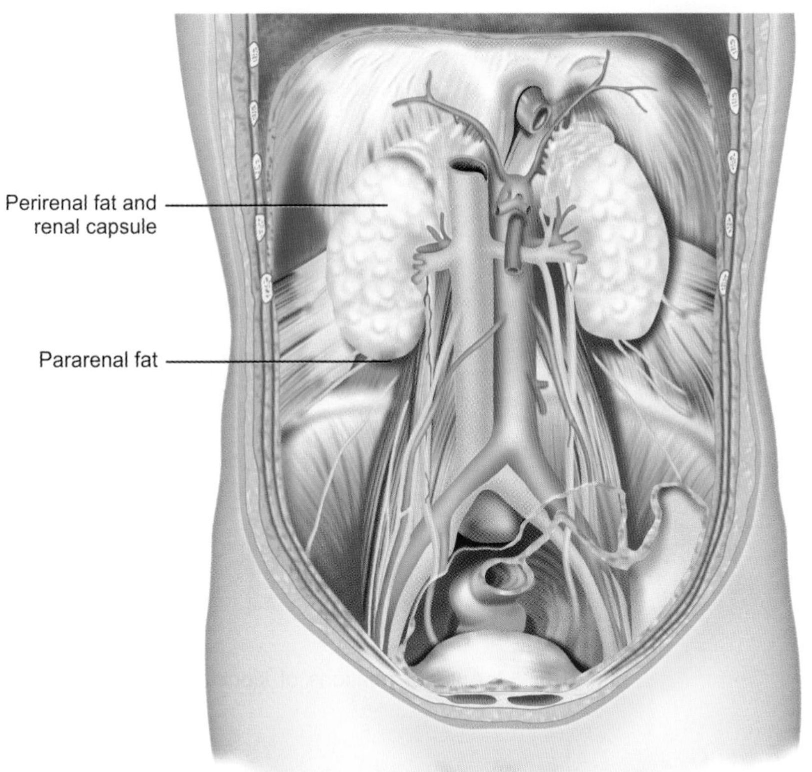

FIGURE 53 Renal fasciae

Renal Fasciae (Fig. 53)

The suprarenal glands, the kidneys and the ureter along with the major blood vessels occupy the position in front of the posterior abdominal wall. The kidney and the suprarenal are enclosed in a thick fascia. This is called ***renal fascia***. The kidney is held in position by thick fat, called the ***perirenal fat***. This is covered by a thin sheet of connective tissue called the ***renal capsule***. There is a good amount of fat deep to the kidney, called the ***pararenal fat***. All the above fasciae along with the intra-abdominal pressure help to retain the kidney in position.

Dissection: Look at the fat around the kidney. Touch it and realize that it is a thick identifiable layer. Note that it is covered by a thin sheet of fascia. It is the renal capsule. The fat deep to it is the perirenal fat. Remove the fat carefully and note the renal fascia. Note that superiorly it encloses suprarenal gland, medially continuous with the blood vessels and laterally merges with the psoas fascia. Slit it along the lateral border of the kidney lift the kidney and note the pararenal fat.

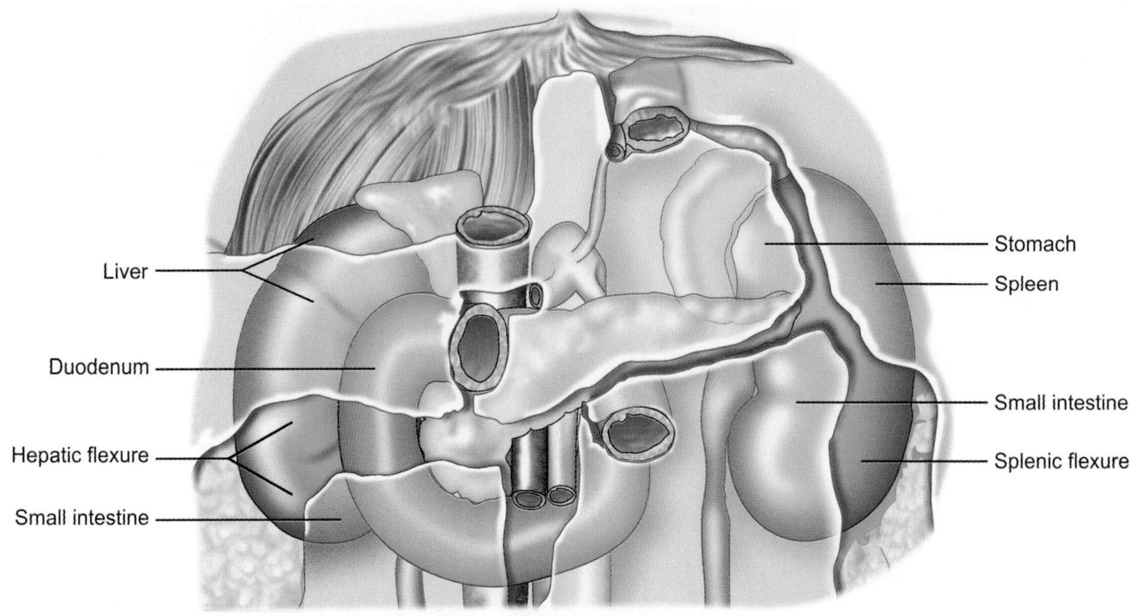

FIGURE 54 Anterior relations of kidney

KIDNEY, SUPRARENAL AND BLOOD VESSELS (Figs 54 and 55)

KIDNEY

The kidneys are bean-shaped organs of the urinary system. Note that it extends from the 12th thoracic vertebra to 3rd lumbar vertebra. The upper poles are nearer to the midline than the lower poles. They are placed on the sloping surface of the vertebral column infront of the posterior abdominal muscles. The hilum of the kidney lies opposite to the L1 vertebra.

Anterior Relations of Kidneys

All these organs in front of the kidney are already removed. Look at the diagram and recollect your memory. Right kidney is directly related to the ***hepatic flexure*** of colon in its middle. Superiorly it is related to the ***liver*** inferiorly to the ***small intestine*** and near the hilum to the ***duodenum*** separated by the peritoneum. The left kidney is directly related to the ***splenic flexure*** and ***pancreas***, and is separated by peritoneum from the ***stomach and small intestine***.

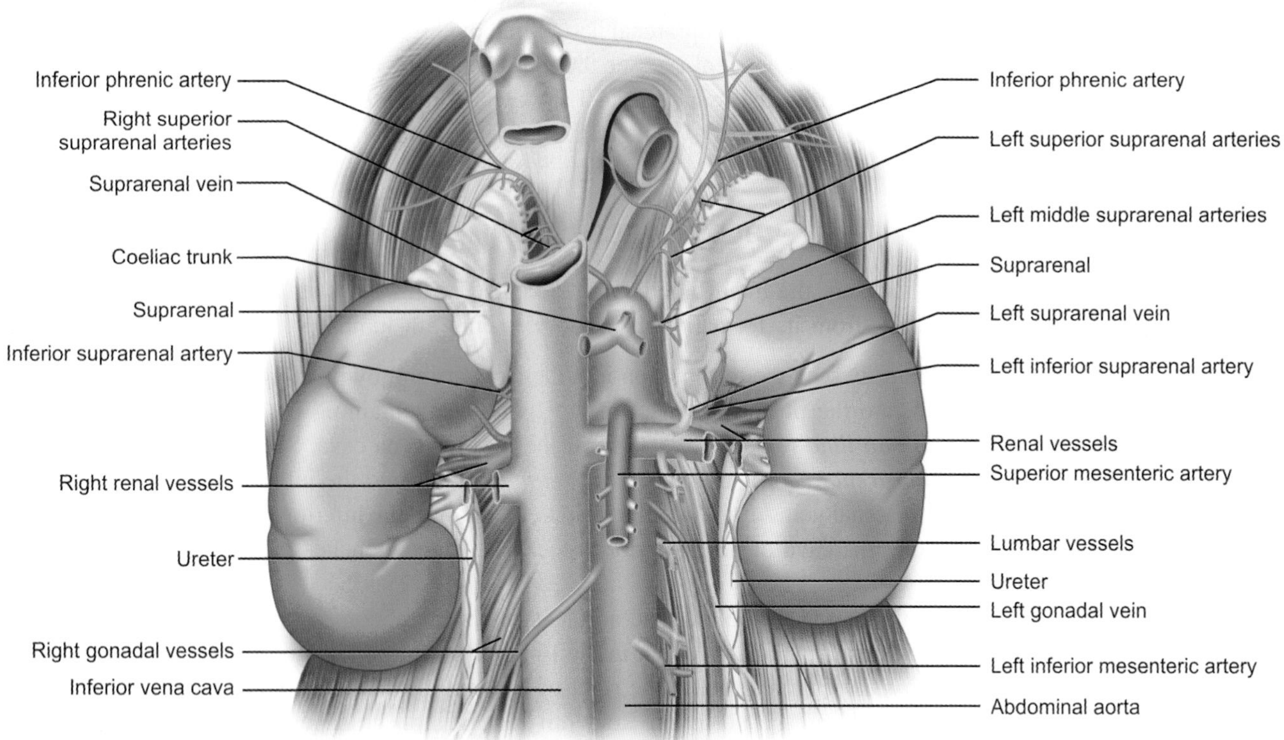

FIGURE 55 Kidney, suprarenal and blood vessels

Blood Vessels

The renal vein is superficial in position compared to the renal artery. Identify this, cut a small segment of the vein to appreciate the renal artery. The kidney is supplied by the renal artery. It is given off at the level of L1 from the abdominal aorta. Note that each renal artery divides into two divisions—an anterior division infront of the ureter and a posterior division behind the ureter. The anterior division divides into four branches as it enters into the kidney. The posterior division is a single branch. Like the lung and the liver, the kidney also can be divided into segments, made use in renal surgery. There can be accessory renal arteries given off directly from the abdominal aorta. When present it supplies the inferior segment. It crosses in front of the ureter.

URETER

The ureter is a muscular tube connecting the kidney to the bladder. It lies over the musculature of the posterior abdominal wall, crosses the pelvic brim enters the pelvis to reach the urinary bladder. The vessels which reach the gut and gonads cross the ureters.

Blood supply: The ureter is supplied by branches from the renal artery, gonadal artery and direct branch from the abdominal aorta, though not very constant.

SUPRARENAL

The suprarenal glands are endocrine glands located on the superior pole of the kidney. Identify them.
Right suprarenal is triangular in shape, located on the superior border of the right kidney. Slit the renal fascia and note that the renal capsule encloses the kidney and the suprarenal independently.

Relations: Note that the ***inferior vena cava*** has grooved the anteromedial aspect of the right suprarenal, the remaining part of the anterior surface is related to the bare area of the ***liver***. Its base lies on the ***kidney*** and its posterior surface lies on the ***diaphragm***. Along the medial border see the ***coeliac ganglion*** and the ***inferior phrenic artery***.

Left suprarenal gland: It is semilunar in shape. It is placed along the medial border of the left kidney.

Relations: Its base lies on the ***kidney,*** anterior surface is related to ***stomach*** and ***pancreas,*** posterior surface is related to the ***diaphragm,*** and medial border is related to the ***coeliac ganglion*** and the ***inferior phrenic artery***.

Blood supply: The suprarenal glands are far bigger in size during development and have a rich blood supply. Even in the adult life though the branches are small in size the suprarenal is supplied by three arteries. Identify the main suprarenal artery from the abdominal aorta, given off at the level of L2. See the inferior phrenic artery gives off number of branches to the suprarenal. The third branch arises from the renal artery. The venous drainage is by only one vein, leaving the center of the anterior aspect of the gland. Note that the right suprarenal vein drains into the inferior vena cava and the left suprarenal vein drains into the renal vein.

BLOOD VESSELS

Inferior vena cava and abdominal aorta are the main blood vessels located in this region to supply all the abdominal organs. Identify the inferior vena cava from its formation at the level of the 5th lumbar vertebra. Trace it up.

The inferior vena cava: You had already seen the termination into the right atrium, by piercing through the diaphragm. Its upper part is almost embedded into the posterior aspect of the liver. The remaining part lies to the right of the abdominal aorta. Note the ***two common iliac veins*** joining to form the inferior vena cava. See the ***right gonadal vein, right and left renal veins, right suprarenal vein*** and ***the phrenic veins*** draining into the inferior vena cava. Note also that the left gonadal vein and the suprarenal veins drain into the renal vein, not into the inferior vena cava. The ***segmental lumbar veins*** drain into the inferior vena cava on its posterior aspect. The right branches pass behind the abdominal aorta.

The abdominal aorta is the continuation of the thoracic aorta. It enters the abdomen through the median arcuate ligament at the level of 12th thoracic vertebra. It runs down in the midline up to the level of L4 where it divides into two common iliac arteries. At the division it is slightly to the right of the midline. The abdominal aorta gives off three sets of branches—the ventral, the lateral and the posterior. Reidentify the ventral branches.

The coeliac trunk at the level of T12, the **superior mesenteric** at the level of L1 and the **inferior mesenteric** at the level of L3, these supply the foregut, midgut and the hindgut correspondingly. See the lateral branches, the ***inferior phrenic artery,*** the ***suprarenal,*** the ***renal*** and the ***gonadal arteries***. Trace the inferior phrenic artery to the diaphragm. The suprarenal artery is given at the level of L1 vertebra, the renal artery is given off at the level of L1 vertebra, the gonadal artery is given off at the level of L2 vertebra. They supply the organs of their name. These organs are located laterally in the abdomen. Pull the aorta forwards, see the branches given off from its posterior aspect. These are ***four lumbar arteries***, and a ***median sacral artery***. The lumbar arteries move laterally, enter the wall and supply the musculature. See the median sacral artery from the posterior aspect of the aorta in the midline. It descends down to the sacrum. It supplies the area on either side.

The blood vessels are surrounded by the sympathetic plexus of nerves. It is contributed by the splanchnic nerves from the sympathetic chain.

***Relations*:** Note that the pancreas, third part of duodenum, the mesentery and the small intestine (which were removed) lie in front of the big vessels.

Note that the renal vein crosses infront of the abdominal aorta. The left suprarenal vein and the gonadal vein drain into the renal vein. The lumbar veins reach the inferior vena cava behind the abdominal aorta. They do so as these are systemic veins draining the body wall. Note that the gonadal artery of the right side crosses the inferior vena cava to reach the right gonad. Note that the right lumbar veins reach the varieties behind the inferior vena cava.

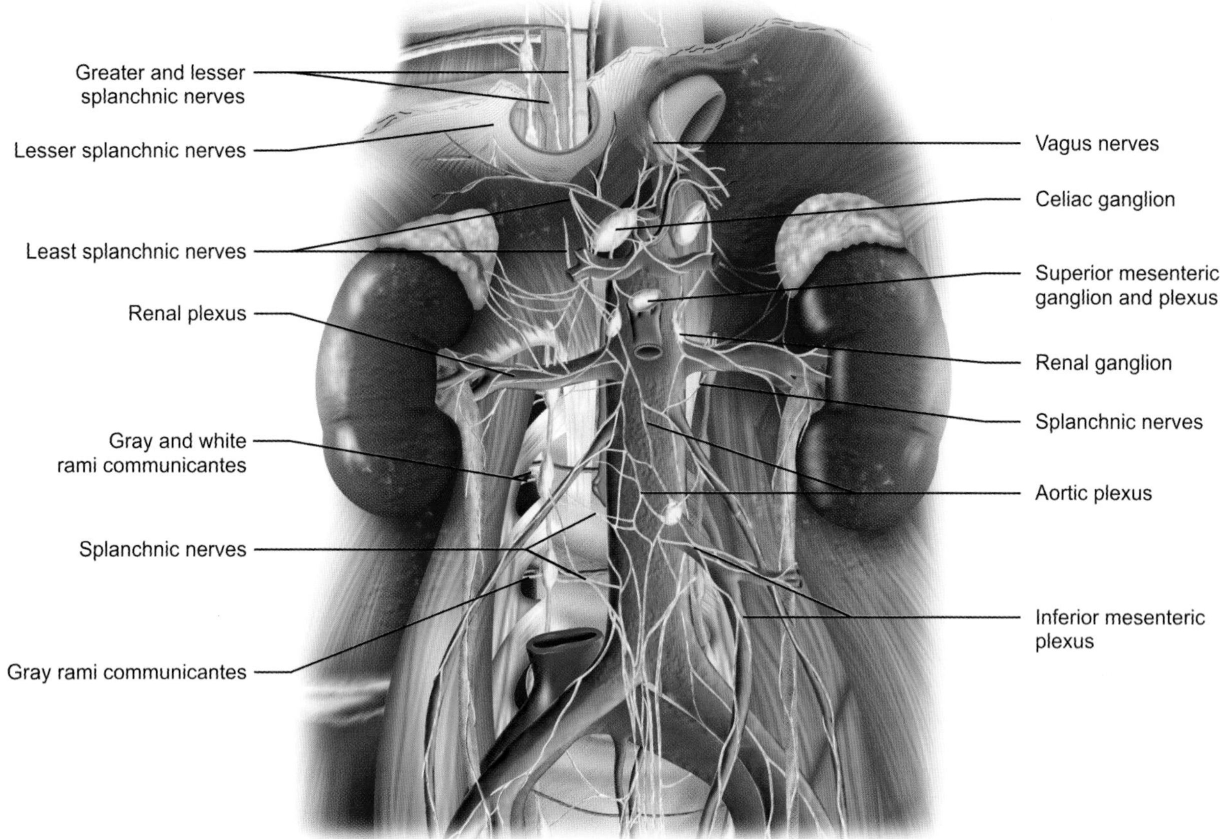

FIGURE 56 Autonomic nerve plexuses

AUTONOMIC NERVE PLEXUSES (Fig. 56)

Dissection: Cut the inferior vena cava at its lower end near its formation. Cut off its tributaries, the right suprarenal vein, the right and left renal veins, the right gonadal vein and the lumbar veins and remove the inferior vena cava. Note the vein arising from the posterior aspect of the inferior vena cava. It is the beginning of the azygos vein. Clean the sympathetic chains and trace the branches arising from them. Identify the autonomic plexuses on the aorta and its branches.

The vagal nerves: Identify the vagal trunks on the esophagus and trace their contribution to the coeliac ganglion. This is the parasympathetic contribution to the vascular plexus. Relatively it is a very small contribution compared to the sympathetic contribution.

Sympathetic chain: Note the right sympathetic chain deep to the inferior vena cava. Identify the ganglia and the intermittent sympathetic chain. The sympathetic chain on the left side lies to the left of the aorta.

Rami communicantes: Note that the upper two ganglia are connected to the spinal nerves by both gray and white rami communicantes. The ***white rami communicantes*** are preganglionic fibres from the spinal nerves to the sympathetic ganglia. In the lower two ganglia they are connected by only ***gray ramus communicantes***. These are the postganglionic fibres. They accompany the spinal nerves, supply vasoconstrictor fibres to the peripheral blood vessels, motor fibres to arrectores pilorum and secretomotor fibres to sweat glands in the skin.

Splanchnic nerves: From each ganglion one or two splanchnic nerves arise from the medial side and contribute to the vascular plexus. These are postganglionic fibres.

The vascular plexus here has prevertebral sympathetic ganglia and plexuses accompanying the blood vessels. All these are vasomotor to the blood vessels.

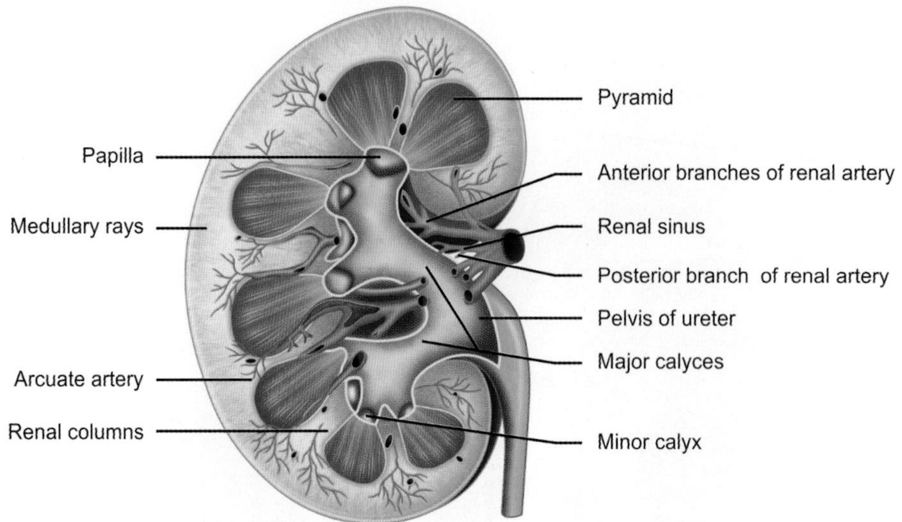

FIGURE 57 Kidney interior

Coeliac ganglion: Identify this definitive, flat irregularly shaped, spider like ganglion on either side of the coeliac artery. Trace the greater and lesser splanchnic nerves arising in the thoracic sympathetic ganglia. They pierce through the crura of the diaphragm to reach the coeliac ganglia.

Renal ganglion: These are small ganglia on either side of the aorta just above the renal arteries. They receive the least splanchnic nerve from the 12th sympathetic ganglion.

Superior mesenteric and inferior mesenteric ganglia are condensation of cell bodies near the respective arteries.

Plexuses: Aortic, renal, coeliac, superior mesenteric, inferior mesenteric plexuses are the names given to the plexuses around the respective arteries. The hypogastric plexus descends down over the pelvic brim.

Dissection: Cut the renal arteries near the abdominal aorta and the ureter near the pelvic brim and remove the kidney and ureter out of the body. Cut the kidney longitudinally through its center and continue the cut into the ureter, see its interior. Peel the adventitia of the ureter and its musculature.

Kidney Interior (Fig. 57)

Put your fingers around the ureter into the kidney. You realize that it is in a space, called ***renal sinus***. Renal sinus lodges the ***pelvis of ureter***, blood vessels, lymphatics and nerves. See the upper end of the ureter. It is expanded and is called pelvis of the ureter. The pelvis divides into two to three divisions, called the ***major calyces***. Each major calyx divides into three to four ***minor calyces***. Each minor calyx receives two to three ***papillae***. Each papilla is a pyramidal shaped projection, which is cribriform in nature. These are the openings of the collecting tubes which pour the urine formed in the nephron to the pelvis of the ureter.

The part covering the calyces is called the ***medulla***. Note the papilla expands into the medulla as the ***pyramid***. It consists of the loops of Henle and the collecting tubes. The area between the pyramids is filled with the ***renal columns***. These are the extensions of the cortical tissue into the medulla.

The ***cortex*** is that part which covers the medulla. This is filled with glomeruli, proximal and distal convoluted tubules of the nephron. Note that there are white lines extending into the cortex. These are the ***medullary rays***, made up of the collecting tubules of the medulla extending into the cortex. The capsule covers the cortex. Push it and see the sheet of connective tissue. The renal pyramid with its covering cortex constitutes a lobe of the kidney.

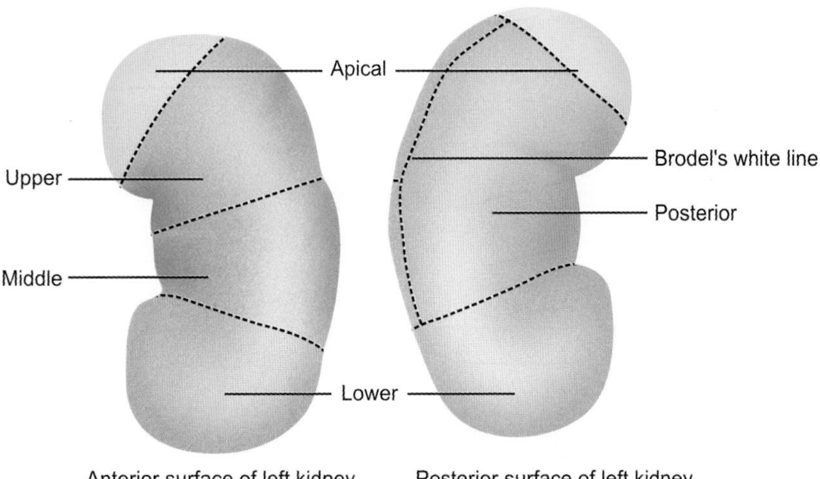

FIGURE 58 Renal segments

Renal Segments (Fig. 58)

These are vascular segments. Trace the renal artery into the renal sinus of the kidney. Note that it divides into four anterior and one posterior segmental arteries. Put the kidney into a mild solution of hydrogen peroxide for a day, and slowly remove the soft tissue along the pathway of the blood vessels. Identify the ***apical***, ***upper***, ***middle*** and ***lower segments***. These segments extend even on to the posterior aspect. The ***posterior segment*** occupies a central area on the posterior aspect. Each segmental artery divides into lobar and interlobar arteries. The interlobar arteries give rise to the radially running arcuate arteries, running between the cortex and medulla. See that the veins accompany the arteries. There is no anastomosis between the anterior and posterior segments. It is called the Brodels' white line. This is made use by the surgeon.

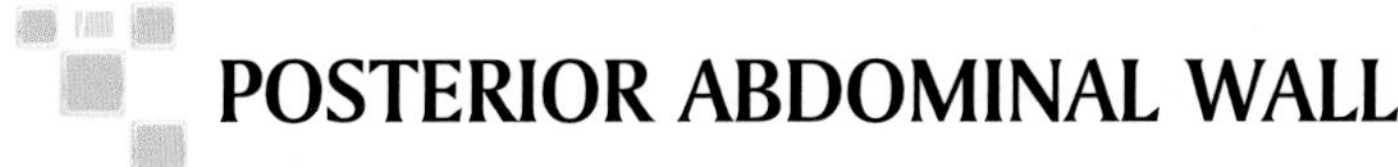

POSTERIOR ABDOMINAL WALL

MUSCLES AND NERVES (Fig. 59)

Dissection: Clean all the connective tissue and fat from the posterior abdominal wall and identify the structures. Cut and remove the diaphragm between the T12 and L4 vertebrae.

Diaphragm: You have seen the costal and sternal origins of the muscle. Now you see the lumbar part of the origin. ***Right crus***—see this arising from the ventral aspects of the upper three lumbar vertebrae. This is tendinous at its origin. Trace these fibres towards its insertion to the central tendon. Identify the fibres looping around the esophagus. ***Left crus***—see this arising from the ventral aspects of the upper two lumbar vertebrae. From ***median arcuate ligament***—identify the median arcuate ligament formed by the union of right and left crura infront of the abdominal aorta. From ***medial arcuate ligament***—identify the upper end of the psoas fascia which is thickened up to form a ligament. From ***lateral arcuate ligament***—this is the upper thickened part of the fascia over the quadratus lumborum muscle. The diaphragm takes origin from all the above ligaments.

Structures passing deep to the diaphragm: ***Detach the diaphragm from the above origins and see the following structures.*** The greater, lesser and least splanchnic nerves—they reach the abdomen to join the autonomic plexus either passing through the muscle or deep to the muscle.

Aortic opening: Lift the aorta and see the ***cisterna chyli,*** the beginning of the thoracic duct. It is 5 cm long, 4 cm wide white structure lying between the aorta and vertebral column. You trace this down from the thorax, where you have already identified this. It receives the intestinal trunk and two lumbar trunks. The ***ascending lumbar vein*** originates from the back of the renal vein, joins with the subcostal vein to form the azygos vein.

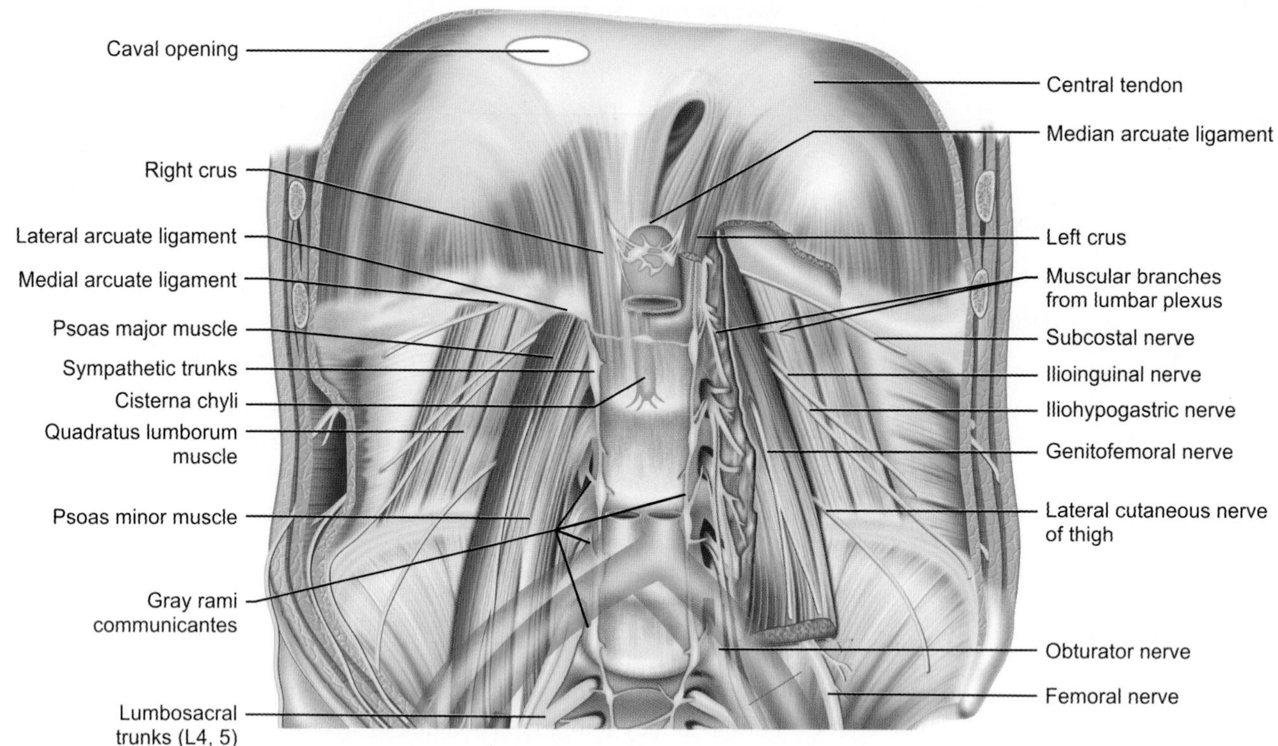

FIGURE 59 Posterior abdominal wall muscles and nerves

Azygos vein: It is a communication between the superior vena cava and the inferior vena cava. This lies lateral to the cisterna chyli and the aorta in the aortic opening.

Esophageal opening: See that esophagus is clasped in the fibres of the right crus of the diaphragm. The ***right and left vagus nerves*** accompany the esophagus.

Sympathetic trunk: Extends from the cervical level to the coccygeal level. See its entrance into the abdomen deep to the medial arcuate ligament.

Subcostal nerve: See this nerve deep to the lateral arcuate ligament.

Psoas major muscle: It is a muscle of the lower limb. It migrates, up into the abdomen for its origin. It extends from T12 vertebra to the 5th lumbar vertebra. See its slips arising from the lateral aspects of the bodies and the anterior aspects of the transverse processes. ***Cut the left crus to see this.*** Note the fibrotendinous arches formed over the lumbar blood vessels between the slips of origin. They are at the level of the intervertebral discs. It is supplied by the lumbar nerves. It is a powerful flexor and a medial rotator of the thigh. It is inserted into the lesser trochanter of the femur along with the iliacus.

Psoas minor muscle: Many a times there is an extra slip of origin from T12 and L1 vertebrae. When it is present it is called psoas minor and gets attached to the pelvic brim in its middle.

Quadratus lumborum muscle: See this quadrilateral muscle lateral to the psoas major muscle. See its origin from the iliolumbar ligament and the inner segment of the iliac crest. It is supplied by subcostal and first three lumbar nerves. It is a lateral rotator of the lumbar part of the vertebral column, flexes the body when acting together and also is a fixator of the 12th rib in deep inspiration.

Iliacus muscle: It is a muscle of the lower limb. Identify its origin from the iliac fossa and ala of the sacrum. It joins with the psoas major and gets inserted into the lesser trochanter of the femur. It is supplied by the femoral nerve.

Lumbar plexus: It is formed by the ventral rami of L1 to L4 nerves. The lumbar nerves as they emerge from the intervertebral foramina enter the psoas major muscle. They form a plexus within the substance of the muscle and emerge out around the periphery of the muscle. This plexus supplies the lateral aspect of the abdomen and ventral and medial aspect of the thigh.

Dissection: Slit the muscle fibres vertically and try to identify the nerves. Locate the nerves near the outer border of the psoas major muscle and trace them to their emergence from the ventral roots.

Iliohypogastric nerve: Locate this nerve immediately below the medial arcuate ligament. Trace it distally across the quadratus lumborum muscle to enter into the transversus abdominis muscle. Trace it proximally to L1 nerve. This is a mixed nerve. It supplies the lateral musculature and becomes cutaneous to the lower lateral skin of the abdomen.

Ilioinguinal nerve: Trace this nerve running parallel and below the ilioinguinal nerve. Trace it distally across the quadratus lumborum to cross the iliac crest to enter into the transversus abdominis. Trace it proximally to the L1 ventral ramus. This is a mixed nerve. It supplies the lateral musculature and becomes cutaneous to the lower lateral skin of the abdomen.

Lateral cutaneous of thigh: Trace this nerve at the lateral border of the psoas major muscle near the iliac crest. Trace it forwards across the iliacus muscle deep to the inguinal ligament, to reach the front of the thigh. This is a sensory nerve to supply the lateral skin of the thigh. Trace it proximally to ventral roots.

Genitofemoral nerve: Identify this nerve on the ventral aspect of the psoas major muscle. It runs longitudinally on the muscle. Trace it distally and note that the genital branch enters the deep inguinal ring, whereas the femoral nerve leaves the abdomen under cover of the inguinal ligament, to reach the thigh.

Femoral nerve: Locate this nerve between the iliacus and psoas major muscle.

Trace it down into the thigh.

Obturator nerve: Identify this nerve medial to the psoas major muscle. Trace it into the pelvis where it leaves through the obturator canal.

Lumbar plexus: It is formed by the ventral rami of L1 to L4 nerves. The lumbar nerves as they emerge from the intervertebral foramina enter the psoas major muscle. They form a plexus within the substance of the muscle and emerge out around the periphery of the muscle. This plexus supplies the lateral aspect of the abdomen and ventral and medial aspect of the thigh.

Dissection: Slit the muscle fibres vertically and try to identify the nerves. Locate the nerves near the outer border of the psoas major muscle and trace them to their emergence from the muscle.

Iliohypogastric nerve: Locate this nerve immediately below the medial arcuate ligament. Trace it distally across the quadratus lumborum muscle to enter into the transversus abdominis muscle. Trace it proximally to L1 nerve. This is a mixed nerve. It supplies the lateral musculature and becomes cutaneous to the lower lateral skin of the abdomen.

Ilioinguinal nerve: Trace this nerve running parallel and below the iliohypogastric nerve. Trace it distally across the quadratus lumborum to cross the iliac crest to enter into the transversus abdominis. Trace it proximally to the L1 ventral ramus. This is a mixed nerve. It supplies the lateral musculature and becomes cutaneous to the lower lateral skin of the abdomen.

Lateral cutaneous of thigh: Trace this nerve at the lateral border of the psoas major muscle near the iliac crest. Trace it towards across the iliacus muscle deep to the inguinal ligament to reach the front of the thigh. This is a sensory nerve to supply the lateral skin of the thigh. Trace it proximally to ventral roots.

Genitofemoral nerve: Identify this nerve on the ventral aspect of the psoas major muscle. It runs longitudinally on the muscle. Trace it distally and note that the genital branch enters the deep inguinal ring whereas the femoral branch leaves the abdomen under cover of the inguinal ligament to reach the thigh.

Femoral nerve: Locate this nerve between the iliacus and psoas major muscle.

Trace it down into the thigh.

Obturator nerve: Identify this nerve medial to the psoas major muscle. Trace it into the pelvis where it leaves through the obturator canal.

CHAPTER 5

PELVIS AND PERINEUM

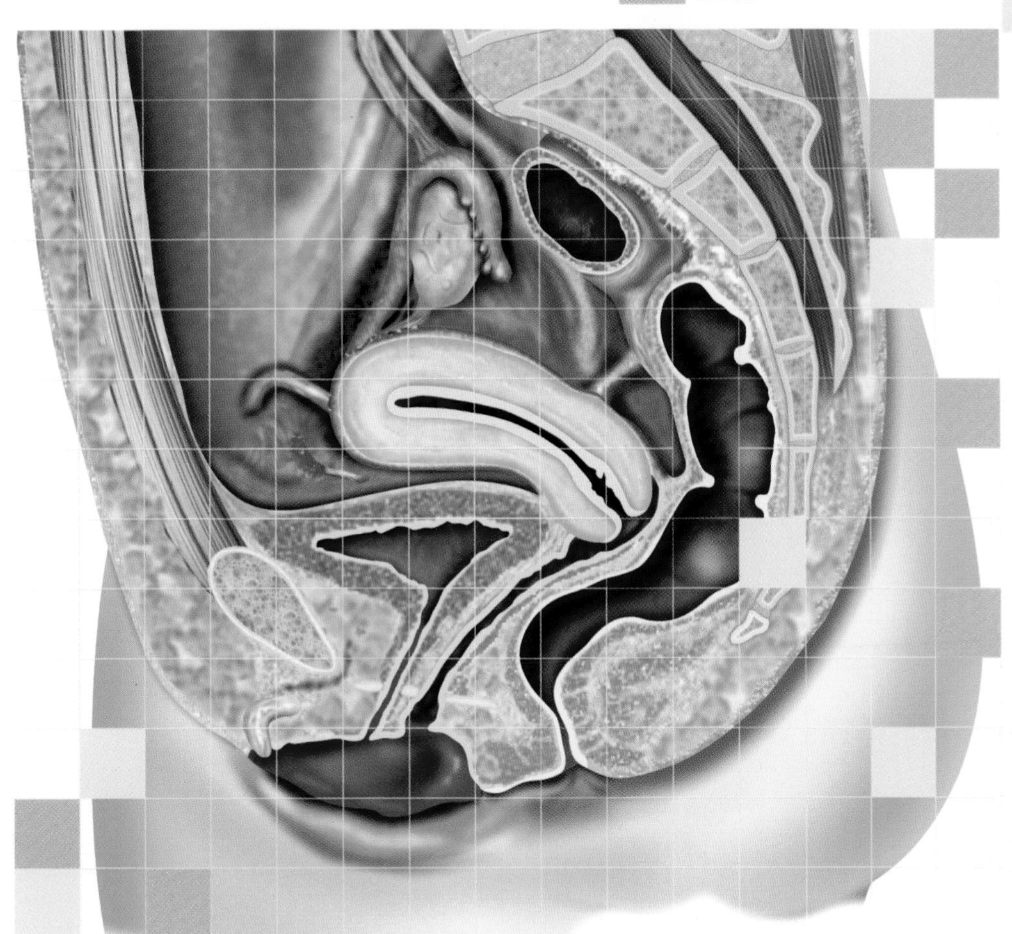

PELVIS

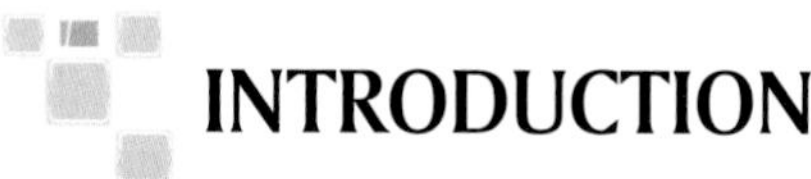

INTRODUCTION

The bony pelvis is made up of two hip bones and a central sacrum. The sacral canal lodges the sacral nerves. The sacrum gives attachment to the erector spinae group of muscles posteriorly. The hip bones give attachment to muscles of the lower limb externally and pelvic musculature internally.

Pelvic cavity is a continuation of the abdominal cavity. It is supported by the bony pelvis, which presents two parts—the true and false pelvis. The false pelvis supports the lower abdominal viscera, whereas the true pelvis lodges the pelvic organs of the urogenital system and the rectum and anal canal of the gastrointestinal tract. Inferiorly the pelvic cavity is limited by the pelvic diaphragm. The part between the pelvic diaphragm and the skin is called perineum. It has the last parts of urogenital and gastrointestinal tract. They open to the exterior.

SKELETON

BONY PELVIS

Go to an articulated skeleton and look at the position and the tilt of the pelvis in the body. Note that the basin like pelvis faces forwards and not upwards. The ischiopubic ramus faces downwards not forwards. The ischial tuberosity faces downwards and backwards. The anterior superior iliac spine and the pubic tubercle are in the same vertical plane.

Take a pelvis preferably with ligaments and note the following **(Fig. 1).**

The bony pelvis is made up of ***two hip bones***—right and left and the ***sacrum*** and ***coccyx*** at the back. The sacrum and coccyx are mostly united in the older individuals, though in young they articulate by a secondary cartilaginous joint like the other vertebrae. The hip bone articulates posteriorly with two to three pieces of sacrum called the alae of the sacrum. This is the ***sacroiliac joint***. The articulation is a plane synovial joint. The two hip bones articulate anteriorly by a secondary cartilaginous joint called ***pubic symphysis***. Minimal movement takes place in these joints. During pregnancy and delivery, in female the hormones soften the ligaments.

Note that the sacrum is made, up of ***five sacral vertebrae,*** the ***anterior*** and ***posterior sacral foraminae.*** The anterior sacral foraminae transmit the anterior primary rami of the sacral nerves which participate in the formation of lumbosacral plexus. Posterior sacral foraminae transmit the dorsal rami of the same nerves. One or two coccygeal nerves may come out through the coccyx. The two hip bones present three parts—the ilium is expanded and forms ***iliac fossa.*** This forms the false pelvis and supports the abdominal viscera. ***Inlet of pelvis*** is formed by the ***sacral promontory, alae of the sacrum, arcuate line, iliopubic eminence, pecten pubis, pubic tubercle, pubic crest and the pubic symphysis.***

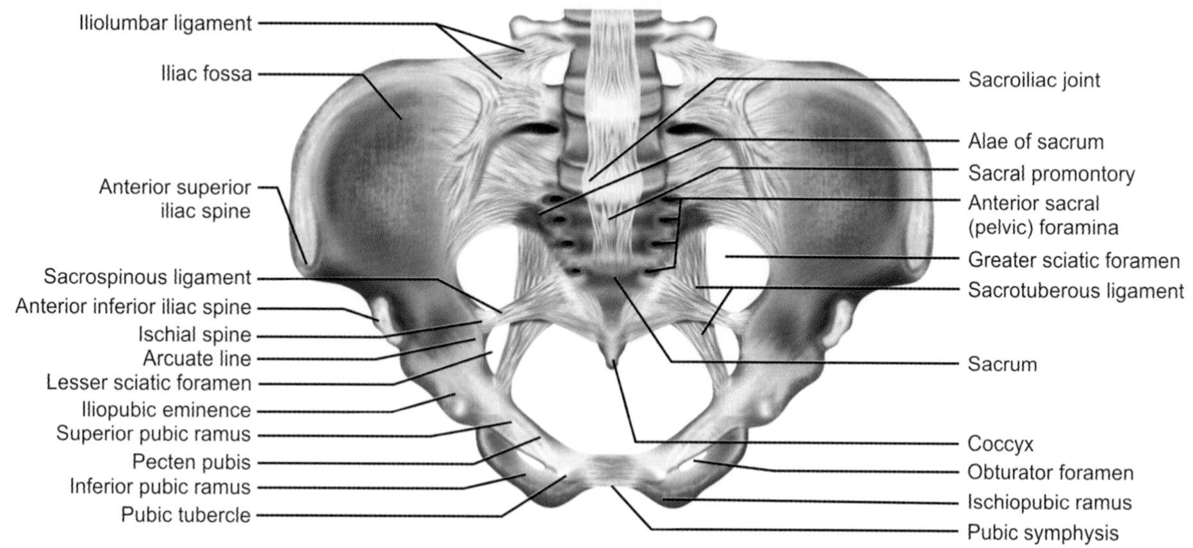

FIGURE 1 Bony pelvis

Ischiopubic ramus is widely separated and constitutes the urogenital region of the perineum. It lodges the external openings of the urinary and genital organs.

Obturator foramen is a big gap in the bony pelvis, but is closed by the obturator membrane in the living, except for a small opening superomedially. This permits the obturator artery and nerve. It gives attachment to muscles on either side. The sacrotuberous and sacrospinous ligaments convert the greater and lesser sciatic notches into ***greater and lesser sciatic foraminae. Sacrotuberous ligament*** extends from sacrum to the ischial tuberosity. The ***sacrospinous ligament*** extends from the ischial spine to the last piece of sacrum and the coccyx. The gap between the two sacrotuberous ligaments constitute the anal part of the perineum and lodge the anal canal and the anus.

A detailed study of the bony pelvis with the differences between the male and female pelvis and metric measurements of the female pelvis is to be undertaken separately.

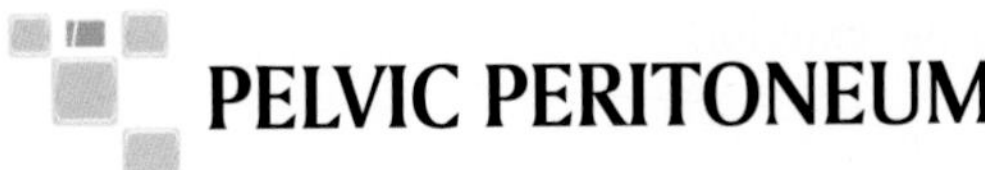

PELVIC PERITONEUM

Pelvic peritoneum is the continuation of the peritoneum of the abdomen and covers the superior surface of all the pelvic organs and dips in between them. It should be studied both anteroposteriorly, as well as laterally.

See the transverse as well as the sagittal section of the pelvis and identify the location of the organs. Note the bladder behind the pubic symphysis, and see the rectum taking the concavity of the sacrum. The part between the two is the urogenital septum. It is occupied by the seminal vesicles and vas deferens in the male. In the female it is filled with vagina, uterus, uterine tube and ovary.

STUDY OF THE PELVIC PERITONEUM

Anterior abdominal wall: Run your fingers along the inner surface of the anterior abdominal wall once again and note the median elevation caused due to the fibrosed urachus called the median umbilical ligament. Feel the hardness of the ligament. The fold of the peritoneum over the median umbilical ligament is the median umbilical fold. Run your fingers laterally if possible locate the medial umbilical folds overlying the medial umbilical ligaments. These are the fibrosed parts ***of the obliterated umbilical arteries. Relocate the inferior epigastric artery and note that the peritoneum raises a fold over this artery called the lateral umbilical fold (these were already identified while opening the abdominal cavity).***

Bladder: Press your fingers downward from the anterior abdominal wall and note upper surface of the urinary bladder. Clasp it between your fingers and feel the sides of the bladder and note that the peritoneum covers the surface of the bladder and passes on to the side wall of the pelvis. The depression that you see by the side is the paravesical fossae.

The part between the urinary bladder and rectum is called the urogenital septum and lodges the genital organs. As they differ in both sexes, make sure you see both male and female bodies.

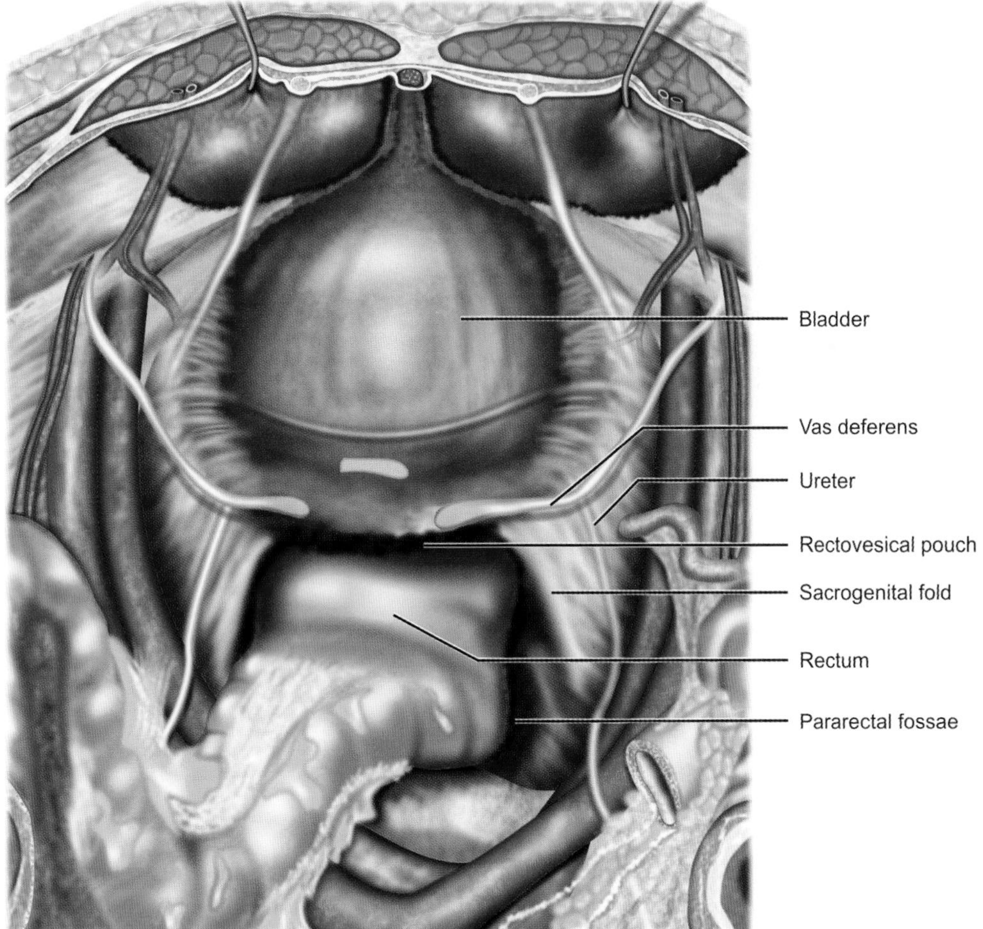

FIGURE 2 Pelvic peritoneum—male

MALE (Fig. 2)

Run your fingers on the posterior aspect of bladder and press it. You can feel the ***seminal vesicle.*** Pull the bladder forwards and see, the raised fold of peritoneum running between the bladder and the sacrum. This is the ***sacrogenital fold.*** The blood vessels from the internal iliac artery raise this fold. Put your fingers in the depression between the bladder and rectum, that is ***rectovesical pouch.*** Trace it up posteriorly and feel the ***rectum.*** Feel the rectum and the sides of the rectum. Note the depressions on either side, the ***pararectal fossae.***

Run your fingers along the lateral wall. You can generally identify two structures, the ***ductus deferens*** anteriorly, from the deep inguinal ring to the posterior aspect of the bladder, and the ***ureter*** posteriorly crossing the internal iliac vessels to the bladder.

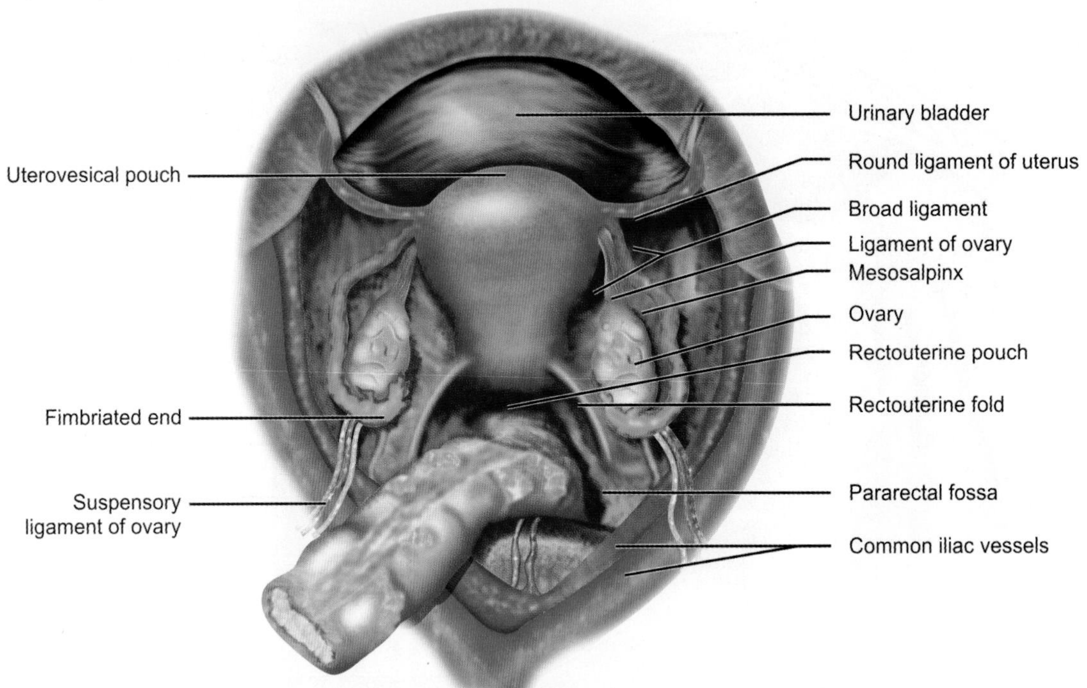

FIGURE 3 Pelvic peritoneum—female

FEMALE (Fig. 3)

In the female you can identify the female genital system between the bladder and the rectum in the genital septum. Clasp the central projecting part ***uterus.*** This is a hard projecting part. Peritoneum between the uterus and the bladder forms ***uterovesical pouch.*** Peritoneum between the uterus and rectum forms ***rectouterine pouch of Douglas. Pararectal fossae*** lie to the sides of the rectum.

Run your fingers laterally and clasp the *broad ligament* extending from the uterus to the lateral pelvic wall. Identify the following in the broad ligament.

Uterine tube: Feel its total extent, and identify the isthmus, the ampulla and fimbriated end in the upper free margin of the broad ligament.

Ovary: Feel thin almond shaped structure in the posterior layer of broad ligament. Clasp the ovary and feel the part of the peritoneum connecting the ovary to the posterior layer. It is the ***mesovarium.*** Clasp the part of the broad ligament between the ovary and the uterine tube. It is the ***mesosalpinx.*** Feel the part of the broad ligament below the ovary. It is the ***mesometrium.***

Round ligament of ovary: Pull the broad ligament posteriorly and note the raised round ligament of uterus extending from the uterus to the deep inguinal ring.

Ligament of ovary: Pull the ovary laterally and note the ligament extending between the ovary and the uterus. Both, ligament of ovary and round ligament of uterus are parts of the embryonic gubernaculum.

Suspensory ligament of ovary: Run your fingers laterally between the ovary and the lateral pelvic wall. You can feel the blood vessels entering into the broad ligament here.

Rectouterine fold: The blood vessels which pass from the internal iliac artery to the uterus raise this fold.

STUDY OF PELVIC ORGANS

It is convenient to study and dissect the pelvis in two bodies, i.e. students of at least two tables come together and study. In one body, cut a sagittal section of the pelvis, see the interior of the organs and dissect the neurovascular bundle. In the other body, study the organs in detail, detach them from the body and study their interiors.

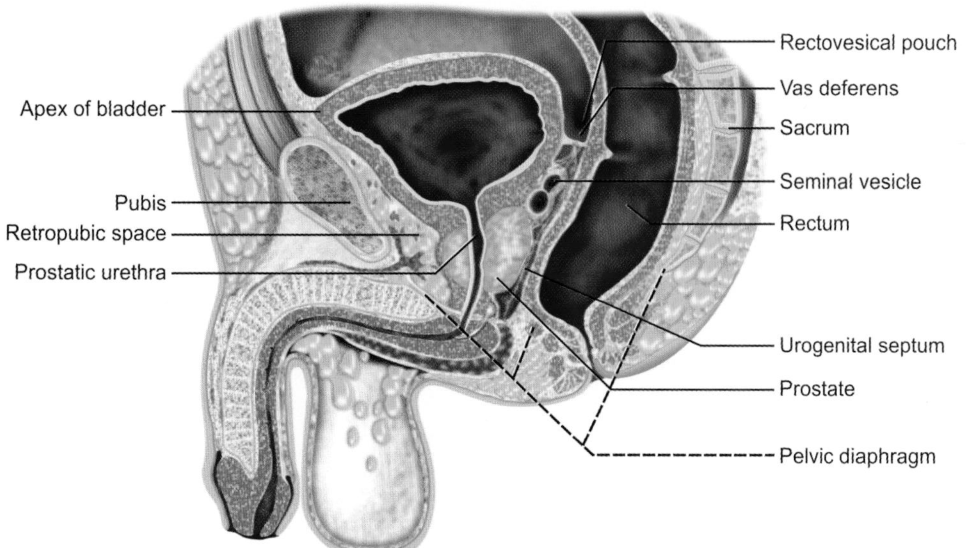

FIGURE 4 Sagittal section—male pelvis

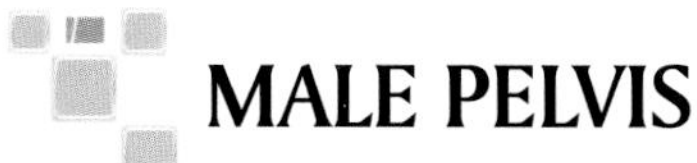

MALE PELVIS

MIDSAGITTAL SECTION (Fig. 4)

In a midsagittal section, identify the following structures anteroposteriorly. See the ***bladder*** behind the pubis. The space between the bladder and the pubis is called the ***retropubic space.*** Identify the apex of the bladder, continuous with the median umbilical ligament. See the neck of the bladder inferiorly. The ***urethra*** begins here. Note the ***prostate*** enveloping the urethra. Put your hand along the sides and feel the ***pelvic diaphragm.*** The part below the pelvic diaphragm is the perineum. See the rectovesicle pouch behind and between the urinary bladder and rectum. See the ***urogenital septum*** behind the bladder. This is occupied by the ***seminal vesicles, vas deferens and ureter.*** Observe that the ***rectum*** takes the curve of the sacrum and coccyx. Feel the pelvic diaphragm and note that the rectum passes through that to enter into the perineum.

RECTUM

Dissection: In the pelvis specimen reidentify the pelvic mesocolon which was attaching the sigmoid colon to the sacrum and lateral pelvic wall. Clean the peritoneum and study the organs.

The ***rectum*** is a part of the large intestine. It is 13 cm long, extends from the 3rd piece of sacrum to the coccyx. It follows the curves of the sacrum and coccyx which can be better appreciated in the sagittal section. It is a tubular organ, but shows an enlargement called rectal ***ampulla.*** It is located above the levator ani muscle. Feel the rectum throughout its extent up to the pelvic floor and realize that the first 1/3rd is covered by peritoneum, the second 1/3rd is covered by peritoneum only anteriorly and the last 1/3 is the ampulla, it is devoid of peritoneal covering. The rectum presents three curvatures—two to the right side one to the left side. Note the prominent flexure of rectum on the right side. The curvatures of the rectum are due to the mucosal valves. They are two on the left and one on the right. These are best seen in the interior of the rectum. Identify there.

Relations: Note that it is related to the curved ***sacrum and coccyx posteriorly***. Posterolaterally it is related to the muscles—the ***levator ani, Coccygeus and piriformis;*** the blood vessels—***median*** and ***lateral sacral vessels***; ***the nerves—S3, 4, 5,*** and ***coccygeal nerves*** and the terminal part of ***sympathetic chain***. Anteriorly it is related to the ***structures forming the urogenital septum.*** The first and second parts of rectum is separated from the organs by the peritoneum and related to the coils of intestine. The third part is related to the ***bladder, seminal vesicle and vas deferens*** in male and in female to the ***vagina***. Laterally note the connective tissue connecting the rectum to the lateral pelvic wall. These are called lateral ligaments.

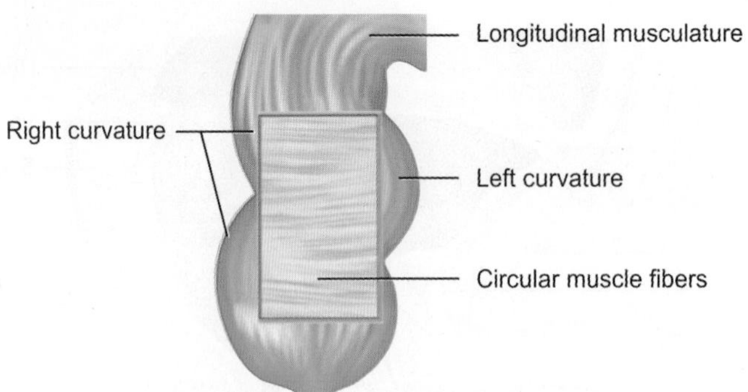

FIGURE 5 Musculature of the rectum

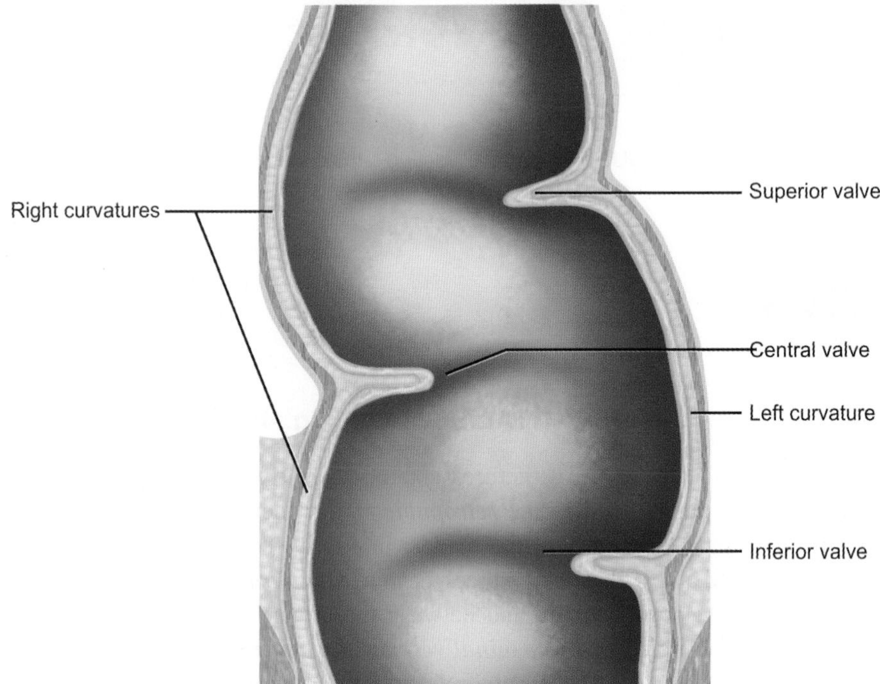

FIGURE 6 Interior of the rectum

Blood supply: Note that the rectum gets blood supply from three sources. Clean and see the ***superior rectal artery*** in the sigmoid mesocolon. See its entry into the rectum. Trace the ***middle rectal branch*** from the internal iliac artery. See its entry by pulling the rectum to one side. It is also supplied by the ***inferior rectal artery,*** a branch from the internal pudendal artery. This will be studied in the ischiorectal fossa dissection.

Interior of Rectum (Figs 5 and 6)

Dissection: Take the rectum out of the body by cutting near the levator ani muscle. Peel the peritoneum and see the longitudinal musculature covering the entire surface of the organ, unlike the other parts of large intestine. Separate the longitudinal layer and see the circular muscle. Make a coronal cut and see the interior. Identify the valves –they are one right and two left. They create one left curvature and two right curvatures.

Pelvic part of ureter: Ureters are 25 cm long tubes. They extend from pelvis of the ureter in the kidney to the trigone of the bladder. Identify the ureters as they enter the pelvis crossing the pelvic brim. Trace them to the bladder. Note that in the pelvis it lies infront of the external and internal iliac vessels as it enters the pelvic cavity. In the male it is crossed by the ductus deferens near the ischial spine. In the female it crosses above the uterine artery near the lateral fornix of the vagina. Identify these relations. It reaches the superolateral angle of the bladder, pierces obliquely through the wall of the bladder to reach the superolateral angle of the trigone of the bladder.

Urinary Bladder—Male

Dissection: Clean the peritoneum from the bladder and study the organ.

External features: Identify the urinary bladder behind the pubic symphysis. Clasp the urinary bladder and realize it is tetrahedral in shape. See its superior surface, two ***inferolateral surfaces and a posterior surface or base***. The ***lateral border*** is sharp and separates the superior surface from the inferolateral surface. The ***posterior border*** separates the superior surface from the base. Identify the ***apex*** where the two lateral borders meet. However, when the bladder is full it looks more spherical with an anterior and posterior surface. Feel the neck of the bladder which lies inferiorly.

Relations: Note that the superior surface is related to the ***coils of small intestine*** (removed in the specimen). Put your fingers between the anterior border and the pubic bone. It is called the ***cave of Retzius, or retropubic space.*** It is filled with fat. Put your fingers along the sides and note that it is closely related to the lateral pelvic wall. Run your fingers posteriorly and identify the central ***vas deferens*** and lateral ***seminal vesicles.*** Clasp the bladder totally and identify the neck of the bladder.

Note: The hard ***prostate gland*** beneath the neck of the bladder.

Ligaments: Note that the inferior part or the neck of the bladder is connected to pelvic wall—anteriorly by ***puboprostatic ligament,*** laterally the ***true lateral ligaments*** and posteriorly to the ***posterior ligaments.*** These ligaments hold the bladder tight inferiorly so that the other part can be distended when it gets filled with fluid.

Blood supply: Reidentify the medial umbilical ligament with the obliterated umbilical vessels and trace it backwards. Note the superior vesical artery. This is the unobliterated part of the vessel. It supplies the upper part of the bladder. Clean the posterior ligament of the bladder. It lodges the inferior vesical blood vessels coming from the internal iliac vessels. Trace the branches of both the blood vessels into the urinary bladder, prostate and seminal vesicle.

Male Genital Organs (Fig. 7)

Prostate: It is an accessory male sex gland and it manufactures nutritive fluid for the sperms. The ducts open by minute openings into the sinus of the urethra. Note the chestnut shaped hard organ below the bladder. Feel the ***anterior surface.*** It is rounded and lies behind the pubic symphysis. ***Base*** is flat and abuts the neck of urinary bladder and is separated from it by a narrow groove. The bladder and the base of the prostate are connected to the neighboring wall by the puboprostatic and lateral ligaments. ***Inferolateral surface*** or the side of the prostate is clasped by the sloping levator ani muscle. ***Apex*** is the inferior part of the prostate and abuts the superior layer of urogenital diaphragm as levator ani is deficient here. Urethra leaves the prostate at the junction of the apex and anterior margin. Clean the connective tissue around the prostate. It is called the false capsule of the prostate. It is the thickened pelvic fascia. When you remove this and you can see the plexus of veins. ***Prostatic plexus of veins*** lie laterally between the false and true capsule. It drains bladder, prostate and the dorsal vein of penis.

Dissection: Cut through the prostate very near the levator ani muscle. Cut the blood vessels entering into it. Lift the bladder, prostate with the seminal vesicle and vas deferens out of the body.

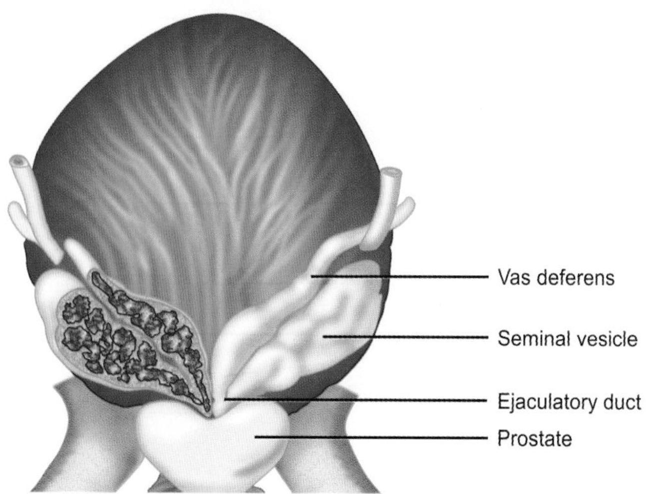

FIGURE 7 Male genital organs

Seminal vesicle: Turn to the posterior aspect of the bladder. Clean the connective tissue and identify the seminal vesicle. It is an accessory male sex gland. It produces nutritive fluid to add to the semen. It is a highly coiled tube wrapped by a thick fascia. It looks oval in shape and the bulging coiled tube is quite visible through the fascia, identify its narrow duct which pierces the base of the prostate. It opens into the prostatic urethra after joining with the ductus deferens.

Vas deferens: Vas deferens of both sides approximate in the midline and lie between the seminal vesicles. Ampulla is its lower enlarged part.

Ejaculatory duct: Ejaculatory duct is formed by the union of the vas deferens and the duct of seminal vesicle beyond the ampulla. It pierces the prostate and opens into the prostatic urethra. Ductus deferens transfers the sperms from the epididymis to the prostatic urethra.

Interior of Bladder and Prostate (Fig. 8)

Dissection: Make a coronal section of bladder and the prostate dividing it into an anterior and posterior halves. Open it to see the interior. You may trim it further to get a clear picture of the posterior aspect of both the organs. Note the openings of the ureter. They are like small slits along the superolateral corners. Put a probe into it and confirm the passage. Inferiorly put a probe and see the urethral opening. Uvula of the bladder is the lower bulging part of the bladder near the trigone.

Trigone: The triangular area between the urethral and the ureteric openings is called trigone**.** Identify the slit like superolateral ***ureteric openings.*** The bladder forms a circular opening at the neck and this is the ***internal urethral orifice.*** The trigone looks different from the rest of the interior. Here the mucous membrane is adherent to the deeper muscle, whereas the mucous membrane can be easily pulled at the lamina propria in the rest of the bladder as it is loosely attached. In the cut part see the thick, the musculature of the bladder goes in a circular, longitudinal manner and is called ***detrusor*** muscle.

Prostatic urethra: It is the widest part of the urethra around 3 cm long. In a section it is semilunar the shape. ***Urethral crest*** is the central posterior bulging part of the urethra. ***Colliculus seminalis*** is the central enlarged part of the middle of the urethra crest. The ***prostatic utricle*** is a blind sac with an opening on to the colliculus seminalis. The ***sinus*** is the depression on either side of the urethral crest. You can see the glandular part of the gland and cut parts of the ejaculatory ducts.

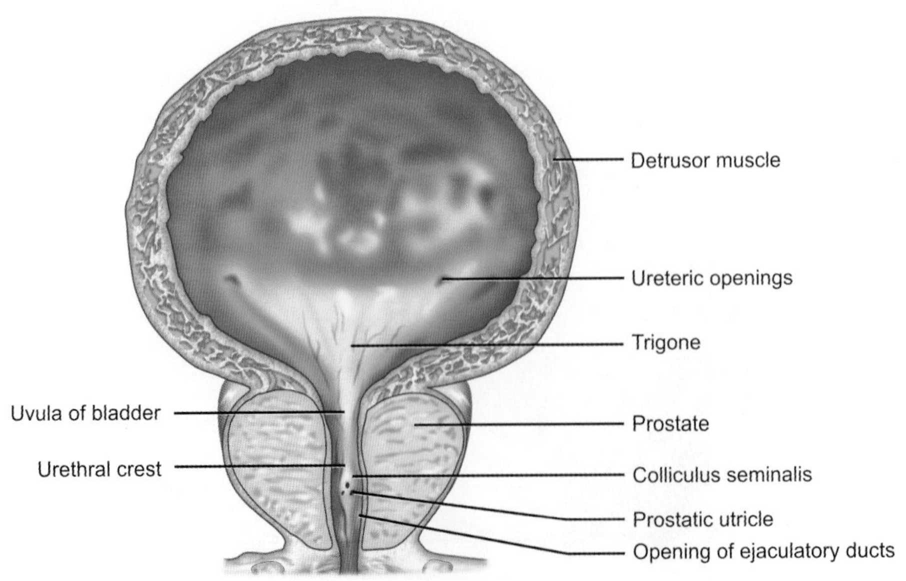

FIGURE 8 Interior of bladder and prostate

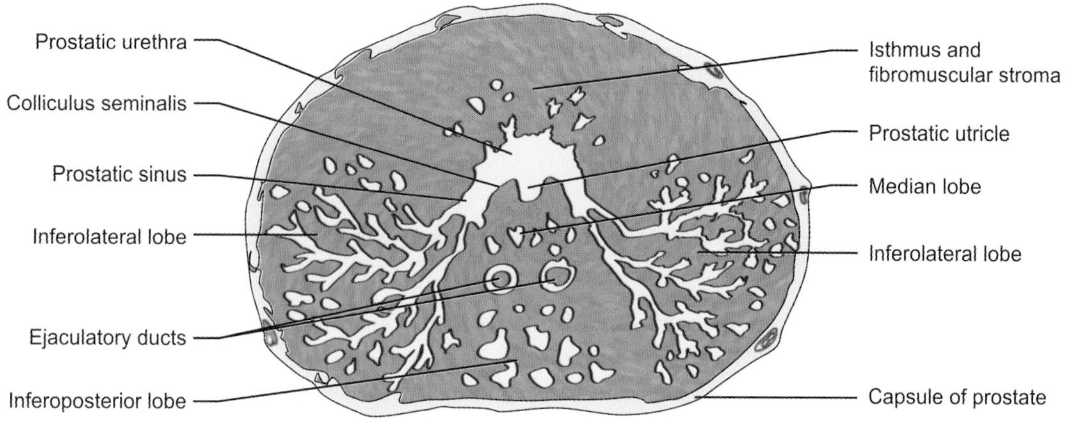

FIGURE 9 Interior of prostate

Ejaculatory ducts open on to the sides of the utricle. Put a fine probe and identify them **(Fig. 9)**.

Dissection: Cut a prostate transversely and see the prostatic urethra and the ducts by putting fine probes.

FEMALE PELVIS

MIDSAGITTAL SECTION (Fig. 10)

In a midsagittal section identify the ***urinary bladder*** immediately behind the pubis. See the ***retropubic space***. It is filled with fat. Note the body, isthmus and cervix of the ***uterus; uterine tube, ovary* and *vagina*** in the urorectal septum. These are the organs of the female genital system. Note that these organs are connected to the lateral pelvic wall by the ***broad ligament.*** Identify the passage of the ***ureter*** from the posterior wall to the anterior aspect to reach the

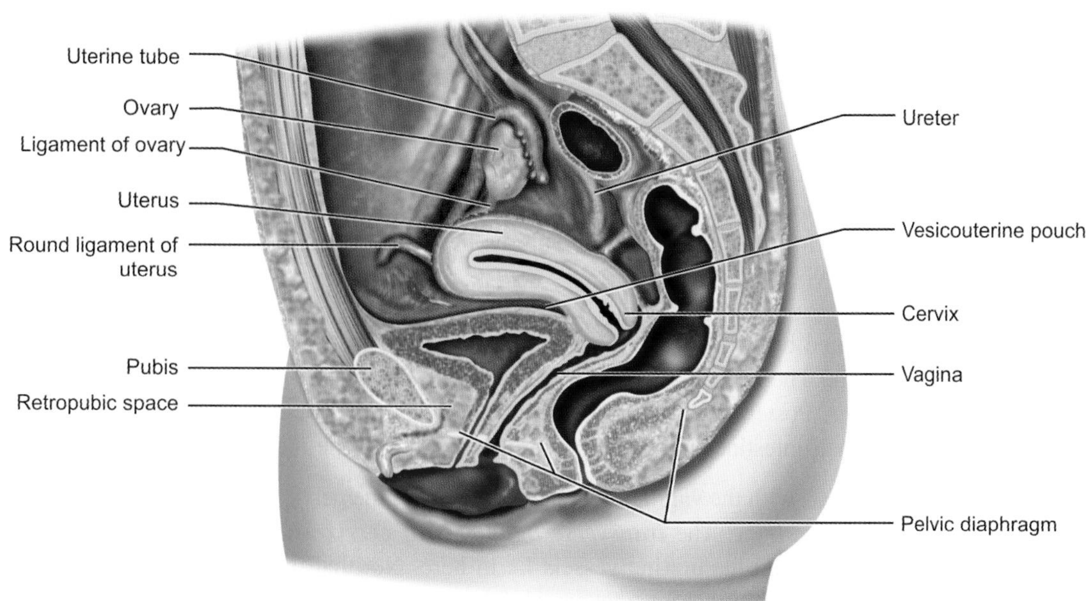

FIGURE 10 Midsagittal section—female pelvis

bladder. See the ***rectum*** behind the uterus and vagina. Note that it takes the curve of the sacrum. Identify the ***pelvic diaphragm*** from the lateral sides to the midline. Note that the pelvic diaphragm is pierced by the urethra, vagina and the rectum. Identify the ***round ligament of uterus*** extending from the deep inguinal ring to the uterus. Note the ***ligament of ovary*** between the ovary and the uterus.

OVARY

Dissection: Clean the peritoneum and study the ovary, uterus and vagina in the full pelvis as well as in the sagittal section.

Ovary is an almond shaped structure measures approximated 3 cm long. 1.5 cm wide and 1 cm thick it is attached to the posterior layer of broad ligament by the ***mesovarium***. It has a superior end, where it is connected to the pelvic wall by the ***suspensory ligament***. Clean this area and locate the ovarian vessels and nerves which enter the hilum of ovary. The ovarian artery is a branch of the abdominal aorta. The lower end is called the uterine end. Here it is connected to the uterus by the ***ligament of ovary***. The ***medial surface*** is related to the coils of small intestine, and the ***lateral surface*** is related to the ovarian fossa.

Ovarian fossa: It is the area between the ureter, external iliac vein and obturator nerve in which the ovary lies in nullipara. Ovaries produce the ova and liberate them into the pelvic cavity. The fimbriated end of the uterine tube collects them and passes it on through the uterine tube.

UTERINE TUBE

It is approximately 10 cm long presents an ***intramural part***—this lies within the wall of uterus, an ***isthmus***—this the narrow part outside the uterus, the expanded ***ampulla*** and the terminal ***infundibulum*** with ***fimbriae***. The fimbriae are finger shaped processes, overlapping the ovary. Ostium lies at the end of the ampulla. The fimbriae help in picking the liberated ovum and pass it on to the uterine tube. Slit it and note the longitudinal folds of mucous membrane.

UTERUS

The uterus is a muscular organ, situated between the bladder and rectum. It is pear shaped and flattened anteroposteriorly. In nullipara it is 7-8 cm long, 5 cm wide and 2.5 cm thick. During pregnancy it enlarges 10 times.

Normal position of the uterus is described as anteverted a forward bend at right angles to the vagina (90º) and anteflexed (55º) a forward bend of the body of the uterus at the isthmus. The uterus in a nulliparous woman is around 7 to 8 cm long. It presents three parts—the ***fundus*** is the portion above the opening of uterine tube, the middle body and a lower cervix. The ***cervix*** and ***body*** are separated by the isthmus. The cervix fixes itself into the anterior wall of vagina.

VAGINA

Vagina is the soft tube which extends from the uterus to the exterior. It opens into the urogenital region of the perineum. The vagina passes upwards and backwards at an angle of 60 degrees to the horizontal. The length of the anterior wall is around 7.5 cm and the posterior wall is around 10.5 cm. As the uterus juts into the vagina, a gap is identified between the uterus and vagina. This is called fornix. The part of the uterus inside the vagina is called the vaginal cervix and the part above is the supravaginal cervix.

Relations*:** Note that the fundus and body of the uterus are separated from the bladder by the ***uterovesical pouch and coils of ***small intestine*** lie in here. The cervix is directly related to the ***superior surface of the bladder***. The vagina is related to the ***base of the bladder***. Posteriorly the uterus is separated from the ***rectum*** by the ***rectouterine pouch*** and this is filled with the coils of small intestine. Vagina is posteriorly related to the rectum.

Ligaments: The uterus at its junction with the vagina is connected firmly to the pelvic wall on all sides. The ***pubocervical ligaments*** connect them to the pubic bone. The ***transverse ligaments of cervix/Mackenrodt's ligament*** connect them to the lateral pelvic wall. The ureter and the uterine vessels lie in here. Not that the artery is superficial to the ureter. In a vaginal examination these are the two structures that can be felt through the lateral fornix. The ***uterosacral ligaments*** connect them posteriorly to the sacrum. Identify the ***ligament of ovary*** extending from the medial end of the ovary to the uterus, below the attachment of the uterine tube. Trace the ***round ligament of uterus*** from the same position to the deep inguinal ring.

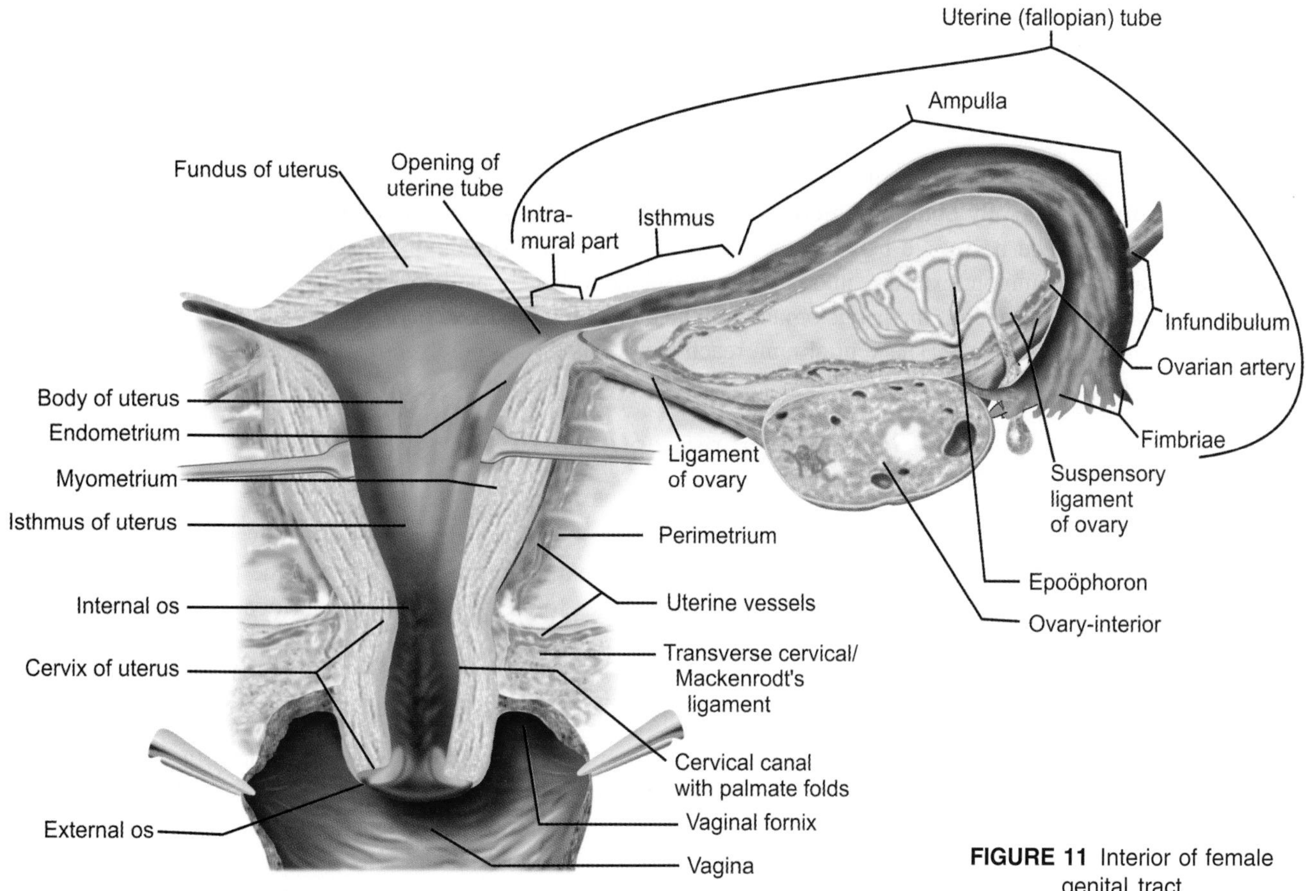

FIGURE 11 Interior of female genital tract

INTERIOR OF FEMALE GENITAL TRACT (Fig. 11)

Dissection: Cut the vagina near the pelvic diaphragm and remove the uterus vagina, uterine tube, by cutting along the lower border of uterine tube and lateral border of uterus and vagina. Cut the uterus, vagina and the tube in a coronal plane and see the interior.

Note the layers of uterus. Identify the mucous membrane in the interior. This is the ***endometrium.*** See the thick ***myometrium*** or the muscle wall. Uterus has the thickest of muscles in the body. See the adventitia around called the ***perimetrium***. Look at the lumen of the uterus. See the opening of the uterine tube into the uterus. The part of the uterus above the opening the uterine tube is called the ***fundus*** of the uterus. The part below is called the ***body***. Its lumen of the body is triangular slit in nonpregnant uterus. Lumen of the cervix is spindle shaped and is called cervical canal. The junction of the ***uterine cavity*** and the ***cervical canal*** is called the ***internal os***. See that the outer opening of the cervical canal is also slit like, and it is called ***external os***. Identify the oblique ridges on the cervical canal. This appearance is described as the palmate in appearance, resembling palm leaves. When the anterior and posterior walls meet, it closes the cervical canal tight. Identify the cervix projecting into the vagina. The circular gap of the vagina around the cervix is normally described as 4 ***fornices*** the anterior, posterior and two lateral. Note that the anterior fornix is much smaller compared to the posterior fornix which in very deep. This is mainly due to the fact that the uterus bulges into the anterior wall of the vagina than at its middle. See the cavity of the uterine tube. Note that the intramural part is very thin and passes through the wall of the uterus. See the isthmus connecting the intramural part with the ampulla. ***Ampulla*** is relatively wider part. The fertilization takes place in this part. See the wide fimbriated end and the finger shaped ***fimbriae***.

Look for the ***epoophoron*** and ***paroophoron,*** the vestigial structures between the two layers of the ***broad ligament.*** Try to dissect the blood vessels within the broad ligament. Identify the ovarian artery in the ***suspensory ligament*** and the uterine artery near the cervix of the uterus.

Cut and see the interior of the ovary. You may identify a ***corpus luteum.*** The structure is better studied in a histological preparation.

Cavity of the vagina is much wider and shows mild mucosal folds.

Female urethra is better seen in the perineum.

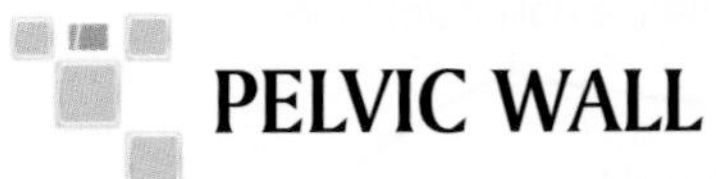

PELVIC WALL

The pelvic wall is made up of musculature, blood vessels and nerves. The muscles forming the pelvic wall are—posteriorly piriformis, laterally obturator infernus and inferiorly by the pelvic diaphragm.

The blood vessels and nerves lie between the wall and the organs. The blood vessels lie inner to the nerves. The blood vessels are the common, external, internal iliac vessels and their branches. The external iliac supplies the lower limb and the internal iliac supplies the pelvic organs and the gluteal region. ***Five sacral nerves*** and ***two to three coccygeal nerves*** are seen within the pelvis. The ventral rami reach the pelvis through the ventral sacral foraminae, unite together to form the sacral plexus.

VESSELS OF PELVIS (Figs 12 and 13)

Dissection: Try to do this dissection on the sagittal section. Remove the peritoneum totally from the superior surface of the visceral organs. You realize all the organs are extraperitoneal, i.e. outside the peritoneum. Trace the common, external, internal iliac vessels and their branches to their destinations and identify them.

Identify the ***common iliac artery*** at the division of the aorta at the level of the 4th lumbar vertebra. Trace the common iliac artery to its division into internal and external iliac arteries at the level of the sacroiliac joint.

External iliac artery is the main artery of supply to the lower limb. It passes along the pelvic brim to reach under surface of the inguinal ligament and at the midinguinal point it continues into the lower limb as femoral artery. ***Inferior epigastric artery*** and ***deep circumflex iliac*** (both dissected in the anterior abdominal wall dissection) arteries are its branches. Reidentify them. The veins accompany the arteries. The internal iliac artery is the artery of supply to all organs within the pelvis, perineum and the gluteal region. Each branch is named according to the organ or the area it supplies.

Trace the internal iliac artery to its division into an anterior and a posterior division.

Posterior division of internal iliac artery: This artery sticks to the sacrum and supplies the musculature. See the ***iliolumbar artery*** which goes deeper to psoas major, supplies psoas major, iliacus and quadratus lumborum muscle.

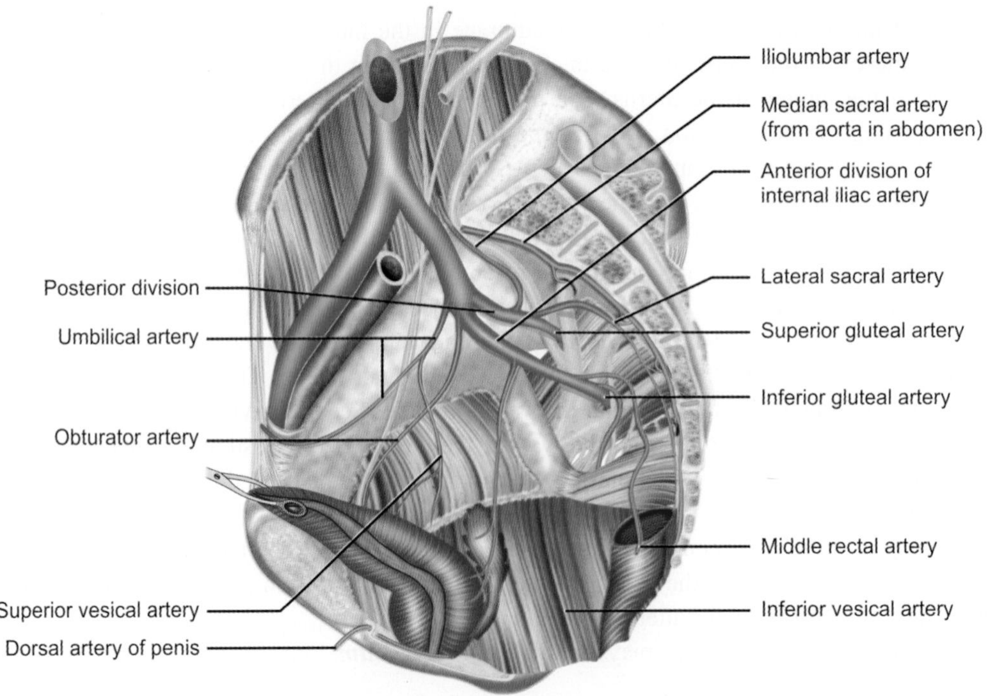

FIGURE 12 Vessels of pelvis—male pelvis

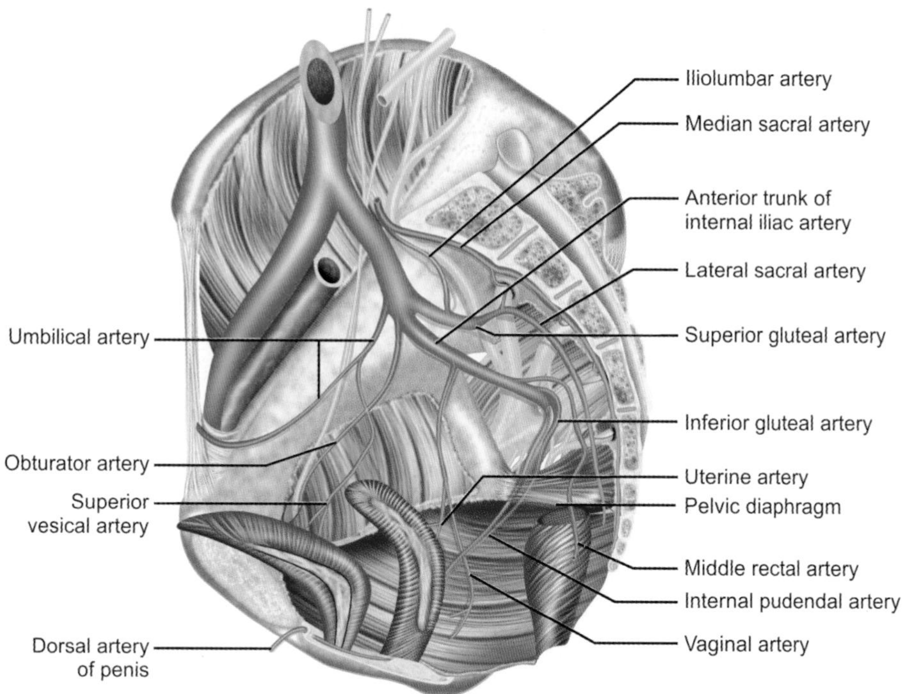

FIGURE 13 Vessels of pelvis—female

Lateral sacral artery is a medial branch. This runs along the lateral border of anterior sacral foramina. See the branches entering into the foramina to supply the sacral nerves within the sacrum. The ***superior gluteal artery*** is the continuation of the posterior division. See it leaves the pelvis through the greater sciatic foramen between the psoas major and piriformis muscle to supply the gluteal muscles.

Anterior division of internal iliac artery: The ***superior vesical artery*** is the most anterior branch. It runs along the lateral wall of the pelvis to reach the superolateral surface of the urinary bladder and it supplies the bladder. The lateral lumbrical ligament is the fibrosed continuation of the superior vesical artery. It is functional in the fetal life. The corresponding umbilical vein reaches the liver through the falciform ligament. It is called ligamentum Teres. The ***obturator artery*** is the next branch. Trace the obturator artery along the lateral wall of the pelvis above the obturator internus muscle to reach the obturator foramen. In the pelvis it supplies the structures nearby otherwise it is the artery of the adductor compartment of thigh.

In the males, trace the ***inferior vesical artery*** to supply the lower part of the bladder seminal vesicles and prostate. In the females, the ***uterine and vaginal arteries*** may arise by a common trunk or separately. They reach the lateral wall to supply the vagina and uterus. Note that the uterine arteries lie lateral to the lateral fornix and is above the ureter. Note that the uterine artery is tortuous in its course along the lateral border of the uterus. This straightens out when the uterus expands during pregnancy. Trace the ***middle rectal artery*** to the middle part of the rectum. The ***internal pudendal artery*** and the ***inferior gluteal artery*** are the terminal divisions of anterior division. They leave the pelvis through the greater sciatic foramen below the piriformis muscle. The internal pudendal artery lies medial to the inferior gluteal artery. Trace them upto the greater sciatic foramen.

The superior rectal artery: It is a continuation of the inferior mesenteric artery. Trace it on to the upper 3rd of rectum. Trace the ***median sacral artery***. It is a posterior branch at the level of division of the abdominal aorta. It runs down along the midline of sacrum. It gives small branches to supply the neighbouring structures.

Veins: All the arteries are accompanied by the veins. The superior rectal vein drains into the portal system. It forms an anastomosis with the middle and inferior sacral veins within the wall of rectum. The veins in general form plexuses within the organs and drain out, accompany the arteries and ultimately drain into internal iliac veins.

Lymph nodes: Numerous lymph nodes are seen along with the blood vessels draining the organs. They are named according to the vessels they accompany.

NERVES OF THE PELVIS (Fig. 14)

Dissection: Clean the nerves that emerge out of the ventral sacral foraminae. Here they lie over the piriformis and coccygeus muscles. These are ***five sacral nerves*** and two to ***three coccygeal nerves.*** They form the sacral plexus. All these nerves leave the pelvis through the greater sciatic foramen, the superior gluteal nerve above and all the other nerves below the piriforms. If the lower limb is already dissected identify them in the gluteal region and see their continuity in the pelvis.

Sympathetic chain: It is a part of the autonomic nervous system. Locate it, medial to the ventral pelvic sacral foraminae to the coccyx where the chains of both sides join to form the ganglion impair. It presents four sacral ganglia. Each ganglion communicates with the spinal nerves by the gray ramus communicantes given off from the lateral sides. Sacral splanchnic nerves are given off from the ventral aspect of the ganglia and contribute to the formation of inferior hypogastric plexus. The ***parasympathetic*** contribution comes from S2, 3, 4 ventral rami as the pelvic splanchnic nerves. The plexus accompanies the pelvic blood vessels supplies the blood vessels as well as the internal organs.

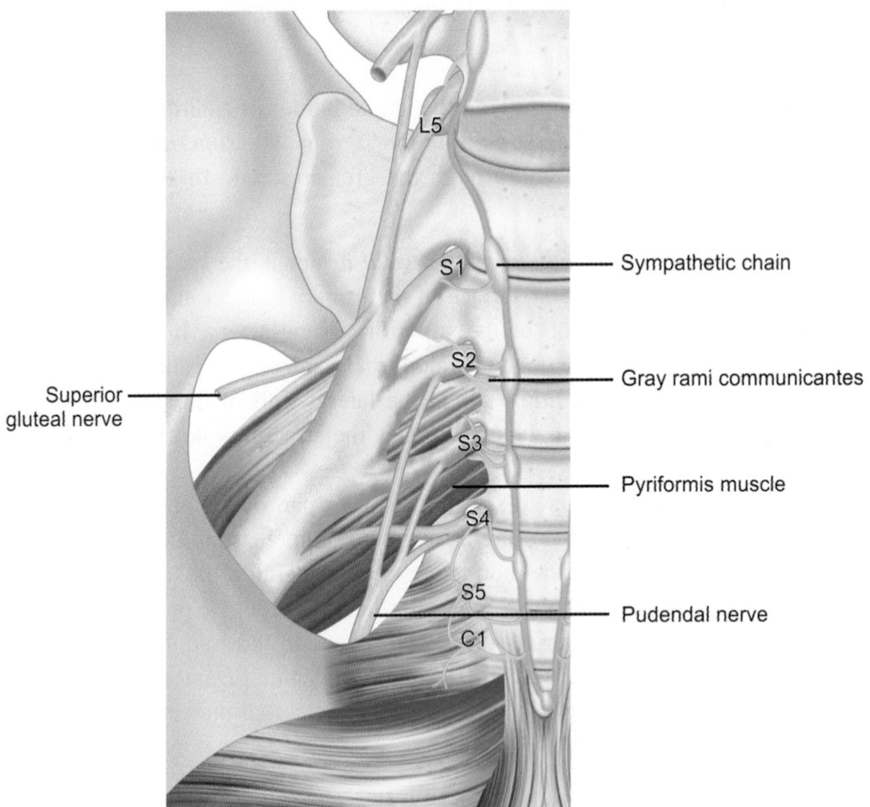

FIGURE 14 Nerves of pelvis

MUSCLES OF PELVIS

The total bony true pelvis is packed by musculature on all sides—posteriorly piriformis, laterally obturator internus and inferiorly by the pelvic diaphragm **(Figs 15 and 16)**.

Dissection: Use the pelvis where you removed all the organs. Now clean all the blood vessels from the pelvis and clean the musculature. In the female, note the lower cut ends of the urethra, vagina and the rectum. In the male, note the lower cut ends of the urethra and the rectum.

Piriformis: This muscle arises from the anterior aspect of the 2nd, 3rd, and 4th sacral vertebrae. The muscle leaves the pelvis through the greater sciatic foramen to be inserted into the greater trochanter. It is a lateral rotator of the femur. It is supplied by sacral ventral rami on its ventral aspect. Trace the muscle and its nerves.

Obturator internus: This covers the side wall of the pelvis. It forms the lateral boundary to pelvis and perineum. It arises from the pelvic surface of the obturator membrane and the bordering bone. It leaves the pelvis through the lesser sciatic foramen to be attached to the greater trochanter. It is a lateral rotator of femur. It is supplied by the nerve to the obturator internus on its internal surface to which it reaches through the lesser sciatic foramen (identified in gluteal region). Fascia covering the obturator inturnus is called obturator fascia.

Pelvic diaphragm: This supports the pelvic viscera inferiorly in the erect posture and bridges the gap between the two hip bones. It is made up of muscle extending from the pubic bone to the coccyx. This is generally described as two muscles—the ***levator ani*** and ***coccygeus***. It is covered by fascia on either side and is called superior and inferior fascial layer of the pelvic diaphragm. Clean the superior layer and study the muscle.

Between the pubic bone and the bladder, the place is small and narrow. In this space, you see the ***inferior pubic ligament, transverse perineal ligament*** and ***deep dorsal vein of penis*** passing between the two. See them.

Levator ani: This muscle arises from the back of the body of the pubis anteriorly, to the spine of the ischium posteriorly. Between these two points it crosses the obturator internus muscle where it takes origin from a fibrotendinous ring called arcuate ligament. Muscles of both sides meet in the midline, support and merge with the pelvic organs, while letting them pass through it.

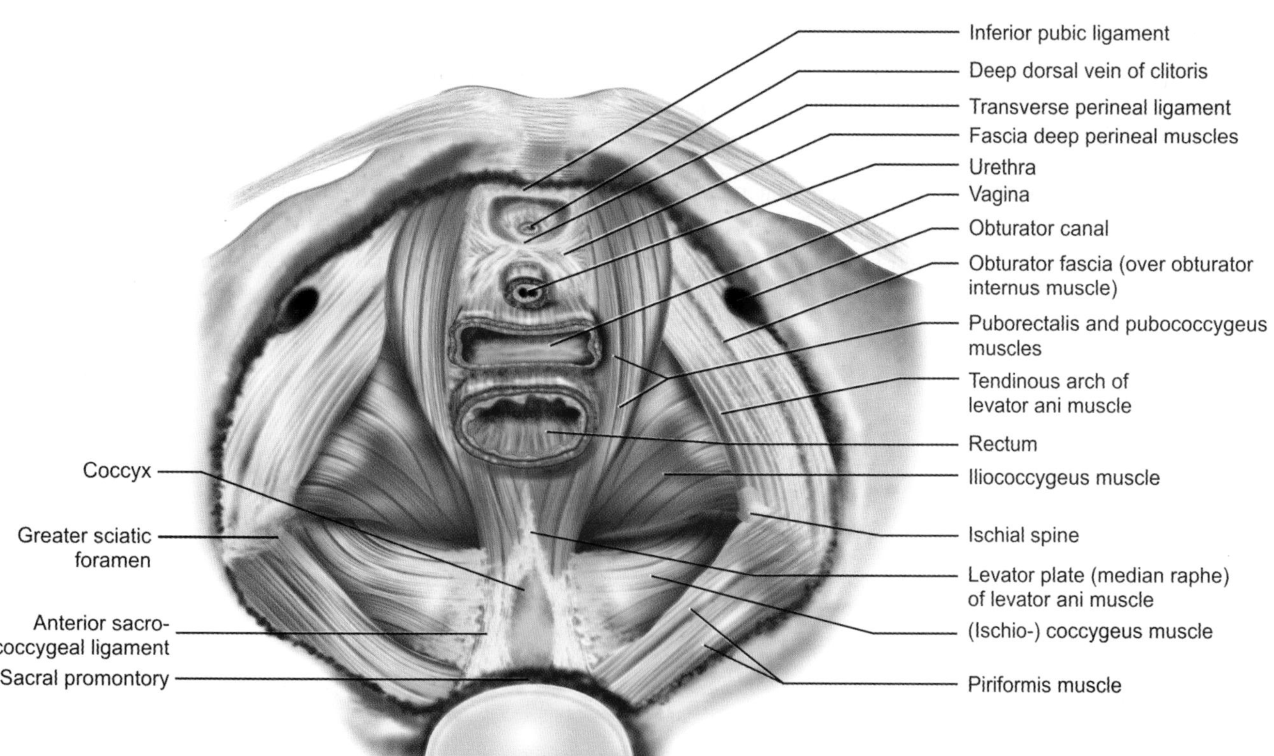

FIGURE 15 Pelvic diaphragm—female

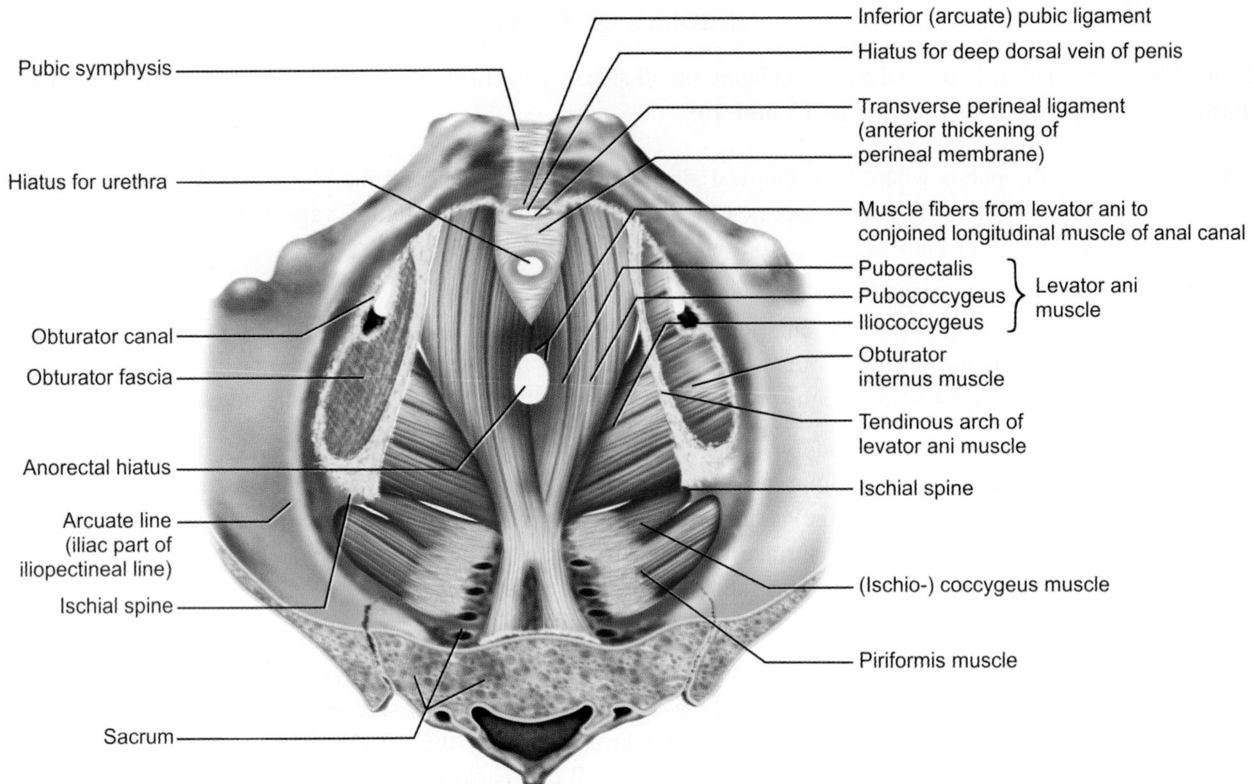

FIGURE 16 Pelvis diaphragm—male

So conventionally the levator ani forms loops around the organs starting from the pubis. So the muscle is further named according to the organ it loops. Between the pubic symphysis and the bladder it is deficient where the gap is filled by pubovesical (F)/puboprostatic (M) ligament. Levator prostate or puboprostaticus (M) – fibres loop from pubis to posterior to the prostate. Pubovaginalis (F) the first fibres from pubis loop behind the vagina. Puborectalis—lateral fibres from pubis loop around the rectum and pull it forwards. Pubococcygeus and iliococcygeus extend to the anococcygeal ligament and coccyx. Between the rectum and coccyx the muscle is more tendinous and forms the ligament. Levator ani is supplied by ventral rami of sacral nerves on its superior surface and by inferior rectal nerves on its inferior aspect.

Coccygeus or **ischiococcygeus:** It is a triangular muscle, arises from the last piece of sacrum and first piece of coccyx it is attached to the spine of the ischium. It is well developed in animals with tail and is the muscle which pulls the tail between the hindlimb. It is supplied by the sacral and coccygeal nerve on its ventral aspect. Its dorsal part is fibrosed to form sacrospinous ligament.

PERINEUM

Dissection: Perineum dissection is given here as it is customary to study it together, because of the continuity of structures. However, it is convenient to undertake this dissection as the last dissection is the body after completing the lower limb dissection. So the description that is given here describes this as the last part of dissection.

Preferably see a pelvis model with ligaments and identify the inferior pelvic aperture. It is a diamond shaped gap formed anteriorly by pubic symphysis, anterolaterally ischiopubic ramus, laterally ischial tuberosity, posterolaterally sacrotuberous ligament and posteriorly coccyx (Fig. 17).

As we have already seen, this gap is closed by the pelvic diaphragm superiorly except for the passage of the organs.

The space between the pelvic diaphragm and the skin is the perineum. The urethra, vagina and the anus open on to the exterior. Here for the convenience of description it is divided to an anterior urogenital region and a posterior anal region. The urogenital region differs in both sexes.

ANAL TRIANGLE

This is the posterior part of the perineum. It lodges the anal canal of the gastrointestinal tract. It opens on to the exterior as anus. The area around the anal canal is called the ischiorectal fossa.

Boundaries of the ischiorectal fossa (Fig. 17): This is ***superiorly*** bounded by the inferior surface of the pelvic diaphragm, ***laterally*** by the obturator muscle with its fascia and ischial tuberosity, ***inferiorly*** by the skin. The area on all the sides of the anal canal is filled with fat. This is a part of the extension of the superficial fascia. The blood vessels and nerves of the perineal region pass through the pudendal canal located in the lateral wall of the ischiorectal fossa.

Dissection: Turn the body to the prone position. Remove the skin located around the anus, and between the gluteus maximus, ischial tuberosity and the perineal membrane. Reidentify the sacrotuberous ligament. See the superficial fascia filled with fat. Remove this fat with care. Trace the inferior rectal vessels and nerves traversing this area from lateral to medial side. Note that it extends deep into the sloping surface between the levator ani and obturator internus muscle. Clean the area around the external opening and the anal canal and see the muscle.

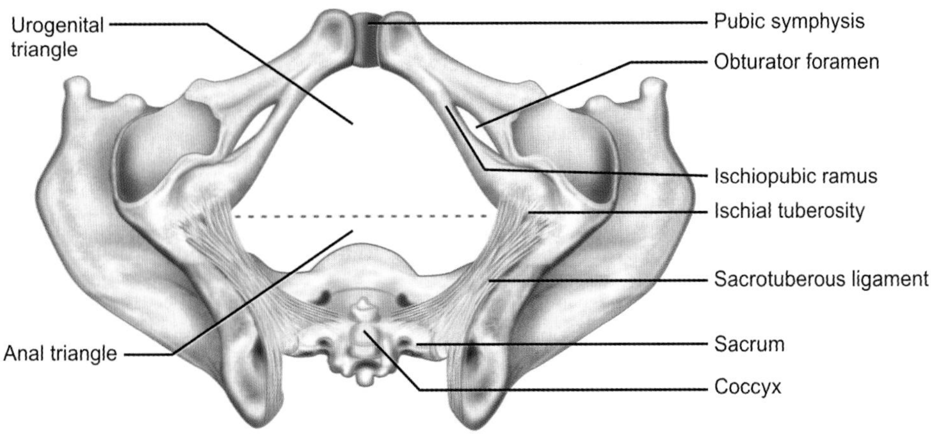

FIGURE 17 Bony boundaries of perineum

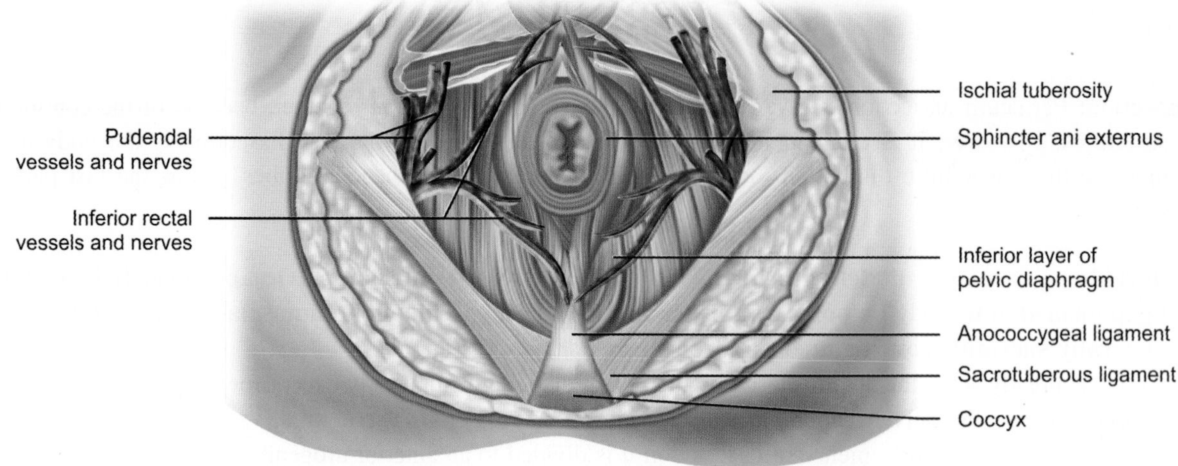

FIGURE 18 Ischiorectal fossa—boundaries and blood vessels

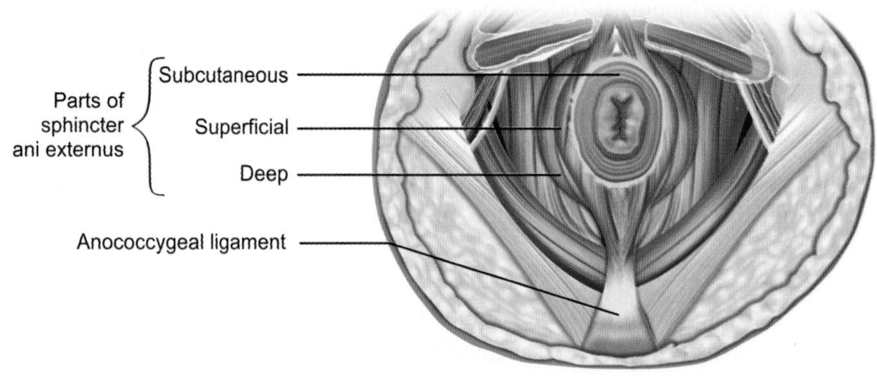

FIGURE 19 Sphincter ani externus

Pudendal vessels and nerves (Fig. 18): Identify the inferior rectal vessels and nerves traversing from the lateral wall to the side of the anus. These are branches of the pudendal vessels and nerves. They run horizontally from the lateral wall to the anus. Pudendal vessels and nerve were identified in the pelvis dissection. They traverse from the pelvis via the gluteal region to the perineum. In their course they lie between the sacrotuberous and sacrospinous ligament. Trace it all the way. In the lateral wall of the perineum they are protected in a fibrous sheath called pudendal canal. Slit it to see them. You will see their branches entering into the urogenital region.

Sphincter ani externus (Fig. 19): It is the muscle around anal canal. Note that it has three layers, the subcutaneous, superficial and deep layers. The subcutaneous part is immediately beneath the skin. It has no bony attachment. Note the superficial part extends from the anococcygeal ligament behind to the perineal body infront. The deep part is around the anal canal and has no bony attachment.

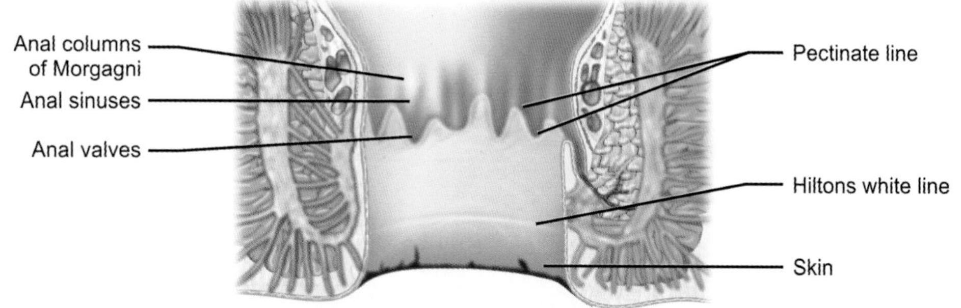

FIGURE 20 Interior of anal canal

Interior of anal canal (Fig. 20): Study this in a sagittal section. You can make out three parts here. The upper third shows vertical mucosal folds. These are called ***columns of Morgagni.*** The vertical mucosal folds are interconnected by raised ***anal valves***. The depressions above the anal valves are called the ***anal sinuses*** and deeply placed mucosal glands open here. The line below the anal valves is called the ***pectinate line***. The middle part is featureless, but under microscope you can visualize that it is made up of nonkeratinized epithelium. Embryologically it corresponds to the anococcygeal membrane. In the adult anatomy it is called anal pectin. The middle part continues with the skin. The line of junction is called the anocutaneous line or ***Hiltons white line***. This is a mucocutaneous junctional zone. Below this the skin with hair follicles are clearly visible.

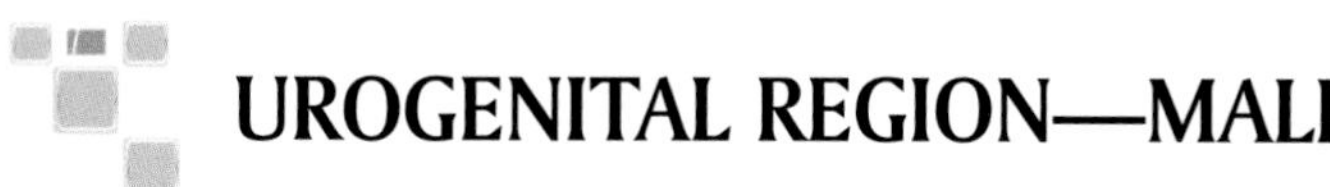

UROGENITAL REGION—MALE

Urogenital region is the anterior half of the perineum. It lodges the terminal parts of the urinary and genital system. It is divided into two layers, superficial to deep. They are called superficial perineal pouch and deep perineal pouch. The superficial perineal pouch lodges the root of the penis in the male. In the female, it lodges the root of the clitoris. The deep perineal pouch lodges the membranous part of the urethra.

Dissection: Make the body supine, lift up the pelvic region by supporting it with a block. Reflect the skin that is seen between the thighs and anterior abdominal wall infront of the ischial tuberosities, by making a midline incision along the median raphae This includes the reminents of the scrotal skin and the skin over the penis.

Superficial fascia: Note that the superficial fascia here is continuous with the superficial fascia of the back of the scrotum. Clear the loose areolar tissue of the superficial fascia and identify the cutaneous scrotal nerves and vessels. These are branches of the pudendal vessels and nerves.

SUPERFICIAL PERINEAL POUCH—MALE

It is the space between the membranous layer of superficial fascia and perineal membrane. Laterally, it is limited by the ischiopubic ramus. Posteriorly, the membranous layer of the superficial fascia and the perineal membrane are united. Anteriorly the membranous layer of the superficial fascia is continuous with the membranous layer of anterior abdominal wall. In other words, the superficial perineal pouch is continuous with the anterior abdominal wall. During extravasation of urine it ascends up into the anterior abdominal wall. Superficial perineal space in male lodges the root of the penis.

Dissection: Clear the superficial fascia and reidentify the scrotal vessels and nerves. Identify the thick membranous layer of the superficial fascia. It is glistening white in color and tightly closes the root of the penis. You can identify the bulging bulb and crura of the penis. Carefully remove the membranous layer, cutting along the ischiopubic ramus. You can keep checking the thin muscles lying over this cavernous tissue. Identify the root of penis and the blood vessels supplying it. The blood vessels and nerves lie superficial here, so trace and identify them entering into the musculature.

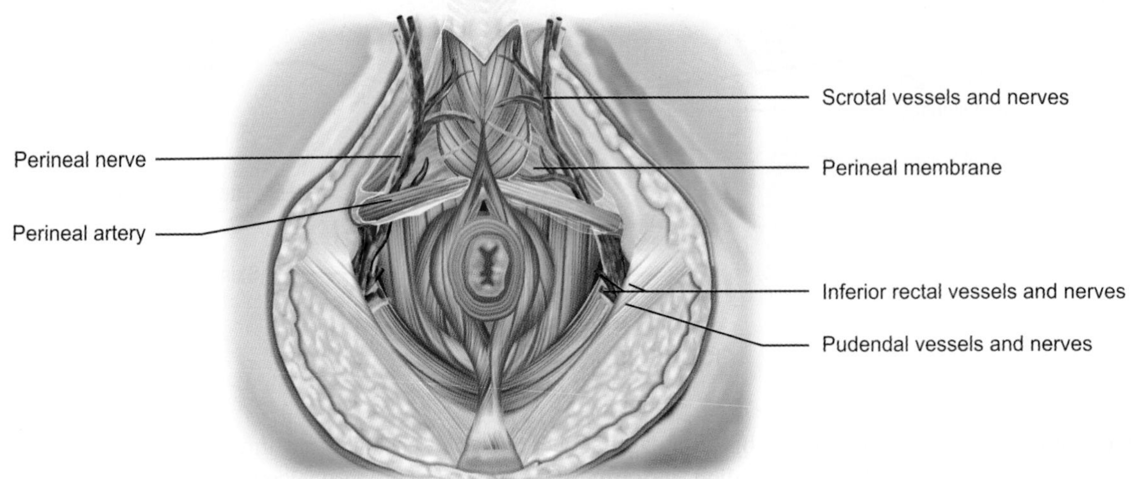

FIGURE 21 Superficial perineal pouch—male blood vessels and nerves

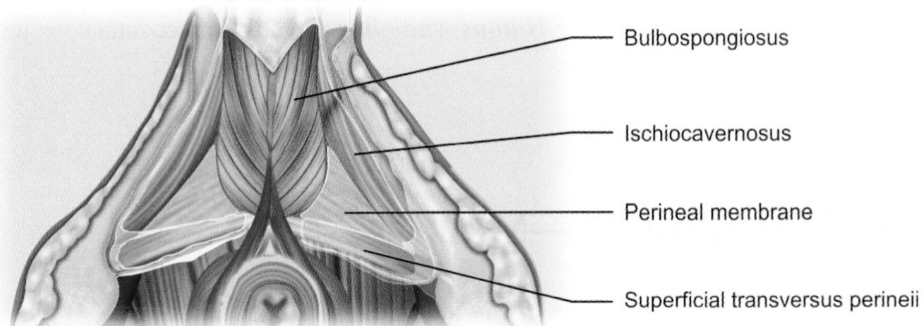

FIGURE 22 Superficial perineal pouch musculature

Nerve and blood supply (Fig. 21): All the muscles of the superficial perineal pouch are supplied by the ***perineal nerve***. This pierces the membranous layer of superficial fascia nearer to the ischial tuberosity and reaches the superficial space. Trace it from the pudendal nerve. The perineal artery and veins accompany the nerve.

Root of penis (Fig. 22): The penis is madeup of cavernous tissue. It is described as having a root, a body and a glans. The root is made up of two crura and a bulb. These are covered by musculature. Identify the musculature over the root. Then remove the musculature to appreciate the root of the penis.

Crura: Press and feel the bulging crus attached to the ischiopubic ramus and the perineal membrane It is covered by ***ischiocavernosus muscle***. See the brown muscle fibres on it. The ischiocavernosus arises from the ischiopubic ramus winds round and is inserted into the corpus cavernous. It compresses the crura to expel the blood from the cavernous tissue. ***Bulb of the penis:*** Identify this centrally located part. This is covered by the ***bulbospongiosus muscle***. It arises from a median raphae and the perineal body, winds round the bulb and is inserted into the deeper aspect of the bulb. This compresses the bulb.

Superficial transversus pereneii muscles: These are two transversely placed muscles extending from the ischial tuberosity to the perineal body. This pulls and tightens the perineal body.

Perineal membrane: It is the facial sheath deep to the root of the penis and forms the roof for the superficial perineal space. The bulb and crura are attached on to it.

Dissection: Identify the perineal membrane between the crura and bulb. Remove the musculature and identify the crura and the bulb. Detach the crura and bulb from the perineal membrane. While cutting them near their attachment, note the arteries entering into them. They are arteries of the bulb into the bulb and deep artery into the crura. Note the urethra entering into the bulb. Remove the root of the penis along with the body. Reflect the skin over the body of the penis and note features of the skin of the prepuce.

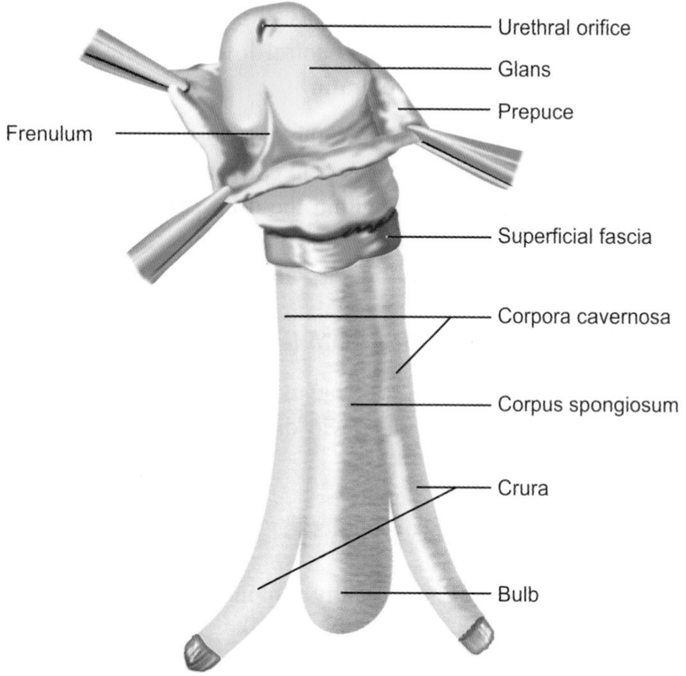

FIGURE 23 Penis

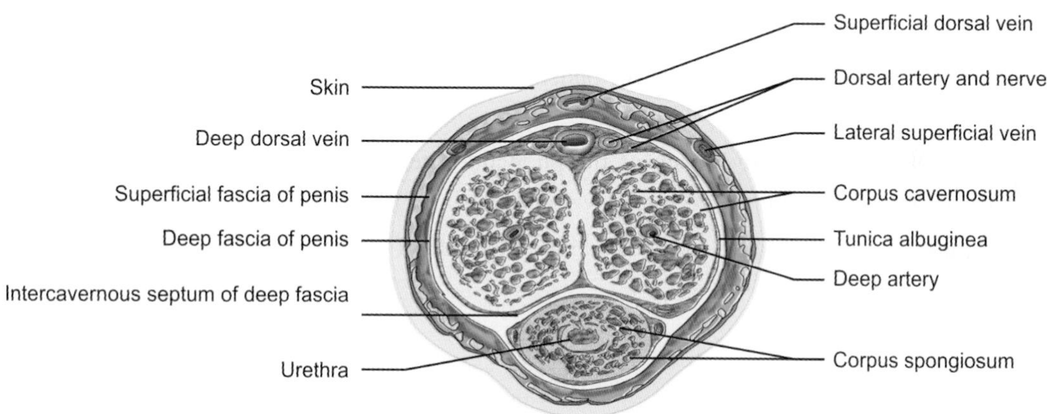

FIGURE 24 Transverse section of penis

Body and glans penis (Fig. 23) is cylindrical in shape. Note that the body is made up of three parts—ventral ***corpus spongiosum,*** the continuation of the bulb of the penis, two dorsal ***corpora cavernosa*** the continuations of crura of penis. ***Glans penis*** is the enlarged part near the tip. It is the corpus spongiosum which enlarges to form the glans. Note that the corpora cavernosa fall short here. ***Prepuce*** is the retractable skin covering the glans. ***Navicular fossa***—is the gap between the skin and prepuce. ***Frenulum*** is the fold of the skin that stretches between the glans and prepuce.

Dissection: Cut through the body of the penis transversely and note the following.

Section of Penis (Fig. 24)

Skin is the outer covering. ***Superficial fascia*** is the loose areolar tissue. Look for the ***deep dorsal vein*** located in the center of the penis on the dorsal surface. This drains into prostatic plexus of veins by passing between the perineal membrane and pubic symphysis. ***Dorsal arteries*** are two in number, one on either side of the deep vein. These are terminal branches of pudendal artery. ***Dorsal nerves*** are two in number. They lie on the lateral side of the artery. These are terminal branches of the pudendal nerves. They supply the skin over the penis. Tunica ***albugenia*** is the thick facial covering deep to the superficial fascia. This is firmly adherent to the spongy bodies corpora cavernous and corpus spongiosum. ***Corpora cavernosa*** lie on the dorsal surface. These are the continuations of the crura. They lie in the midline. They are made up of erectile spongy tissue. This gets filled with blood during penile erection.

Deep artery of the penis: This lies in the substance of the penis. It is the terminal division of the pudendal artery. This supplies the corpora cavernosa. ***Corpus spongisum*** is the central lower erectile body. This is the continuation of the bulb of the penis. Note the horizontally cut central urethra in it.

Urethra in the male carries both urine and seminal fluid to the exterior. It is 20 cm long. This starts at the lower end of the bladder and opens on the tip of the glans penis. It is conventionally divided into three parts—the ***prostatic part,*** this lies within the prostate, the ***membranous part*** lies within the deep perineal pouch, the ***spongy part*** lies within the corpus spongiosum and the glans penis. Try to put a flexible probe into the urethra and note its passage. This is a common procedure followed to drain the urine in bedridden patients.

DEEP PERINEAL POUCH/UROGENITAL DIAPHRAGM (Fig. 25)

This is a closed space formed by the superior and inferior facial layers with the sphincter urethra and deep transverses perineii muscles within its substance. Inferior layer of pelvic diaphragm or perineal membrane is the sheet of fascia separating superficial and deep perineal pouch.

Dissection: Remove the remnants of the perineal membrane to see the deeper structures.

Deep transversus pereneii: These are two small horizontally running muscles one on either side of the perineal body. They take origin from the ischial tuberosity and get inserted into the perineal body in the midline. It helps to fix the perineal body. It is supplied by the pudendal nerve.

Sphincter urethrae: It is a thick circular muscle. It extends from the ischiopubic ramus to the perineal body. It encircles the urethra. It is a voluntary muscle supplied by a branch of the pudendal nerve. This muscle expels the last drop of urine. This is normally closed. This relaxes at the time of urination.

Deep artery of penis: It is a terminal division of the pudendal artery. This runs along the inner border of the ischiopubic ramus. This enters the crura by piercing through it.

Artery of the bulb: It is a transverse branch of the pudendal artery. This traverses to the center and pierces the perineal membrane to supply the bulb of penis.

Bulbourethral glands: These are small glands placed on either side of the urethra inferiorly. Ducts of the gland pierce the perineal membrane and open into urethra.

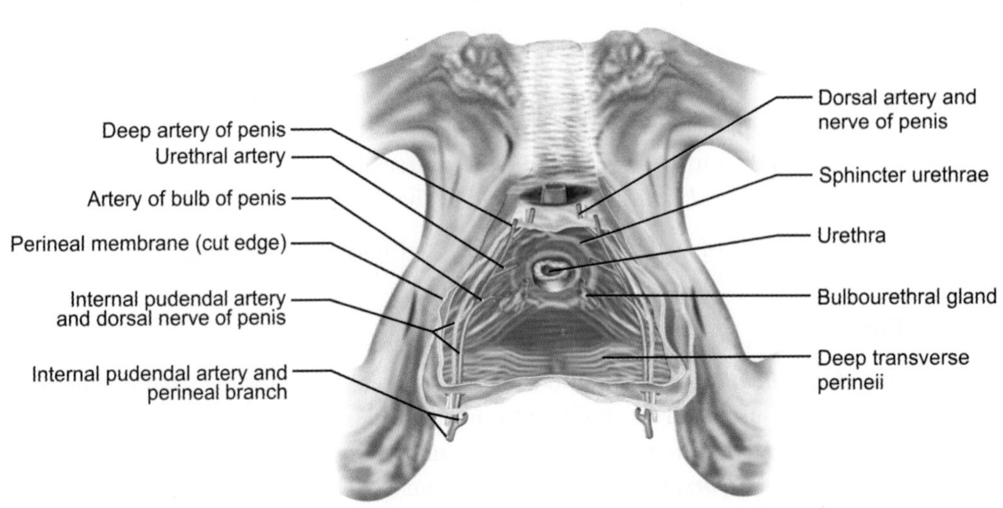

FIGURE 25 Deep perineal pouch—male

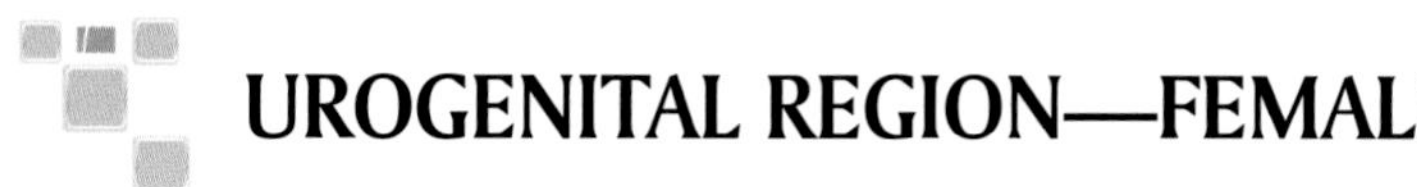

UROGENITAL REGION—FEMALE

FEMALE EXTERNAL GENITALIA (FIG. 26)

Identify the following on a female body.

Mons pubis is the hairy skin over the pubic bone. This region feels hard due to heavily laden fat beneath it. ***Labium major*** is the fold of skin that extends from the mons pubis to the area infront of the anus where both the labia majora unite in the midline. ***Pudendal cleft*** is the area between the two labia majora. The labia majora presents a smooth surface towards the inner side due to openings of the sebaceous glands. ***Labia minora*** are thin red folds of nonhairy skin. This encloses the clitoris superiorly and meets each other inferiorly. ***Clitoris*** is the cavernous organ. It corresponds to the penis. The ***glans of the clitoridis*** can be seen as a small projection. It is enclosed in suspensory ligament. Inferiorly it forms the ***frenulum. Vestibule*** is the space between the two labia minora. Urethral orifice is smaller and is an anterior orifice. The vaginal orifice is a wider posterior orifice.

Dissection: Remove the skin from the perineal region totally.

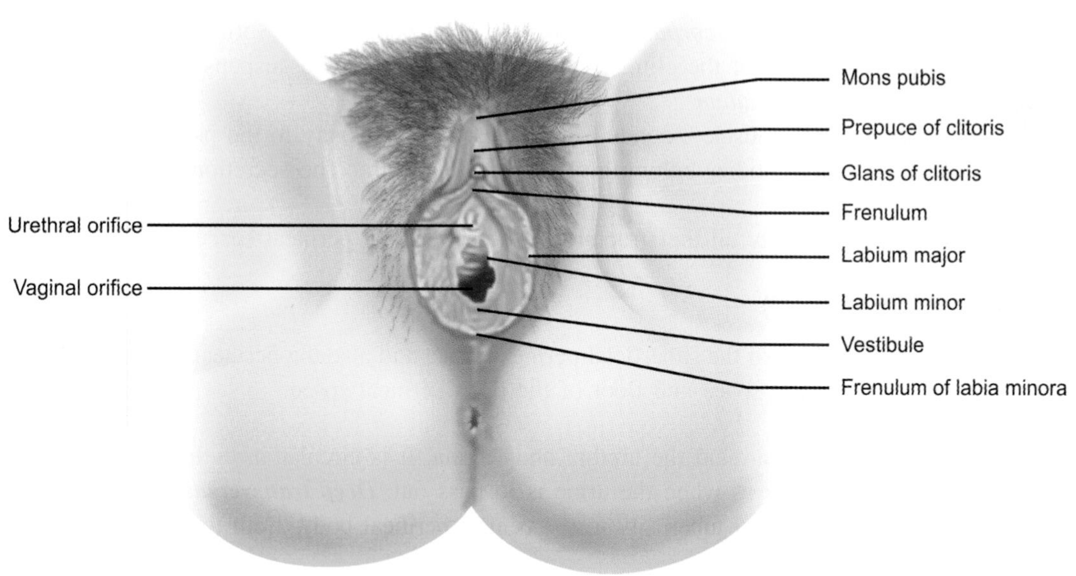

FIGURE 26 Female external genitalia

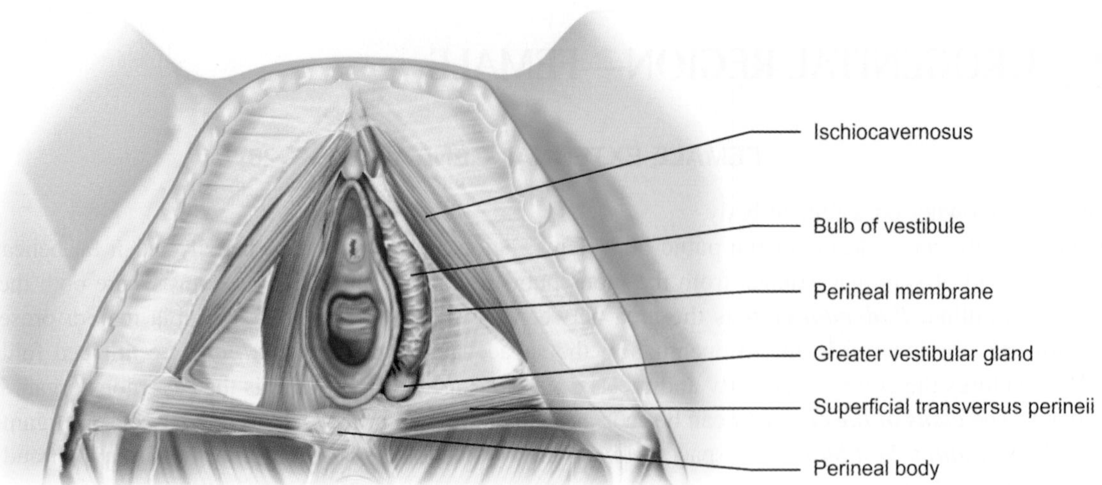

FIGURE 27 Superficial perineal pouch—female

Superficial perineal pouch (Fig. 27) in female though has the same structures as the male, it is smaller in size as the clitoris is much a smaller structure.

Identify the following.

Crura are attached to the ischiopubic ramus. The ***ischiocavernous muscle*** takes origin from the ischiopubic ramus and is inserted into the crura. ***Bulb*** is split in female and is seen around the vestibule, i.e. around the vaginal and urethral orifice.

See the ***bulbospongiosus muscle***. It arises from the perineal body and the perineal membrane and is inserted into the sides of the bulb. The crura continue as ***corpora cavernosa*** and the two parts of the bulb join together at the ***commissure of the vestibule*** and form the ***corpus spongiosum.*** They both unite to form the ***body of the clitoris.*** The body is very short and ends as *glans* of the clitoris. The glans is enclosed in suspensory ligament. Inferiorly the connection can be identified as the *frenulum.*

Superficial transversus pereneii muscle extends from the ischial tuberosity to the perineal body in the midline. Greater ***vestibular glands*** are small bodies below the bulb of the urethra. The secretions pour into the side of the vestibule.

Perineal vessels and nerves supply all the structure in the superficial perineal space.

DEEP PERINEAL SPACE (Fig. 28)

Dissection: Remove the structures of the superficial perineal space and also the perineal membrane which forms the roof of the superficial perineal space and floor of the deep perineal space.

Sphincter urethrae is the muscle around the urethra and vagina. It is circular in outline and a voluntary muscle supplied by the perineal nerve. It relaxes when the urine is to pass out. ***Deep transversus pereneii*** is a horizontally placed muscle extending from the ischial tuberosity to the central perineal body. Both these muscles are supplied by the perineal nerve.

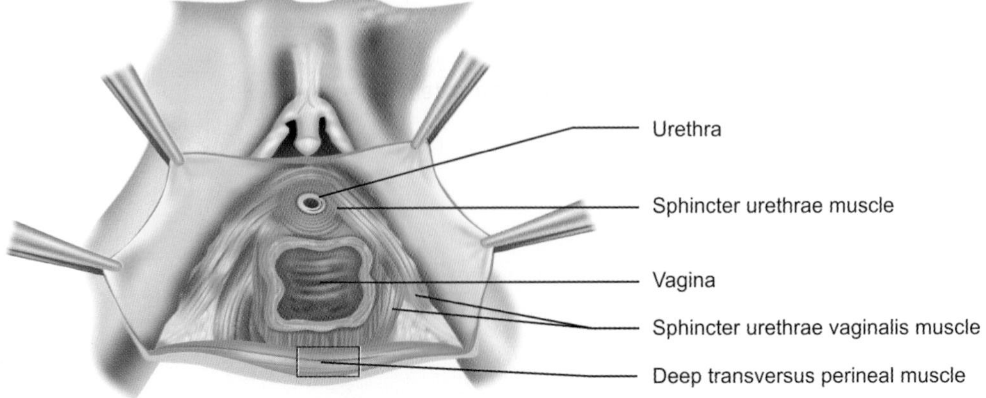

FIGURE 28 Deep perineal pouch—female

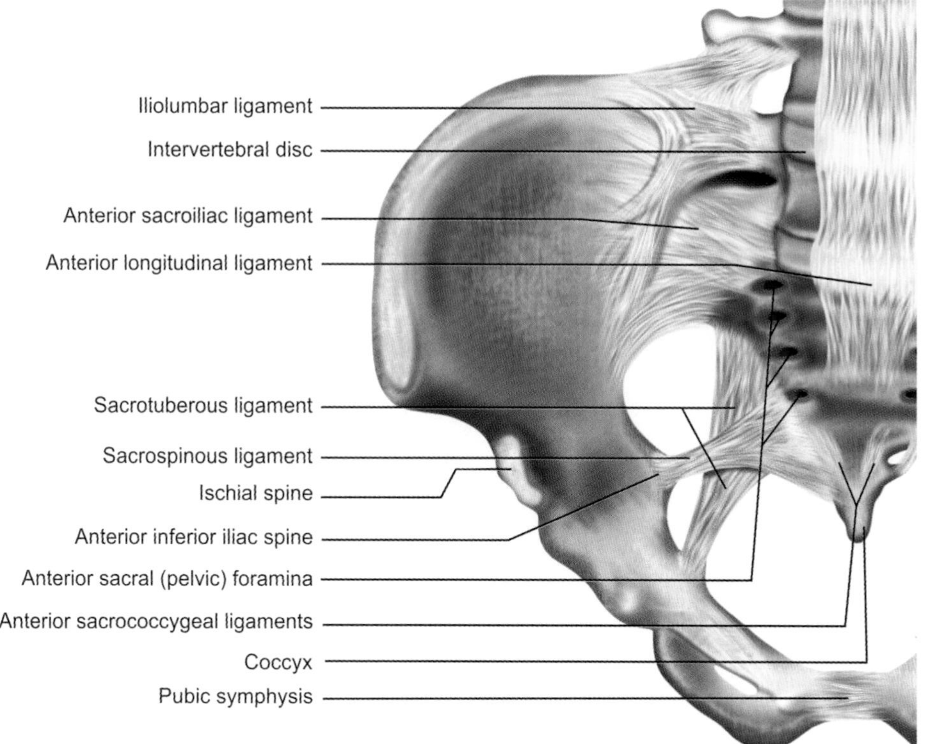

FIGURE 29 Joints of pelvis

JOINTS OF PELVIS (Fig. 29)

See the articulated skeleton and note that the sacrum and the two hip bones form the pelvis. The sacrum articulates with the ilium laterally at the sacroiliac joint. The two hip bones articulate in front at the pubic symphysis. The sacrum articulates superiorly with the 5th lumbar vertebra and inferiorly with the coccyx.

Dissection: Clean the areas of the joints and try to see the ligaments. It is not essential to open up the joints to see the interiors.

The sacroiliac joint is a plane synovial joint. Observe the joint surfaces on dry bones. Note that they are reciprocally curved to fit into each other. The bones are united together by capsule and are supported by dorsal ventral and interosseous ligaments.

Pubic symphysis is a secondary cartilaginous joint. See the articulating surfaces on a dry bone. In living they are covered by hyaline cartilage. These are further united together by fibrocartilage. They are supported by superior and inferior pubic ligaments.

Lumbosacral joint is a secondary cartilaginous joint. A fibrocartilaginous intervertebral disc is placed between the 5th lumbar vertebra and the sacrum. The anterior and posterior longitudinal ligaments connect the vertebrae, the ligamentum flava connects the two laminae, the interspinous ligaments connect the spines of the vertebrae. Iliolumbar ligament is an accessory ligament connects the transverse process of the 5th lumbar vertebra to the inner lip of the iliac crest. It is a very strong ligament.

Sacrococcygeal joint is a secondary cartilaginous joint. The bones are united by the fibrocartilage. Generally it is ossified.

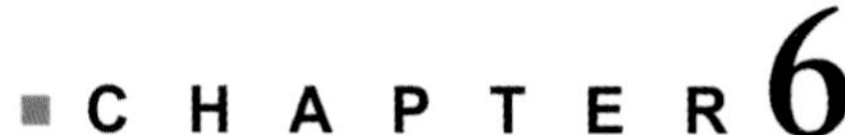

CHAPTER 6

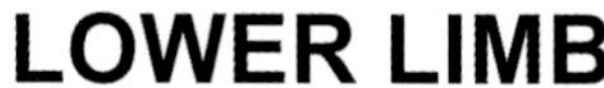

LOWER LIMB

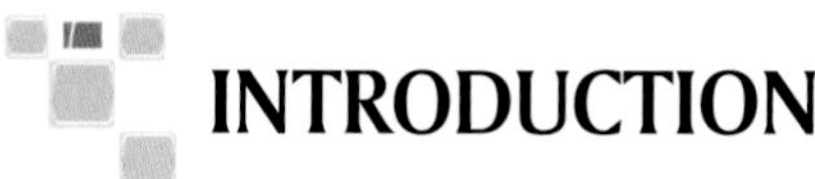

INTRODUCTION

The lower limb is another appendage of the trunk. Functionally it bears the weight of the body, and propels it. So the bones of the lower limb are bigger and are heavily laden with musculature. Though its arrangement is similar to the upper limb with four parts—the pelvic girdle, thigh, leg and foot, the arrangement of bones and joints are such that they are specialized for weight transmission, and relatively the movement is limited.

The lower limb is attached to the trunk by the ***pelvic girdle***. Unlike the pectoral girdle, which is located on the thoracic cage the pelvic girdle directly articulates with the sacral part of the vertebral column, forms the pelvis and protects the pelvic organs. The external surface of the pelvic girdle gives attachment to the musculature of the thigh. This region is called ***gluteal region***. It lodges the extensors and lateral rotators of the thigh.

Thigh is the proximal part of the lower limb. ***Femur*** forms its skeleton. The thigh has an anterior junctional region—***femoral triangle***. This lodges the flexor muscles of the thigh and the neurovascular bundle. The thigh is in general divided into anterior **(Fig. 1)**, medial and posterior compartments by intermuscular septa **(Fig. 2)**. The adductors of the thigh occupy the medial and posterior aspect of thigh. The extensors of leg occupy the anterior, medial and lateral

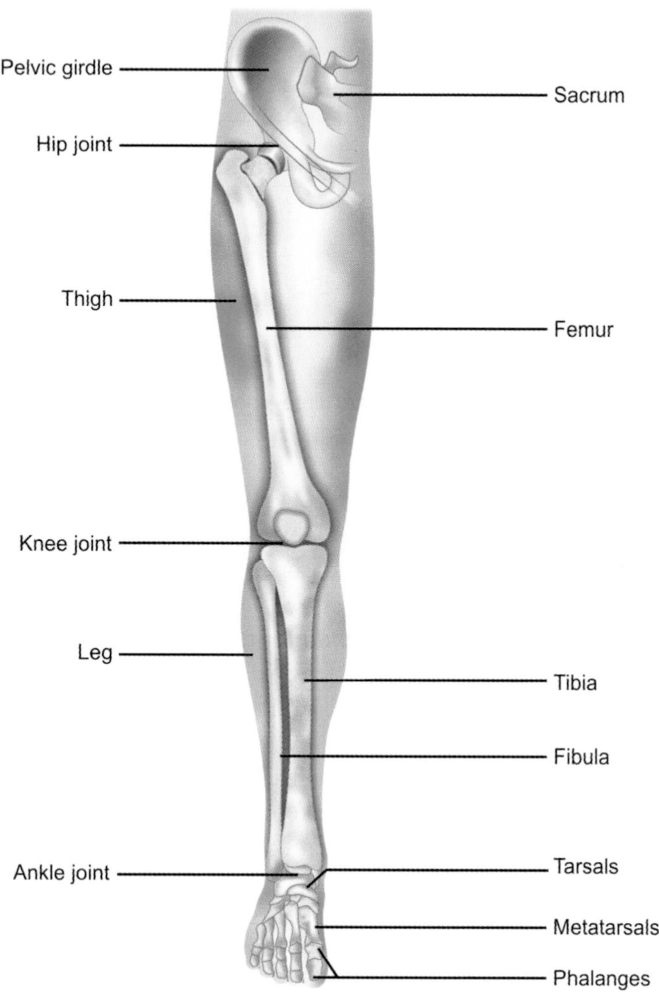

FIGURE 1: Lower limb—anterior view

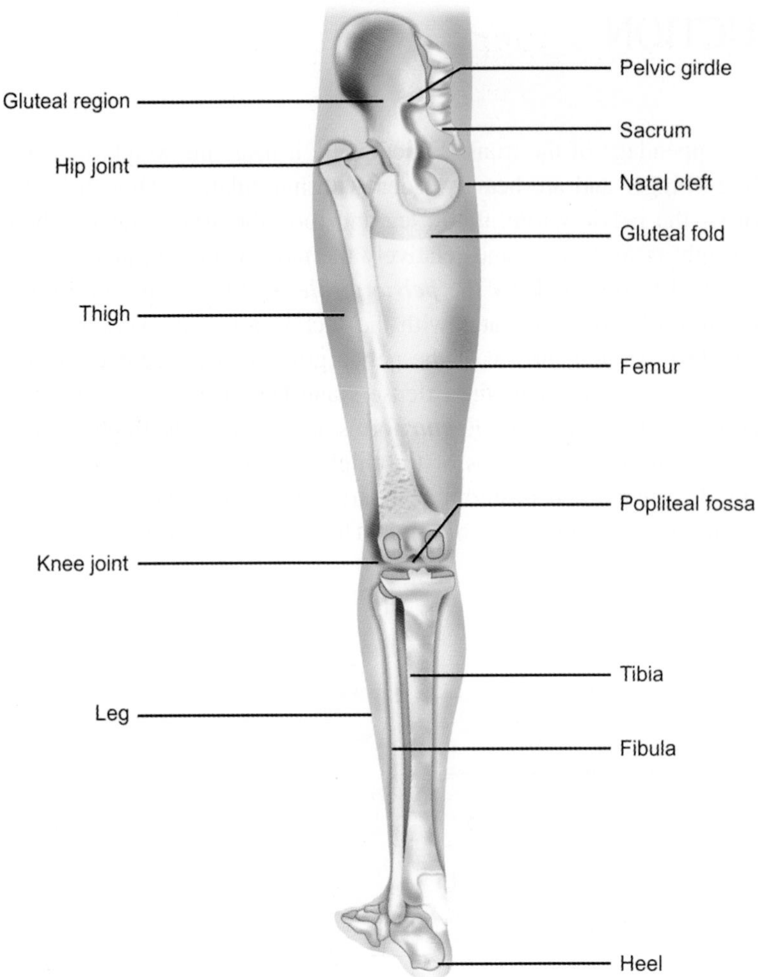

FIGURE 2 Lower limb—posterior view

aspect of thigh; this is a single quadriceps femoris muscle. Flexors of the leg occupy the posterior aspect of the thigh. Some of them ascend up to the pelvis so as to act as extensors of thigh. These are called hamstrings. The ***popliteal fossa*** lies behind the bend of the knee.

Leg is the next part of the lower limb. The ***tibia*** and ***fibula*** form the skeleton of the leg. The interosseous membrane unites these two bones to each other and movement is not feasible. Proximally it receives the insertions of the muscles acting on the knee joint. It lodges the muscles of the foot, in three compartments—anteriorly the extensors, laterally evertors, posteriorly flexors and invertors.

Foot is the distal part of the lower limb. It is located perpendicular to the other part. It is arranged in an arched form. Its main function is weight bearing and accommodates the foot to the uneven surfaces on which it has to walk. Its skeleton if formed by the ***tarsals, metatarsals*** and ***phalanges.*** It lodges the intrinsic muscles of the foot within its concavity.

The lower limb articulates with the trunk at the ***hip joint***. It is a polyaxial joint. Though movement is possible in all directions, it is very much restricted and the importance is given to the stability of the joint. Thigh articulates with the leg at the ***knee joint.*** This articulation is between the lower end of the femur with the upper end of the tibia. The robust articulating surfaces effectively transmit the weight. The leg articulates with the foot at the ***ankle joint.*** The ***subtalar*** and ***mid tarsal joints*** of the foot are of great importance. All these joints act in unison to move the foot in all directions and help it to accommodate to the uneven surfaces of the ground. The ***intertarsal, tarsometatarsal, metatarsophalangeal*** and ***interphalangeal*** joints form the joints of the foot.

See cross sections of thigh and leg to understand the compartments.

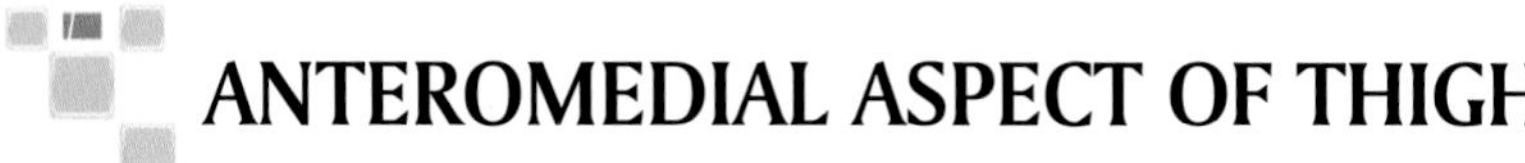

ANTEROMEDIAL ASPECT OF THIGH

Bony Points (Fig. 3)

Go to an articulated skeleton and note the ***pelvic girdle, femur*** and the ***upper part of tibia.***
Identify the following bony points on the hip bone—*anterior superior iliac spine, anterior inferior iliac spine, iliac crest, iliac tubercle, iliopubic eminence, superior ramus of pubis, pubic crest, body of the pubis, pubic tubercle, ischiopubic ramus* and *the ischial tuberosity.*

Note the position of the ***acetabulum*** facing laterally.

On the femur note the ***head, neck*** and ***greater trochanter, lesser trochanter*** and ***the intertrochanteric line.*** Look at the shaft of the femur, note its anterior convexity. Note that the shaft is smooth on all the surfaces except for the posterior thick ***linea aspera.*** At the lower end of the femur identify the expanded femoral condyles. See the adductor tubercle above the medial condyle. Note the ***patellar articulating surface*** on the anterior aspect of the femur.

See the upper end of the tibia. It is expanded to form the ***tibial condyles.*** These articulate with the femoral condyles. The tibial tuberosity which lies below the condyles receives the ligamentum patellae.

See the position of fibula. It lies below the tibia. It articulates with the undersurface of the tibia.

Note that the femur is obliquely located in the body. The upper end of the femur is widely separated by the positioning of the pelvis between the two femurs whereas the lower ends approximate each other.

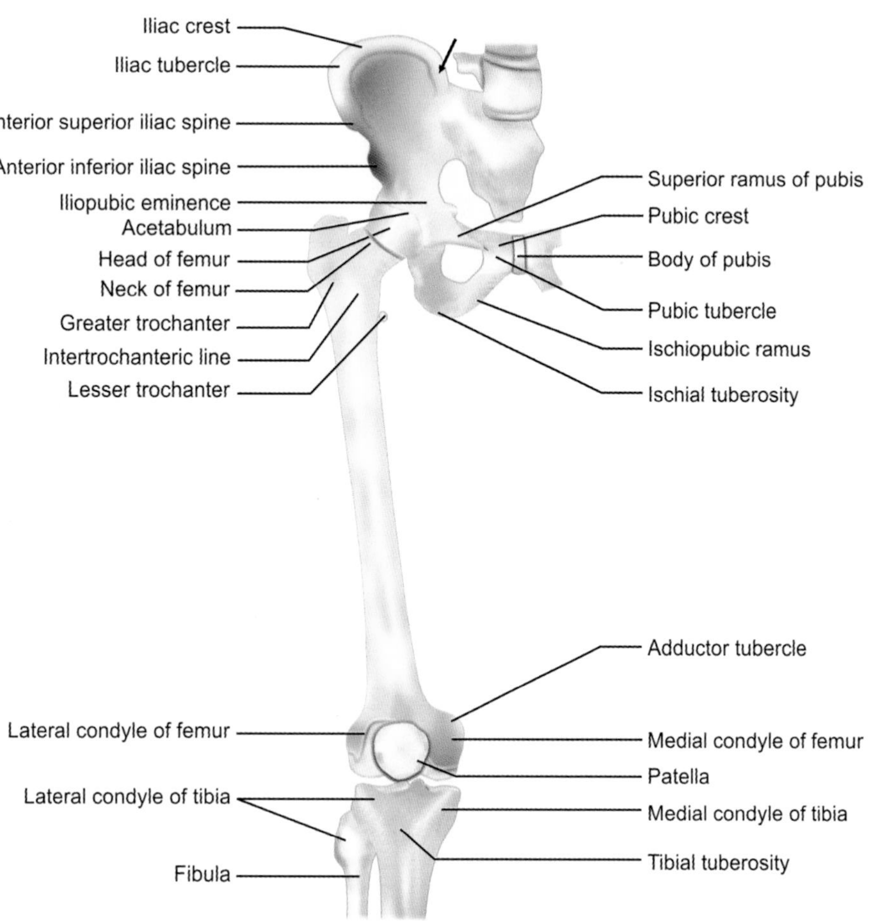

FIGURE 3 Bony points

SURFACE AND LIVING ANATOMY (Fig. 4)

Identify the following on the living body and the cadaver

Feel the following bony points—***the anterior superior iliac spine, the iliac crest, iliac tubercle, ischiopubic ramus*** and ***the ischial tuberosity.*** Note that the anteromedial aspect of the thigh is occupied by very thick musculature. In a muscular body identify the ***tensor fascia lata, adductor muscles, quadriceps muscle*** and ***the femoral triangle*** between the two bulging muscle masses.

The junction between the abdomen and the thigh is called the ***groin.*** Feel the resilient inguinal ligament extending between the anterior superior iliac spine and the pubic tubercle along the groin.

Feel the pulsations of the ***femoral artery*** at the midinguinal point, midway between the anterior superior iliac spine and pubic symphysis against the tendon of psoas major.

At the lower end, identify the ***femoral condyles, tibial condyles, tibial tuberosity*** and ***patella.***

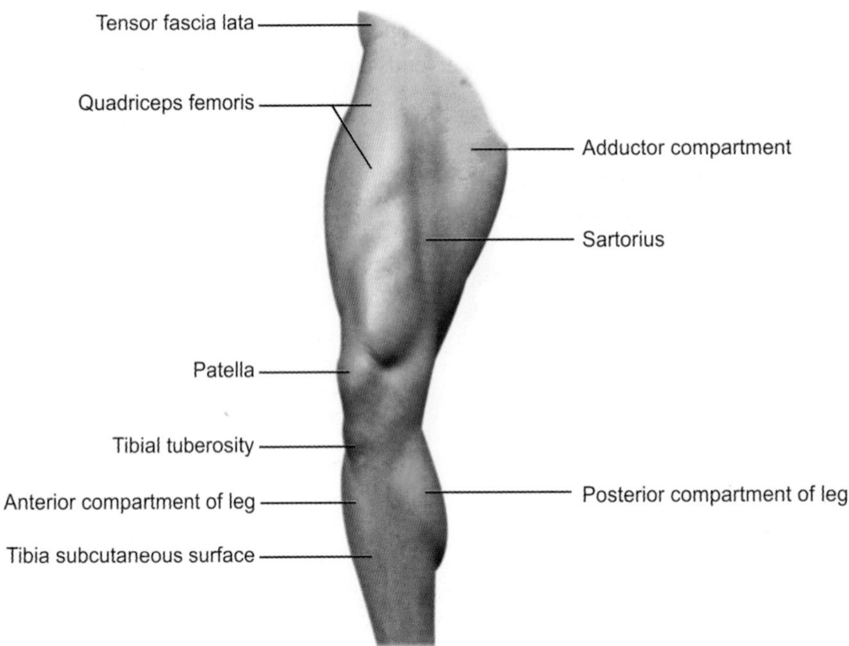

FIGURE 4 Surface and living anatomy

Skin Incision (Fig. 5)

Dissection: Make the following skin incisions: A superior incision from the anterior superior iliac spine to the pubic tubercle, pubic tubercle to the pubic crest below the rectus sheath, Pull and turn the limb laterally, identify the ischial tuberosity and make the following incision - from pubic crest to ischial tuberosity along the ischiopubic ramus, Make a superolateral incision from the anterior superior iliac spine along the iliac crest to the tubercle of ilium. Make a lateral vertical incision from the tubercle of the ilium to the leg below the tibial tuberosity, on the lateral side. Make a medial vertical incision from the ischial tuberosity along the medial side of the thigh to reach the leg below the tibial tuberosity. Make a horizontal incision connecting medial and lower vertical incisions.

In the bodies where abdomen is dissected you need to make only lower incisions.

Reflect the total skin starting from the medial side of the thigh and reflect it towards the lateral side. Skin here is thin needs a careful dissection, but it can easily be stripped off, as the subcutaneous tissue is loose. Generally it is laden with fat. The prominent structure seen in the fat is the great saphenous vein.

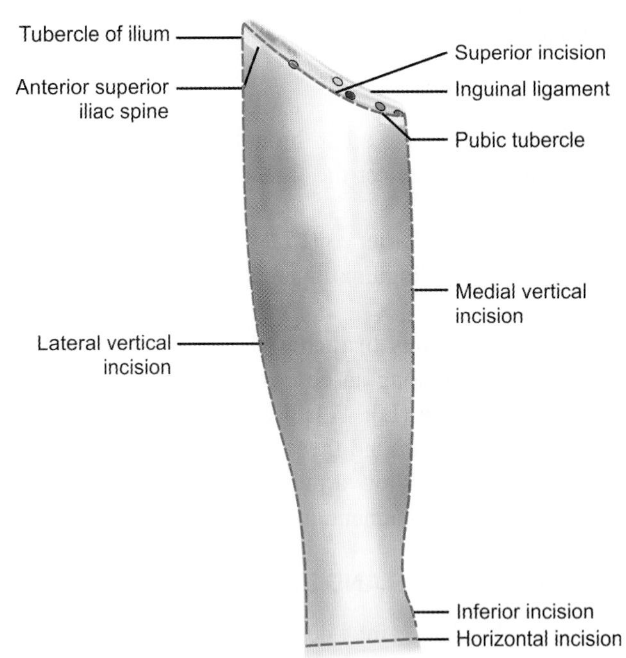

FIGURE 5 Skin incision—Anterior side of thigh

CUTANEOUS STRUCTURES (Fig. 6)

The subcutaneous tissue is heavily laden with fat here. In the subcutaneous connective tissue identify and clean the cutaneous veins, arteries and the nerves. The superficial veins in the lower limb play a very important role in draining the blood against gravity. They drain all the superficial structures. The arteries are few and small in caliber compared to the veins. They do not accompany the veins. The cutaneous nerves pierce the deep fascia at definitive points, thick and can easily be identified.

Cutaneous Nerves

Identify the cutaneous nerves in two rows—one row along the lower border of the inguinal ligament. These are the terminal branches of these nerves and are very fine. They are difficult to identify. ***Femoral branch of genitofemoral nerve*** supplies the skin over the middle of the upper end of the thigh. Identify the following cutaneous nerves along an

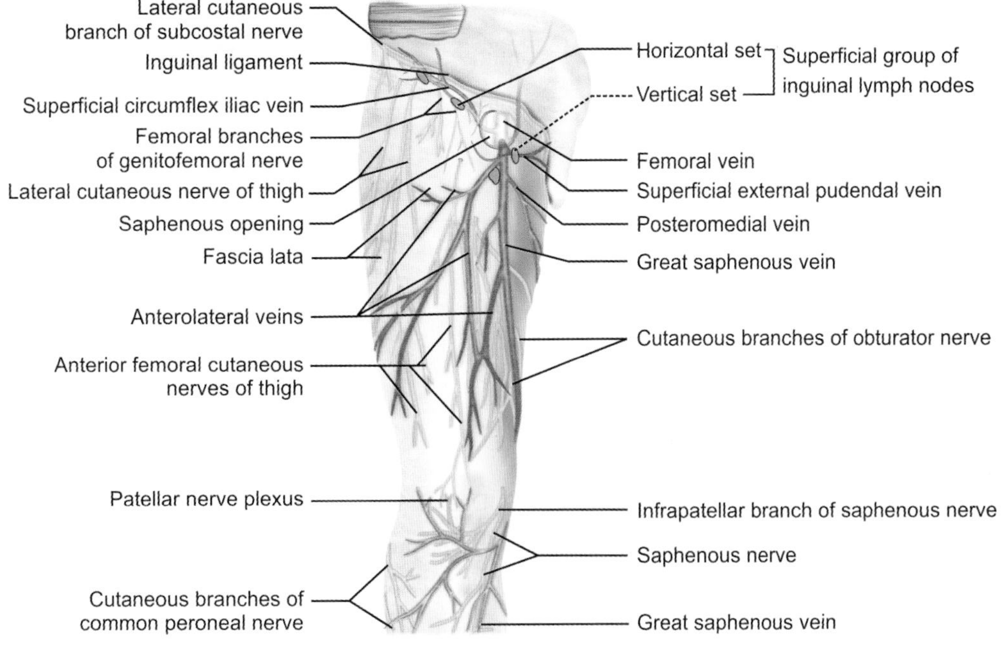

FIGURE 6 Cutaneous structures

oblique line from below the anterior superior iliac spine to the medial side of thigh, they pierce the deep fascia at the points indicated, lateral to the great saphenous vein.

Dissection: Make a cut through the fat along the anterior superior iliac spine to the middle of the thigh on the medial side. Reflect the fascia downwards, while doing so note the cutaneous nerves piercing the deep fascia.

Lateral cutaneous nerve (L2,3) is a direct branch from the lumbar plexus. This pierces the deep fascia below the lateral end of the inguinal ligament divides into branches and supplies the skin on the lateral aspect of the thigh up to the patella.

Anterior cutaneous branches (L2, 3) are branches of femoral nerve. They are lateral and medial branches, pierces and deep fascia along an oblique line and supply the anterior aspect of the skin of the thigh and leg.

Saphenous nerve (L3, 4) is a branch of the femoral nerve, its infrapatellar branch pierces just above the patella and supplies the skin around the patella on its medial side.

The above nerves show a plexiform arrangement in front of the patella and is called prepatellar plexus. This supplies the skin over the ligamentum patellae.

BLOOD VESSELS AND LYMPHATICS

Great saphenous vein: Locate this thick vein on the anteromedial aspect of the thigh. It is a very prominent structure here. It begins at the dorsum of the foot and drains most of the superficial structures on the medial side of lower limb. Locate its tributaries in the thigh—the ***anterolateral vein, the posteromedial vein.*** Trace the great saphenous vein superiorly till it disappears into the saphenous opening.

Arteries: *Superficial circumflex iliac, superficial epigastric and superficial external pudendal arteries* and veins are small cutaneous blood vessels—reaching the corresponding regions and supplying the skin over those areas. Try to identify the small arteries near the termination of the great saphenous vein. Try to identify the corresponding veins entering into the great saphenous vein.

Superficial inguinal lymph nodes: Try to see the lymph nodes in the upper part of thigh. There are two sets of lymph nodes in the superficial fascia along the inguinal ligament. One set is called ***horizontal set*** and that lies along and parallel to the inguinal ligament, the ***vertical set*** lies perpendicular to the horizontal set along the long saphenous vein. The horizontal set drains lymph the area of skin and superficial fascia below the level of umbilicus; the vertical set drains lymph from the superficial fascia and skin of the lower limb.

The position of great saphenous vein, and its tributaries is of great importance while operating on varicose veins in lower limb.

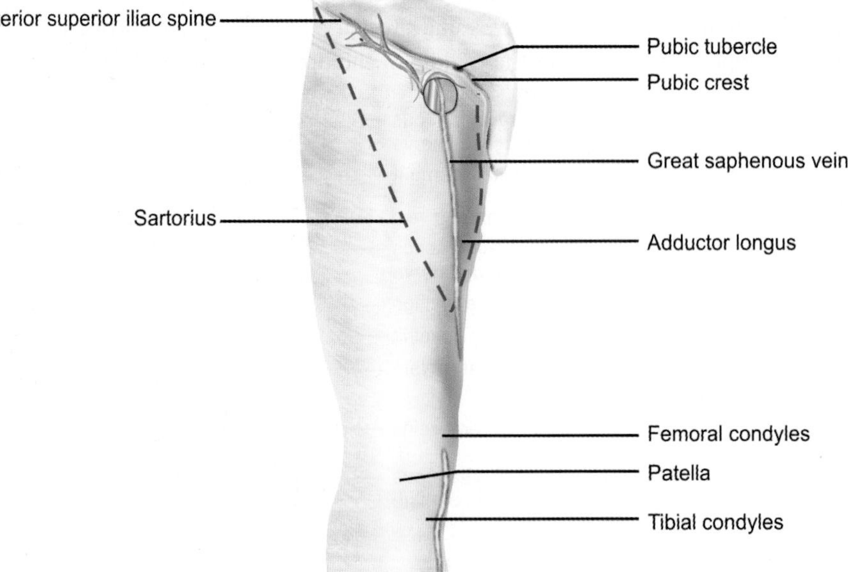

FIGURE 7 Deep fascia/fascia lata. Incision and reflection of deep fascia

DEEP FASCIA—FASCIA LATA (Fig. 7)

Fascia lata is a sleeve of deep fascia, covers all the muscles of thigh and gets attached to the bony points proximally and distally. Before proceeding further confirm the following details on the skeleton and on the body.

Proximal attachment: Take a pelvis, preferably with ligamentous attachments, and confirm the points of attachments of the fascia lata-anterior superior iliac spine, inguinal ligament, pubic tubercle, pubic crest, ischiopubic ramus, ischial tuberosity, sacrotuberous ligament, posterior inferior iliac spine, posterior superior iliac spine and iliac crest.

Distal attachment: Go near a skeletal and identify the following points, superior border of patella, femoral condyles along the sides, tibial tuberosity, tibial condyles—infront and along the side, and head of the fibula.

The fascia lata is thinner nearer to the medial side of thigh. The fascia is thick and encloses two muscles in the lateral aspect by splitting into two parts. Here it is called iliotibial tract (It will be seen at a later dissection).

The fascia lata sends in three septa to reach the linea aspera of femur. It divides the thigh into three compartments–the anterior extensor compartment, the medial adductor compartment and the posterior flexor compartment.

Patellar bursae are subcutaneous bursae present, infront (prepatellar) and below (subcutaneous infrapatellar) the patella. These help in the free movement of the skin over the patella and tibia.

Saphenous opening and cribriform plate: Locate the great saphenous vein near its termination. Clean the sharp margin of the deep fascia lateral to the veins. Lift the vein put your fingers deep to it. The gap between the lateral margin and the medial deeper part is the saphenous opening. It is a sickle shaped gap within the deep fascia. The great saphenous vein, cutaneous arteries pass through this gap. The interstices is filled with connective tissue, so it is called cribriform plate—a sieve like area is with the passage of structures.

Dissection: Make a triangular incision in the deep fascia along the lines shown in the figure. The deep fascia is to be removed to expose the triangle. It is very thick over the lateral aspect and thinner over the adductor longus. Trace the cutaneous nerves proximally, to their origin. Lateral cutaneous nerve of thigh lies between sartorius and deep fascia, femoral cutaneous nerves from the femoral nerve lie in a deep groove between iliacus and psoas major lateral to the femoral artery. Note that the fibres of the deep fascia run longitudinally. Carefully remove the deep fascia from the structures deep to it.

FEMORAL TRIANGLE

Boundaries (Fig. 8)

This shows the position of the muscles in this sloping muscular triangle. The neurovascular bundle occupies the slope. The deep fascia along with the cutaneous structures studied so far forms ***roof*** of the femoral triangle. The medial border of the adductor longus muscle forms ***medial wall.*** The medial border of the ***sartorius*** forms ***lateral wall.*** The inguinal ligament forms ***base. Apex*** is the point where sartorius and adductor longus meet. The iliopsoas, pectineus and the adductor longus form the sloping floor of the triangle.

The structures will be studied as you encounter them in the body. Identify the structures in the following order:

Inguinal ligament: It is the thick lower margin of the external oblique muscle of the abdomen.

Sartorius muscle: This is a long muscle extending from the anterior superior iliac spine to the medial aspect of the shaft of the tibia. This muscle crosses the hip joint anteriorly and is a flexor of hip joint. Note that it crosses the knee joint on its posterior aspect and so also it is a flexor of knee joint. As it crosses from lateral to the medial aspect it rotates the tibia laterally. This muscle is called tailor's muscle, the position assumed by a tailor while stitching. It is a muscle with parallel fibres.

Adductor longus: It has a rounded tendinous origin from the body of the pubis, spreads out to form a triangular muscle, passes deep, to reach the posterior aspect of the femur on to the linea aspera. Feel this muscle from origin to insertion.

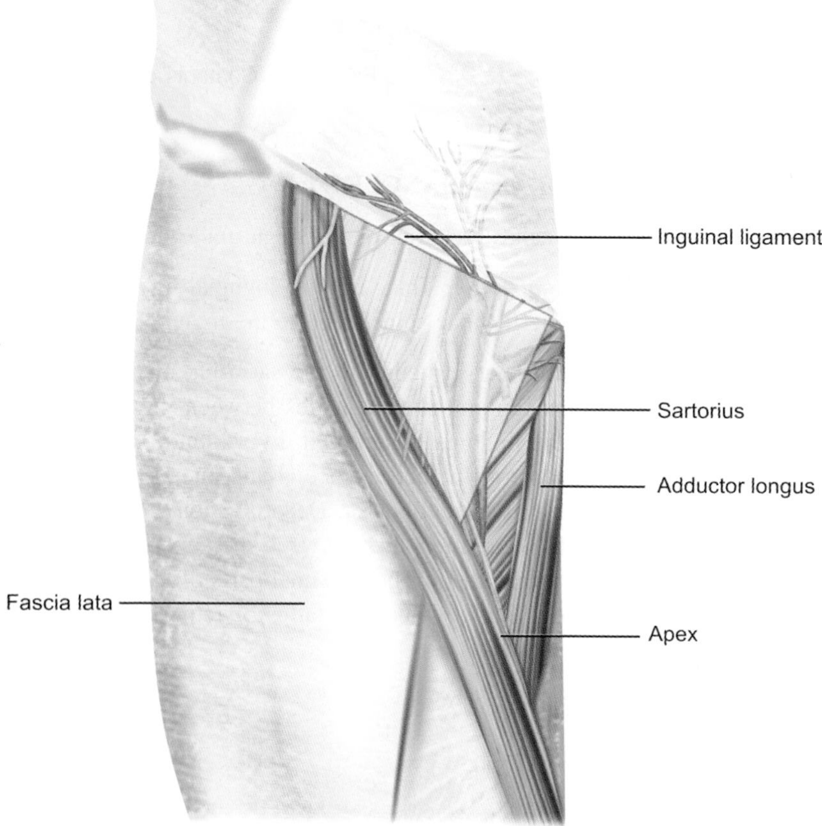

FIGURE 8 Boundaries of femoral triangle

Note that all these muscles slope, go deep to reach the back of femur.

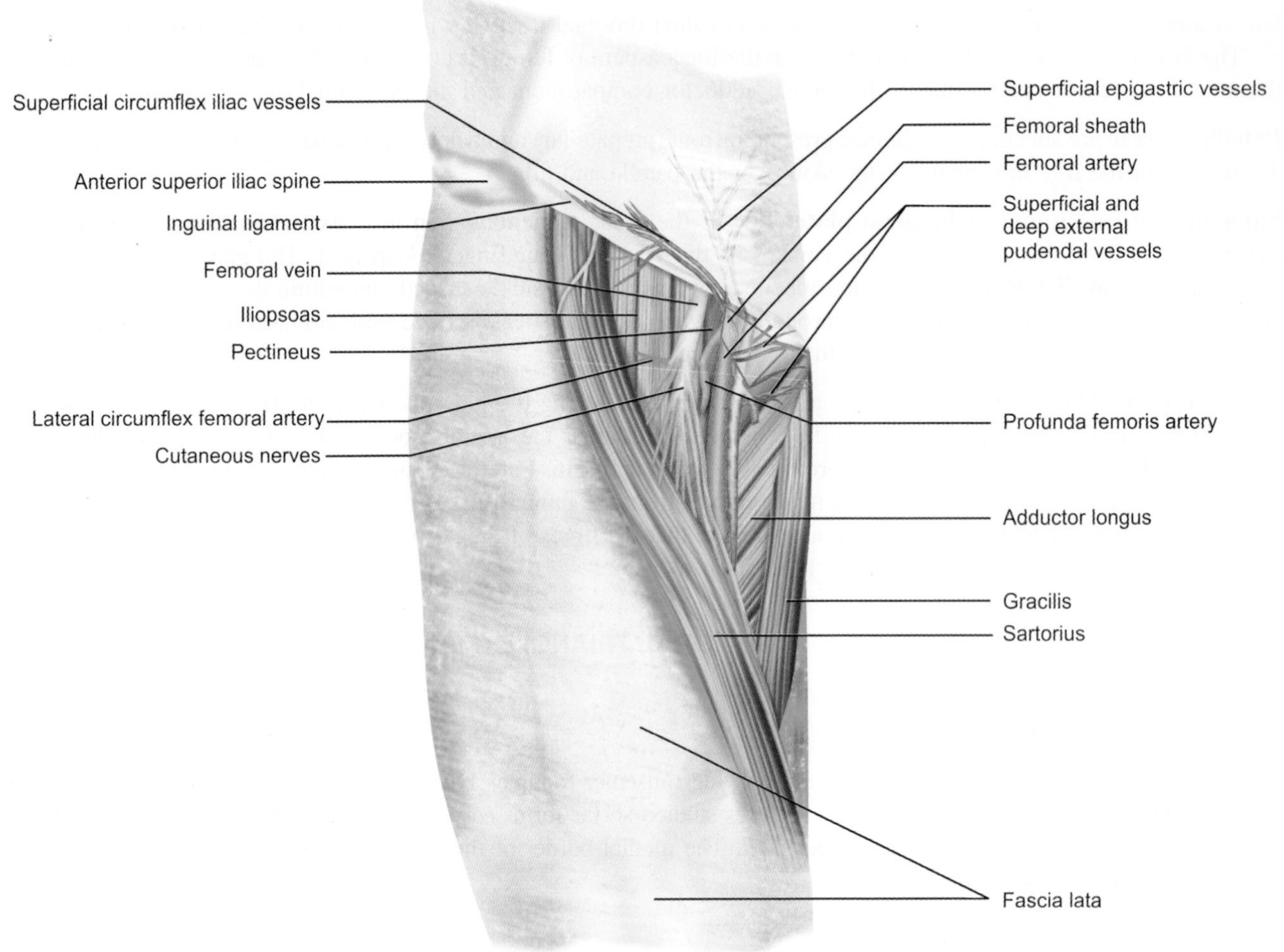

FIGURE 9 Contents of femoral triangle

CONTENTS OF FEMORAL TRIANGLE (Fig. 9)

Neurovascular bundle reaches the front of the thigh under cover of the inguinal ligament. They are:

Lateral cutaneous nerve of thigh: Trace it up to inguinal ligament. You already have the cutaneous part of it; trace it medial to the anterior superior iliac spine, deep to the inguinal ligament.

Femoral nerve: Trace this nerve medial to the sartorius muscle. It lies deep to the inguinal ligament. It is a thick nerve, seen lateral to the femoral sheath. It lies between the iliacus, which is muscular, and psoas major, which is tendinous. 2 cm below the linguinal ligament it divides into a superficial and a deep division. The superficial division gives off the anterior cutaneous branches (medial and lateral) and nerve to sartorius. Trace the nerve to the sartorius. It enters the muscle along its medial border. Deep division is predominantly motor, this can be traced at a later stage. The lateral circumflex femoral artery lies between the superficial and deep divisions of the femoral nerve. It can be taken as a guide to distinguish them. The proximal parts of femoral artery and femoral vein are enclosed in the femoral sheath. Branches of femoral artery, and tributaries of femoral vein pierce the sheath.

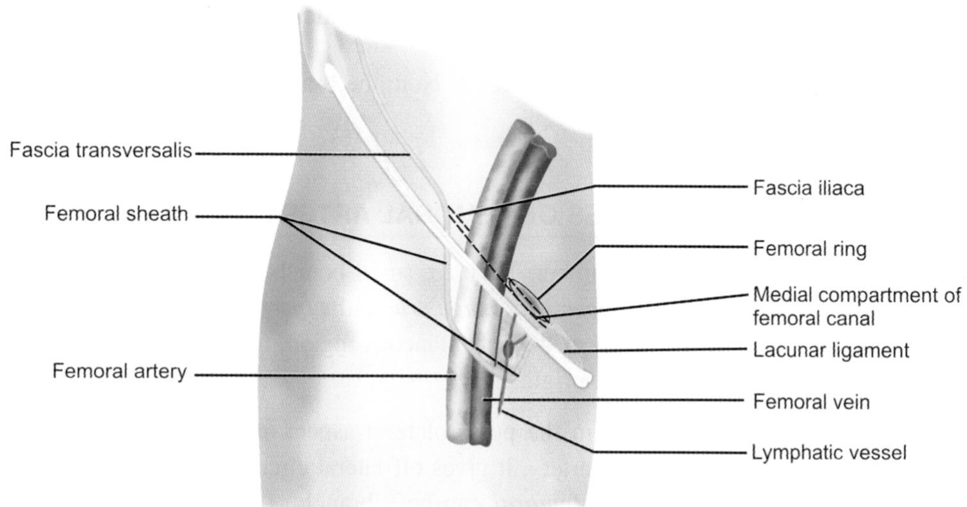

FIGURE 10 Femoral sheath (diagrammatic representation)

Femoral Sheath (Fig. 10)

Femoral sheath is a thick connective tissue sheath covering the blood vessels in this region. When the blood vessels enter the thigh, they pass between the anterior and posterior walls of the abdomen. This is formed by ***fascia transversalis***, the fascia on the undersurface of the anterior abdominal wall musculature and ***fascia iliaca*** which covers the posterior abdominal wall musculature. The blood vessels drag these coverings and get enclosed by them. It is seen as a triangular shaped femoral sheath. The fascia thins out and merges with the adventitia of the blood vessels an inch and half below the inguinal ligament. Three compartments separated by septa can be identified in this sheath. ***Lateral compartment*** lodges the femoral artery. ***Intermediate compartment*** lodges the femoral vein. ***Medial compartment*** is called femoral canal. It is filled by fat and Cloquet's lymph node.

Femoral hernia—herniation of the abdominal contents through the femoral canal is called femoral hernia. It is a common occurrence in females due to wider pelvis.

Dissection: Femoral branch of genitofemoral nerve–if possible trace this small branch in front of the femoral artery. This supplies a small area of the skin here. Clean the anterior wall and identify the artery and vein. Slit the medial part of the sheath and identify its boundaries. Put a finger and push it up towards the abdomen and note the boundaries of the upper end called femoral ring. Medially it is bounded by lacunar ligament, posteriorly by pectinate ligament and pectin pubis, anteriorly by inguinal ligament and laterally by septum. The femoral canal is a dead space and it helps in the enlargement of femoral vein. An abnormal obturator artery can sometimes pass through this.

Presence of this artery is to be borne in mind during surgical correction of the femoral hernia.

See the following muscles from lateral to medial side. These form the floor of the femoral triangle.

Iliopsoas: Locate this most lateral muscle mass under cover of the inguinal ligament. The iliacus and psoas major muscles are ***flexors of the thigh.*** The iliacus takes origin from the pelvic surface of the ilium and the psoas major arises from the ventral aspect of the vertebral column. They are bulky muscles crossing the femur anteriorly to reach their insertion. They descend down under cover of the inguinal ligament. The iliacus is fleshy and located laterally. It joins tendon of the psoas major muscle to be inserted into the lesser trochanter of the femur, which lies at a depth. Put your finger press and ***feel*** the lesser trochanter.

Pectineus: It is a fleshy muscle which lies medial to the psoas major. It arises from the superior ramus of the pubis and is inserted into the pectineal line on the posterior aspect of the femur. Trace the nerve supply to this muscle from the ***femoral nerve,*** which reaches this muscle passing deep to the femoral artery. It is a ***flexor*** and ***an adductor of thigh.***

Adductor longus: This is in line with the pectineus. It is a muscle of adductor compartment.

Dissection: Cut the sartorius near its middle and reflect it. Note the branch of the femoral nerve entering into the medial border of this muscle near its origin.

BRANCHES OF FEMORAL ARTERY

Superficial cutaneous branches—are three in number. They are small branches given off from the anterior aspect of the artery. ***The superficial external pudendal, superficial epigastric*** and ***superficial circumflex iliac*** supply the areas as per their names. These were already identified in the subcutaneous region, reidentify them and trace them to their origin. These branches generally have a common origin.

Profunda femoris is a big branch, given off from the posterolateral aspect of the femoral artery. Pull the femoral artery medially and identify the profunda femoris artery. It gives off lateral circumflex femoral artery. This artery goes deep to the sartorius muscle. ***Medial circumflex femoral*** can be a branch of the femoral artery or can be a direct branch from the femoral.

Origin of the branches of the femoral artery is variable.

Femoral vein: Locate this vein medial to the femoral artery. Trace the great saphenous vein termination into the femoral vein.

Deep external pudendal artery: Pull the femoral artery laterally and identify this small branch passing under cover of the femoral vein to reach the scrotum. It lies over the pectineus muscle.

Deep inguinal lymph nodes: These are 3 to 4 in number. Trace them along the femoral vein. They drain the deeper structures of the thigh and the leg. The afferents pass from here to the external iliac nodes.

Note ***the exit of the following structures from the femoral triangle.***

Lateral circumflex femoral artery between the sartorius and rectus femoris.

Medial circumflex femoral artery between the psoas major and pectineus.

Profunda femoris artery between the pectineus and adductor longus.

Femoral artery and vein between the vastus medialis and adductor longus under cover of the sartorius.

SUBSARTORIAL CANAL /ADDUCTOR CANAL (Fig. 11)

Dissection: Clean the connective tissue deep to sartorius stretching between the quadriceps femoris muscle and adductor muscles. Note the boundaries of subsartorial canal.

It extends from the apex of the femoral triangle to the lower one-third of thigh.

Laterally: It is bounded by vastus medialis.

Medially: Adductor longus and magnus

Roof: The fascia deep to the sartorius. Identify the contents

Femoral artery: Entering the canal at the triangle.

Femoral vein: Deep to the artery.

Saphenous nerve: The cutaneous branch of the deep division of the femoral nerve. This lies superficial to the vessels. Note that in the lower part it pierces the roof, and becomes cutaneous. Here it lies posterior to the sartorius. ***Nerve to vastus medialis***—it lies lateral to the vessels. Trace this nerve into the muscle.

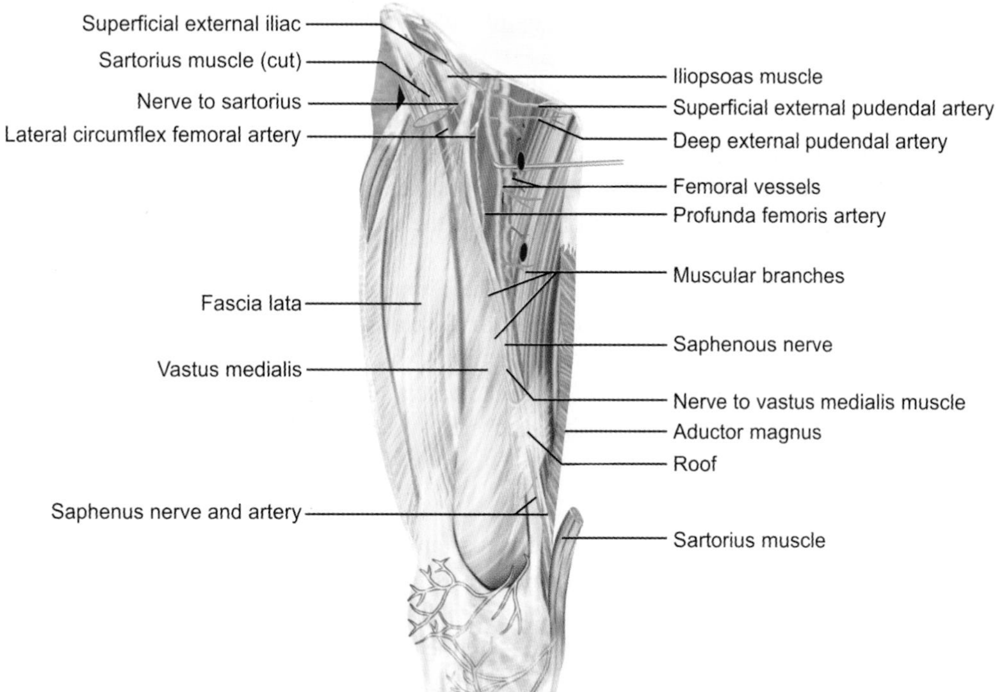

FIGURE 11 Femoral artery and subsartorial canal

ANTERIOR MUSCULATURE/QUADRICEPS FEMORIS (Fig. 12)

Iliotibial tract is the part of the deep fascia on the lateral aspect of thigh. It extends from the iliac crest to the tibia. It splits into two layers in its upper 1/3rd to enclose two muscles—the gluteus maximus and tensor fascia lata. These two muscles get inserted into the tibia through the iliotibial tract. It exerts an antigravity force to support the leg during walking and running.

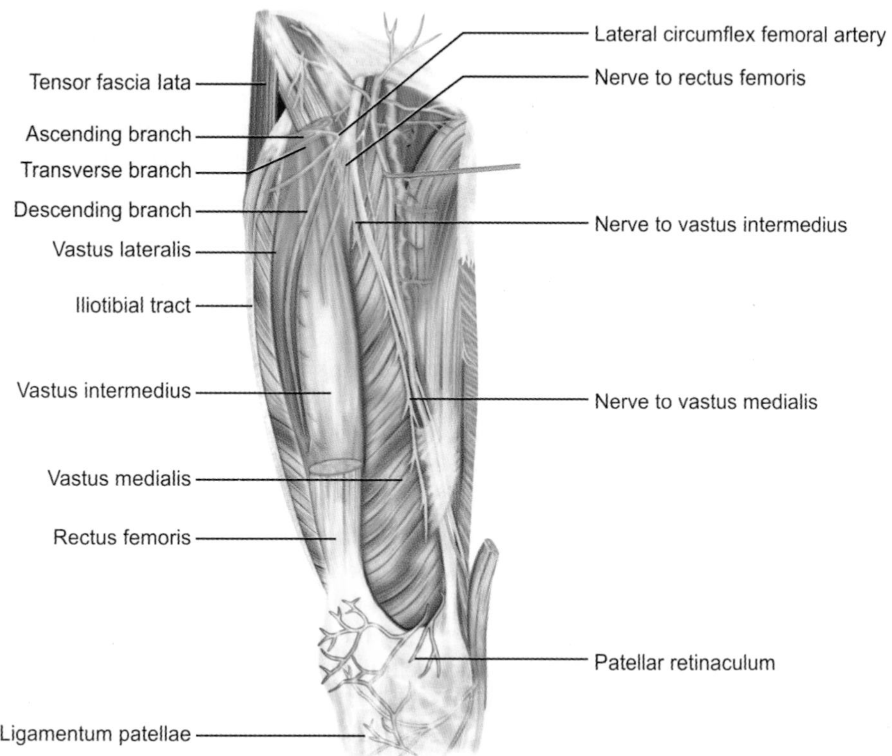

FIGURE 12 Quadriceps femoris muscle

Dissection: Cut the femoral vein from the level of the inguinal ligament to the apex of the femoral triangle and note the following:

Put your fingers deep to the deep fascia lateral to the sartorius muscle and feel its thickness. You would note that it has enclosed a muscle between its layers. This muscle is the tensor fascia lata. Pass your fingers down up to the lower end, to the tibia. The fascia is attached here to the anterior surface of the lateral condyle of tibia. Pull the deep fascia down and note that it has sent another extension posteriorly to the hipbone. Here it encloses the gluteus maximus muscle (This will be seen in the gluteal region dissection).

Dissection: Feel the iliac crest, identify the tubercle of the ilium on its middle. Detach the superficial layer of the iliotibial tract carefully and expose the muscle **tensor fascia lata**. This muscle takes origin from the iliac crest between the iliac tubercle and the anterior superior iliac spine. By pulling this muscle identify the iliotibial tract. Detach the muscle from its origin and cut the deep fascia along its anterior border up to the tibia. The muscle that you see now is the quadriceps femoris muscle.

Quadriceps Femoris

The anterior compartment is occupied by a single quadriceps femoris muscle. It is a thick four-headed muscle. The rectus femoris is the part of the quadriceps muscle, which arises from the hip bone, the remaining three parts occupy major part of the thigh—anteriorly, medially and posteriorly. Femoral nerve is the nerve of supply and lateral circumflex femoral is the artery of supply. It is an extensor of the leg at the knee joint.

Dissection: Note the deep fascia covering the quadriceps femoris muscle. Carefully remove the deep fascia between the sartorius anteriorly and tensor fascia lata and iliotibial tract posteriorly without damaging the quadriceps femoris muscle. Study its four heads

Rectus femoris: Identify this head lying deep to the iliotibial tract. It has two heads of origin. Locate the straight head from the anterior inferior iliac spine. It has a reflected head from the groove above the acetabulum. Both the heads are tendinous at their origin. It is easy to identify the heads by pulling them where both the heads join. Note that the combined part lies over the vastus intermedius.

Dissection: Cut the rectus femoris muscle near its middle and reflect the parts.

Vastus medialis is the medial head. It arises from the intertrochanteric line, spiral line, linea aspera and the medial supracondylar line. ***Vastus lateralis*** is the lateral head. It arises from the root of the greater trochanter along the lateral margin of the linea aspera to the lateral supracondylar line. Vastus ***intermedius*** is the Intermediate head. It arises from the front and lateral surface of the body of the femur, leaving lower 1/4th free. ***Articularis genu*** constitute few of the detached fibres of the vastus intermedius and are inserted into the synovial membrane. (It will be seen at a later dissection).

Insertion of quadriceps femoris: The whole muscle gets inserted onto the patella. It is a flat tendon reaching the top of the patella and aponeurotic on lateral and medial sides called ***patellar retinacula.*** The patella is a sesamoid bone in the passage of quadriceps muscle. The combined tendon from the lower part of the patella reaches the tibial tuberosity as ***ligamentum patellae.*** A bursa is interposed between the tendon and the upper part of tibial tuberosity. This is called deep infra patellar bursa. ***Nerve supply—***the ***femoral nerve*** supplies all the heads of quadriceps femoris muscle by its deep division. Trace the branches into the muscle. The rectus femoris is supplied on its deeper aspect by 2 branches; upper of the two branches supplies the hip joint. Trace the nerve to the vastus lateralis between the rectus femoris and vastus intermedius to the vastus lateralis which it supplies on its anterior surface. It is accompanied by the descending branch of the lateral circumflex femoral artery. The vastus intermedius is supplied by 2 to 3 branches on its anterior aspect; medial of these branches supplies the articularis genu muscle and knee joint. Nerve to the vastus medialis was already identified in the subsartorial canal dissection. It supplies the muscle on its medial side. ***Arterial supply***—the quadriceps femoris muscle is supplied by branches of the ***lateral circumflex femoral artery***. The lateral circumflex femoral is a branch of the profunda femoris artery. Trace them and note, that they accompany the branches of the femoral nerve into the muscle. ***Action—***As the rectus femoris muscle arises from the hip bone and crosses the hip joint anteriorly, it is a ***flexor of the hip joint.*** The total muscle is an ***extensor of the leg at the knee joint***.

MEDIAL SIDE OF THIGH/ADDUCTOR COMPARTMENT

The adductors of the thigh occupy medial side of thigh; they are five muscles—the ***pectineus, adductor longus, brevis, magnus*** and ***gracilis***. The gracilis is a long superficial muscle of this compartment. The others extend from the pubis and ischium to the posterior aspect of the thigh. Observe the direction of these muscles on an articulated skeleton. You would note that these muscles pass from the hipbone to the femur laterally and posteriorly. The obturator externus though does not belong to the adductor group of musculature lies deep in the compartment.

The nerve of this compartment is the ***obturator nerve*** and the artery is the ***medial circumflex femoral artery*** and the profunda femoris artery. The muscles are arranged in layers with the neurovascular bundle running between them. The pectineus and adductor longus forms the anterior layer of the muscles. The adductor brevis forms the intermediate layer. The profunda femoris artery and the anterior division of obturator nerve lies between the two. The obturator externus and the adductor magnus forms the deep layer. The deep division of the obturator nerve lies between the intermediate and deep layer of muscles. The medial circumflex femoral artery reaches the back of the thigh above the pectineus muscle. The branches from the medial circumflex femoral accompany the deep division of obturator nerve.

Superficial Dissection (Fig. 13)

Dissection: Turn the limb laterally and tie it to the table. This exposes the medial side of thigh. Clean the superficial layer of muscles seen in here. Cut the femoral artery and vein from the level of the inguinal ligament to the apex of the femoral triangle and note the following:

Pectineus: This is a quadrangular composite muscle both adductor and flexor. It arises from pectin pubis, slopes backwards and posteriorly to be inserted into the pectineal line on femur. Trace this muscle.

Adductor longus: This is a triangular next muscle in line with the pectineus. It lies below the pectineus. It arises from the body of the pubis by a rounded tendon below the pubic crest. Trace it down to its insertion into the linea aspera.

Dissection: Cut the pectineus and adductor longus near its insertion and reflect it. Study the intermediate layer of muscle and the neurovascular bundle.

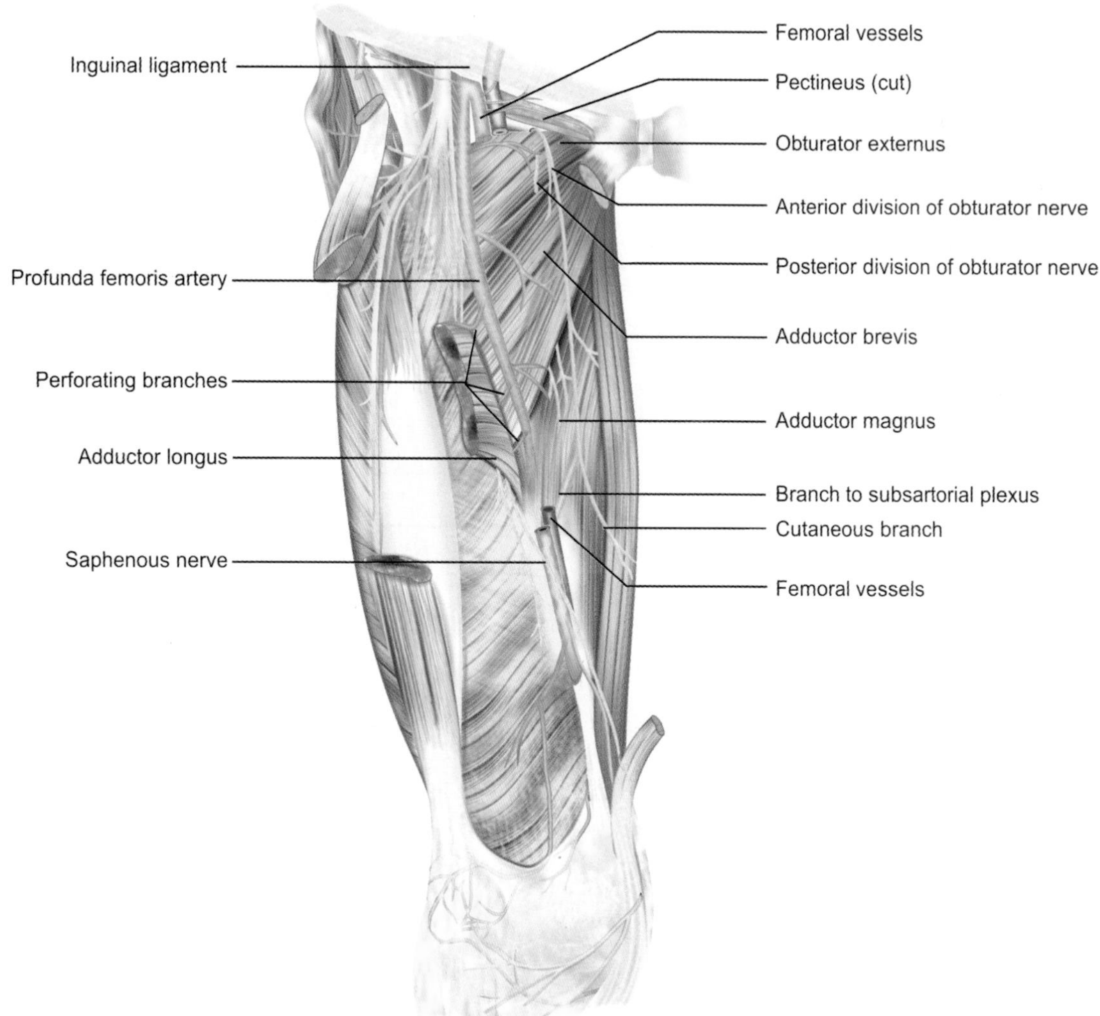

FIGURE 13 Superficial dissection of obturator compartment

Profunda femoris artery and vein passes over the pectineus, deep to the adductor longus, between the longus and brevis initially and longus and magnus lower down.

Medial circumflex femoral artery and vein is a branch of the profunda femoris artery. The medial circumflex femoral artery passes above the pectineus muscle.

First perforating artery is given off from the profunda femoris artery above the adductor brevis. It anastomoses with descending branch of medial circumflex femoral deep to the adductor brevis.

Second perforating artery is given off while the profunda artery lies over the adductor brevis.

See the continuation of profunda femoris artery on its anterior aspect and locate the ***perforator branches,*** 3rd and 4th terminal branch penetrating the adductor magnus muscle.

Obturator nerve. See the ***anterior division*** of obturator nerve between the adductor longus and brevis. Trace its muscular branches into the adductor longus which it supplies on its deeper aspect, adductor brevis which it supplies on its anterior aspect, pectineus on its lateral aspect and the gracilis in its middle. It is variable at its termination. It contributes to the subsartorial plexus, gives a small vascular branch to supply the femoral artery in the adductor canal and leaves the adductor region to become cutaneous to the medial side of thigh.

Adductor brevis: This forms the intermediate layer of muscle. It is deep to the adductor longus. It takes origin from the ischiopubic ramus. It is also a triangular muscle descends posteriorly to be inserted into the linea aspera posterior to the adductor longus.

Deep Dissection (Fig. 14)

Dissection: Cut the anterior division of obturator nerve over the adductor brevis. Cut through the adductor brevis near its insertion and reflect it. Study the deep layer of muscles and neurovascular bundle. Pull the adductor longus, adductor brevis and gracilis towards their origins and identify the deeply located obturator externus muscle.

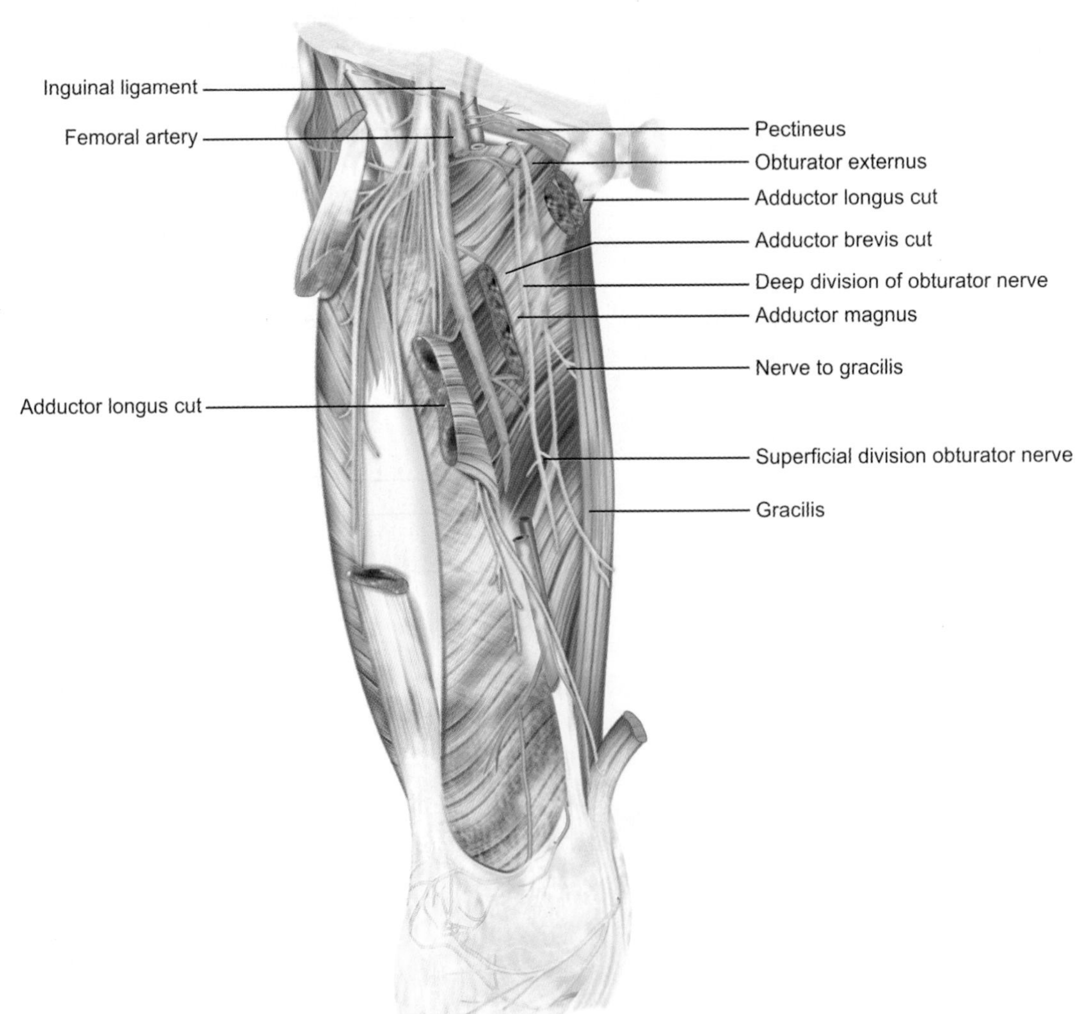

FIGURE 14 Deep dissection of obturator compartment

Obturator externus is flat muscle at its origin sticking to the external surface of the obturator membrane and the adjoining bony margin. It quickly becomes tendinous and should be seen in the gluteal region dissection for its insertion. The anterior division of obturator nerve passes above the obturator externus and the posterior division pierces through the muscle.

Obturator nerve posterior branch: Locate this nerve piercing through the obturator externus muscle. Trace it down between the adductor brevis and adductor magnus. It supplies obturator externus, adductor brevis and adductor magnus. It sends a branch to the knee joint through the adductor magnus muscle.

The muscular branches of the medial circumflex artery accompanies the branches of the obturator nerve deep branch into the muscles adductor brevis and adductor magnus.

Adductor magnus: This is a thick composite muscle made up of both adductor parts from ischiopubic ramus and hamstring part from ischial tuberosity. It is continuous at its origin though said to have two parts. Trace the muscle to its insertion. The muscle runs across and obliquely downward to reach the linea aspera, medial supra condylar line to the adductor tubercle on the medial condyle of femur.

Gracilis: It is the most medial and most superficial of the adductor group of musculature. Locate its origin from the medial border of the ischiopubic ramus. Trace the muscle to the medial surface of the shaft of the tibia behind the insertion of the sartorius (the insertion can be seen at a later dissection). Nerve supply—Trace its nerve supply from the anterior division of the obturator nerve.

GLUTEAL REGION

Turn the body to the prone position. Identify the following regions—the gluteal region, the back of thigh, the popliteal fossa and the back of leg.

Gluteal region occupies the upper end of the posterolateral aspect of the lower limb. Superiorly, it extends up to the iliac crest, inferiorly the gluteal fold, medially the vertebral column and natal cleft and laterally a vertical line from the anterior superior iliac spine to the greater trochanter. It lies external to the hipbone. The anterosuperior part gives attachment to the abductors of the thigh, which cross the hip joint to get inserted to the greater trochanter. The posteroinferior part gives attachment to the lateral rotators of the thigh, which run horizontally to cross the hip joint to be attached to the greater trochanter. The gluteus maximus is the biggest muscle of this region, it covers all the other structures, extends from posterosuperior aspect to the anteroinferior aspect. It is a powerful extensor and lateral rotator.

The musculature of the gluteal region gets its neurovascular bundle from the pelvis through the greater sciatic foramen. The neurovascular bundle of the perineum takes a deviated route along the gluteal region before passing through the lesser sciatic foramen.

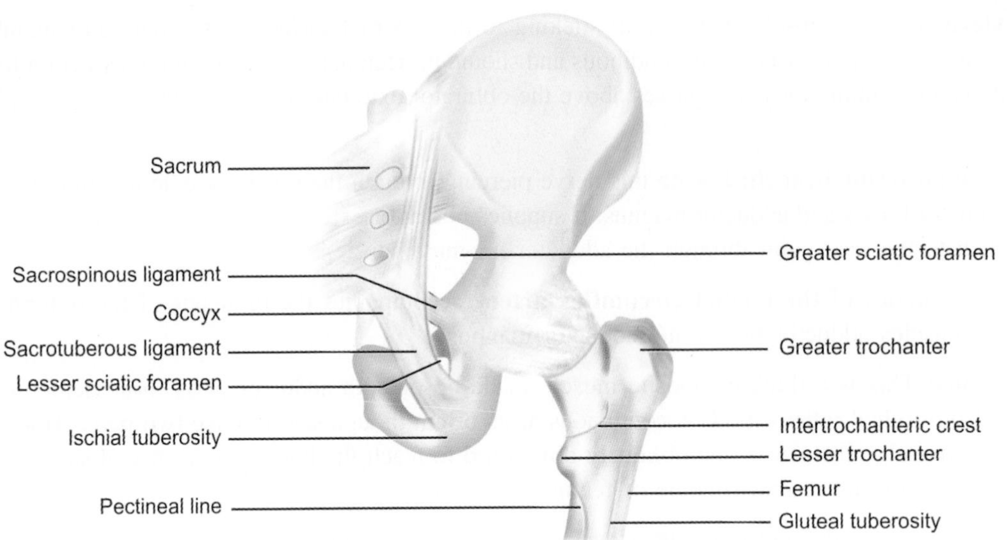

FIGURE 15 Gluteal region—skeleton

SKELETON (Fig. 15)

Go to an articulated skeleton with ligaments and identify the following bony points.

Sacrum: It is the lower part of the vertebral column. It is made up of 5 vertebrae. The anterior and posterior sacral foramina are seen between the vertebrae. Feel the median, medial and lateral sacral crests.

Coccyx: It is the last piece of the vertebral column, made up of three coccygeal vertebrae. It presents a hiatus posteriorly.

Locate the anterior superior iliac spine, iliac crest, iliac tubercle, posterior superior iliac spine, greater sciatic notch, posterior inferior iliac spine and the lesser sciatic notch on the hip bone.

Ischial tuberosity: Identify this on the ischial part of the hipbone.

Femur: Identify the head, neck, greater trochanter, lesser trochanter and the intertrochanteric crest on the back of the femur. On the posterior aspect of the shaft of the femur note the pectineal line, the spiral line and the gluteal tuberosity.

Sacrotuberous ligament: See this extending from ischial tuberosity to the sacrum and coccyx.

Sacrospinous ligament: This lies under cover of the sacrotuberous ligament. It extends from the spine of the ischium to the last piece of sacrum and first piece of coccyx.

Greater sciatic foramen: It is formed by greater sciatic notch, lateral border of sacrum, sacrotuberous ligament and sacrospinous ligament.

Lesser sciatic foramen: It is formed by the lesser sciatic notch, sacrotuberous and sacrospinous ligament.

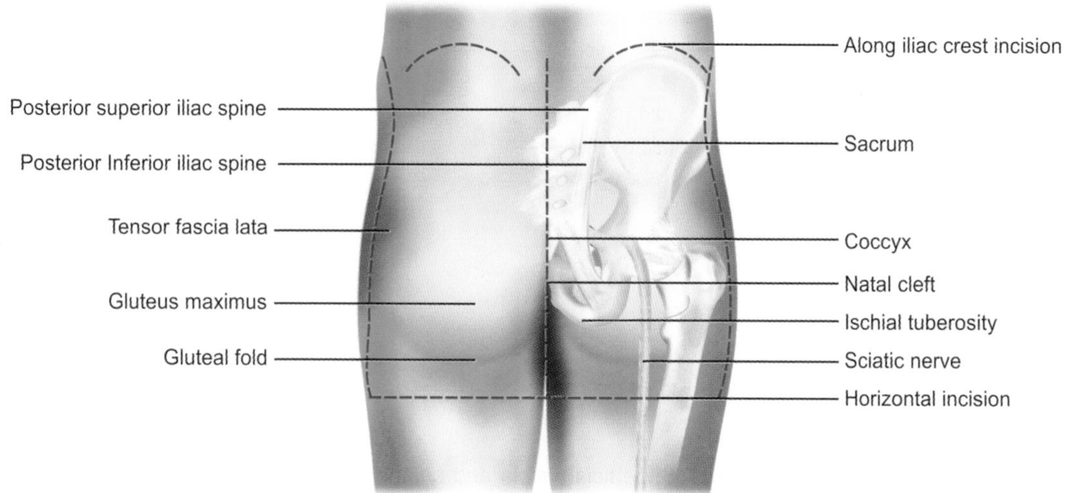

FIGURE 16 Surface and living anatomy and skin incision

SURFACE AND LIVING ANATOMY (Fig. 16)

Identify the following bony points on the living body and the cadaver.

Natal cleft: Note this as the gap between the two gluteal regions.

Feel the ***anterior superior iliac spine, iliac crest, iliac tubercle*** and the ***posterior superior iliac spine***, all of which are subcutaneous. The tight adherence of subcutaneous tissue near the posterior superior iliac spine causes a dimple on skin. A horizontal plane passing through the posterior superior iliac spine cuts through the 2nd sacral vertebra. This is an important landmark as the subarachnoid space ends here.

Feel the ***median sacral crest*** and the ***coccyx*** in the midline.

Feel the ***ischial tuberosity***, the elevation in-line with the posterior superior iliac spine, below the coccyx. This is the elevation on which we sit.

Greater trochanter of the femur can be easily felt through the muscles as a bony prominence a hands breadth below the tubercle of ilium.

Gluteal fold—it is the skin fold seen on the inferior aspect. It is due to the abrupt absence of the big muscle gluteus maximus, as it gets inserted below this level. Note the prominence of the gluteus maximus posteriorly, the tensor facia lata anteriorly and the depression of the iliotibial tact in between.

Skin Incision

Dissection: Make the following skin incisions—along the iliac crest, posterior superior and inferior iliac spines, natal cleft to the medial side of thigh. Make a horizontal incision in the mid thigh. The skin was already reflected on the lateral and medial sides. Remove the skin from the posterior aspect. Skin over here is very thick.

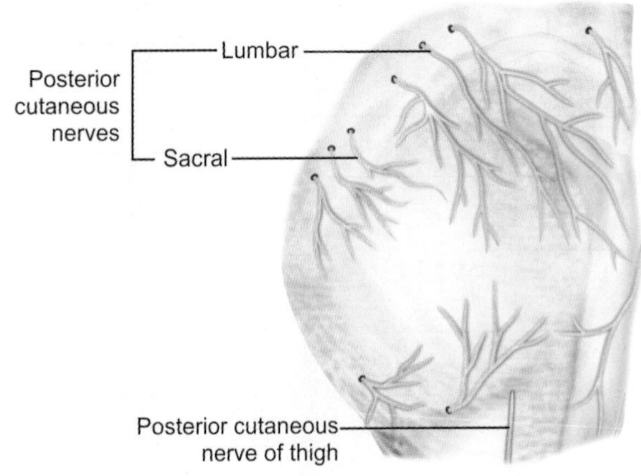

FIGURE 17 Superficial fascia and cutaneous nerves

SUPERFICIAL FASCIA (Fig. 17)

Superficial fascia is heavily laden with fat, particularly in female bodies. Clean the fat. The cutaneous vessels and nerves are located in this fat. As the branches are very fine and mingling with the fascia it is difficult to locate them, but study from the diagram.

Cutaneous nerves: Study the position of the cutaneous nerves—anterolaterally the ***lateral cutaneous branches of subcostal*** and ***iliohypogastric nerve, laterally lumbar nerves, posteriorly sacral nerves, inferiorly posterior cutaneous nerve.***

Clean the superficial fascia. Identify the thick glistening deep fascia splitting into two layers and enclosing the gluteus maximus muscle. Define the boundaries of the muscle. Remove the superficial layer of the deep fascia over the gluteus maximus to expose the muscle. Note that the muscle takes origin from the undersurface of the deep fascia. Note that at the distal end of the muscle the two layers of deep fascia enclosing the muscle join to form the iliotibial tract. It receives the insertion of the tensor fascia lata muscle.

Gluteus Maximus (Fig. 18)

Gluteus maximus is a powerful multipennate muscle. Study its origin from the external surface of the ileum behind the posterior gluteal line, back of sacrum, coccyx and sacrotuberous ligament. Note that bulk of the muscle suddenly dips deep, to be inserted into the gluteal tuberosity on the posterior aspect of the femur. A superficial part of the muscle becomes aponeurotic, joins with the tensor fascia lata, together they form the iliotibial tract. The gluteus maximus receives its neurovascular bundle from the ***inferior gluteal nerve*** and the ***inferior gluteal artery*** and vein on its undersurface. ***Action***—Note that this bulky muscle crosses the hip joint from medial to lateral and superior to inferior direction. It is an ***abductor, extensor*** and ***lateral rotator***. It is a powerful antigravity muscle particularly while getting up from sitting position, and climbing stairs.

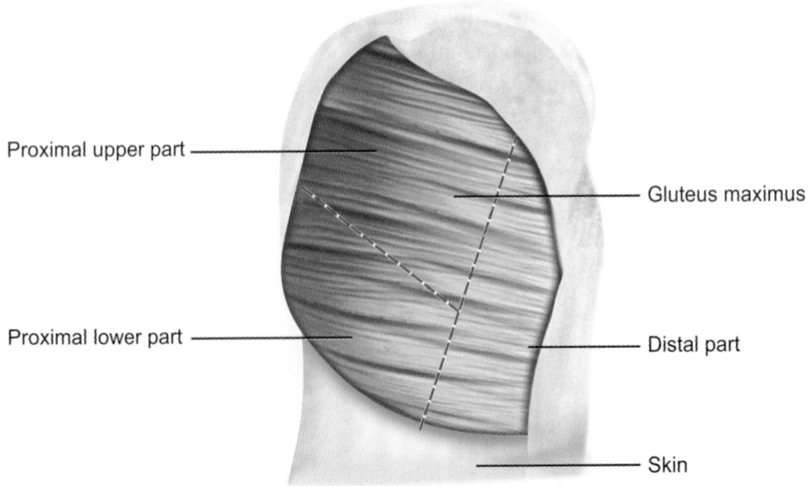

FIGURE 18 Gluteus maximus muscle

Dissection: Gluteus maximus muscle has to be reflected with utmost care as all the structures of this region lie under cover of this muscle. Locate the upper and lower borders of the gluteus maximus muscle. Push your fingers deep to the muscle. Feel the freedom that you would experience over the greater trochanter and over the ischial tuberosity. These two bony areas are separated from the gluteus maximus by the bursae. Push your fingers down to feel the insertion of the muscle on the gluteal tuberosity.

Carefully cut through the muscle vertically from the lower border to the upper border medial to the greater trochanter. Lift the muscle from below, pull the distal part downwards. Note the ***trochanteric bursa*** between this muscle and the greater trochanter. Trace it further down to reach the insertion on the gluteal tuberosity. Feel the insertion on the bone. Lift the proximal part and carefully, cut it horizontally as shown in the Figure and try to reflect it towards the origin. Note the structures entering the lower half in its undersurface—the ***inferior gluteal vessels*** and ***nerve*** enter near its lower border, as you further lift it note the sciatic and other nerves related to its deeper surface. Trace the upper part medially to its origin from the ilium behind the posterior gluteal line. Here you note the superficial branch of the ***superior gluteal artery*** entering into it. Note its origin from the sacrotuberous ligament and carefully separate the muscle from it, and push the muscle as much as possible to the medial end of hip bone. Note the ischial bursa between the ischial tuberosity and the gluteus maximus muscle.

STRUCTURES UNDER COVER OF GLUTEUS MAXIMUS MUSCLE (Fig. 19)

The structures under cover of the gluteus maximus can be divided as two parts—the anterosuperior part constituting the deeper gluteal abductor muscles and the posteroinferior short rotators. Both are accompanied by their neurovascular bundle.

Dissection: Turn the body to a midprone position and study the deeper gluteal muscles.

Superficial branch of superior gluteal artery: Trace this artery and its branches. This branch runs between the gluteus maximus and medius. It supplies both the muscles. Trace it to the parent trunk above the piriformis muscle.

Gluteus medius muscle: This is the most anterior thick muscle extending between the anterior and posterior of gluteal lines. It is inserted into the posterior aspect of the external surface of the greater trochanter. (Locate these parts on the articulated skeleton). Clean the muscle from origin to insertion. Note that the muscle extends from above downwards. It is an ***abductor***.

Dissection: Put your fingers above the piriformis, beneath the gluteus medius, lift the muscle and cut through the gluteus medius muscle in a semicircular manner, nearer to its insertion. Pull the tendinous part and identify its insertion into the greater trochanter. Lift the muscular part towards its origin. See the neurovascular bundle between it and the gluteus minimus. It is the superior gluteal vessels and nerve.

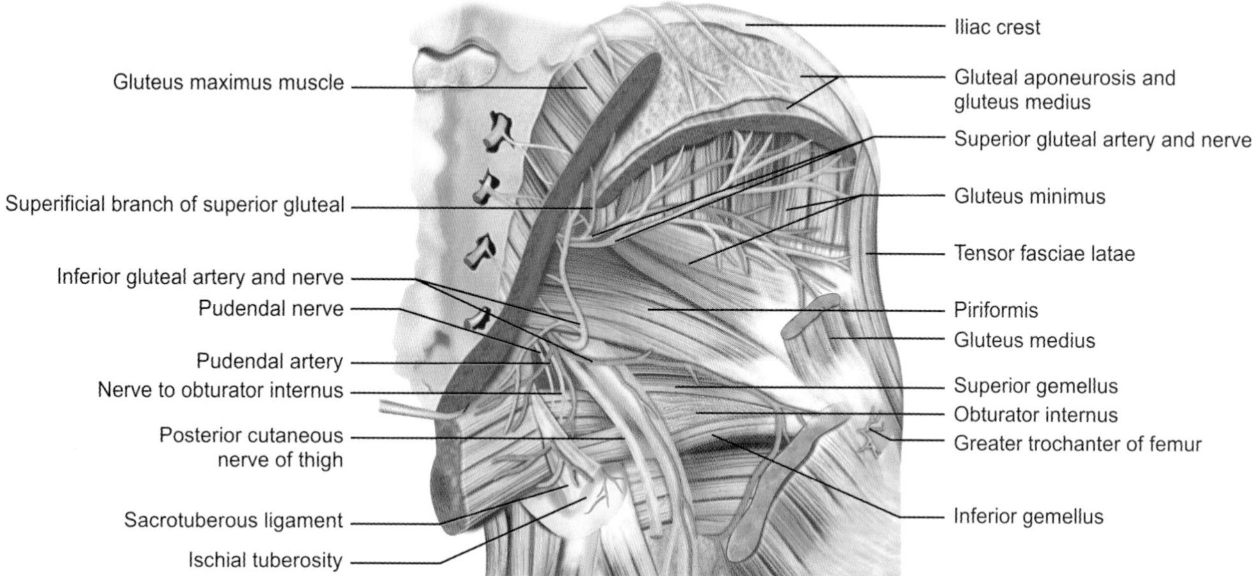

FIGURE 19 Structures under cover of gluteus maximus

Deep branch of the superior gluteal artery and superior gluteal nerve: Trace this neurovascular bundle into the gluteus medius, gluteus minimus and tensor fascia lata.

Gluteus minimus muscle: Lies deeper to the gluteus medius. Identify this muscle extending between the anterior and inferior gluteal lines. See its insertion into the anterior aspect of the external surface of the greater trochanter. Confirm both on a dry skeleton. Note that this muscle also extends from above downwards. It is also an *abductor.* Both gluteus medius and gluteus minimus are postural muscles, during walking they act from their insertion to the origin and pull the hip downwards.

GREATER SCIATIC FORAMEN AND STRUCTURES PASSING THROUGH IT

Superior gluteal vessels and nerves: The superior gluteal artery is a continuation of the posterior division of the internal iliac artery; the nerve arises from the lumbosacral plexus. The branches of this neurovascular bundle are already dissected. Trace them to the place above the piriformis muscle.

Piriformis muscle: This forms the key muscle of this region. It is muscular here and presents a small tendon near its insertion. This distal part is to be identified in this region. (The muscle arises from the ventral aspect of the 2,3,4th sacral vertebrae. Leaves the pelvis through the greater sciatic foramen, crosses the hipbone and is inserted into the medial border of the greater trochanter. The sacral nerves on its pelvic surface supply it).

Sciatic nerve: It is 5 cm wide nerve leaves the lower border of the piriformis muscle. This nerve supplies the back of thigh, total leg and foot. Trace it down. See that it lies superficial to the other muscles.

Inferior gluteal vessels and nerves: The artery is the terminal branch of the anterior division of internal iliac artery. See this neurovascular bundle entering into the gluteus maximus muscle.

Posterior cutaneous nerve of thigh: It is the thin nerve seen on the surface of the sciatic nerve. It pierces the deep fascia near the popliteal fossa. Locate this nerve on the surface of sciatic nerve and trace it down till it pierces the deep fascia.

Nerve to obturator internus pudendal vessels and nerve: These three structures leave the greater sciatic foramen and enter into the lesser sciatic foramen, of them the nerve to obturator internus is lateral, the artery intermediate and the pudendal nerve medial in position. Locate all these structures and trace them into the lesser sciatic foramen.

STRUCTURES THROUGH LESSER SCIATIC FORAMEN

Tendon of obturator internus and gemelli occupy this space. The tendon of obturator internus lies in the center and it is covered by the gemelli on either side.

Tendon of obturator internus: Locate this tendon below the piriformis muscle. (The obturator internus muscle takes origin from the obturator membrane on its pelvic side and the adjoining bone, it takes a sharp U bend leaves through the lesser sciatic foramen to get inserted into the medial aspect of the greater trochanter).

Superior gemellus: This muscle takes origin from the lesser sciatic notch above the obturator internus tendon.

Inferior gemellus: Takes origin from the lesser sciatic notch below the tendon of obturator internus.

Both superior and inferior gemelli get inserted into the tendon of obturator internus above and below. These muscles pull the tendon of obturator internus in line with the obturator internus muscle.

Quadratus femoris: Locate this muscle below the previous group of muscles. It is a quadrilateral muscle extending from the lateral border of the ischial tuberosity to the quadrate tubercle between the greater and lesser trochanter on the posterior aspect.

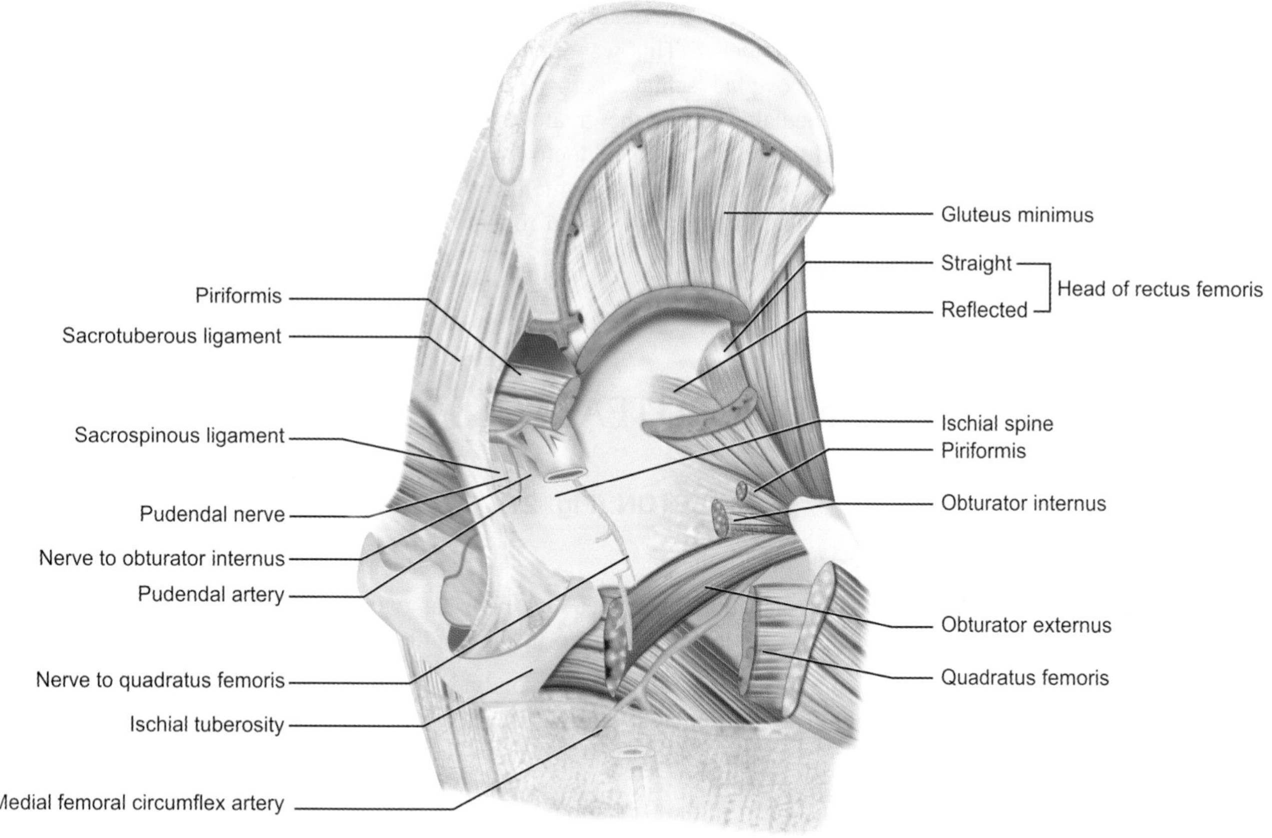

FIGURE 20 Deep structures of gluteal region

DEEP STRUCTURES OF GLUTEAL REGION (Fig. 20)

Dissection: Detach the gluteus maximus from its origin and see the sacrotuberous ligament.

Sacrotuberous ligament: See its extent from the posterolateral surface of sacrum and coccyx to the medial side of ischial tuberosity.

Sacrospinous ligament: Trace this from the deeper aspect of the sacrotuberous ligament. It extends from the last piece of sacrum and first piece of coccyx to the spine of the ischium.

Structures passing from greater sciatic foramen to lesser sciatic foramen: See the structures passing from greater sciatic foramen to the lesser sciatic foramen. They cross the ischial spine and sacrospinous ligament, under cover of sacrotuberous ligament. These are ***pudendal vessels, pudendal nerve*** *and* ***nerve to obturator internus***. The artery and its venae commitantis lie in the middle with the nerve to obturator internus to the lateral and the pudendal nerve medial to it.

The pudendal vessels and the nerve reach the perineum to supply the perineal structures.

Dissection: Cut the gluteus minimus muscle in a midway between its origin and insertion, pull them apart and see the origin of the straight and reflected heads of rectus femoris. Look for the nerve supply to the above muscles. Cut vertically through the obturator internus tendon, gemelli and quadratus femoris nearer to their insertion. Lift the muscles and pull them towards their origins. See the nerve to the superior gemellus from the nerve to the obturator internus before it enters the lesser sciatic foramen. It enters the muscle on its superior surface. The nerve to the quadratus femoris lies in contact with the ischium, Trace it into the undersurface of the muscle. See its small branch entering into the inferior gemellus.

Origin of rectus femoris: This muscle is a part of the anterior compartment of thigh. It is a deeply placed muscle. The straight head of rectus femoris arises from the anterior inferior iliac spine. Look for the reflected head of rectus femoris muscle. It arises from the groove above the acetabulum. See that soon they join together.

Locate the tendon of obturator externus deep to the quadratus femoris. ***Obturator externus*** muscle takes origin from the external surface of the obturator membrane. This was identified in the medial compartment dissection. The tendon of this muscle grooves the ischium above the ischial tuberosity and on reaching the gluteal region it is tendinous and reaches the trochanteric fossa on the medial aspect of the greater trochanter. Locate the medial circumflex femoral artery between the quadratus femoris and upper border of adductor magnus.

All the small muscles the piriformis, obturator internus gamelli, obturator externus and the quadratus femoris extend from the medial side to the lateral side. They are all lateral rotators of the thigh at the hip joint.

Study the cruciate and trochanteric arterial anastomosis in the gluteal region. It is very fine to dissect.

BACK OF THIGH AND POPLITEAL FOSSA

SKELETON (Fig. 21)

Study the bony architecture of the back of the thigh.

Shaft of the femur. Note the central raised elevation—the linea aspera. It has two lips. All the muscles of this region get attached here. The linea aspera widens in its lower part to form the popliteal surface of femur.

Condyles of femur are the bulges on the lower end. The medial condyle shows the adductor tubercle. Look at the smooth articulating surface of the femur. These articulate with the tibial condyles to form the knee joint.

Upper end of the tibia shows enlargement called the tibial condyles.

Head of the fibula: Note that it does not take part in the formation of the knee joint. It articulates with the undersurface of the tibia.

SURFACE AND LIVING ANATOMY (Fig. 22)

Locate the thick posterior aspect of the thigh and the bend of the knee. Feel the muscle mass and note that as you reach down the muscle mass diverges medially and laterally, leaving a depression in the middle. This depression is called the popliteal fossa. Flex the knee against resistance and feel the muscle mass superolaterally and superomedially. The medial muscle mass is made up of gracilis, semitendinosus and semimembranosus; the lateral muscle is biceps femoris. Feel the bony prominence below this. It is the head of the fibula. Run your fingers slightly below and feel the cord like common peroneal nerve. It is subcutaneous here and can easily be damaged during accidents.

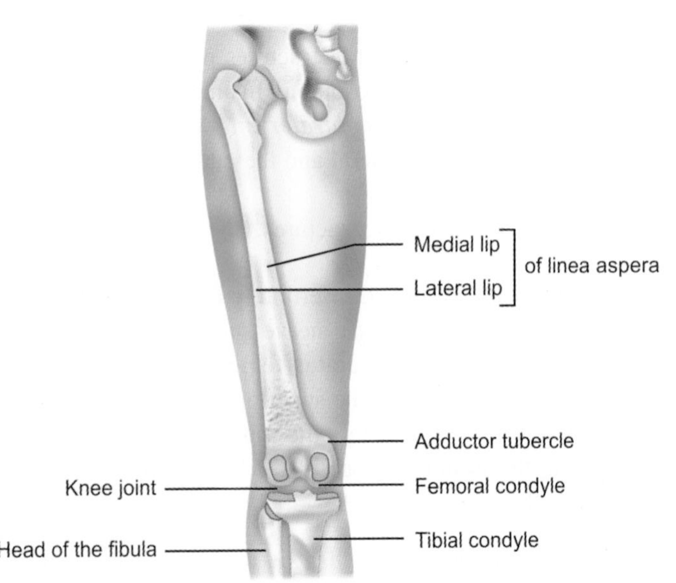

FIGURE 21 Skeleton of back up thigh and popliteal fossa

Gluteal fold
Horizontal incision
Vertical incision
Popliteal fossa
Horizontal incision
Medial side
Lateral side

FIGURE 22 Surface anatomy—skin incision back of thigh and popliteal region

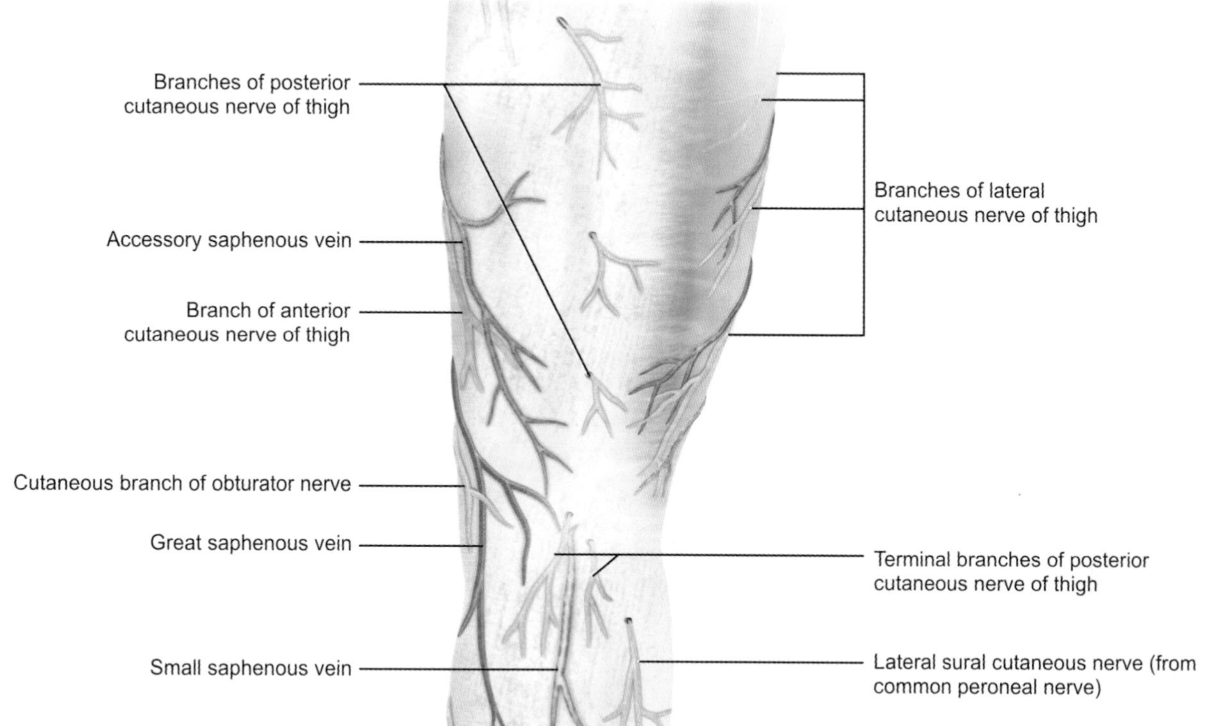

FIGURE 23 Cutaneous structures

CUTANEOUS STRUCTURES (Fig. 23)

Dissection: Make a vertical incision from the cut end of the gluteal skin up to the level of the anterior incision below the tibial tuberosity. Make a horizontal incision in line with the anterior incision. Reflect the skin on either side and remove it and identify the cutaneous structures.

Posterior cutaneous nerve of thigh: It is seen in the midline. It becomes cutaneous by piercing the deep fascia near the lower half of thigh. Trace it down.

Small saphenous vein and the sural nerve are seen in the midline at the bend of the knee. Small saphenous vein pierces the deep fascia to enter into popliteal vein here.

Sural nerve: It is a cutaneous nerve which accompany the short saphenous vein. See that it pierces the deep fascia near the skin reflection.

Common peroneal nerve: It is one of the terminal divisions of the sciatic nerve. Note it along the medial border of the biceps femoris.

Sural communicating nerve: It is one of the cutaneous branches of the common peroneal nerve.

Lateral cutaneous nerve of calf: It is the other cutaneous branch of common peroneal nerve. Trace these two cutaneous nerves. They pierce the deep fascia at a lower level.

Sural nerve: This is the cutaneous branch of tibial nerve. It accompanies the small saphenous vein.

The lower part of femur, back of knee joint and the fascia form floor of the fossa over the popliteus muscle. These can be seen at a later dissection.

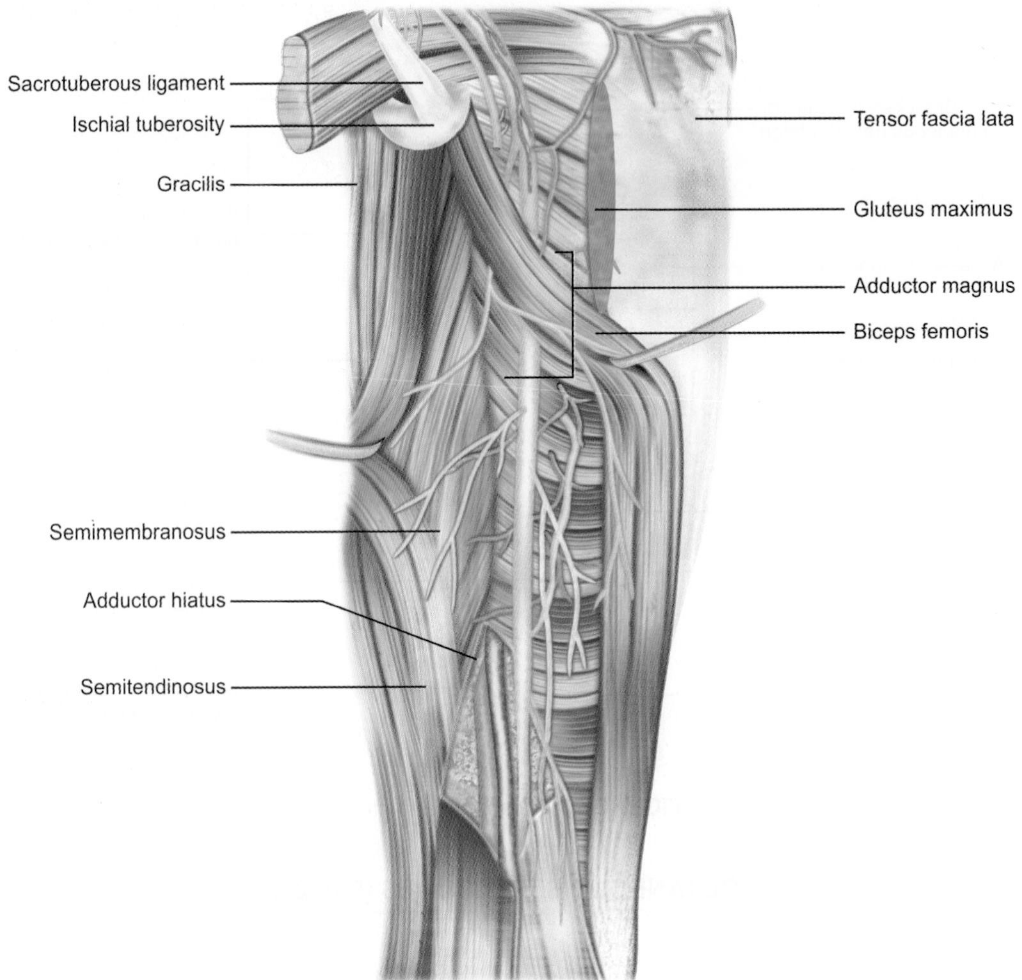

FIGURE 24 Muscles of back of thigh and boundaries of popliteal fossa

MUSCLES OF BACK OF THIGH (Fig. 24)

Back of thigh lodges the hamstring muscles, they extend from the ischial tuberosity above, to the tibia and fibula below. Sciatic nerve is the nerve of this compartment and the muscles are supplied by anastomosis of the perforating arteries.

Dissection: Clean the muscle from their fascia, trace them to their origins and towards the insertions, but the actual insertions can be studied at a later stage.

Semitendinosus: This is the medial most of the posterior group of muscles. Note that it arises from the medial part of the ischial tuberosity along with the long head of biceps. It becomes tendinous in the lower part of the back of the thigh.

Semimembranosus: Lies deeper and lateral to semitendinosus, it arises from the lateral part of the ischial tuberosity. It is flat and membranous at its origin.

Biceps femoris: The long head of biceps femoris muscle arises in common with the semitendinosus. Trace it down. Realize that this muscle deviates to the lateral side. ***Short head of biceps***—Pull the biceps towards you and note the deep short head that arises from the linea aspera between the vastus lateralis and the adductor magnus muscle. It joins with the long head and forms a combined muscle mass. This deviates to the lateral side to reach the head of the fibula.

Adductor magnus: Locate this thick muscle on the medial line of the linea aspera up to the adductor tubercle on the medial femoral condyle. This is its insertion. Trace it above to its hamstring origin from the ischial tuberosity.

All the hamstrings cross the hip joint as they arise from the ischial tuberosity. They are all initiators of flexion of the thigh at the hip joint. They cross the knee joint posteriorly, so they are flexors of the leg at the knee joint.

BOUNDARIES OF POPLITEAL FOSSA

Popliteal fossa is the diamond shaped area present on the posterior aspect at the bend of the knee. ***Roof***—is formed by the skin superficial fascia with the cutaneous structures and the deep fascia deep to it. This is what is dissected, and now note its lateral boundaries. The sides are formed by muscles: ***Superolaterally***—the biceps femoris. ***Superomedially***—semitendinosus semimembranosus sartorius and gracilis. ***Inferolaterally***—lateral head of gastrocnemius and plantaris. ***Inferomedially***—medial head of gastrocnemius.

Gastrocnemius: See the origin of lateral and medial head heads. The medial head arises from the medial condyle above the articular surface. The lateral head arises from the lower end of the femur on the lateral aspect. Both are muscular at their origin. Soon join to form a bulky muscle. Which suddenly flattens and becomes aponeurotic on the undersurface.

DEEP DISSECTION OF BACK OF THIGH (Fig. 25)

Dissection: Separate the hamstrings to the sides and identify trace the neurovascular bundle into the muscles.

Sciatic nerve: Separate the muscle masses laterally and medially and try to locate the sciatic nerve, which is already traced up to the quadratus femoris. Trace this nerve downward and identify its muscular branches. Trace them into the respective muscles.

The medial side of the sciatic nerve that will be the tibial part of the nerve supplies semitendinosus, semimembranosus, biceps femoris long head and the hamstring part of the adductor magnus.

The lateral side of the sciatic nerve that is the common peroneal part supplies the short head of the biceps.

Perforating branches of the profunda femoris artery: These pass through the tendinous rings in the adductor magnus and supply the hamstring muscles. These were identified in the medial compartment and trace at least few branches.

Near the lower one-third of the femur the sciatic nerve divides into medial tibial and lateral common peroneal division.

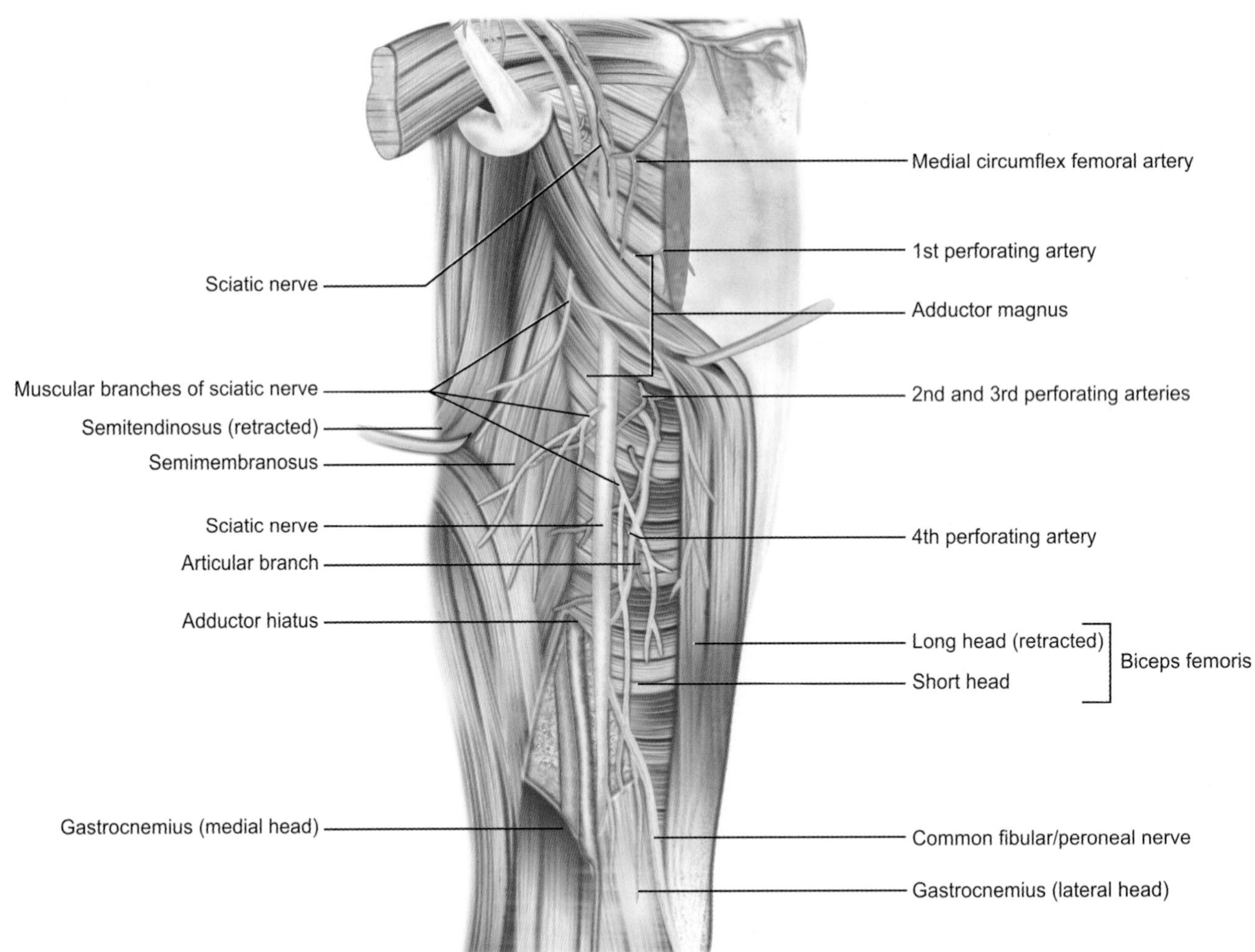

FIGURE 25 Deep dissection of back of thigh

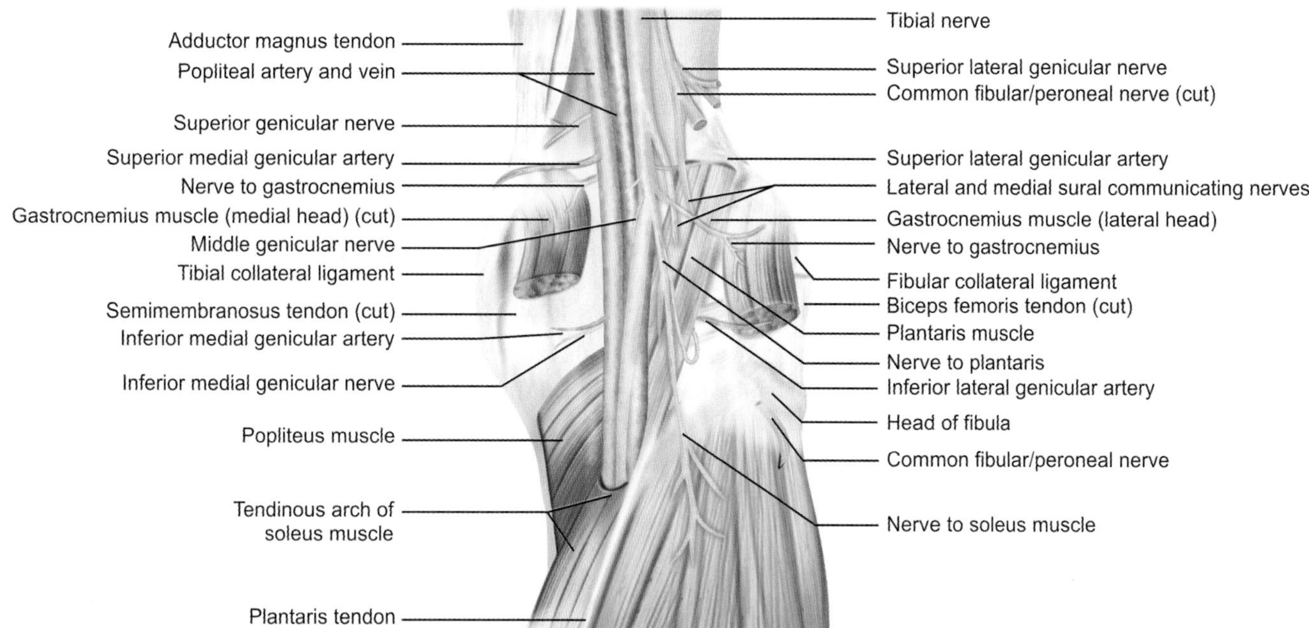

FIGURE 26 Deep dissection of popliteal fossa

DEEP DISSECTION OF POPLITEAL FOSSA (Fig. 26)

Dissection: Cut the hamstrings near their insertions. Pull the hamstring muscles away clean and identify the gastrocnemius muscle. This muscle belongs to the musculature of the leg, which has migrated up for its origin. It is the musculature of the posterior aspect of leg. The musculature of the leg is arranged in three layers, one deep to the other.

Superficial layer: It is made up of gastrocnemius and soleus, they join together, have a common tendon of insertion called the tendocalcaneous or Achilles tendon. It is inserted into the posterior surface of the calcaneum. The total muscle will be studied at later stage of dissection.

Dissection: Lift the gastrocnemius muscle carefully, feel the connective tissue underneath and cut both the bellies below the bend of the knee transversely and lift them up towards their origin, both the bellies get separated off. Trace the nerves entering the deeper surface of the muscles bellies from the tibial nerve. Cut and remove a small segment of common. Peroneal nerve to see the deeper structures clearly.

Plantaris: Locate this small muscle under cover of the lateral head of gastrocnemius. See the origin of this muscle from the popliteal surface of femur above the lateral condyle.

Neurovascular Bundle

This dissection of the back of knee is to expose the neurovascular bundle. Clean the neurovascular bundle and identify the branches. Trace the sciatic nerve from the middle of the thigh. Note that this nerve divides into two branches near the lower one-third of thigh into lateral common peroneal and medial tibial nerves. Trace these nerves and the cutaneous nerves emerging from them (these were already identified in the superficial dissection). These are:

Common peroneal nerve: It is the lateral division of the sciatic nerve will follow the medial border of the biceps femoris muscle to the neck of the fibula. This gives off two cutaneous and two genicular branches—**The sural communicating nerve** is a cutaneous branch given off from the medial side runs down and joins the sural nerve in the lower part of the leg. **Lateral cutaneous nerve of leg** is a lateral branch of the common personal nerve, winds round the lateral aspect and supplies it. **Lateral superior and inferior genicular nerves** accompany the respective arteries.

Tibial nerve lies in the midline between the two heads of gastrocnemius. This nerve gives off one cutaneous branch, all muscular branches and three genicular branches. **The sural nerve** is the cutaneous branch of the tibial nerve, accompanying the small saphenous vein. **The muscular branches** supply both the heads of gastrocnemius, soleus and plantaris. Trace them into the respective muscles. **The genicular branches**—superior middle and inferior genicular branches are given off from the tibial nerve. Trace these branches accompanying the respective arteries.

Popliteal Artery and Genicular Vessels

The popliteal artery reaches the popliteal region by passing through the adductor hiatus in the adductor magnus. Note that the vein lies deeper to the artery here. The blood vessels lie directly on the femur and give off genicular branches to supply the knee joint.

The popliteal artery gives off five genicular arteries–two superior, two inferior and one middle genicular arteries.

Superior genicular vessels and nerve pass deep to the muscles on either side and are above the femoral condyles. They supply the upper aspect of the joint.

Middle genicular branches: They pierce the capsule of the knee joint, to supply the joint.

Inferior genicular vessels and nerve supply the lower aspect of the knee joint capsule. They are given off below the tibial condyle pass under cover of the gastrocnemius muscle to reach the lateral aspect of the capsule.

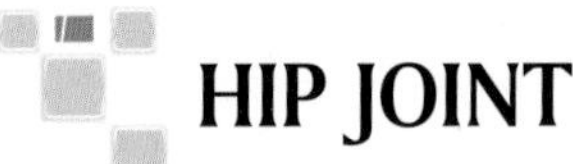

HIP JOINT

Hip joint is a poly axial, ball and socket type of joint. The acetabulum of the hip bone forms the socket and the head of the femur forms the ball. The neck of the femur is enclosed within the joint cavity. The bones are kept in position by thick capsule and powerful ligaments. Most of the muscles acting on the joint are inserted into the greater and lesser trochanter of femur. All the nerves passing around the joint give an articular branch to supply the joint. The medial and lateral circumflex, superior and inferior gluteal arteries and the obturator artery give vascular supply to the joint.

MUSCLES AROUND AND MOVEMENTS

Identify all the muscles around the hip joint, note their origins, insertions and direction of the fibres.These are the following:

Iliopsoas: See this muscle crosses the joint anteriorly and is a flexor of the thigh.

The gluteus medius and minimus cross the joint laterally and are abductors.

The gluteus maximus is a big muscle crossing the joint posteriorly. It is an abductor and a lateral rotator.

All the short muscles of the gluteal region which cross the joint medial to lateral are all lateral rotators. They are piriformis, obturator internus, externus gemelli and quadratus femoris.

The hamstring muscles cross the joint posteriorly so they are extensors of thigh.

The adductor group of muscles cross the joint medially and anteroposteriorly. They extend to the total length of femur. They are adductors and medial rotators.

Dissection: The body is in the prone position. Most of the muscles on the posterior aspect were cut transversely in their regional dissection. Now detach the muscles on the posterior aspect of the hip joint to get a clear view of the joint. Try to trace the articular branches from the nerve to quadratus femoris and superior gluteal nerve. Trace the medial circumflex femoral artery and its branches along the distal border of the neck of the femur. This was already identified along the lower border of quadratus femoris muscle.

POSTERIOR VIEW (Fig. 27)

Capsule and ischiofemoral ligament: The ischiofemoral ligament extends from the ischium of the hip bone external to the acetabular margin to the neck of the femur Identify this and note that its fibres spiral towards the greater trochanter. Insert a hook between the distal margin of the ligament and the neck of the femur and note that the *ligament is not attached to the neck of the femur here.*

Dissection: Make a curved cut into the ischiofemoral ligament nearer to the acetabular margin. Note that it is very thick here. It has got both the ligament and the capsule. Turn the body to the supine position. Cut the iliopsoas very near the inguinal ligament. Detach the rectus femoris and pectineus from their origins and dissect the neurovascular bundle on the anterior aspect. Clean and identify the ascending branch of the lateral circumflex femoral artery and its branches along the intertrochanteric line. The lateral and medial circumflex femoral arteries anastomose near the upper end of the neck of the femur.

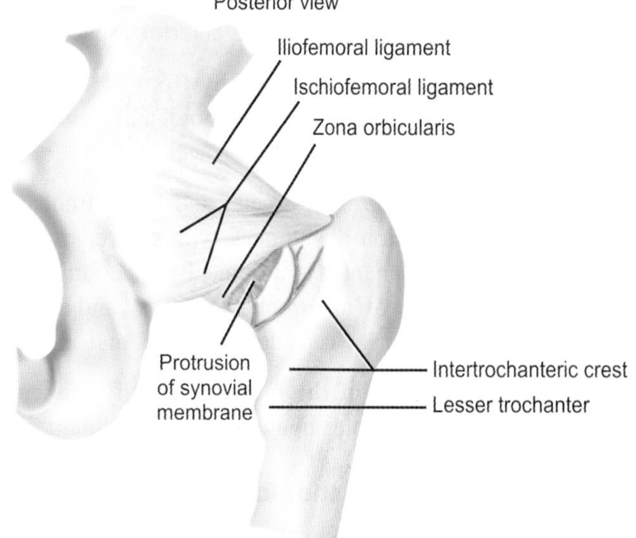

FIGURE 27 Hip joint—posterior aspect

ANTERIOR VIEW (Fig. 28)

Iliofemoral ligament: Identify this thick ligament. It is inverted y shaped ligament. Note its attachment from the anterior inferior iliac spine to the intertrochanteric line.

Dissection: Raise the body with the support of a block kept under the sacral region. Reidentify the obturator externus muscle from the obturator membrane. Cut the tendon nearer to the femur. Pull the muscle medially and identify the arterial anastomosis of the obturator artery deep to the muscle. Trace a branch of the artery deep to the pubofemoral ligament. This is the artery of the ligament of the head of the femur.

Pubofemoral ligament: It is a triangular ligament. It extends from the iliopubic eminence and obturator membrane to the lesser trochanter of the femur.

Note: The gap between the iliofemoral and pubofemoral ligaments. In this gap the synovial membrane of the joint cavity communicates with the bursa under cover of the iliopsoas muscle. Many a times you may feel the sticky synovial fluid here.

Dissection: Cut through the anterior part of the capsule and ligaments by a oblique cut extending from the anterior superior iliac spine to the inferior acetabular margin. Pull the femur down. This would separate the two bones and totally exposes the interior of the joint.

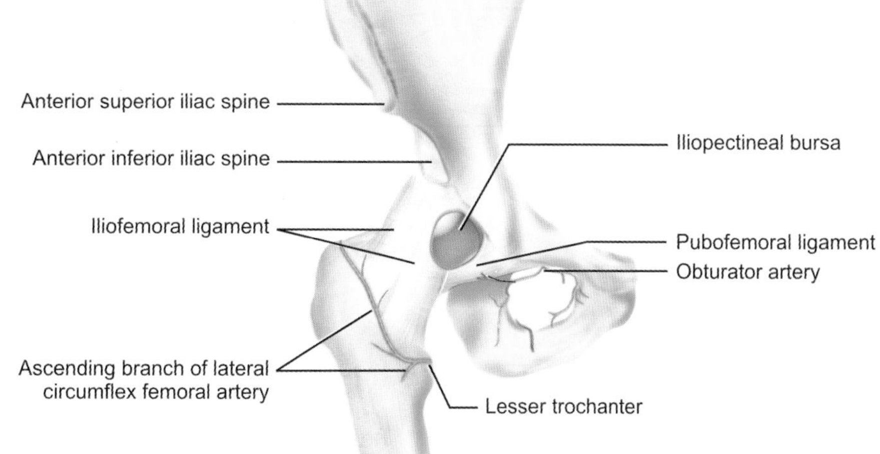

FIGURE 28 Hip joint—anterior view

INTERIOR OF THE JOINT (Fig. 29)

Acetabulum of the hip bone is a deep cup placed laterally. Lunate surface is the smooth inverted u shaped articulating surface of the acetabulum. It is wider at its upper part where the pressure of the body weight falls. The lower deep rough surface is non articular. The acetabular notch is the inferior deficiency in the acetabular margin.

Upper end of the femur: Head of the femur is two-third of a sphere and is the articular surface of the femur. The articular surface is extensive on the anterior aspect. Pit or fovea is the central medially located part.

Neck of the femur: Extends laterally from the head and joins with the shaft at an angle of 125 degrees. It is not articular, but intracapsular. Its upper border is shorter compared to its lower border. It presents vascular grooves and foraminae parallel to the direction of neck.

Upper end of shaft: Present greater and lesser trochanters. The greater trochanter is a beak shaped projection at the upper end. The junction of the neck with greater trochanter, in its upper part presents a fossa, called the trochanteric fossa. The lesser trochanter is a conical projection on the inferomedial aspect. The greater and lesser trochanters are connected posteriorly by intertrochanteric crest and anteriorly by intertrochanteric line. The greater and lesser trochanters receive the attachment of capsule, ligaments and insertions of the muscles acting on the hip joint.

Ligament of the head of the femur: Identify this cord like ligament extending from the pit or fovea of the femur to the transverse acetabular ligament. Cut this ligament and this totally frees the femur.

Study the Interior of the Joint

Femur: On the femur see the articular surface , ligament of the head of the femur, neck of the femur blood vessels on the neck, capsule and the synovial membrane lining it.

In the acetabulum: Note the labrum acetabular. It is a thick circular ligament attached to the rim of the acetabulum. It is triangular in cross section, the base is attached to the acetabulum and the apex presents a free border. Identify this. This increases the depth of the acetabulum. The part of the acetabular labrum which bridges the acetabular notch is named as the transverse acetabular ligament.

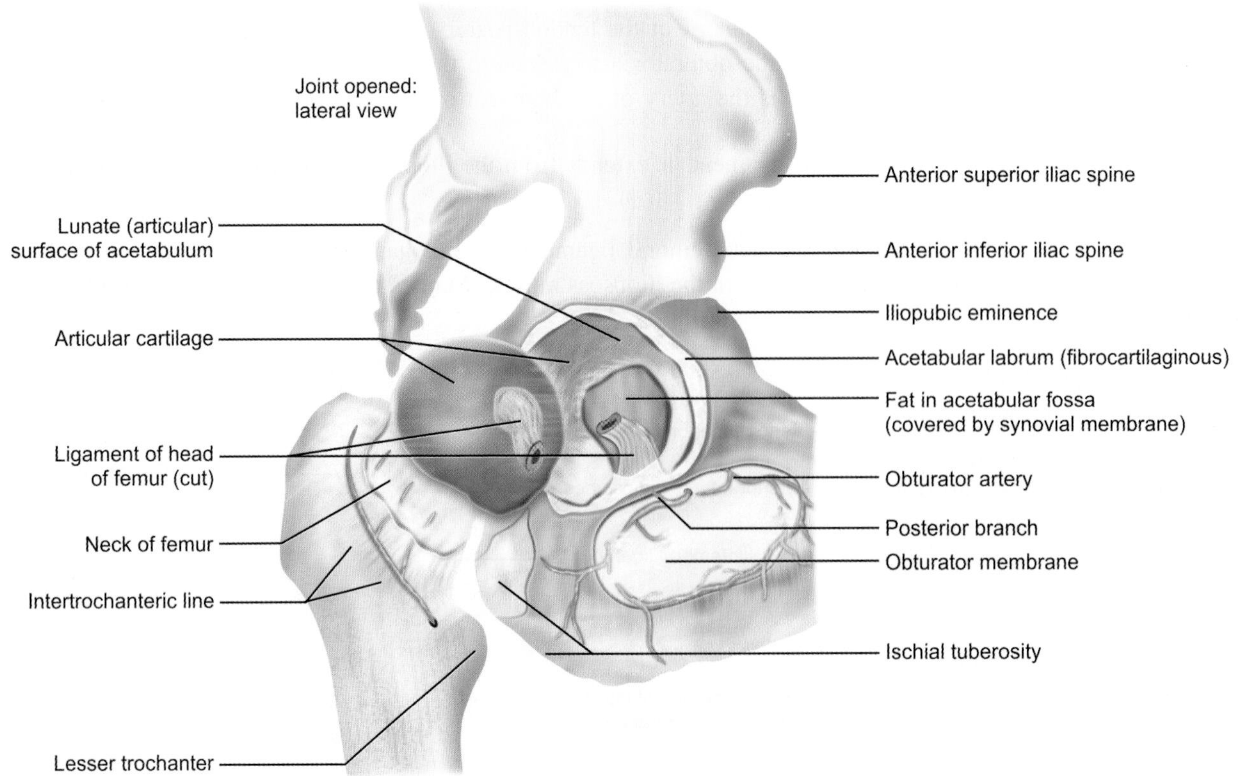

FIGURE 29 Interior of hip joint

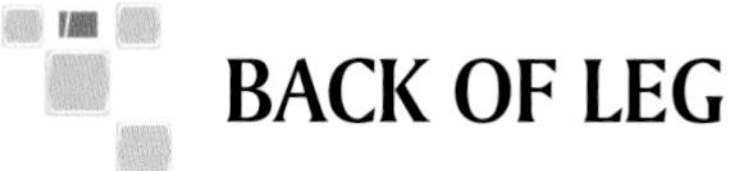

BACK OF LEG

SKELETON (Fig. 30)

Go to a skeleton and identify the posterior aspect of the leg bones.

Tibia is the medial bone. Note that its upper end is enlarged to form the condyles. They articulate with the femoral condyles to form the knee joint. The lower end is enlarged to form the medial malleolus. Note the oblique solely line on the upper aspect of the shaft.

Fibula is the lateral bone. See its upper end. Here it forms the head. Head is followed by neck and shaft. The lower end enlarges to form the lateral malleolus.

The tibia and fibula articulate with each other at three joints. The upper one is a synovial joint, the lower two are fibrous joints.

Talus is the bone below the tibia and fibula. It articulates with them to form the ankle joint.

Calcaneum is the bone to form the heel. It articulates superiorly with the talus.

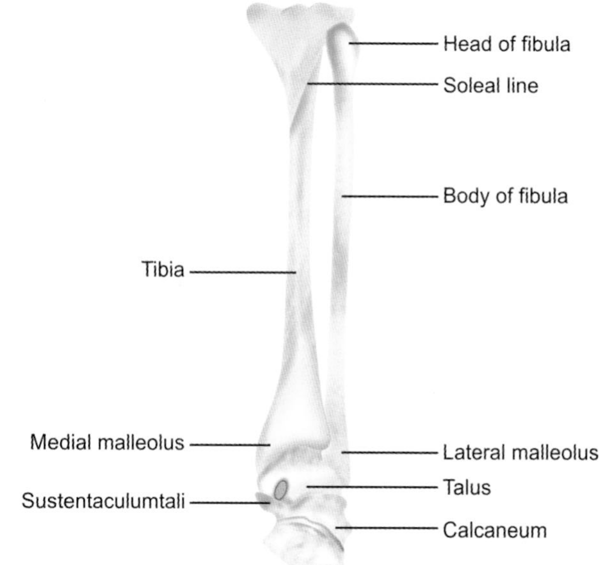

FIGURE 30 Back of the leg—skeleton

SURFACE AND LIVING ANATOMY (Fig. 31)

The back of the leg is made up of three layers of musculature, superficial to deep. Intermuscular septa separate the layers of muscles. The superficial layer is the bulkiest and can easily be identified on the surface. Note that it tapers into a thick tendon near the heel, which can be clasped between the fingers. This is the tendo calcaneus/ tendo Achilles.

Great saphenous vein: It can easily be identified behind the medial malleolus in a living subject.

> **Dissection:** Make a midline incision vertically from cut end of the skin to the heel. Make a horizontal incision near the heel. Reflect the flaps to the medial and lateral sides.

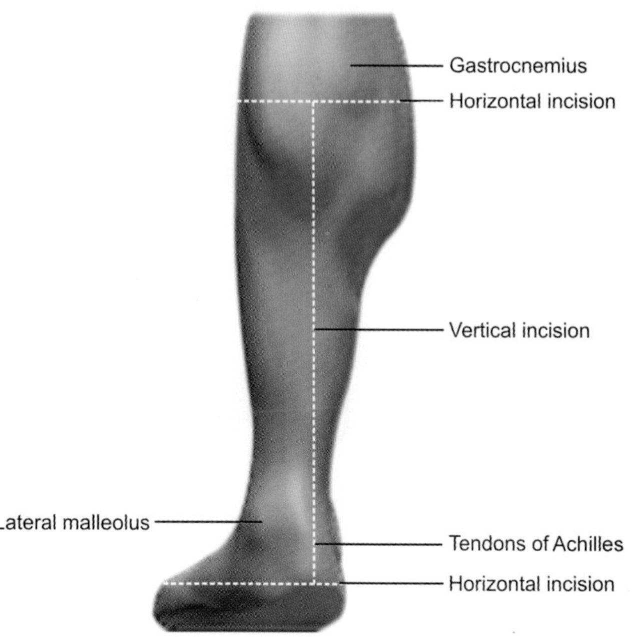

FIGURE 31 Surface and living anatomy—back of leg

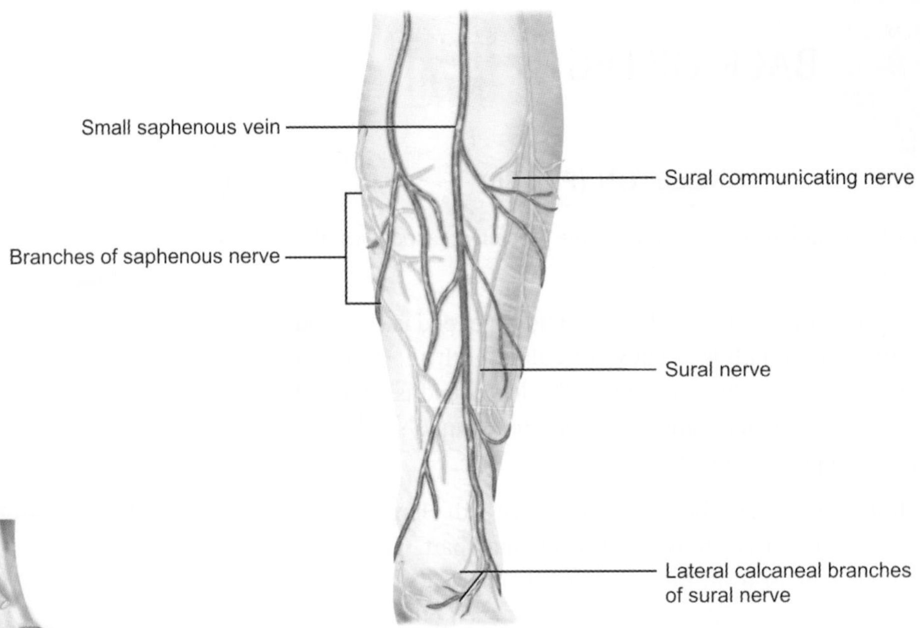

FIGURE 32 Cutaneous structures of back of leg

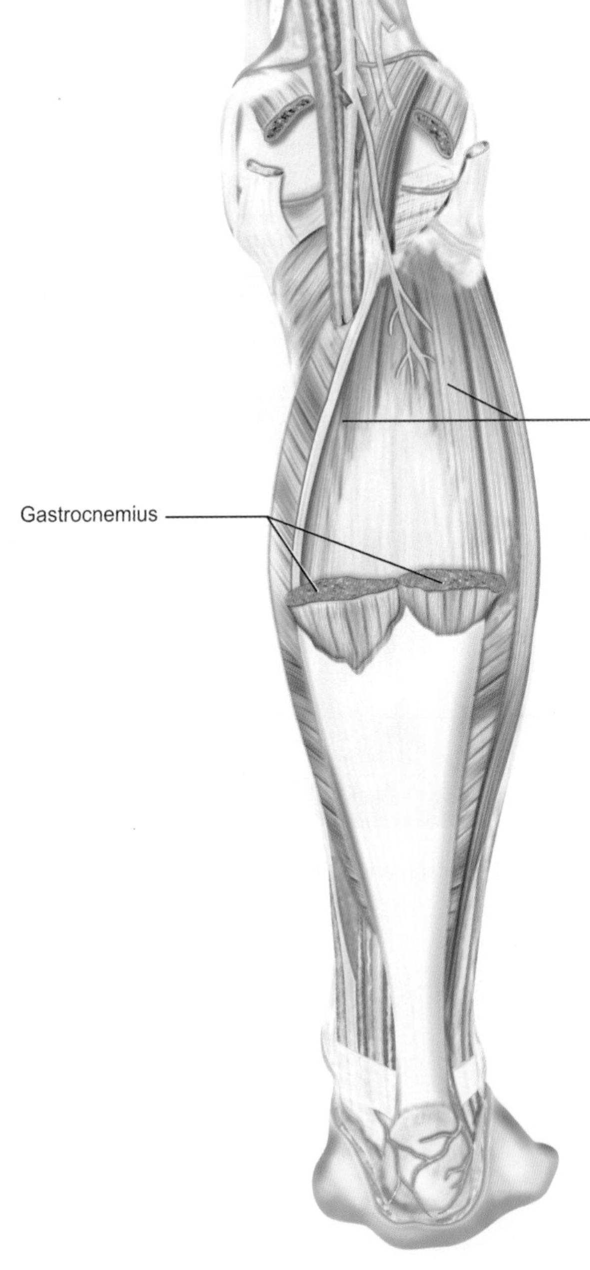

FIGURE 33 Superficial layer of back of leg

CUTANEOUS STRUCTURES (Fig. 32)

Cutaneous structures (Fig. 32) Continue the ***sural nerve and the sural communicating nerve*** to the back of the heel. They communicate with each other at variable level, and supply the skin of the back of the leg.

Short saphenous vein: Trace it down to the posterior aspect of the lateral malleolus.

Dissection: Cut the deep fascia from the posterior aspect of the popliteal fossa upto the lower end of the calcaneum.

SUPERFICIAL LAYER (Fig. 33)

Gastrocnemius: You have already seen the origin and nerve supply of gastrocnemius. See the bulk of the muscle and its insertion into the flat tendon. Reflect the muscle nearer to the insertion into the tendocalcaneus and see the soleus

Soleus: It is the deeper of the superficial layer of muscles. It has two heads of origin. The tibial head arises from the oblique line on the posterior aspect of tibia. The fibular head arises from the head and posterior aspect of the shaft of the fibula. Between the two heads it arises from a tendinous arch. Which covers the neurovascular bundle reaching the deeper aspect of the leg.

Soleus is muscular at its origin develops aponeurosis on the superficial surface of the muscle, joins with the aponeurotic part of the gastrocnemius rounds up forms a thick tendon called the tendocalcaneus.

Tibial nerve and popliteal artery pass deep to the tendinous arch under cover of soleus.

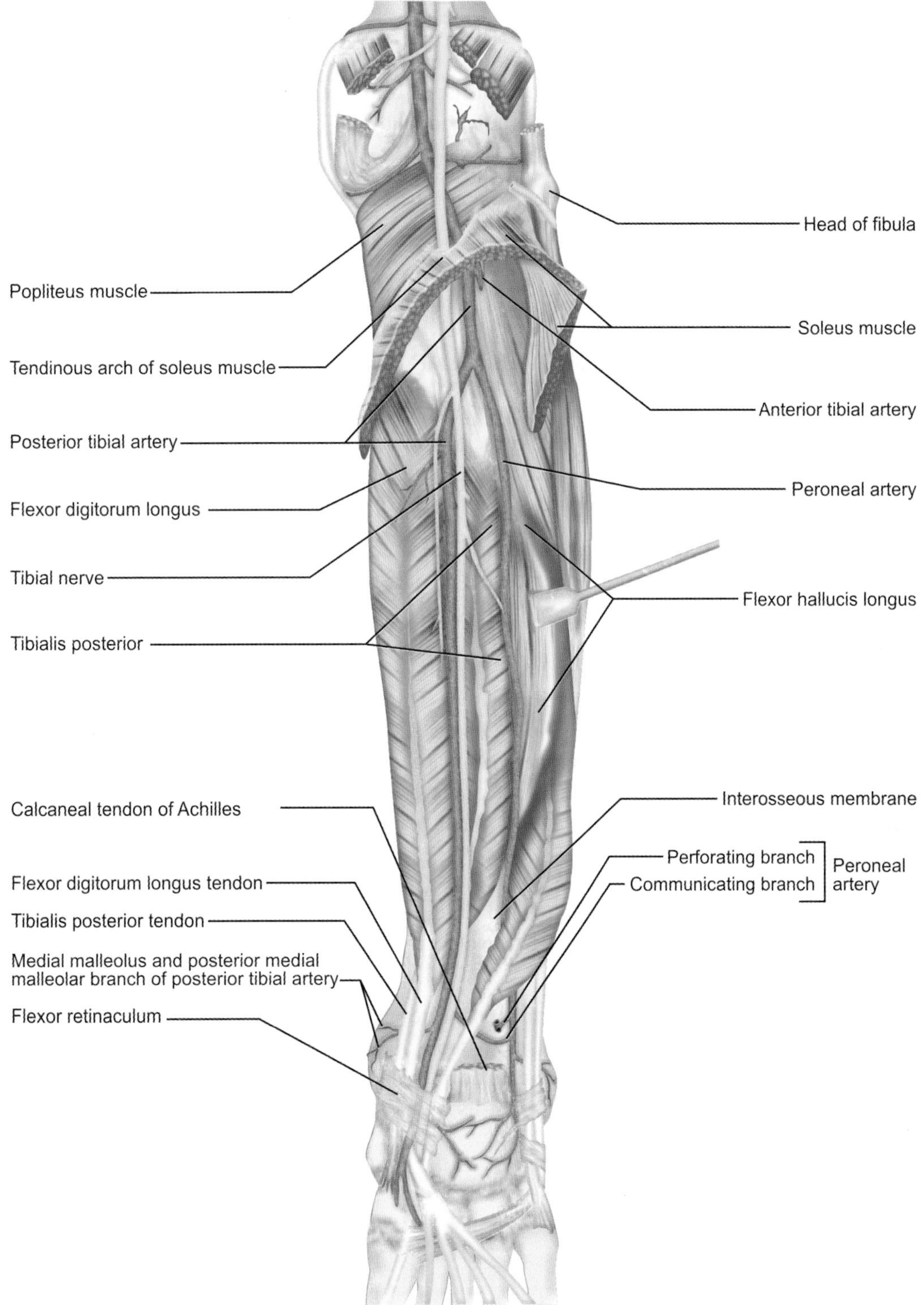

FIGURE 34 Deep structures of back of leg

DEEP STRUCTURES OF BACK OF LEG (Fig. 34)

Dissection: Clean the genicular branches and the neurovascular bundle to the soleus muscle.

Popliteus: At this stage you can see the insertion of the popliteus muscle. It is inserted into the popliteal surface on the back of the tibia.

Action: The gastrocnemius and soleus act together on the foot at the ankle and produces planter flexion as the gastrocnemius crosses the knee joint it acts as a flexor of the knee joint. It is a powerful flexor particularly in running. It is a fast contracting muscle. The soleus acts only at the ankle joint. It is a slow contracting postural muscle.

Dissection: Cut the soleus near the origin and reflect the muscle downwards, leaving a small bit of its origin along with the nerve supply.

Note: The intermuscular septum separating the superficial layer from the middle layer of the leg. The neurovascular bundle passes deep to it. Clean this intermuscular septum and study.

Flexor digitorum longus: It is the medial muscle of this layer. It takes origin from the middle one-third of the posterior surface of the tibia below the insertion of the popliteus. Soon it becomes tendineous, passes towards the medial surface of the ankle region.

Flexor hallucis longus: It is the lateral muscle of this layer, arises from the posterior surface of the middle one-third of fibula, becomes tendinous in its lower part and deviates towards the medial surface of the ankle.

NEUROVASCULAR BUNDLE

The tibial nerve soon continues down between the two muscles and superficial to the tibial posterior the deepest muscle of the layer. This nerve supplies all the three muscles, continues down to the medial side of the ankle between the flexor hallucis and digitorum. This nerve is called posterior tibial, once it crosses the popliteus muscle. It gives off a recurrent branch, which goes deep to the popliteus from its lower border to supply its deeper aspect.

The popliteal artery divides into the anterior and posterior tibial arteries below the lower border of the popliteus muscle. The anterior tibial artery reaches the anterior compartment by passing above the interosseous membrane.

Circumflex fibular artery is given off from the posterior tibial artery. It winds around the neck of the fibula. Trace this artery.

Peroneal artery is the big branch of the posterior tibial artery. Trace this artery from the posterior tibial artery towards the lateral side between the origin of the flexor hallucis longus and the posterior intermuscular septum. It is the artery for the peroneal compartment. It supplies the peroneal compartment by passing through the intermuscular septum as perforating branches. Pull the peroneal artery medially and note these branches. The peroneal artery gives off a perforating branch which reaches the anterior compartment and terminal branches to supply the lateral malleolus and the joints around.

Dissection: Separate the flexor hallucus longus and digitorum to see the 2nd deeper intermuscular septum, which separates the second and third layers of leg. Note the deeper muscles.

Tibialis posterior: It is one of the examples of a circumpennate muscles. It takes origin from the deep intermuscular septum posterior aspects of the tibia and fibula and interosseous membrane. Posterior tibial vessels and nerves supply it. This muscle deviates to the medial aspect of the ankle deep to the other muscles and will be related to the posterior aspect of the medial malleolus. Locate this muscle from its origin to under cover of the flexor retinaculum.

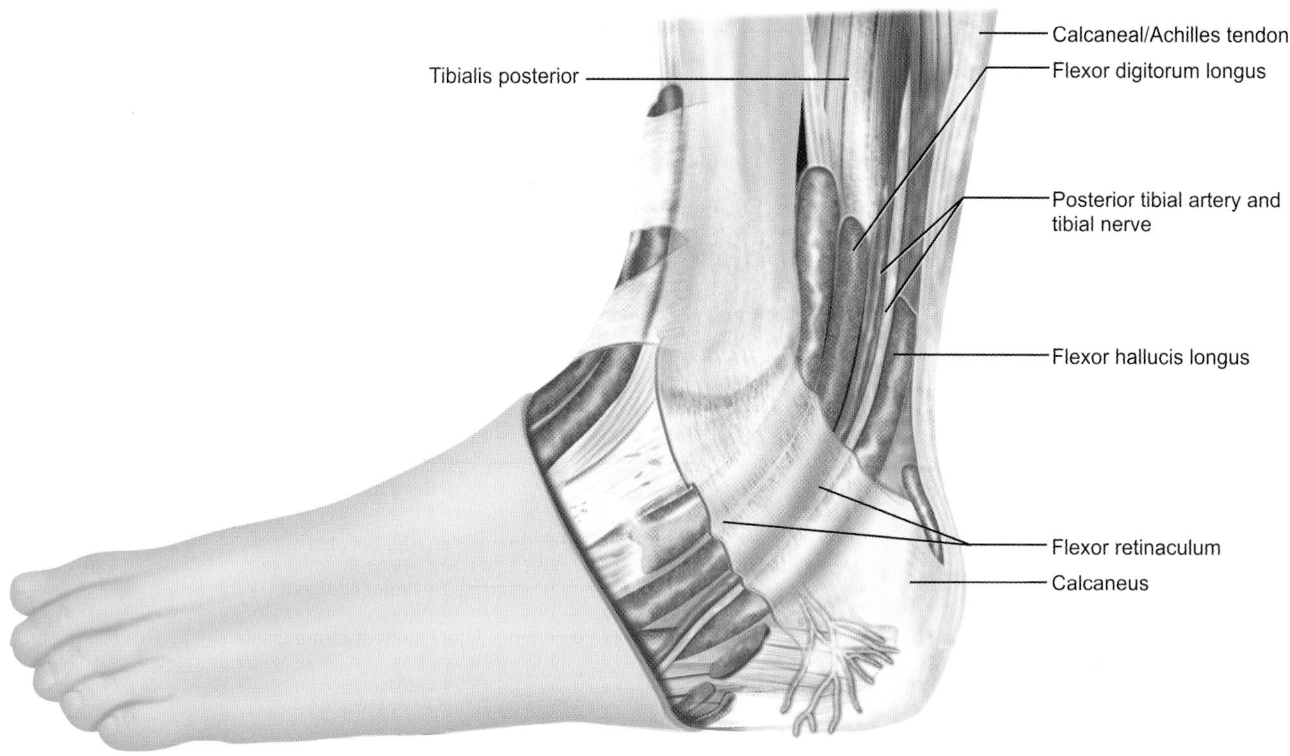

FIGURE 35 Flexor retinaculum

FLEXOR RETINACULUM (Fig. 35)

Flexor retinaculum extends from the lower border of the medial malleolus to the medial side of the calcaneum. The tendons and the neurovascular bundle of the posterior compartment of the leg passes down into the sole of the foot along the medial side of the ankle under cover of the flexor retinaculum. Identify these structures from the medial malleolus to the calcaneum. The ***tibialis posterior***—identify the this tendon grooving the medial malleolus. Trace the tendon into the tuberosity of the navicular bone. It sends in more slips to be inserted into the tarsal and metatarsals. The ***flexor digitorum longus*** is the next muscle. It acquires its tendon low down. The division into four tendons to reach the toes takes place within the sole. Identify the ***posterior tibial artery*** with its venae comitantes. Behind the blood vessels lies the posterior ***tibial nerve***. The last structures in this line is the ***flexor hallucis longus***. All the tendons are covered by the synovial sheaths.

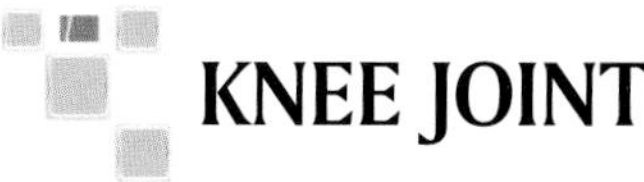

KNEE JOINT

Knee joint is a compound joint. It presents a sellar joint between the patella and the femur. Here the patella slides over the femur. It has a condylar joint between the tibial and femoral condyles. Intra articular menisci are present between the condyles separate the joint into two parts. Flexion and extension takes place in the meniscofemoral compartment and rotation takes place in the meniscotibial compartment.

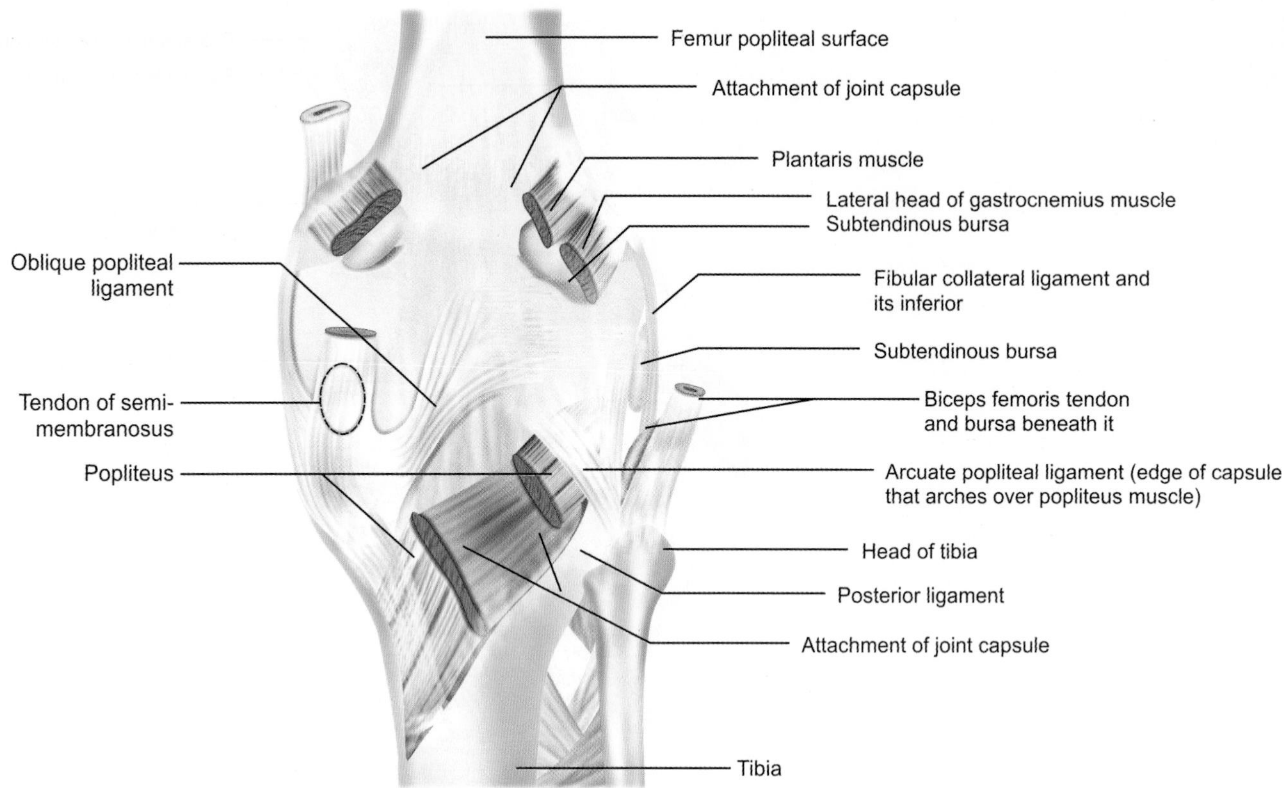

FIGURE 36 Posterior aspect of knee joint

POSTERIOR ASPECT OF KNEE JOINT (FIG. 36)

Dissection: Cut all the muscles around the knee very near their insertion. Clean the capsule ligaments that lie deep to the muscles.

Posteriorly identify ***semimembranosus*** and trace it down along the medial side of the gastrocnemius to the posterior aspect of the tibial condyle. Note that it widens out to be inserted into a groove on the back of the tibial condyle. Identify its extensions by pulling the muscle upwards and medially. You will note that it sends aponeurotic extensions to the capsule of the knee joint as oblique popliteal ligament and on to the popliteus as popliteal fascia.

Posteriomedially identify the tendons of ***semitendinosus, gracilis and sartorius.*** Note that they are posterior here but move forwards to get inserted into the medial surface of the shaft of the tibia. Laterally identify ***biceps femoris*** muscle. It is lateral to the gastrocnemius muscle. Note its cord like insertion into the styloid process of the fibula

Gastrocnemius: Note that both the heads of this muscle arise from the area above the articulating surface of the femur .Note the origin of ***plantaris***, which is also in line with the gastrocnemius.

All these above muscles crossing the joint posteriorly are flexors of the leg over the thigh. The biceps femoris which crosses the joint laterally is a lateral rotator of the femur.

The semitendinosus, gracilis and the sartorius are all medial rotators of the leg.

Note the ***oblique popliteal ligament,*** the extension of the semimembranosus muscle.

Capsule: Cut the popliteus muscle and see the thin capsule on the posterior aspect of the knee joint.

Arcuate popliteal ligament: Note this triangular ligament extending from the head of the fibula to the lateral femoral condyle. Note the popliteus muscle emerging under cover of this.

Fibular collateral ligament: Identify this cord like ligament extending from the lateral epicondyle to the head of the fibula. Note that it is overlapped by the biceps femoris muscle.

Turn the leg anteriorly and identify the muscles on the shaft of the tibia

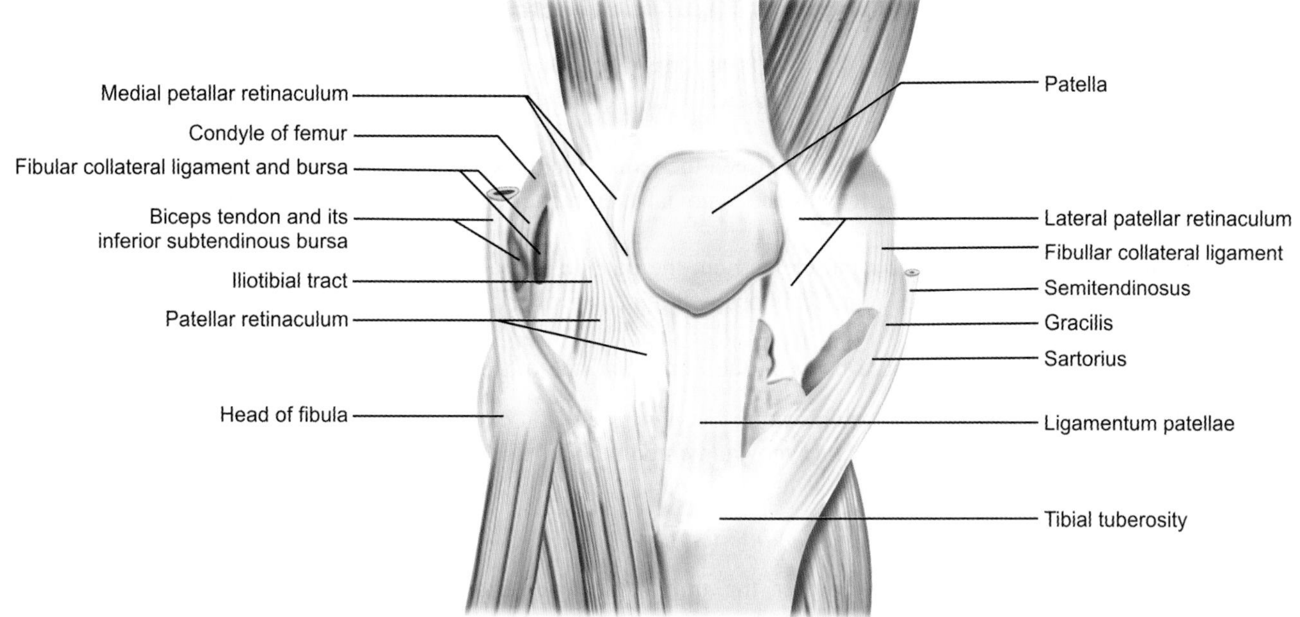

FIGURE 37 Anterior aspect of knee joint

MUSCLES AND LIGAMENTS ANTERIOR ASPECT (Fig. 37)

Anteromedially three muscles—the ***Sartorius*** of anterior compartment, the ***gracilis*** of medial compartment, the ***semitendinosus*** of the posterior compartment converge and get inserted into the upper one-third of the medial aspect of the shaft of the tibia. The sartorius is the most anterior muscle, gracilis lies intermediate in position and the semitendinosus is the most posterior of the muscles. By this insertion they perform medial rotation of the tibia on the femur.

Anteriorly* the *ligamentum patellae and patellar retinacula constitute the insertion of the quadriceps femoris muscle. This forms the anterior part of the capsule. It inserts into the tibia through the patella, which is a sesamoid bone. The vastus medialis reaches the medial aspect of patella and is called medial patellar retinaculum the vastus lateralis reaches the lateral aspect of the patella called lateral patellar retinaculum. Vastus intermedius reaches the flat surface on the upper surface of the patella. This part is more muscular when this reaches the patella. The rectus femoris is tendinous at its insertion and reaches the upper surface of the patella superficial to the vastus intermedius.

Ligamentum patellae: It is the continuation of the above four muscles, it extends from the lower border of the patella to the tibial tuberosity.

Tibial tuberosity: Note this elevation on the anterior aspect of the tibia. It gives attachment to the ligamentum patellae.

Action: The quadriceps femoris is an extensor of the leg at the knee joint.

Laterally and medially the capsule is attached to the femoral and tibial condyles beyond their articular surfaces.

Posteriorly: It is attached to the area beyond the articular surfaces of the tibia and femur.

Tibial collateral ligament: Identify this ligament extending from the medial epicondyle to the shaft of the tibia. It is a wide ligament and runs obliquely.

INTERIOR OF KNEE JOINT (Fig. 38)

Dissection: Cut the quadratus femoris muscle transversely near the lower one-third of femur. Detach the muscle forwards and identify the articularis genu muscle.

Articularis genu: Note this muscle extending between the femur and the synovial membrane. This muscle is a detached part of the vastus intermedius muscle**.** It pulls the synovial membrane during movement of the joint.

Dissection: Cut the articularis genu muscle and cut the patellar retinacula along the sides of the patella. Bend the leg over the thigh at the knee joint. This opens the interior of the joint.

Suprapatellar bursa: This is the space between the femur and the quadriceps femoris muscle above the patella.

Infrapatellar pad of fat and synovial membrane: See this pad of fat extending from the ligamentum patellae to the interior of the joint . Note that it is covered by synovial membrane. This fills the gaps in the joint cavity during movement. Note the lateral extensions of this fat. It is called alar folds.

If necessary cut and separate these and see the interior.

Cruciate ligaments: These are two in number, the ***anterior and posterior.*** See the anterior ligament which extends from the medial side of the front of the tibia to the lateral condyle of the femur in the intertrochanteric notch. A very small part of the lateral cruciate ligament will be seen here in the intertrochanteric notch getting attached to the medial condyle of femur.

Menisci: These two in number—the ***medial and lateral meniscus.*** These are fibrocartilaginous structures. In cross section they are triangular in shape. Observe their shape. The medial meniscus is c-shaped whereas the lateral meniscus is circular in shape. Locate their attachment on the intercondylar eminence. The menisci separate the articulating femoral and tibial condyles. This divides the joint into two sub joints—the menisco femoral and menisco tibial compartments. Flexion and extension takes place in menisco femoral compartment and rotation takes place in menisco tibial compartment.

Synovial membrane and bursae: Run your fingers along the inner side of the capsule and feel the synovial membrane lining it. Note that it covers the synovial pad of fat and the cruciate ligaments and popliteus muscle. Note that they extra synovial though they are intra articular.

Transverse ligament: It connects both the menisci.

Dissection: Turn the part posteriorly and cut the arcuate ligament and see the origin of the popliteus muscle.

Popliteus muscle arises from the groove below the lateral epicondyle, and deeper to the lateral collateral ligament. Trace the muscle to its insertion. Note that this muscle crosses the joint from lateral to medial side. It is a medial rotator of the tibia on the femur when the foot is off the ground. It rotates the femur laterally when the foot is on the ground, thus is a muscle of unlocking. It initiates the flexion of the leg by rotating the femur on the tibia.

Dissection: Cut through the medial and lateral collateral ligaments, cruciate ligaments and separate the two bones.

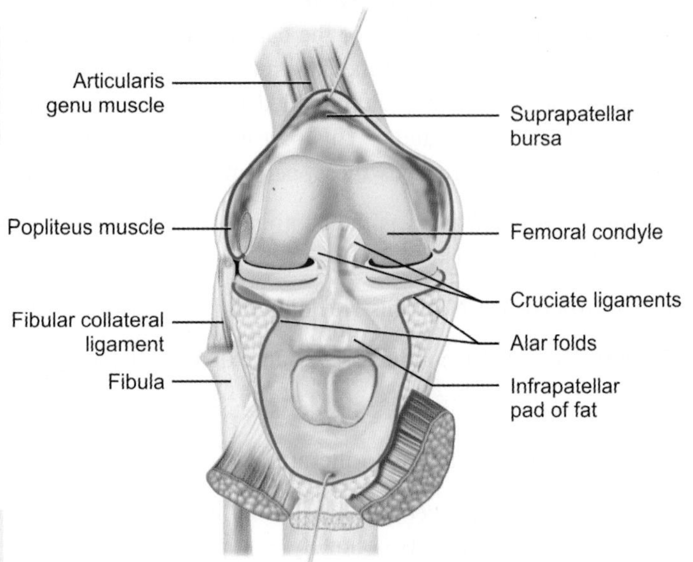

FIGURE 38 Interior of knee joint

ARTICULAR SURFACES (Fig. 39)

Patellar surface of femur: Note that it is a v-shaped depression on the anterior aspect of the lower end of femur. The lateral part is more pronounced than the medial part. It is separated from the condyles of the femur by medial and lateral grooves.

Condyles of femur: Note that the ***medial femoral condyle*** is bigger than the lateral femoral condyle.

Intercondylar notch: Note this gap is on the posterior aspect between the two condyles.

Patella is a sesamoid bone seen within the tendon of quadratus femoris muscle. It is a sead like structure. See that its anterior aspect is rough as it receives the muscle. The posterior surface is wedge shaped and presents articular area which is divided into facets. A central projection divides it into a medial and a lateral part. The medial part is further divided into small medial most flange. This part articulates with femur in extreme flexion. It presents a lower conical projection. This gives attachment to ligamentum patellae.

Upper end of tibia: Note the articular surface of the tibial condyles. The medial condyle presents a c-shaped articulating surface and the lateral condyle presents a circular articulating surface.

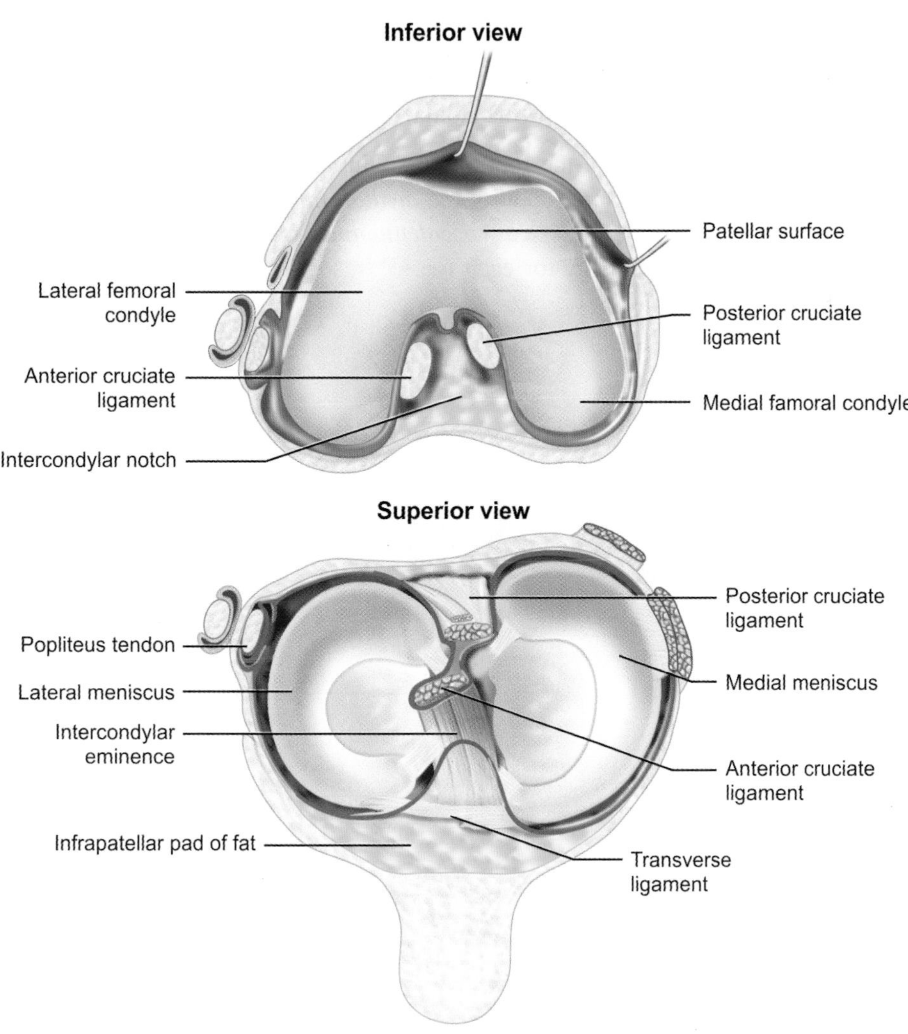

FIGURE 39 Articular surfaces of knee joint

ANTEROLATERAL COMPARTMENT OF LEG AND DORSUM OF FOOT

On an articulated skeleton identify the medial surface of the shaft of the tibia. Feel the same on your body and realize that it is subcutaneous throughout its extent.

SKELETON (Fig. 40)

Go to an articulated skeleton and identify the following:

Anterior sharp margin of the ***tibia***. It is subcutaneous throughout its extent. This margin gradually moves to the medial side to form the ***medial malleolus***.

Superiorly identify the expanded upper end of the tibia. See its massive size and its articulation with the femur. The lower end of the tibia also expands and projects downward medially. It is the medial malleolus.

Fibula note its expanded upper head. Note its articulation with the tibia. Fibula articulates with the undersurface of the expanded upper end of tibia. It forms a plane synovial joint. Fibula though it is a lean bone it is totally surrounded by muscles. It gives attachment to the anterior, lateral and posterior group of musculature.

Identify the anterior border, interosseous border, anterior and medial surfaces of the fibula.

Lateral malleolus is the lower expanded part of the fibula.

Foot: Identify the dorsal aspect of the bones of the foot See the talus articulating with tibia and fibula. Note the head of the ***talus*** articulating with the ***navicular bone***. Identify the ***medial, intermediate*** and ***lateral cuneiform*** articulating with the navicular. Below and lateral to the talus see the ***calcaneum***. Note the ***cuboid*** articulating with calcaneum. Identify the five ***metatarsals***. See the ***phalanges*** for each toe.

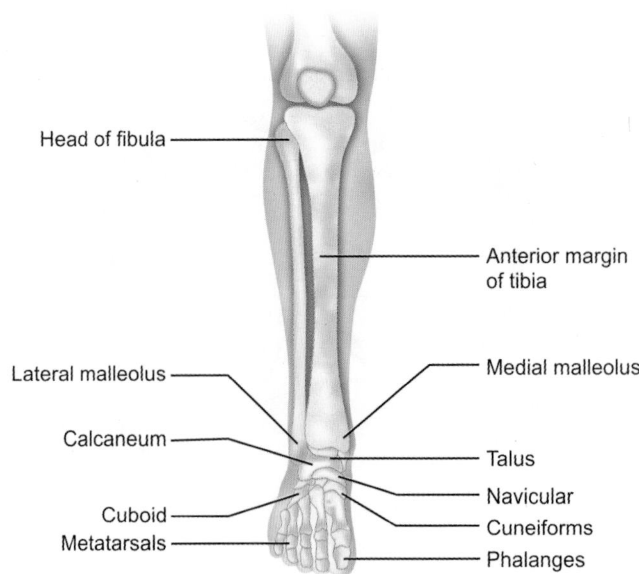

FIGURE 40 Skeleton of leg and foot

SURFACE ANATOMY (Fig. 41)

Feel the area around the ankle. You can feel it that it is bony. Feel ***medial malleolus*** of the tibia and the ***lateral malleolus*** of the fibula**.** ***Identifiable veins,*** You can see the ***dorsal venous arch*** on the dorsum of the foot. Trace the medial end into the ***great saphenous vein,*** note that it passes posterior to the medial malleolus. Trace the lateral end of the dorsal venous arch to the ***small saphenous vein. Arterial pulsations***: you can feel the pulsations of the ***anterior tibial artery*** between the malleoli. You can feel its continuation, the ***dorsalis pedis artery*** in the first interosseous space. ***Tendons*:** by extending the foot you can see the ***tibialis anterior, extensor hallucis longus, extensor digitorum longus tendons*** on the dorsum of the foot. By everting the foot you can see the ***peroneus longus brevis*** and ***tertius*** tendons on the lateral aspect, by plantar flexing the foot you can see the ***tendocalcaneus*** posteriorly. Tendons are deeply placed on the medial side, so it is difficult to see them.

Dissection: Identify the medial and lateral tibial condyles and medial and lateral malleoli. Make a vertical incision from between the condyles, malleoli to the tip of the second toe. Make a horizontal incision between the two malleoli. Reflect the four flaps of the skin to the sides as much as possible. Here the skin is very thin. This would expose the medial, anterior and lateral compartments.

Medial side of the leg: It is formed by the medial surface of the tibia and it is subcutaneous throughout its extent. See it on the body and feel it on yourself.

The ***anterior compartment*** forms the lateral side of the leg in its upper part and the front of the leg in its lower part. It is occupied by the extensor muscles of the foot. ***Lateral compartment of leg*** lies lateral throughout the extent. It is occupied by the peronei. They move posterior to the lateral malleolus. The lateral compartment is separated by the anterior compartment by the lateral intermuscular septum.

The dorsum of the foot is a continuation of the anterior compartment of leg. The tendons of the muscles of the anterior compartment along with the blood vessels continue into the dorsum.

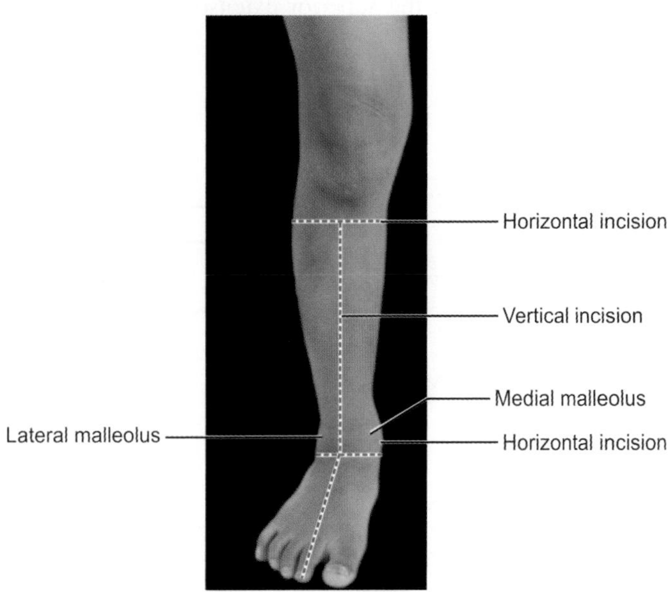

FIGURE 41 Surface anatomy and skin incision

SUPERFICIAL FASCIA (Fig. 42)

Venous arch: Locate the dorsal venous arch and its digital tributaries. The great ***saphenous vein*** is the continuation of the dorsal venous arch on the medial side in front of the medial malleolus. Trace it up, till it goes behind the bend of the knee. The ***small saphenous vein*** begins at the lateral end of the dorsal venous arch. Trace this up to the posterior aspect of the lateral malleolus.

Saphenous nerve: Trace this nerve accompanying the great saphenous vein to supply the skin up to the base of the big toe.

Superficial peroneal nerve: Pierces the deep fascia on the lateral side of the leg near its middle, crosses towards the medial side and supplies up to the digits. Trace these digital branches to the medial side of the big toe, to the webs between the second and third toe, third and fourth toe and fourth and fifth toe. They supply the contiguous sides of the toes.

Sural nerve: Supplies the lateral side of the little toe. Trace it.

Digital branch of deep peroneal nerve: Locate this nerve in the gap between the first and 2nd toes.

Deep fascia: Study the deep fascia of the leg and note that the fibres. They are generally vertically placed, but shows horizontal thickenings near the ankle. These are called retinacula and they hold the deeper tendons in position.

Superior extensor retinaculum: This retinaculum extends between the lower ends of the anterior borders of the tibia and fibula. Connects the lower ends of the fibula and tibia. Clean this thick sheet and see the attachment.

Inferior extensor retinaculum: This is a Y shaped retinaculum. The stem of the Y is attached to the calcaneum, the upper limb of Y to the anterior margin of medial malleolus, the lower limb of the Y merges with the deep fascia on the medial side of sole. Clean this retinaculum and see its attachment.

Dissection: Feel the anterior border of the shaft of the tibia, detach the deep fascia from here and clean the muscles beneath. Identify the structures near the superior extensor retinaculum.

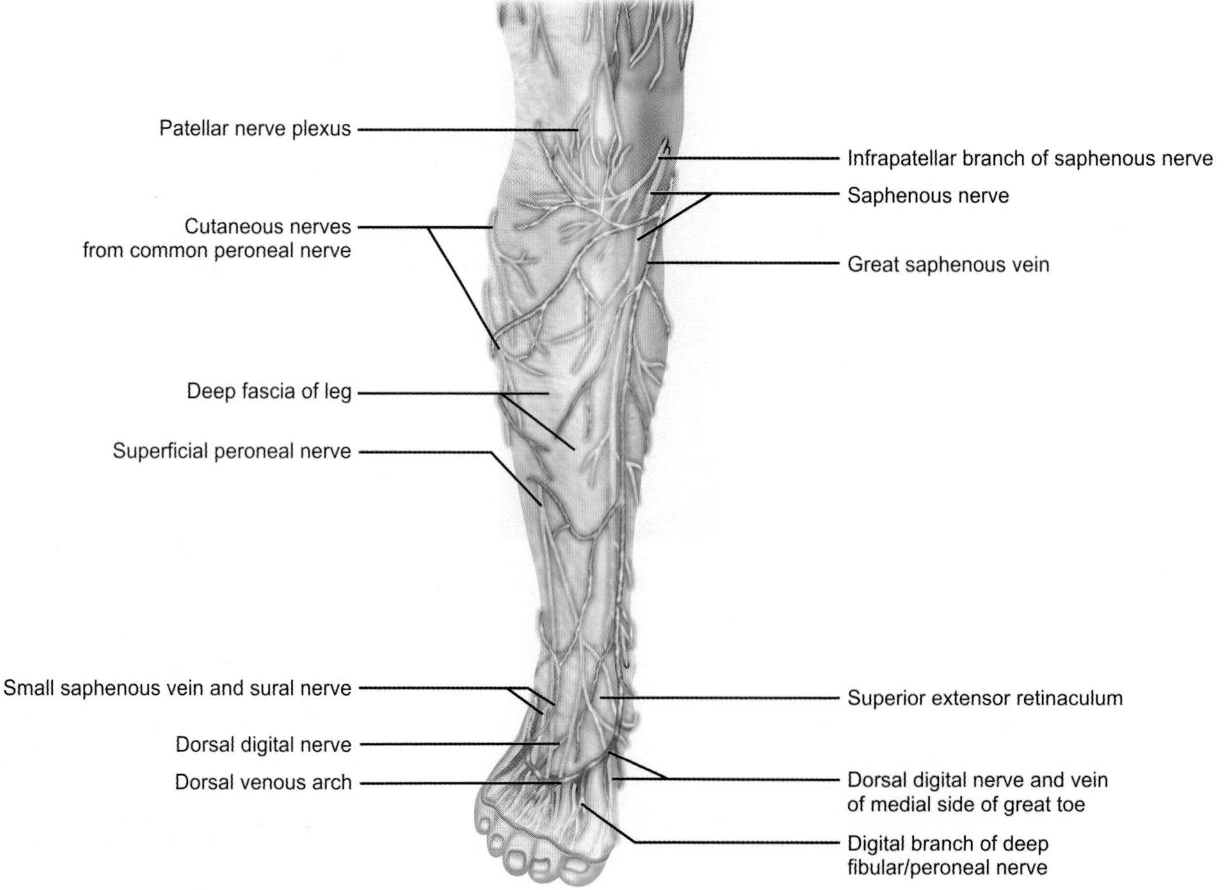

FIGURE 42 Superficial fascia of leg

MUSCLES OF ANTERIOR COMPARTMENT (Fig. 43)

Tibialis anterior: This is the most medial muscle. Trace this muscle above to its origin and note that it arises from the proximal two-thirds of lateral surface of the tibia and the interosseous membrane. Trace it down to its insertion in the medial surface of medial cuneiform bone.

Extensor hallucis longus: It is the next muscle trace it up and see its origin from the interosseous membrane and the middle two-thirds of anterior surface of fibula. Trace it down to its insertion into the base of the distal phalanx of the great toe.

Extensor digitorum longus: It is the medial muscle, which arises from the anterior surface of the fibula. Trace it distally and note that it divides into 4 slips to reach the bases of the lateral four distal phalanx.

Peroneus tertius: It is a small muscle from lower one-fourth of the anterior surface of fibula. This muscle deviates laterally and is inserted into the dorsal surface of the base of the fifth metatarsal bone.

Trace the branches of the neurovascular bundle into each of the muscles. They all enter the center of the fleshy parts of the muscle.

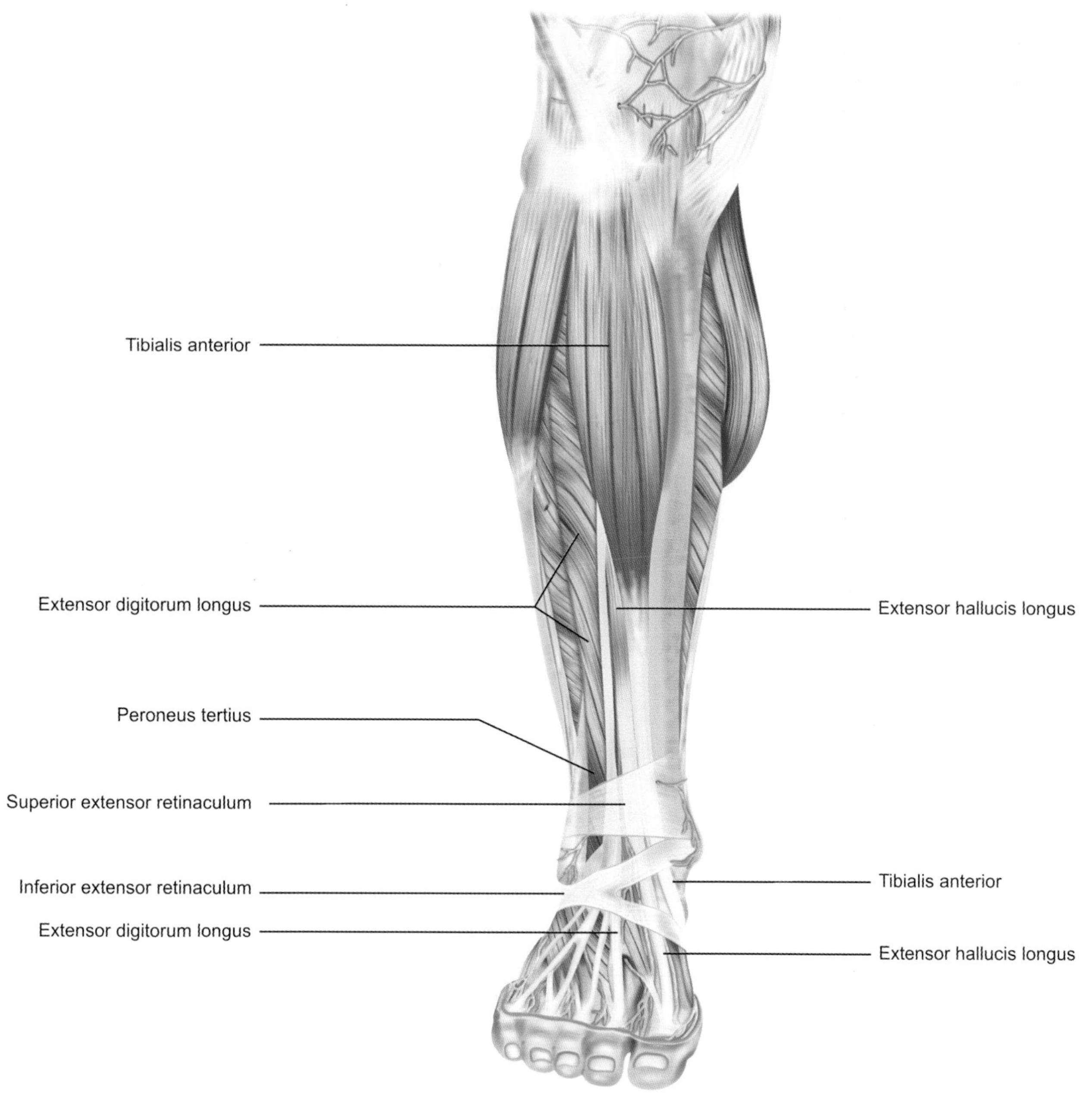

FIGURE 43 Muscles of anterior compartment

MUSCLES OF LATERAL COMPARTMENT (Fig. 44)

Locate this compartment between the anterior and posterior intermuscular septa. Clean the deep fascia over this compartment. The deep fascia is modified as the superior and inferior peroneal retinacula near the lateral side of foot.

Superior peroneal retinaculum: Extends from the posterior aspect of the lateral malleolus to the calcaneum.

Inferior peroneal retinaculum: It lies on the lateral aspect of the calcaneum near the peroneal trochlea. The tendons pass on either side of the trochlea.

Dissection: Locate the tendons of peroneus longus and brevis near the peroneal retinaculum and trace them to their origins.

Peroneus longus: It is the superficial bigger muscle. It arises from the upper two-thirds of the lateral aspect of the fibula. Separate this muscle from the deeper peroneus brevis and feel the origin. Trace it into sole near the cuboid. Its actual insertion can be studied in the dissection of the foot.

Peroneus brevis: Pull it out and see the peroneus brevis. Identify this deeper muscle. It arises from the lower two-thirds of the lateral surface of the fibula. Trace it down to the lateral malleolus. Here, it is held in position by the superior and inferior peroneal retinacula. Trace its insertion to the tubercle on the base of the 5th metatarsal bone. The peronei cross the foot laterally.

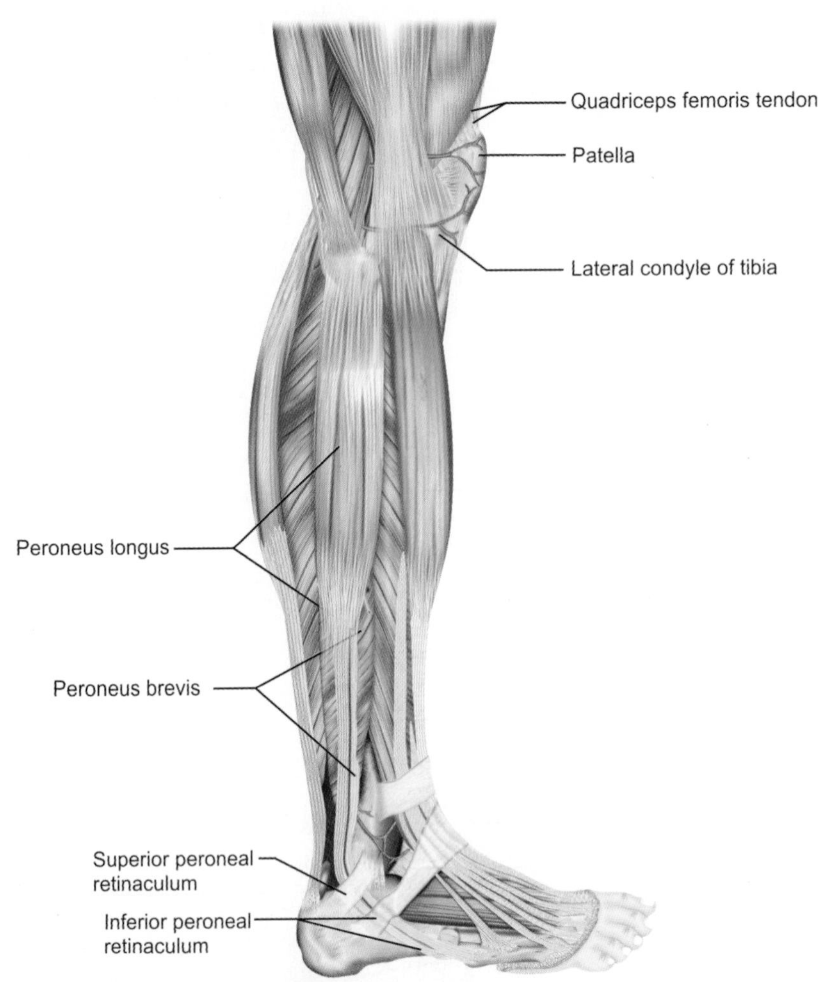

FIGURE 44 Muscles of lateral compartment

MUSCLES OF DORSUM OF THE FOOT (Fig. 45)

Dissection: Slit through the superior, inferior extensor retinacula through the location of the tendons and note that they are covered by synovial sheath. Each synovial sheath has a parietal layer lining the wall and the visceral layer covering the tendons. When they are opened up the open area that can be seen is the synovial cavity between the parietal and visceral layers and many a times you can feel the sticky synovial fluid in this area.

Extensor digitorum brevis: Identify this muscle deep to the tendons of extensor digitorum longus. This arises from the superior surface of the calcaneum. Divides into four tendinous slips. The most medial one gets inserted into the medial side of the base of the proximal phalanx. The remaining three join the extensor expansion.

Extensor expansion: Trace this at least on two or three of the toes. The extensor digitorum longus and brevis join with the interossei and Lumbricales from the side and form an expansion the dorsum of the first phalanx. It divides into three slips the central one attaches on to the base of the second phalanx whereas the two lateral slips join up together and attach by a common tendon into the base of the distal phalanx. This prevents the puckering of the toes between the floor and the foot while walking.

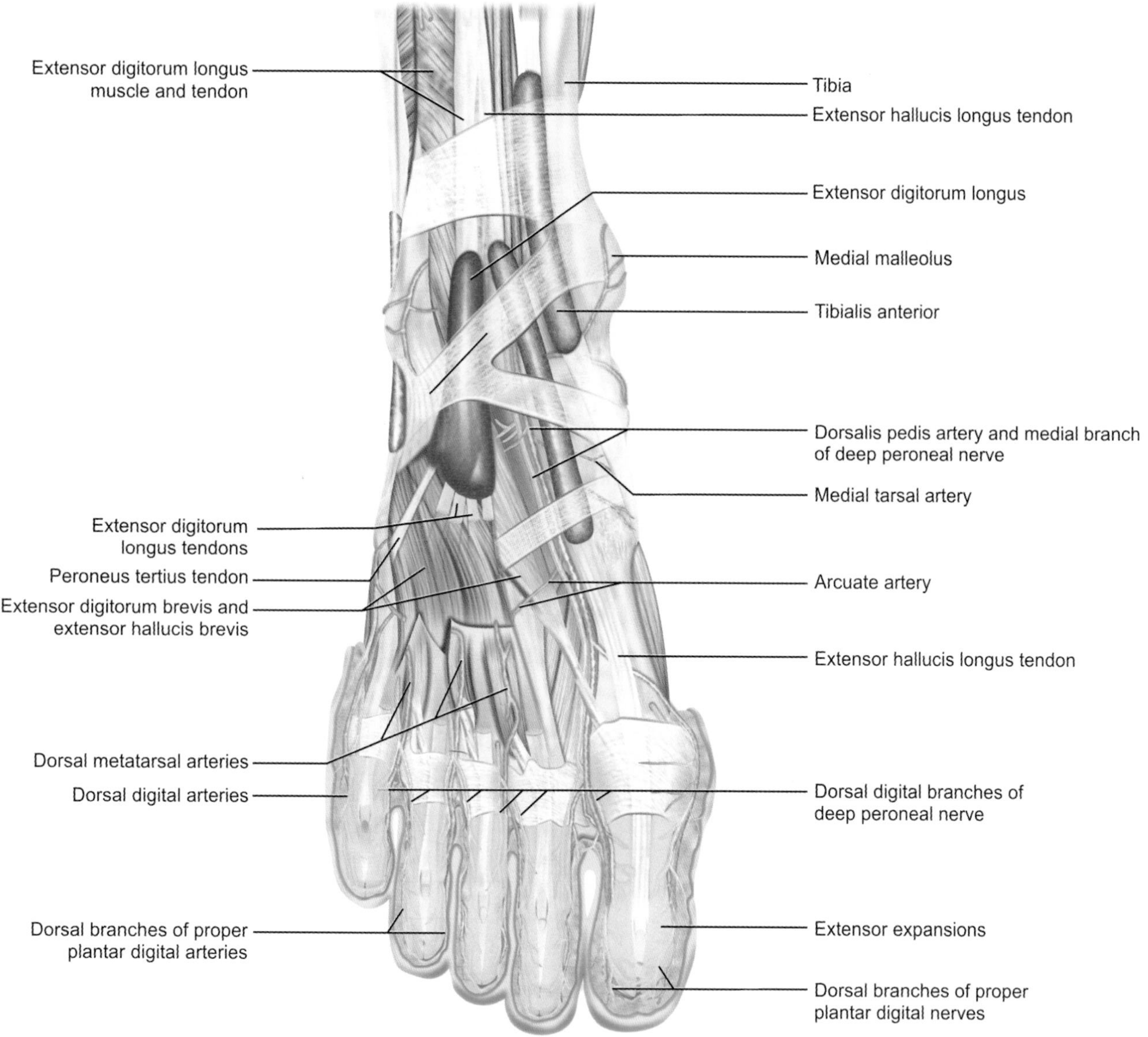

FIGURE 45 Muscles of dorsum of foot

NEUROVASCULAR BUNDLE (Fig. 46)

Common peroneal nerve divides into two branches—the superficial and deep peroneal nerves. The ***superficial peroneal nerve*** supplies the lateral compartment and the ***deep peroneal supplies*** the extensor compartment. The anterior tibial artery accompanies the deep peroneal nerve. The peroneal artery by its perforating branches supplies the peroneal compartment.

Dissection: Cut the peroneus longus, extensor digitorum longus and tibialis anterior nearer to their origin. Catch the common peroneal nerve in the popliteal fossa and trace it. Trace its superficial division into the peroneal compartment and its deep division into the extensor compartment. Identify their branches.

Common peroneal nerve: Locate this nerve posterior to the biceps femoris, trace it laterally to neck of the fibula undercover of the peroneus longus muscle. Locate its branches here.

Recurrent genicular nerve: It is a small branch, passes through the peroneal longus to the anterior compartment to supply the superior tibiofibular joint, and knee joint.

Arteries: The lateral compartment has no specific artery. These muscles are supplied by the perforating branches of peroneal artery. This was already identified in the posterior compartment of leg. See these perforating arteries.

Deep peroneal nerve/anterior tibial nerve: Pierces the lateral intermuscular septum to reach the anterior compartment.

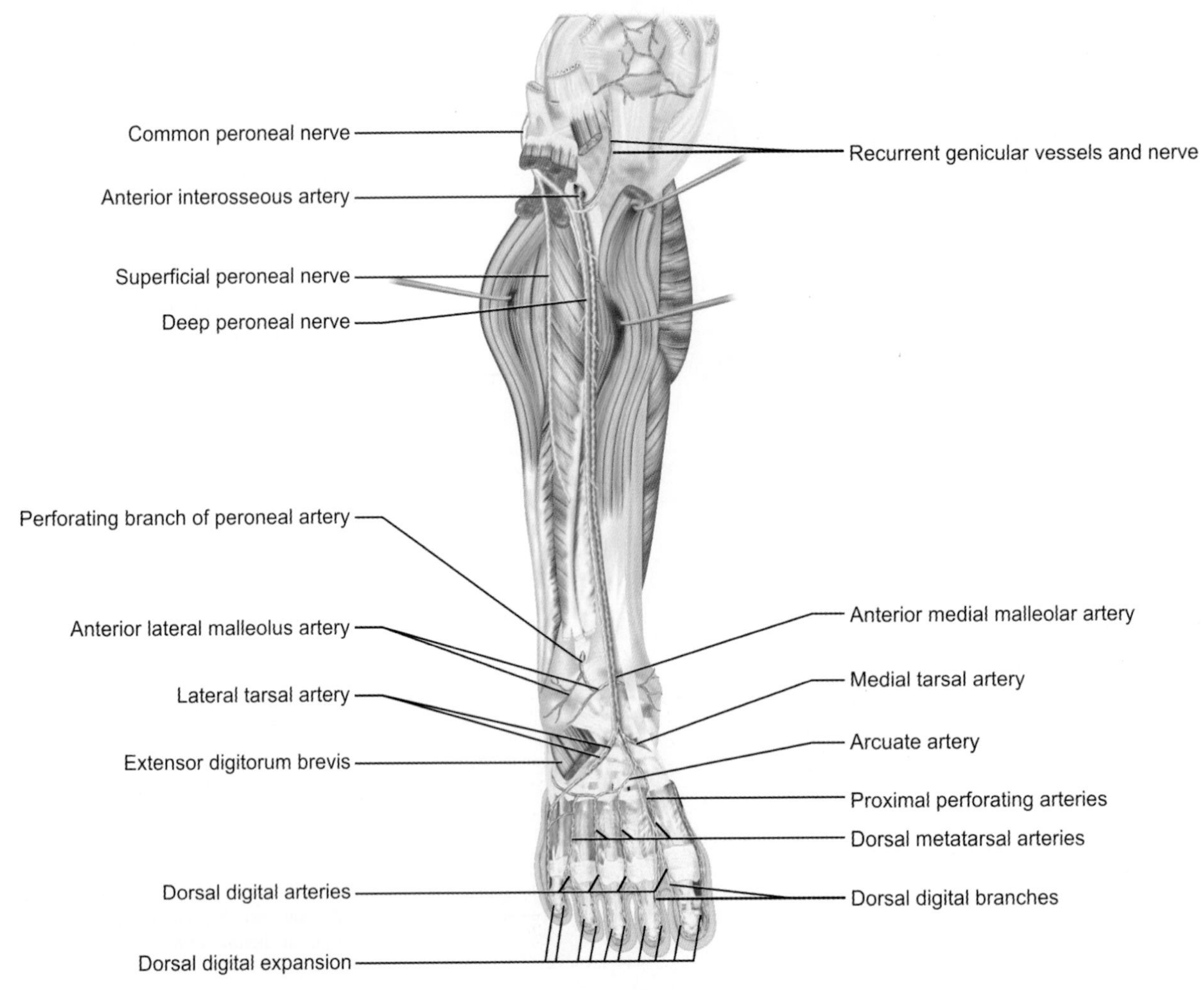

FIGURE 46 Neurovascular bundle

Superficial peroneal nerve or musculocutaneous nerve: This is the nerve of supply to the lateral compartment. It passes between the peroneal muscles. Trace its muscular branches into the peroneal muscles. Note that near the lower one-third of leg it pierces the lateral intermuscular septum to become cutaneous to lower part of the leg and the dorsum of the foot.

Anterior tibial nerve: Reaches from the lateral side to the anterior compartment by winding round the neck of the fibula. It lies lateral to the artery throughout its extent.

Anterior tibial artery: Trace the artery between the extensor digitorum longus and tibialis anterior in the upper one-third, extensor hallucis and the tibialis anterior in the middle one-third and between the extensor longus and hallucis in the lower one-third. Trace it superiorly where it enters the anterior compartment by piercing through the interosseous membrane. It gives number of branches to supply the muscles of this compartment.

Malleolar branches: See these arteries given off near the malleoli. These are medial and lateral malleolar branches. These supply the ankle joint and malleoli.

Perforating branch of the peroneal artery: See this artery reaching the anterior compartment by piercing through the interosseous membrane. It contributes in the supply of the inferior tibiofibular joint.

Neurovascular bundle of dorsum of foot: Cut through the superior and inferior extensor expansion and continue to locate the continuation of the anterior tibial nerve and artery.

Dorsalis pedis artery: The anterior tibial artery beyond the malleoli is called the dorsalis pedis artery. It leaves the dorsum by passing between the two heads of the 1st dorsal interosseous muscle.

Dissection: Divide the muscle the extensor digitorum brevis nearer to its origin and reflecting it towards its insertion. Trace the dorsalis pedis artery, its branches.

Medial and lateral dorsal branches supply the joints.
Four dorsal metatarsal arteries in each of the intermetatarsal areas
Four proximal perforating arteries
Four distal perforating arteries.
Four dorsal digital arteries—supply the adjacent sides of the toes and also the medial side of the big toe and lateral side of the little toe.

The anterior tibial nerve, trace it down and identify the branch to the deep surface of the extensor digitorum brevis.

Cutaneous branch at the web of the big toe and second toe supplies the adjacent sides of the toes.

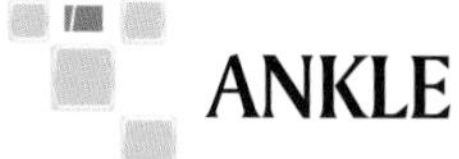

ANKLE

Ankle is the junctional zone between the leg and the foot. It is a common site for sprains, dislocations and fractures, which can involve any of the structures passing around it, reidentify them.

Anterior aspect: The extensor group of muscles for the toes along with the anterior tibial vessels and nerve pass infront, under cover of the extensor retinacula. This is a wide area between the medial and lateral malleolus. Identify the tibialis anterior, flexor hallucis longus, anterior tibial vessels and nerves, flexor digitorum longus and peroneus tertius tendon from medial to lateral side.

Medial aspect: It is occupied by the medial malleolus anteriorly and the flexor retinaculum. Extending between the medial malleolus and tubercle of the calcaneum posteriorly. The deep group of muscles of posterior compartment takes this deviated pathway to reach the sole of the foot. These are the flexor muscles of the toes along with the posterior tibial vessels and nerves. Identify these structures anteroposteriorly, they are—tibialis posterior tendon, this grooves the posterior aspect of the medial malleolus, flexor digitorum longus tendon, posterior tibial artery with venae comitantes, tibial nerve and flexor hallucis longus tendon.

Posterior aspect: This area is occupied by the tendocalcaneus or tendo Achilles. This is a very thick tendon attached to the posterior aspect of the calcaneum.

Lateral aspect: This area is occupied by the lateral malleolus and the peroneal tendons. The tendons pass from the posterior aspect of the lateral malleolus to the sole of the foot under cover of the peroneal retinacula.

FOOT

The foot is located perpendicular to the leg. The leg articulates with the summit of the foot formed by the talus. This is placed more posteriorly resulting in a small thick posterior segment and long wide anterior segment. The bones of the foot are seven tarsals, five metatarsals and fourteen phalanges. The arrangement of bones creates an arched form, with a superior convexity and an inferior concavity. The musculature of the foot is located within this concavity. The dorsal surface of the foot is traversed by the extensor tendons.

SKELETON (Fig. 47)

Skeleton: Go to an articulated skeleton and identify the bones and their features on the plantar surface.

Talus: The talus is a key bone. It is located on the calcaneum obliquely. Note it has a body, neck and a head in that order from posteroanteriorly. Posterior surface of the body shows a medial and a lateral tubercle with a groove in between, which permits the passage of the flexor hallucis longus. The upper trochlear surface of the talus articulates with the distal surface of the tibia, medial malleolus of tibia and lateral malleolus of fibula. The body articulates inferiorly with the upper surface of the calcaneum. See the sinus tarsi between the neck of the talus and calcaneum. See the head dips down to articulate with the navicular bone. See how the head of the talus is supported by the sustentaculum tali of the calcaneum.

Calcaneum: It is the posterior irregular long bone. Superiorly it articulates with the talus at three areas. Identify them. Note the lateral projecting sustentaculum tali. See the thick posterior surface. See the medial and lateral processes of the calcaneal tuberosity on the plantar aspect. See the distal anterior tubercle. See the groove on the undersurface of the sustentaculum tali. This is due to the passage of the flexor hallucis longus tendon. On the lateral side identify the peroneal trochlea,. It separates the peroneal tendons.

Navicular bone: Note this semilunar shaped bone articulating with the head of the talus. See it articulates with three cuneiform bones. Note its medial inferiorly located tuberosity.

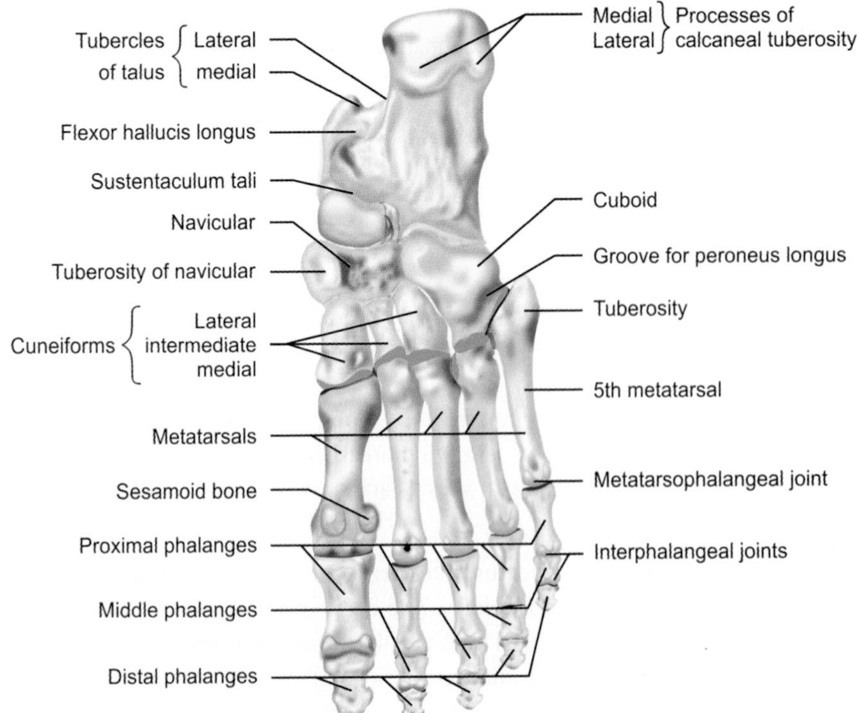

FIGURE 47 Plantar surface of the skeleton of the foot

Cuboid: Note this lateral bone. See its articulation with the calcaneum. See the groove on the undersurface. It lodges the tendon of the peroneus longus. See distally it articulates with fourth and fifth metatarsals.

Cuneiforms: They are three in number—the medial, intermediate and lateral cuneiform. See all of these articulate proximally with the navicular and distally they articulate with the first, second and third metatarsal bones.

Metatarsals: These are five in number. They have an expanded base, triangular shaft and a convex head. They are numbered from medial to lateral. Note the tuberosity on the lateral aspect of the fifth metatarsal bone. The first three articulate with the navicular and the lateral two articulate with the cuboid. The heads articulate with the concave facet on the first phalange.

Phalanges: There are fourteen phalanges. The hallux has two phalanges where as the remaining have three phalanges each. These are short bones with a base.

ARCHES OF THE FOOT (Figs 48 and 49)

Note the articulated foot presents an arch. When the two feet are put together it forms a dome. You can make the arch on the medial side is deeper than the lateral aspect. This fact can be seen when we observe an adult foot imprint. The foot is described as having a medial and a lateral longitudinal arch and a transverse arch. The calcaneum, the talus, the navicular, three cuneiform and three metatarsals constitute the medial longitudinal arch. The calcaneum, the cuboid, the lateral metatarsals constitute the lateral longitudinal arch. The arch formation of the bones is maintained by the ligaments, muscles tendons and plantar aponeurosis.

SOLE OF THE FOOT

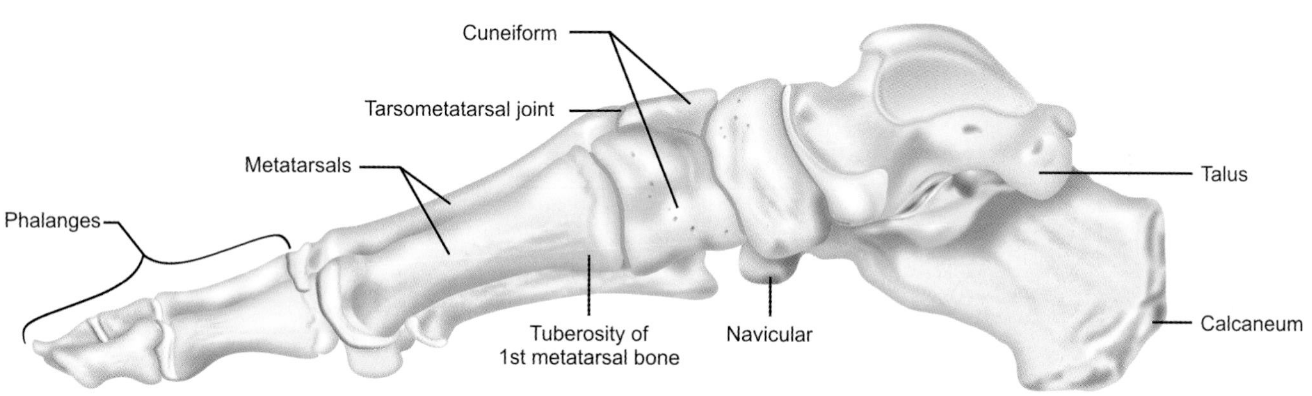

FIGURE 48 Medial longitudinal arch

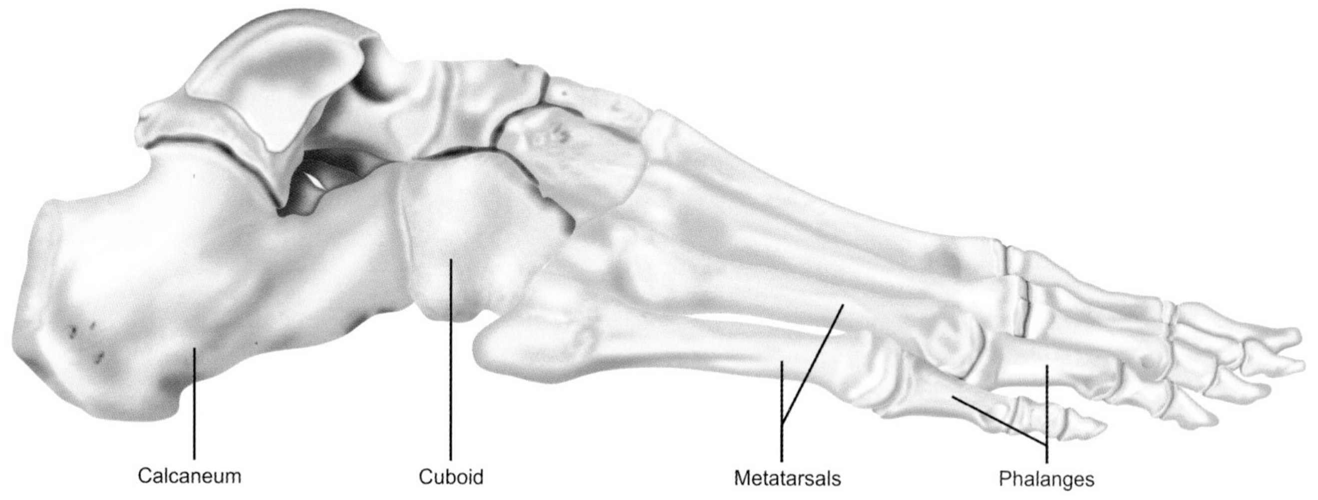

FIGURE 49 Lateral longitudinal arch

Skin: Skin of the sole of the foot is very thick and devoid of hair. It is firmly adherent to the deep fascia by thick connective tissue septa and the interstices between the septa is filled with fat.

Dissection (Fig. 50): Make a vertical incision from the heel to the tip of the second toe. Make a horizontal incision near the bases of the toe. Compared to other parts of the body this skin is very thick and difficult to reflect. Try to remove the skin from the total area of the sole including the side, while doing so make sure that you are not damaging the deeper plantar aponeurosis. Define the plantar aponeurosis.

Cutaneous vessels and nerves: As the skin is reflected the cutaneous vessels and nerves can be located on the sole. Identify the ***medial calcaneal vessels and nerve*** just infront of the calcaneum. See the ***lateral calcaneal vessels and nerves*** lateral to the plantar aponeurosis. Identify the digital vessels and nerves in the inerdigital webs between the slips of the plantar aponeurosis.

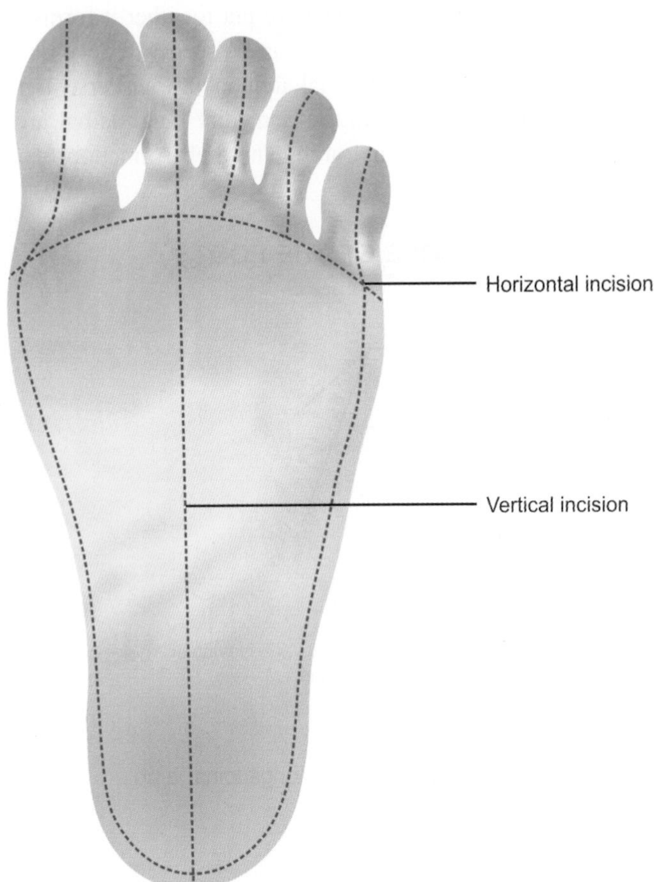

FIGURE 50 Sole—skin incision

PLANTAR APONEUROSIS (Fig. 51)

Plantar aponeurosis is the central part of the deep fascia of the sole it is triangular in shape note its proximal attachment to the medial and lateral calcaneal tubercles.

Distally near the heads of the metatarsals it divides into a five slips. Each slip divides into two parts, encloses the long flexor tendons and reaches the base of the proximal phalanx and transverse metatarsal ligament. The plantar aponeurosis sends in septa both laterally and medially into the deeper aspect. Though facial spaces are described in the sole like the palm they are of less importance.

Functions: It protects the sole from the rough surfaces on which we walk, it protects all the intrinsic muscles and vessels of the sole. Plantar aponeurosis acts as a tie beam in maintaining the arches of the foot. Note that the aponeurosis is stretched when the toes are extended. Feel this in your body.

Deep fascia over the lateral and medial sides of the foot. Note that it is thin over these areas and covers the musculature.

Dissection: Carefully remove the deep fascia. Note that the deep fascia gives attachment to the deeper muscle.

The muscles and neurovascular bundle are arranged in layers from superficial to deep.

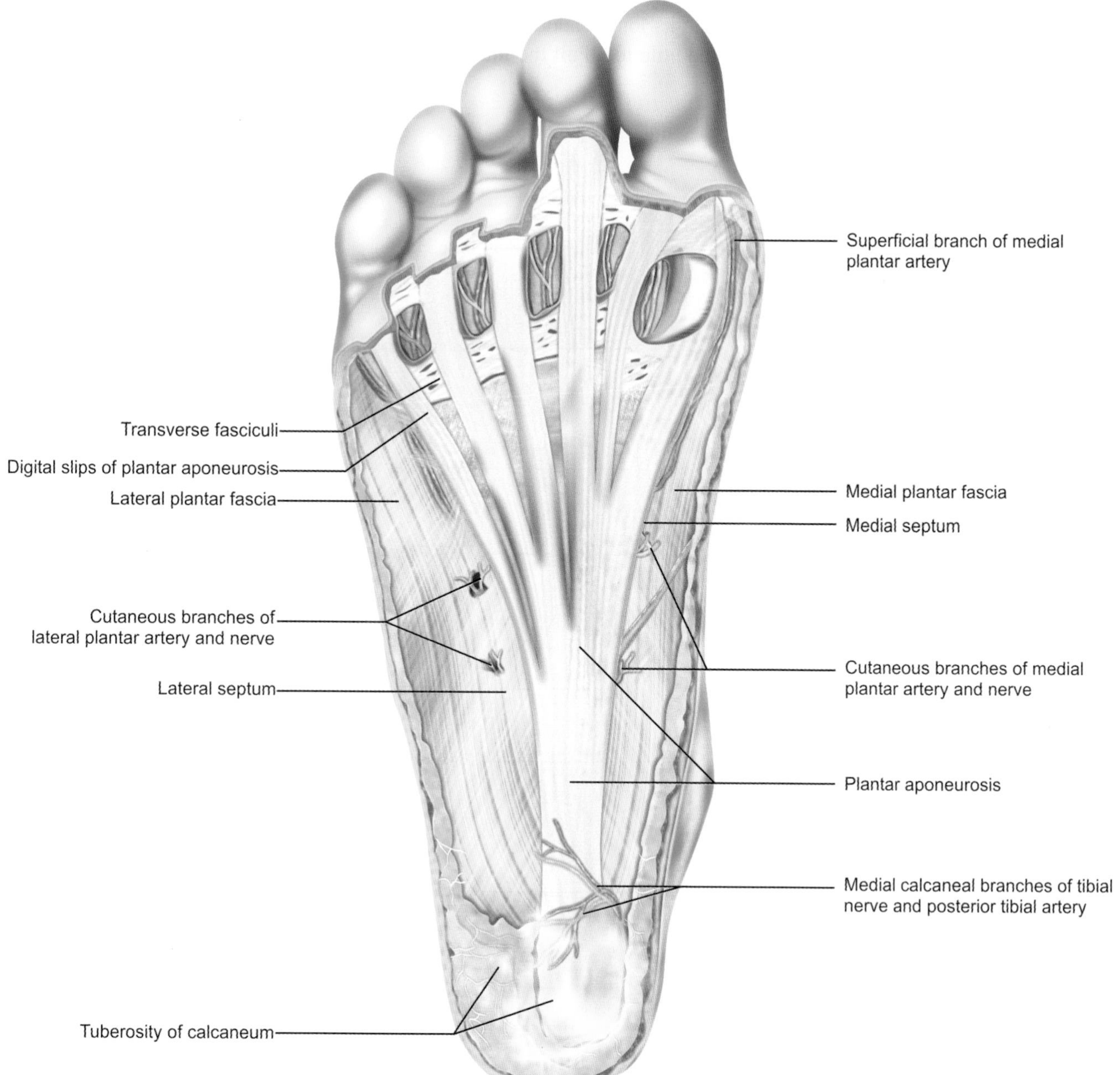

FIGURE 51 Plantar aponeurosis

MUSCLES OF FIRST LAYER OF SOLE (Fig. 52)

This layer has long muscles. They take origin from the calcaneal tubercles. They are muscular at their origin and in their proximal one-third and become tendinous in distally. They are three in number.

Abductor hallucis: This is the big, long muscle on the medial side of sole, trace its origin from the medial tubercle of calcaneum and the flexor retinaculum.

It has a thick fleshy origin, it becomes tendinous half way. Trace its tendon and locate its insertion into the medial side of the base of the proximal phalanx of big toe. Pull this muscle and note its action. It is an abductor of the big toe.

Flexor digitorum brevis: This is a central muscle. Locate its origin from the medial tubercle of calcaneum and plantar aponeurosis. It is fleshy at its origin and near the bases of metatarsals it divides into four tendons. Trace them distally into the toes. Near the base of the proximal phalanx each tendon splits into two parts, pass on either side of the tendon of flexor digitorum longus to be inserted into the base of the middle phalanx of lateral four toes. Pull the muscles and note that they are flexors at the middle phalanx at the proximal interphalangeal joint. The tendons along with the tendons of flexor digitorum longus are enclosed in fibrous flexor sheath. Slit it and trace them to their insertion

Abductor digiti minimi: Identify this long, lateral muscle. It extends laterally from the calcaneum to the little toe. Note its origin from the medial and lateral tubercles of calcaneum. It is muscular at its origin becomes tendinous in the distal one-third of foot. Lift the muscle, locate its long tendon over the flexor digiti minimi and trace its insertion into the lateral side of the proximal phalanx of the little toe. Pull the muscle and note that it is an abductor of the little toe.

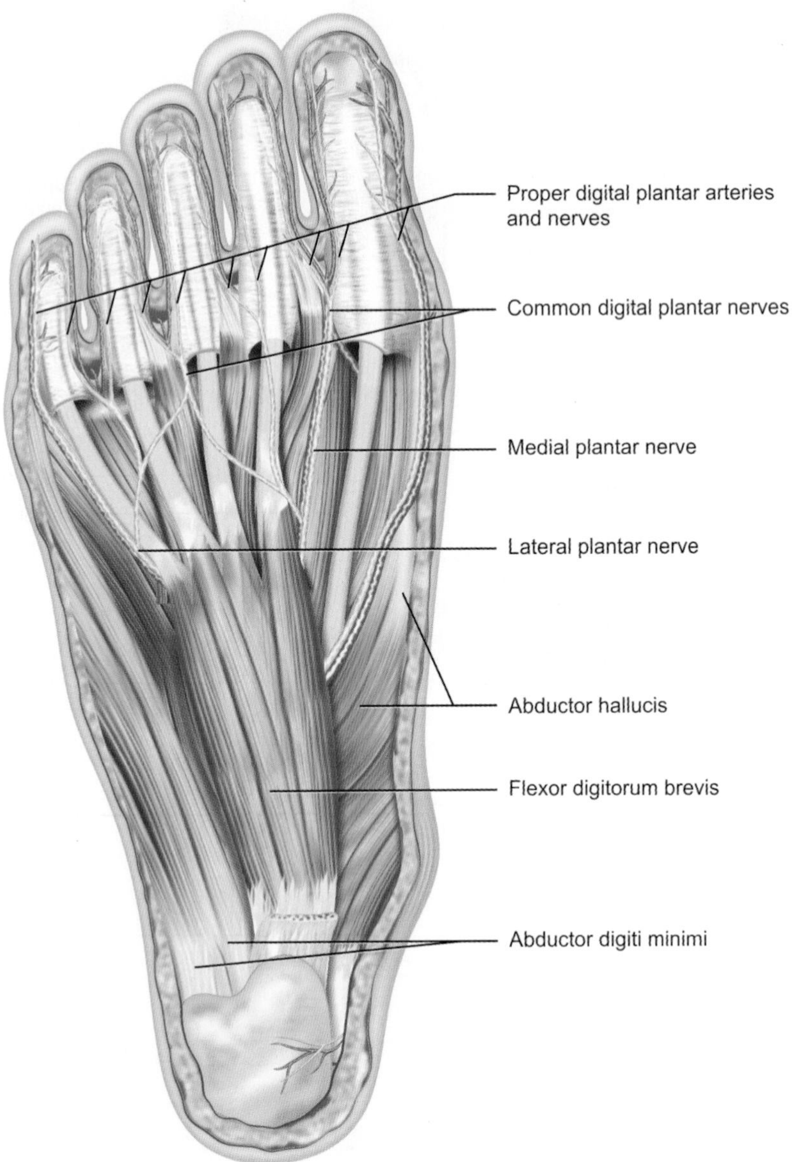

FIGURE 52 Muscles of first layer of sole and cutaneous vessels and nerves

NEUROVASCULAR BUNDLE (Fig. 53)

Neurovascular bundle: The neurovascular bundle enters the sole near the heel between the first and second layer muscles. It is made up of medial and lateral plantar vessels and nerves. Medial plantar nerve supplies the abductor hallucis, flexor digitorum brevis, flexor hallucis brevis and the first lumbrical, it is cutaneous to the medial three and half digits. The lateral plantar nerve supplies the abductor digiti minimi, adductor hallucis, lateral three lumbricals, all the plantar and dorsal interossei. It is cutaneous to the lateral one and half toes.

Medial Plantar Nerve and Vessels

Dissection: Cut the muscular part of abductor hallucis in its middle. Reflect the distal part to its insertion and lift the proximal part medially and trace the nerve supply from the medial plantar nerve into its undersurface. After identifying the nerve carefully reflect this part up to the calcaneum.

Cut the muscular part of flexor digitorum brevis midway. Reflect the distal part towards their insertion. Lift up the proximal part, trace the nerve supply into the undersurface from the medial plantar nerve. Reflect the muscle to the calcaneum. Trace the nerve forwards between abductor hallucis and flexor digitorum brevis. As it passes it gives off the proper digital nerve to the medial side of great toe, and three common plantar digital nerves to the webs of medial four toes. These divide into proper digital branches and supply the toes. The muscular branch to the flexor hallucis brevis comes from the digital nerve to the medial side of big toe. The nerve to the 1st lumbrical comes from the first plantar digital nerve. Note that the medial plantar vessels and nerves supply the medial 31/2 toes.

Lateral plantar vessels and nerves trace it near its origin under cover of the flexor retinaculum. Trace it course from medial to lateral aspect to the base of the 5th metacarpal bone, passing deep to abductor hallucis and flexor digitorum brevis. Locate it between the flexor digitorum brevis and abductor digiti minimi. Trace its muscular branches into flexor accessories and the abductor digiti minimi. Note that lateral side of the skin of the sole and the lateral 11/2 toes are supplied by the lateral plantar vessels and nerves through their digital branches.

Generally the branches of medial and lateral plantar nerves communicate. Try to identify these nerves. The blood vessels accompany the nerves.

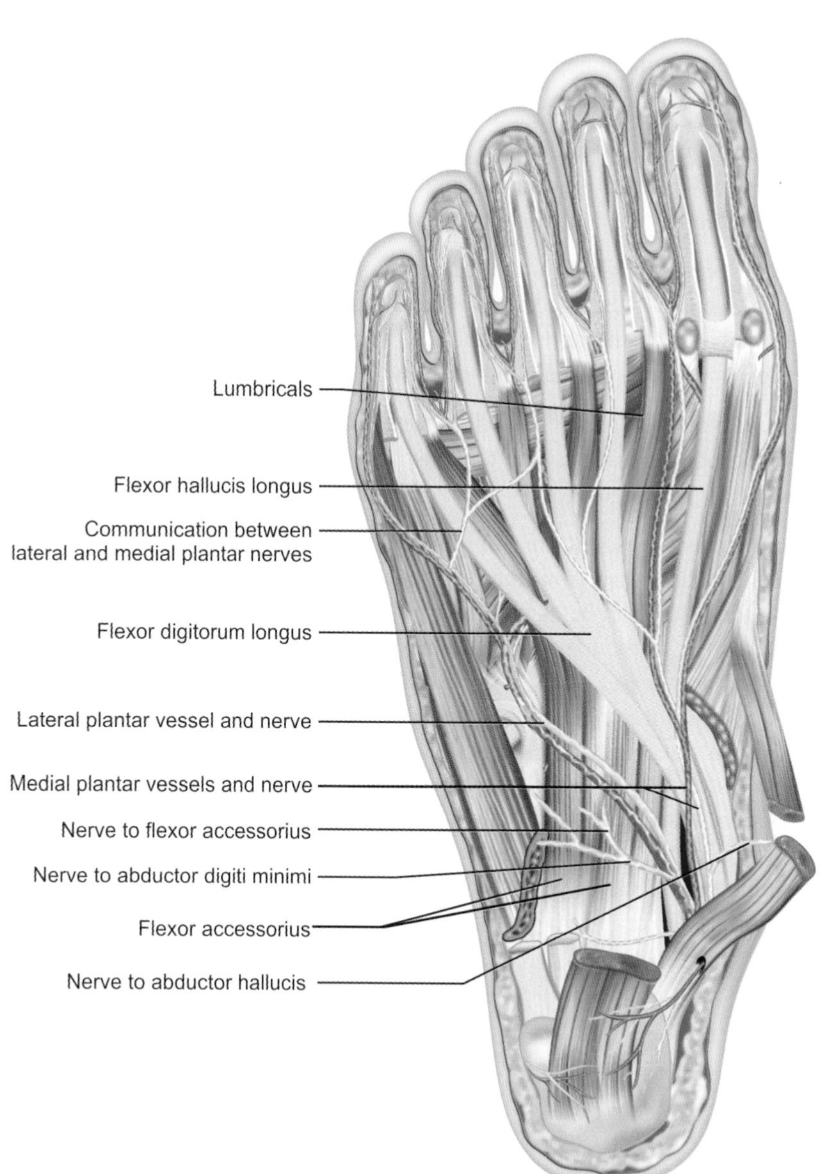

FIGURE 53 Superficial neurovascular bundle and second layer of sole

MUSCLES OF SECOND LAYER OF SOLE

This layer occupies the central area of the sole and is made up of the long tendons of the digits. The flexor hallucis longus and flexor digitorum longus arise from the posterior aspect of the bones of the leg deviate to the flexor retinaculum and reach the sole. These muscles loose their direction of control due to this deviated route. The flexor accessories is an extra muscle added in the group to align the flexor digitorum longus. Lumbricals are the other muscles of this layer. Identify and study them.

The flexor hallucis and flexor digitorum enter the sole under cover of the flexor retinaculum. Locate these tendons, the tendon of flexor digitorum longus lies medial and the flexor hallucis longus lies lateral near the flexor retinaculum. Note the neurovascular bundle between the two:

Flexor hallucis longus: Tendon deeply grooves the sustentaculum tali (observe it on the calcaneum) passes deep to the flexor digitorum tendon to reach the hallux. It is inserted into the base of the distal pharynx. It is enclosed in a synovial sheath.

Flexor digitorum longus: Trace this tendon from medial side of the sole. It divides into four tendons for the lateral four toes. They reach to their insertion into the base of the distal phalanx. Note that the flexor digitorum brevis tendons split and clasp the longus tendon. Note that these tendons together are enclosed in a fibrous flexor sheaths and covered by the synovial sheath.

Turner's slip: Lift both the tendons near their crossing and identify the fibrous slip that passes from the flexor hallucis longus to the flexor digitorum longus. This helps in transferring a part of the muscle power to the digitorum It is also responsible for the united action of the all the five toes.

Flexor accessorius: This is an accessory muscle for the flexor digitorum. It is a strong muscle with two heads of origin. Identify these medial and lateral heads from the medial and lateral aspect of the calcaneum. Combined muscle soon joins to be inserted into the lateral border of the flexor digitorum longus. Many a times it clasps the digitorum tendon and may even be continuous with the lumbricals. Reidentify its nerve supply from the lateral plantar nerve.

Action: Note that it is a powerful muscle. And pulls the flexor digitorum longus tendon laterally to counter its medial deviation. So that it puts the tendons in line with the origin of the muscle in the back of the leg to its insertion to the distal inter phalangeal joint.

Lumbricals: These are four in number. The medial most muscle is a unipennate muscle. The other three are bipennate muscles. They arise from the tendons of flexor digitorum longus. Trace them distally to the webs of the toes. They cross the metatarsophalangeal joint on the medial side of the lateral four toes. They join the extensor expansion on the dorsal aspect of the toes. Trace the nerve supply to the medial lumbrical from the medial plantar nerve on its superficial surface. The lateral three lumbricals are supplied by the lateral plantar nerve on their deep surface. Note that these muscles cross the metatarsophalangeal joint on their ventral aspect and the interphalangeal joints on their dorsal aspect. These are flexors at the metatarsophalangeal joint and the extensors at the interphalangeal joint.

Dissection: Cut the muscles and tendons of the second layer transversely near the bases of the first phalanges and near the distal end of the calcaneum. Remove the central part totally. Remove the medial plantar nerves and blood vessels. Note that the lateral three lumbricals get their nerve supply on their deeper aspect. Reidentify the fibrous flexor sheaths, tendons of flexor digitorum longus and brevis enclosed in the synovial sheaths.

MUSCLES OF THIRD LAYER (Fig. 54)

Short flexors of the big toe, little toe and the adductor of the big toe constitute this layer. They occupy the distal half of the plantar surface of the foot.

Flexor hallucis brevis: Note the origin of this muscle from the cuboid and cuneiform. Trace its thick belly distally. Note that it divides into two parts, the medial part joins with the abductor hallucis tendon and gets inserted into the medial side of the base of the proximal phalanx, the lateral part of flexor hallucis joins the tendon of adductor hallucis and gets inserted into the lateral side of the base of the proximal phalanx of big toe. Note its nerve supply from the digital nerve to the medial side of big toe. It is a flexor of the proximal phalanx of the big toe. Pull it and see the action.

Dissection: Cut the tendons of this muscle proximal to the metatarsophalangeal joint and reflect it distally. Note that sesamoid bones are placed in both the slips and they slide over the head of the metatarsal and prevent the tendon from rubbing against the bone.

Adductor hallucis: This muscle occupies the central part of the sole. It has two heads of origin. Trace the oblique head arising from the bases of the middle three metatarsals and fascia over cuboid. Note that the transverse head arises from the deep transverse metatarsal ligaments and plantar ligaments of the lateral four metatarsophalangeal joints. Note its combined insertion into the lateral side of the base of the proximal phalange of the big toe combining with the flexor hallucis brevis. It is supplied by lateral plantar nerve. Pull the muscle and note its action as an adductor on the big toe.

Flexor digiti minimi brevis: Identify this muscle in the lateral side of the foot in the distal half. Note its origin from the base of the fifth metatarsal bone. It is fleshy and becomes tendinous near its insertion. Trace the muscle to its insertion into the lateral side of the base of the proximal phalanx of the little toe. Note its nerve supply from the lateral plantar nerve. It is a flexor of the little toe at the metatarsophalangeal joint pull the muscle and check its action.

Dissection: Trace the muscular branches from the superficial branch of the lateral plantar nerve into the flexor digiti minimi brevis, third plantar and 4th dorsal interosseous in the 4th interosseous space. Detach the adductor hallucis muscle from its origin and reflect it towards its insertion (or remove it totally), while doing so note the nerve supply into the muscle. It is supplied on its deeper surface.

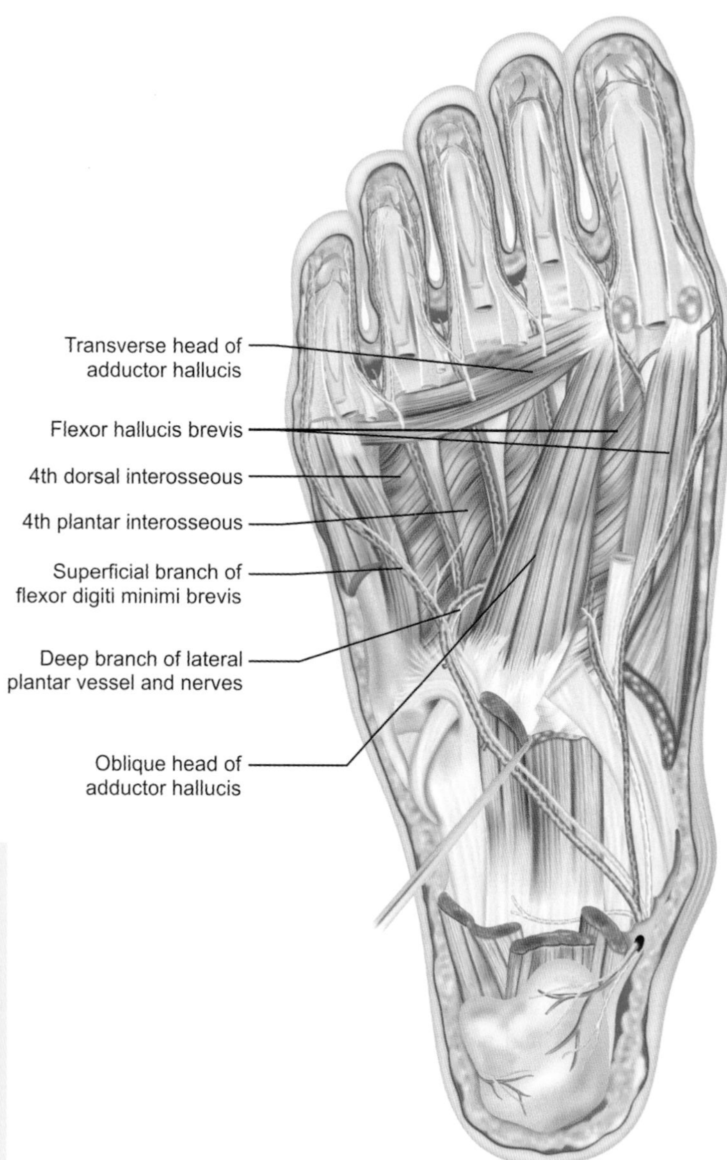

FIGURE 54 Muscles of third layer sole

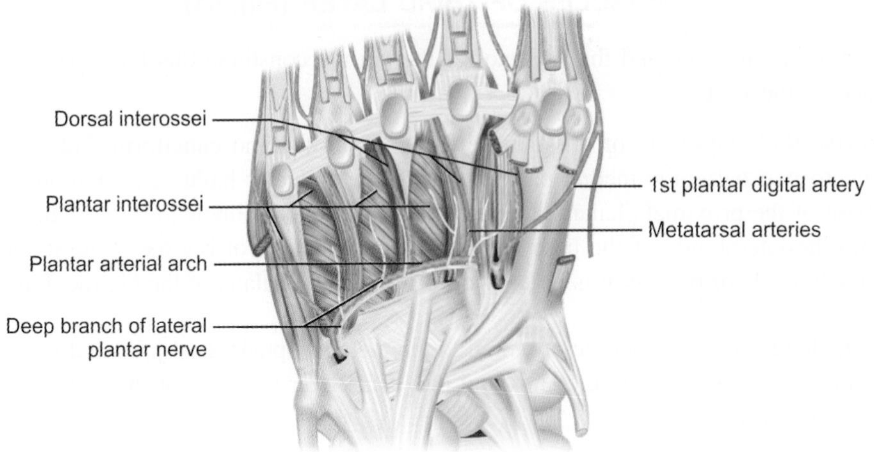

FIGURE 55 Deep neurovascular bundle and muscles of fourth layer

THE DEEP LAYER OF NEUROVASCULAR BUNDLE (Fig. 55)

Deep layer of neurovascular bundle is the lateral plantar nerve and artery, which enters the deeper aspect of the sole between third and 4th layer of musculature. It supplies all the muscles, bones and joints.

Trace this vessel and nerve from the base of the 5th metatarsal to across the bases of the metatarsals to the 1st interosseous space. Note and trace the following muscular branches from the deep branch to their destinations—the branch to the adductor hallucis, (lateral three lumbricals—identified and cut), medial two plantar interossei and medial three dorsal interossei. The lateral plantar nerve sends articular branches to the intertarsal, tarsometatarsal and intermetatarsal joints.

Plantar arch is the continuation of the lateral plantar artery at the base of the 5th metatarsal bone. It is distal to the nerve. Trace its metatarsal arteries to the lateral three intermetatarsal space. In the first space the plantar arch anastomoses with the perforating branch of the arcuate artery. Trace the branches of these arteries into the muscles bones and the joints.

In general plantar metatarsal arteries anastomose with the digital arteries directly and with the dorsal metatarsal arteries through the perforating branches, which pass through each space.

MUSCLES OF FOURTH LAYER

This layer is formed by interossei. They occupy the space between the metatarsals. The long tendons of the leg reach the proximal half of the foot to be inserted into the tarsals.

Study of Interossei

They are three ***plantar interossei***. These are unipennate muscles arising from the ventral aspect of the lateral three metatarsals. Locate them near the proximal phalanx on their medial side. Here, they can be seen as fine tendons crossing the metatarsophalangeal joints to reach the extensor expansion. Trace the tendons back to the origin from the bone. Pull the muscles and note their action as adduction.

Dorsal interossei are bipennate muscles. They arises from adjacent sides of the metatarsal bones in the interosseus spaces. Locate their tendons on either side of the proximal phalanx of the second toe, lateral side of proximal phalanx 3rd and 4th toes. Trace them back to their origins. Pull the tendons and note that they are abductors. Note that all the interossei reach the dorsum deep to the deep transverse metatarsal ligaments which connect the heads of the metatarsal bones.

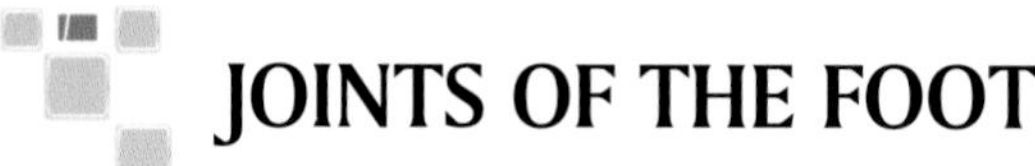

JOINTS OF THE FOOT

ANKLE JOINT (Fig. 56)

Ankle joint: It is a uniaxial hinge joint. Proximally it is a bucket shaped articulation formed by the distal ends of tibia and fibula, distally it is formed by the upper surface of the talus. Dorsiflexion and plantar flexion around the transverse axis are the movements feasible here.

Capsule clean and identify the is thin over the anterior and posterior surfaces, where the movement takes lace. It is supported by ligaments both medially and laterally.

The **medial deltoid ligament (Fig. 56):** See this on the medial side. It is a powerful triangular ligament. Identify its proximal attachment to the medial malleolus and its distal attachment into the tuberosity of the navicular, talocalcaneonavicular ligament, sustentaculum tali and posterior tubercle of talus.

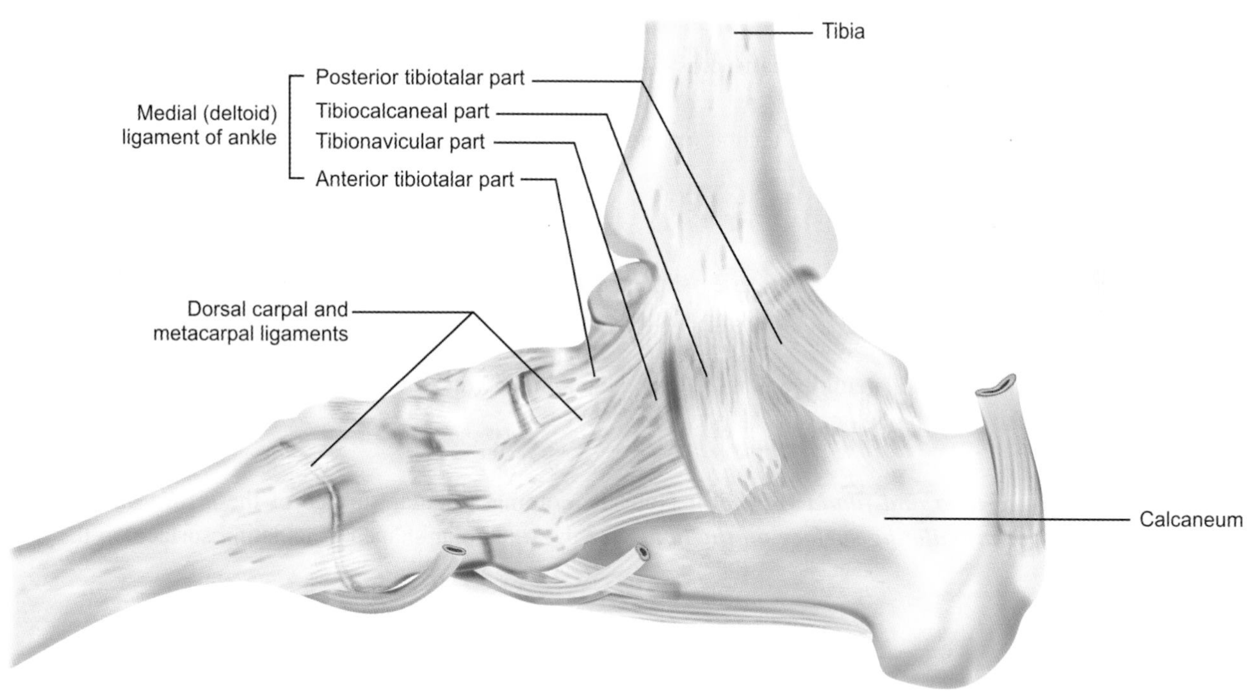

FIGURE 56 Deltoid ligament and other dorsal ligaments

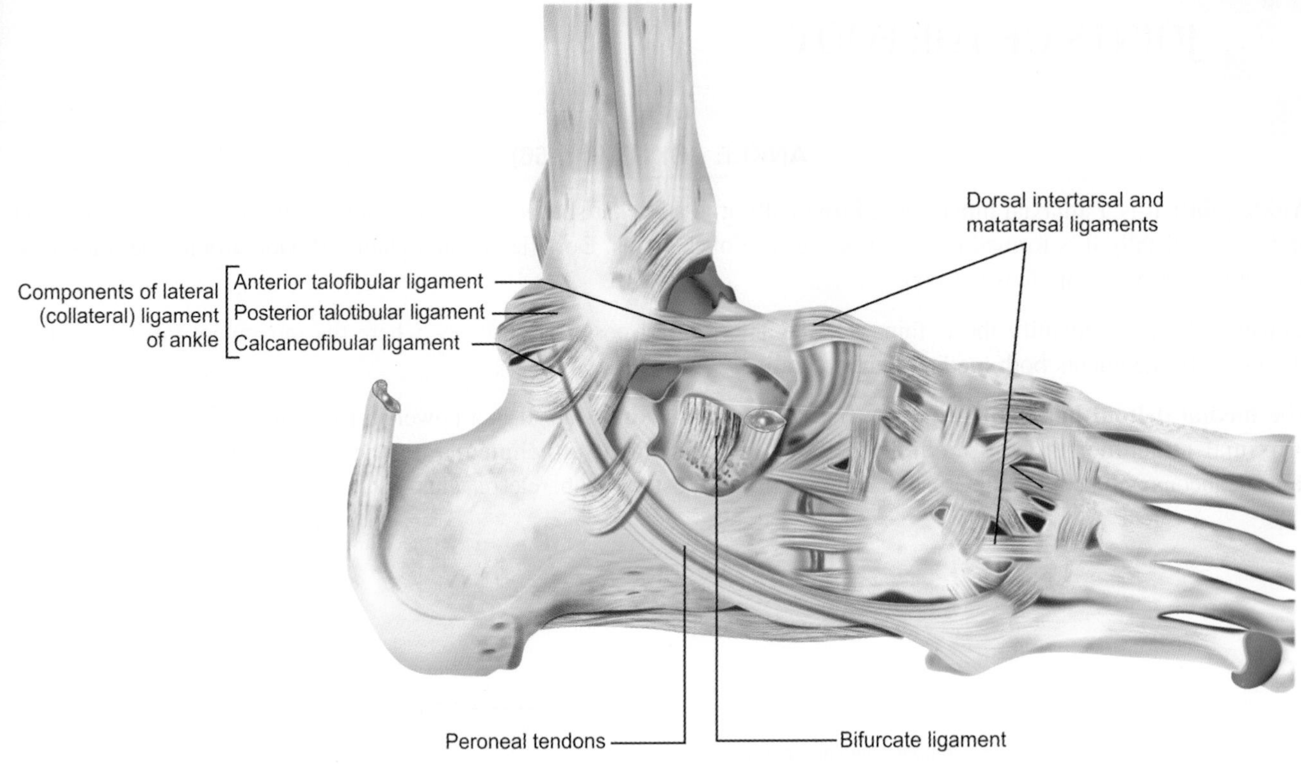

FIGURE 57 Lateral (collateral) ligament and sinus tarsi

The **lateral ligament (Fig. 57)** is divided into three slips and extend from the lateral malleolus to the talus anteriorly and posteriorly whereas the middle part extends up to the calcaneum.

Dissection: Cut the medial and lateral ligaments of the ankle joint and disarticulate the foot from the leg. Observe the articulating surfaces of the ankle joint.

Articulating surfaces of *tibia and fibula* (Fig. 58): Note the comma articular surface of the ***medial malleolus,*** the enlarged curved ***inferior articulating surface on the tibia.*** See the triangular shaped articulating surface on the ***fibular malleolus***.

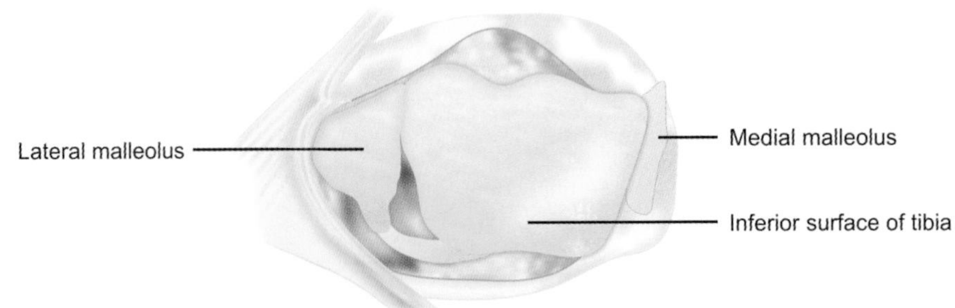

FIGURE 58 Articulating surfaces of tibia and fibula

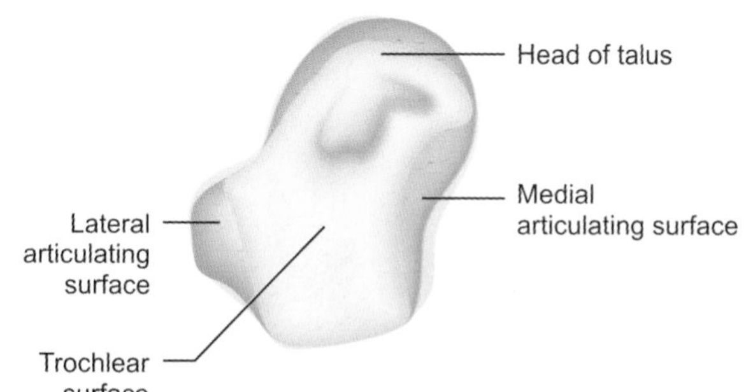

FIGURE 59 Articulating surface of talus

The ***talus*** also shows ***three articulating surfaces*** **(Fig. 59)** corresponding to the tibiofibular articulating surfaces. The superior trochlear surface of the talus is convex and wider in front than behind, the medial articulating surface is comma shaped and the lateral articulating surface is triangular in shape.

Blood supply: The joint is supplied by the malleolar branches of the anterior tibial and peroneal artery. The nerves come from the deep peroneal and tibial nerve.

Movements: Perform the movements dorsiflexion and plantar flexion. Note that in dorsiflexion the foot becomes immobile as air attains a tight packed position. This is because of the wider articulation of the talus fitting into a closed packed position with the superior articulating surface.

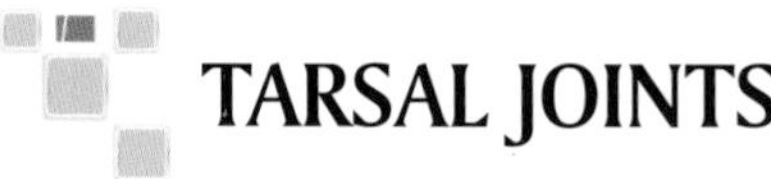

TARSAL JOINTS

Tarsal joints: Except for the talocalcaneonavicular joint all other joints are plane synovial joints. The capsule around the joints is thinner. It is thickened by superior and inferior ligaments. These help in holding the joints together during weight bearing and movements. The talocalcaneonavicular joint is a ball and socket joint. Try to identify the big and important ligaments on the foot.

Subtalar joints: Inferiorly the body of talus articulates with calcaneum and the head of the talus articulates with the navicular and calcaneum.

Capsule: Unites both the bones and it is thin allover.

Dissection: Cut the capsule and separate the talus, identify the interior of the joint cavity and the articular surfaces.

Talocalcaneonavicular joint (Fig. 60)
It is ball and socket type of joint. Observe the articulating surfaces. Note that the proximal curved articular surface of the navicular bone, the sustentaculum surface of the calcaneum and the plantar talocalcaneonavicular ligament forms the concavity of the joint. The head of the talus forms the ball of the joint.

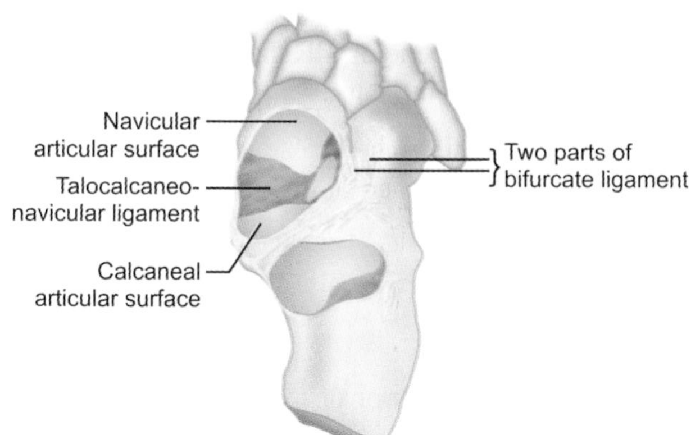

FIGURE 60 Talocalcaneonavicular joint

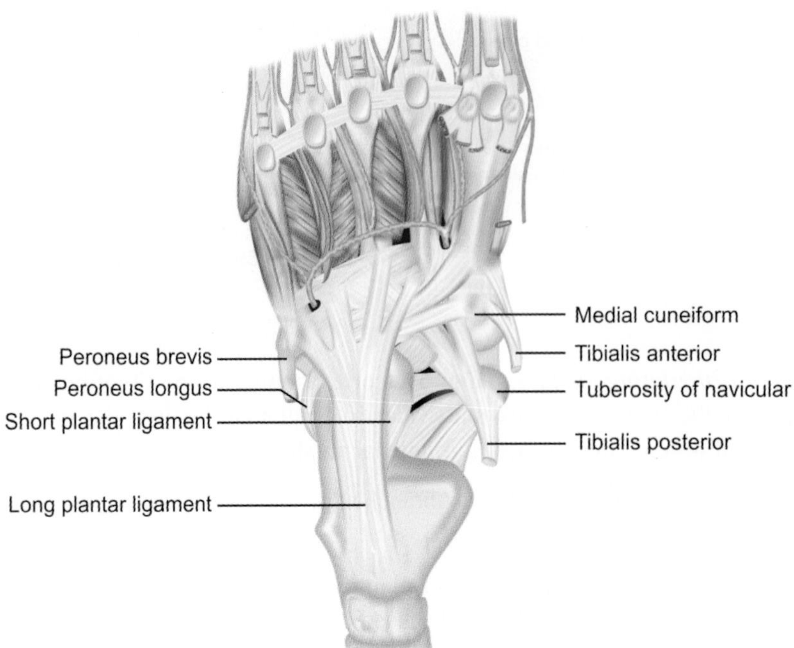

FIGURE 61 Tendons and ligaments—plantar surface

Tendons and Ligaments—Plantar Surface (Fig. 61)

The tendons and ligaments play an important part in maintaining the arches of the foot. They are thick and strong on the plantar surface.

Tendon of tibialis posterior muscle: This muscle belongs to the deep layer of the back of the leg. It reaches the sole deep to the flexor retinaculum. It lies deep to the long tendons of the second layer. Note that its main insertion is into the tuberosity of the navicular bone. It further divides into number of slips to be inserted into the bases of the metacarpals, cuneiform and cuboid. It acts as a strong union between all the bones of the sole, apart from being a inverter of the foot.

Tendon of peroneus longus muscle: Identify this tendon on the lateral side. It enters the sole of the foot near the cuboid bone. It passes across the sole grooving the cuboid bone. The groove is converted into a osseofibrous tunnel by the long plantar ligament.

Long plantar ligament: Note this strong ligament extending from the proximal part of the calcaneum to the cuboid, distal to the groove in the cuboid (identify this groove on a dry bone). Feel the peroneus longus tendon and the long plantar ligament. Cut the long plantar ligament near the groove in the cuboid and see the tendon. Trace the tendon of the petronius longus muscle to its insertion into the lateral side of the medial cuneiform bone and the base of the first metatarsal bone.

Short plantar ligament: Identify this deep to the long plantar ligament: this is wider than the long plantar ligament and extends from the distal end of the calcaneum to the proximal end of the cuboid bone.

Plantar calcaneonavicular or spring ligament: It is thick triangular fibrocartilaginous ligament. It extends from the sustentaculum tali of the calcaneum to the plantar surface of the navicular bone. It fills the gap between the calcaneum and the navicular bone and forms the articulating surface for the head of the talus.

Tarsometatarsal joints: These are biaxial joints. The fibrous capsule is attached close to the articular surface. It is superiorly supported by extensor expansion, laterally by collateral ligament and on the plantar surface by transverse metatarsal ligaments.

Deep transverse metatarsal ligaments: See them near the heads of the metatarsals. They interconnect the heads of the metatarsals.

Dissection: Cut the capsule and see the articulating surfaces and the interior of the joint.

Note the convex head fitting into the concavity of the base of the phalange. Note the sesamoid bones on the ventral aspect of the head of the first metatarsal bone. They are two in number and are seen in the tendon of flexor hallucis brevis.

Ligaments on the Dorsal Surface

Interosseous talocalcaneal ligament: This lies in the sinus tarsi. This is the gap between the talus and the calcaneum on the lateral side. This gap is filled by ligament called the interosseous ligament.

Bifurcate ligament: Identify this ligament between the distal end of the calcaneum to the proximal end of the navicular and cuboid bone.

MOVEMENTS OF THE FOOT

Subtalar and midtarsal joints constitute three joints: The articulation between the talus and the calcaneum, the articulation between the head of the talus and the navicular and between the calcaneum and the cuboid. The invertion and evertion are the movements feasible here around a long oblique axis passing through the neck of the talus. Here, the head of the talus remains stationary and the remaining part of the foot rotates around the neck. Invertion has more range compared to the evertion. The invertion is accompanied by dorsiflexion and the evertion is accompanied by plantar flexion. Perform these movements and appreciate.

Intertarsal joints and tarsometatarsal joints are all plane synovial joints. Gliding movement occurs between them during movements of foot like walking running and weight-bearing.

Metatarsophalangeal joints are biaxial ellipsoidal joist. Flexion and extension and abduction and adduction take place here. The line passing through the center of the second finger forms the midline here. Movement away from this line is abduction and movement towards this central line is the adduction.

Interphalangeal joints are uniaxial condylar joints. Flexion and extension takes place here. Note while walking the metatarsophalangeal joints are extended and interphalangeal joints are flexed. Perform this movement and observe. This is achieved by the contraction of the lumbricals and interossei.

CHAPTER 7

HEAD AND NECK

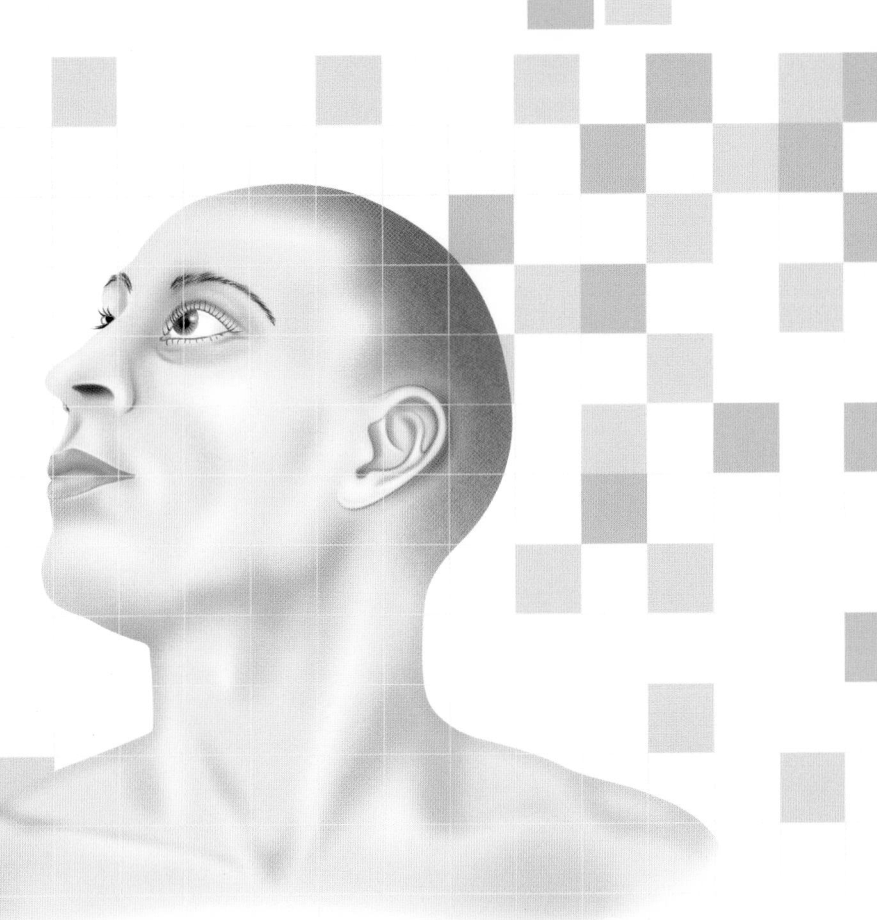

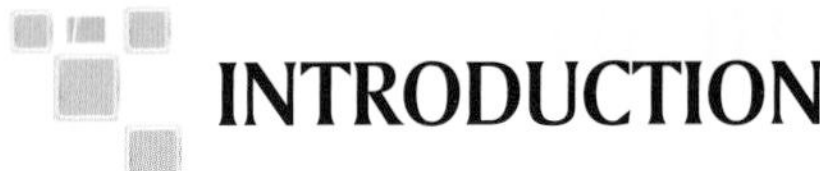

INTRODUCTION

The head and neck is the upper part of the trunk. Skull forms the skeleton of the head. It is a bony box. The main function of skull is protection. The brain is protected in the cranial cavity. The anterior part of the skull forms the facial skeleton. It lodges the sense organs and the receiving ends of the respiratory and digestive system. As you can feel, note that there is a thin area between the skull and the skin. In our dissection we are studying this area under the superficial dissection of the head. The skull has only one movable bone, the mandible. This bone articulates to form the temporomandibular joint. Muscles which act at this joint form the temporal and infratemporal regions. The eye, ear, nose and mouth along with their associated structures are located within the bony box, the skull. All these structures are studied under the heading deep dissection. Most of these being midline structures they are studied in sagittal section.

The neck is the part connecting the head with the thorax below. The cervical vertebrae form the axis for this. The prominent sternocleidomastoid muscle forms as a landmark to separate the neck into two triangles, a posterior muscular part and an anterior visceral triangle. The posterior triangle is made up of musculature spanning from the vertebrae posteriorly to the scapula, clavicle and the ribs laterally and inferiorly. It is wider inferiorly. The viscera are lodged in the anterior triangle. It is wider superiorly and narrower inferiorly. The neurovascular bundle lies between the musculature and the viscera **(Fig. 1)**.

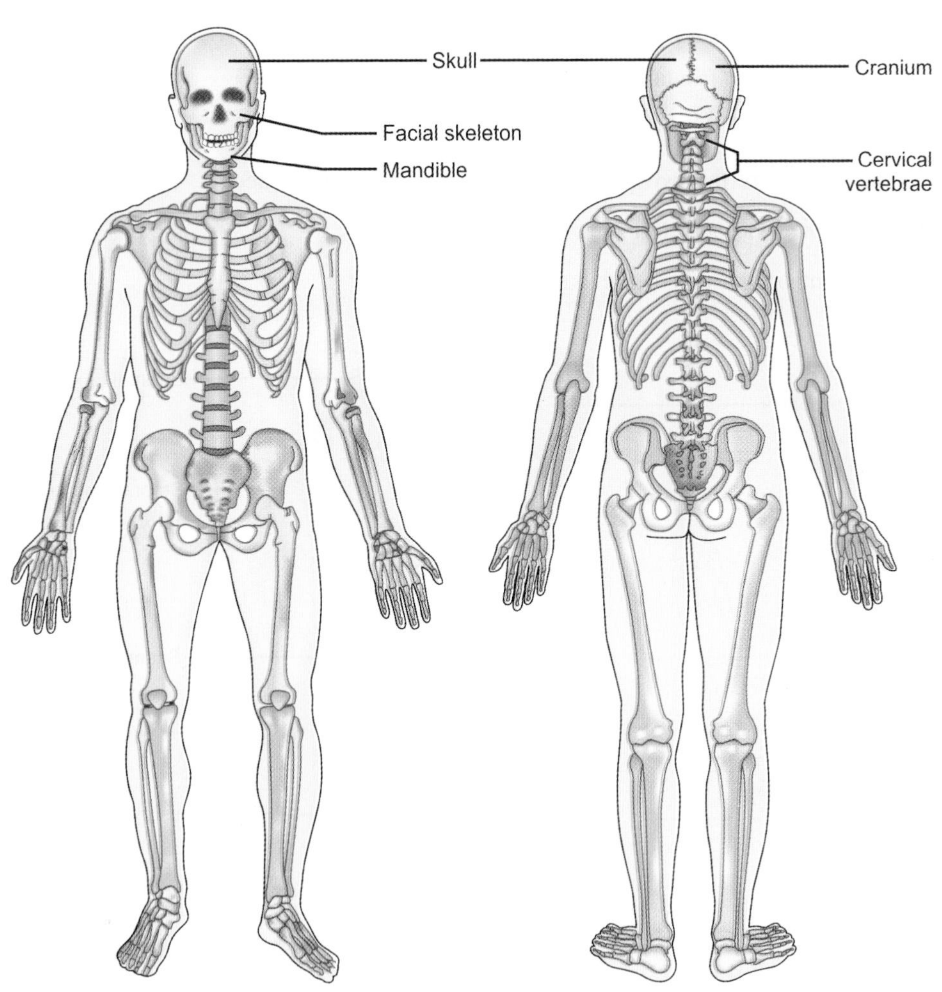

FIGURE 1 Head and neck

SUPERFICIAL DISSECTION OF HEAD

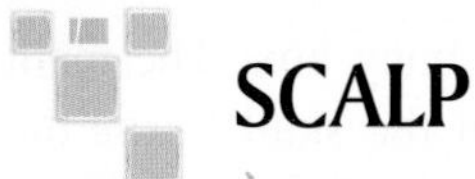

SCALP

Scalp is the region on the top of the skull. ***Anteriorly*** it extends up to the superior orbital margin. Here the forehead is included. ***Posteriorly*** it extends up to the external occipital protuberance and superior nuchal line. ***Laterally*** it extends up to the zygomatic arch. The scalp is made up of five layers – skin superficial fascia with neurovascular bundle occipitofrontalis muscle, loose areolar tissue and the pericranium.

SKELETON

Norma Verticalis **(Fig. 2)**

This is the external surface of the skull, viewed from above. Note the following features:

Frontal bone: This occupies the anterior part of this region.

Frontal tubers: These are the prominent elevations on the front. These are more prominent in females

Parietal bones: They occupy the central part of the norma verticalis. Note the emissary foramen. This permits the emissary veins.

Parietal tubers: They form the lateral prominence on the parietal bone.

Coronal suture: This is where the frontal bone meets the two parietal bones.

Sagittal suture: This is where the two parietal bones meet.

Lambdoid suture: This is where the two parietal and the occipital bones meet.

Occipital bone: This occupies the posterior part of the skull

Vertex: This is the midpoint on the top of the skull.

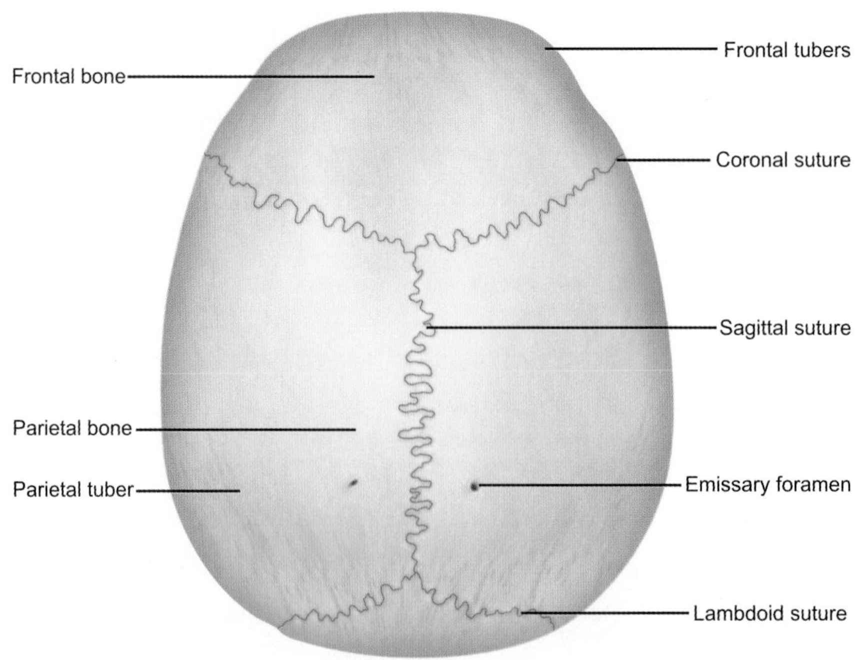

FIGURE 2 Norma verticalis

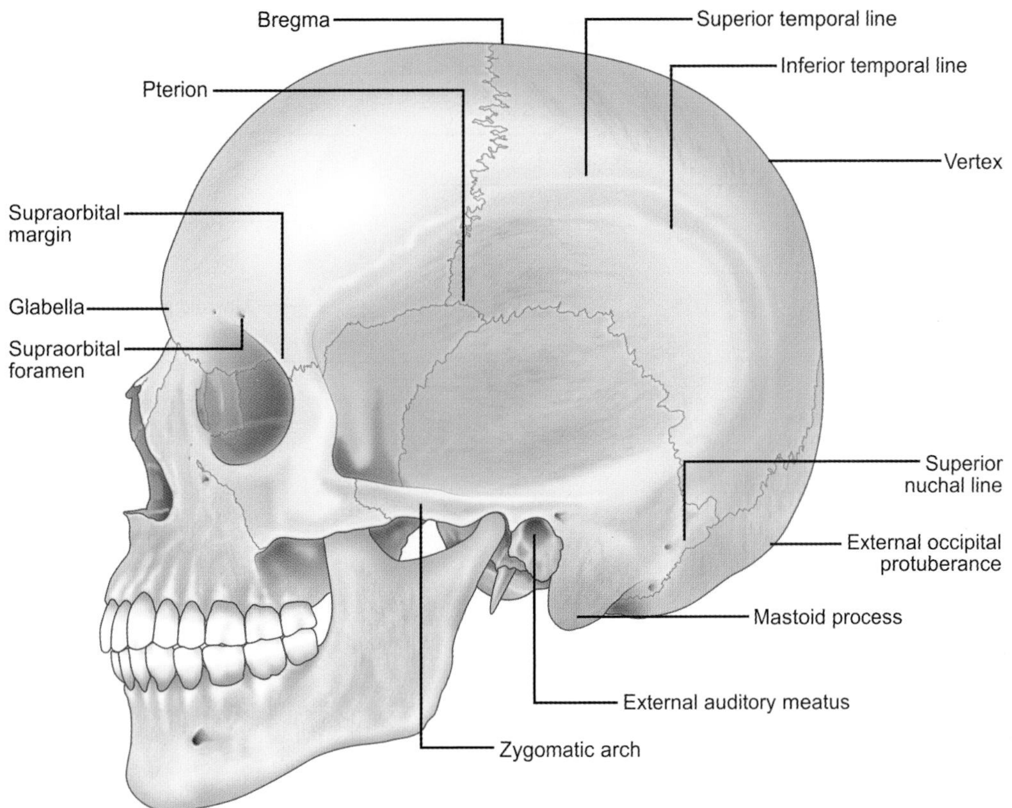

FIGURE 3 External features of skull

Norma Frontalis **(Fig. 3)**

Identify the following features on the skull in the anterior aspect.

Glabella: This is the midline elevation where the superciliary arches meet.

Superciliary arches: These are the elevations above the supraorbital margins.

Supraorbital margins: These are the sharp margins forming the superior border of orbit.

Supraorbital foramen or notch: See this nearer to the medial side on the supraorbital margin. It can be either a foramen or a notch on the skull.

Norma Lateralis **(Fig. 3)**

On the lateral side identify:

Zygomatic arch: This is the bony elevation felt between the lateral margin of the orbit and the pinna of the ear.

Superior temporal lines: Note these superior and inferior temporal lines above the zygomatic arch.

External auditory meatus: Note this opening in front of the mastoid process

Mastoid process: This is the bony prominence seen behind the auditory meatus.

Norma Occipitalis (Fig. 3)

On the posterior side identify:

External occipital protuberance: This is a prominence on the posterior aspect of the occipital bone in the midline.

Superior nuchal line: This is the line radiating from the external occipital protuberance.

Supreme nuchal line: This is the line radiating from the external occipital protuberance, but thinner and above the superior nuchal line.

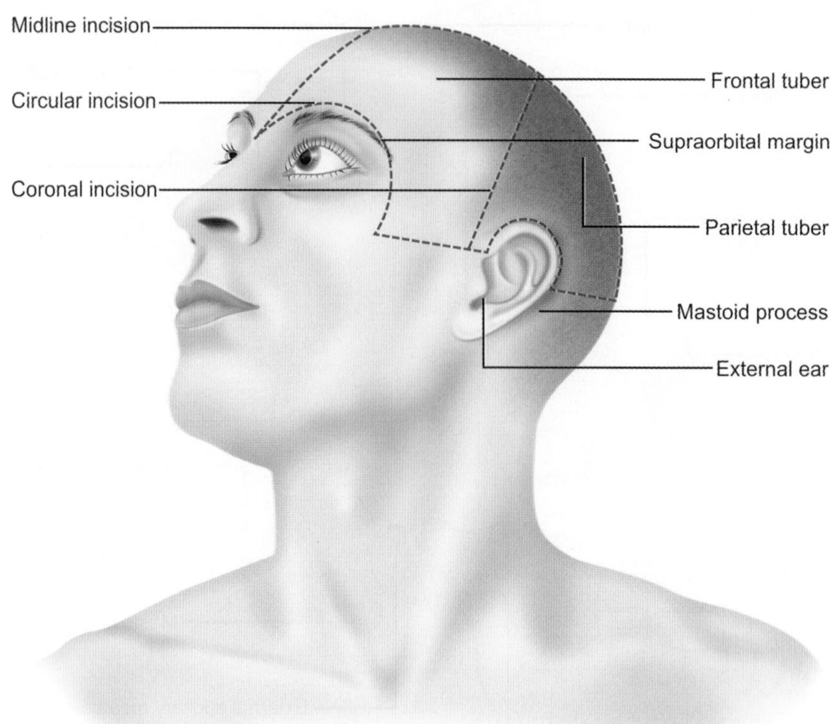

FIGURE 4 Dissection lines and surface anatomy

SURFACE ANATOMY (Fig. 4)

- On the living feel, the ***supraorbital margins***. The ***supraorbital notch*** can be easily felt on the living, but not the foramen.
- Feel the subcutaneous skull throughout the region. Note the ***frontal and parietal tubers***.
- On the lateral side, in front of the external ear feel the ***zygomatic arch***.
- ***Superficial temporal artery*** pulsations can be felt in front of the external ear, above the zygomatic arch.
- Feel the ***mastoid process*** behind the external ear, and the ***external occipital protuberance*** in the midline posteriorly.

Dissection: Raise the neck on a block so that the total scalp can be easily visualized. Make a midline incision from glabella to the external occipital protuberance. A coronal incision from one pinna of the ear to the other. Make a circular incision from glabella—superciliary arches—zygomatic arch—upper part of mastoid process—external occipital protuberance. Remove the total skin upto vertex starting from the periphery. Here the skin is adherent with the deeper muscle layer by connective tissue. This connective tissue lodges the neurovascular bundle of the skin, so special care is to be taken while reflecting the skin. The surface is to be kept wet constantly and the undersurface of the skin is to be checked for protruding hair follicles. They can constantly be felt like bristles to the cutting knife.

SUPERFICIAL FASCIA

The superficial fascia is fibrous, attaches the skin to the occipitofrontalis muscle. It is also firmly attached to the blood vessels. It has the cutaneous neurovascular bundle. They enter the scalp from the periphery and move towards the vertex. Nearer to the circumference they are deeper to the muscle. They pierce through the muscle to reach the superficial fascia. The arteries can easily be identified as they bulge. The veins can be identified by their blue coloration. The nerves accompany the blood vessels.

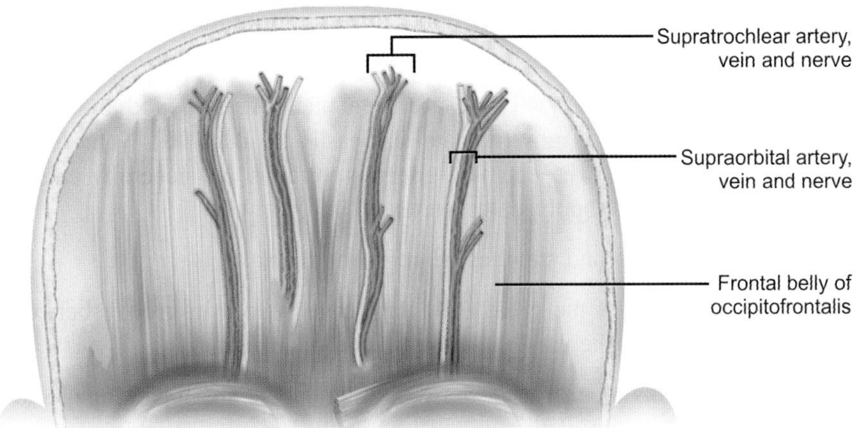

FIGURE 5 Anterior aspect of scalp

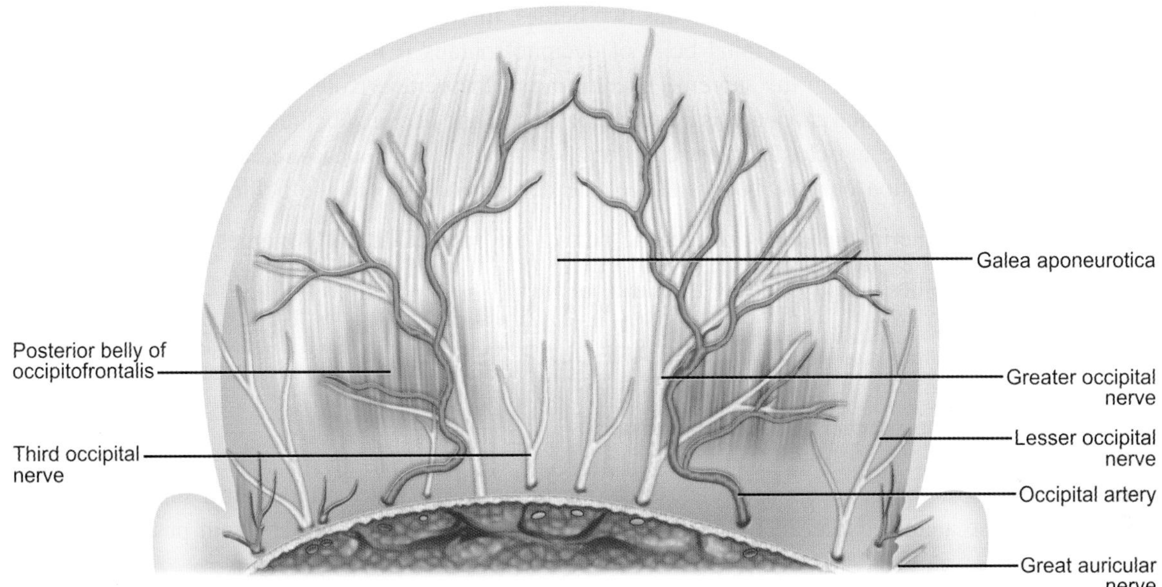

FIGURE 6 Posterior aspect of scalp

Cutaneous Nerves–Anterior Aspect (Fig. 5)

Dissection: The neurovascular bundle pierces through the deeper layers of the scalp to supply the skin. Try to locate the following neurovascular bundle and the frontal belly of the occipitofrontalis muscle in the anterior aspect of scalp.

Supratrochlear nerve and blood vessels: These are fine branches located one finger breadth from the glabella.

Supraorbital nerve and blood vessels: Feel for the supraorbital notch or foramen trace the thick neurovascular bundle through the frontal belly of occipitofrontalis.

Auriculotemporal nerve and superficial temporal blood vessels: Feel the zygomatic arch near the pinna of the ear trace the thick anterior and posterior branches of the neurovascular bundle traversing to the vertex. It is easy to locate the artery, which is bulging and anterior most structure. The nerve is thick, behind the artery and deeply placed.

Frontal belly of occipitofrontalis muscle: This is relatively a thicker belly. It is inserted into the skin near the eye brow. It has two bellies, the right and the left. An aponeurosis can be easily seen between the two bellies.

Cutaneous Nerves—Posterior Aspect (Fig. 6)

Dissection: Turn the body to a prone position and reflect the skin from the vertex up to the external occipital protuberance. Try to locate the neurovascular bundle at the posterior half of the scalp. Identify the deeply placed brown fibres of the occipital belly of the occipitofrontalis muscle fibres.

A wide central area upto the vertex is supplied by the upper three posterior rami. The first cervical branch joins the second to form the greater occipital nerve.

Greater occipital nerve and occipital artery: These are seen one finger breadth from the external occipital protuberance. The greater occipital nerve is 0.5 mm thick and can easily be identified. Note the greater occipital nerve passing through the occipitofrontalis muscle. The occipital artery is tortuous and generally can be easily identified. It runs lateral to the nerve, gives branches to supply up to vertex.

Third occipital nerve: It is a small branch and supplies nearer to midline.

Great auricular nerve: Posterior branch of the great auricular nerve is seen in groove between the pinna and the mastoid process. This supplies the back of the ear lobule and the adjoining scalp.

Lesser occipital nerve: This nerve runs along the posterior border of the sternocleidomastoid muscle. Clean this nerve. It gives branches to the lateral aspect of the skin of the back. Branches of this nerve are seen between the above two nerves.

Occipital belly of occipitofrontalis muscle: This has two bellies, the right and the left. Identify this thin muscle belly arising from the supreme nuchal line. Occipital belly of occipitofrontalis is the muscle of the posterior aspect of the scalp. Trace these thin flat fibres from the supreme nuchal line to the vertex. Note the aponeurosis between the right and left bellies and also the epicranial aponeurosis between the frontal and occipital bellies of the occipitofrontalis muscle. The occipitofrontalis is a single muscle. This muscle along with the galea aponeurotica acts together to raise skin of the forehead. Perform this action on your body and feel the contraction of both the bellies of occipitofrontalis.

Galea aponeurotica: It is the intermediate aponeurotic part of the muscle, laterally merges with the temporal fascia.

Nerve supply: Both the bellies are supplied by the facial nerve.

LOOSE AREOLAR TISSUE

Turn the body back to the supine position and dissect:

Dissection: Cut across the galea aponeurotica from one pinna to the other pinna, put a scalpel beneath and appreciate this loose areolar tissue. In front of the vertex you may see the emissary vein passing through the parietal foramen.

PERICRANIUM

Appreciate the vault of the skull here. It is covered by the periosteum. This periosteum is called the pericranium.

Dissection: Alternatively the posterior part of the scalp can be dissected along with the back dissection. This would avoid turning the body from supine to prone, prone to supine position.

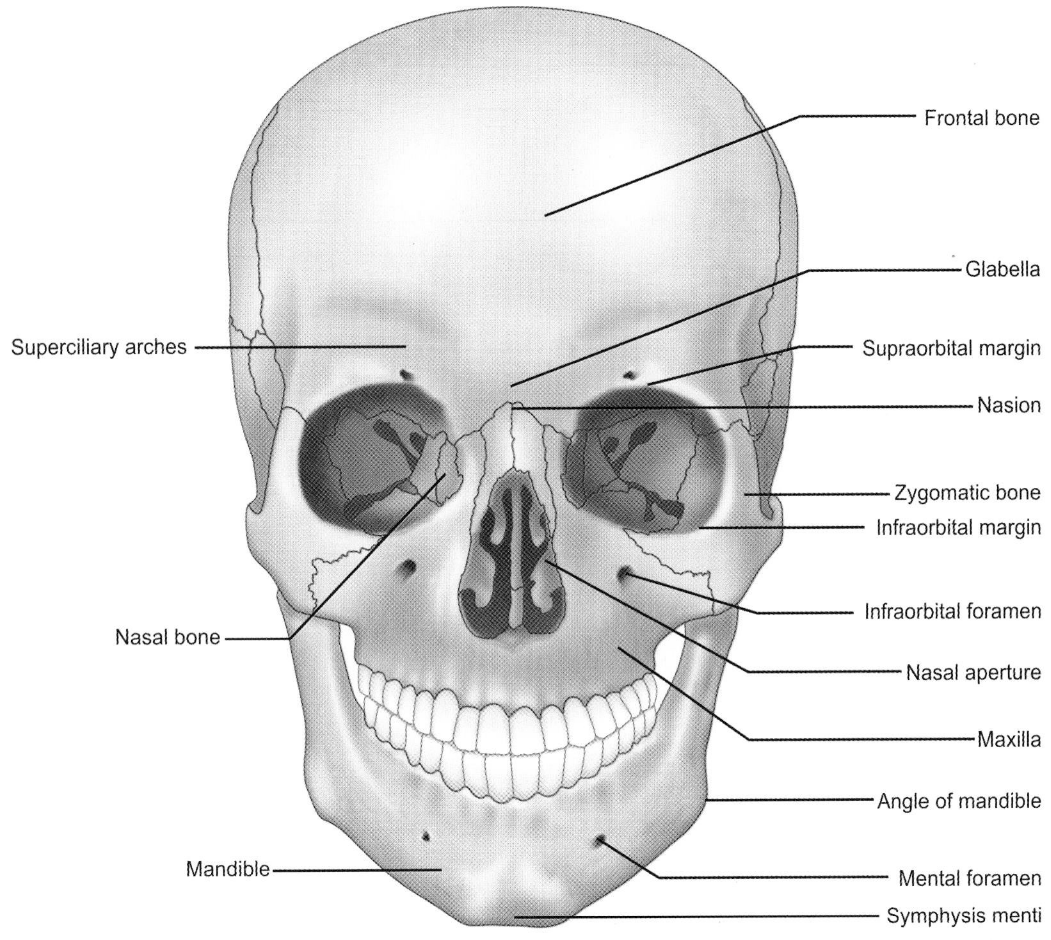

FIGURE 7 Skeleton—anterior aspect

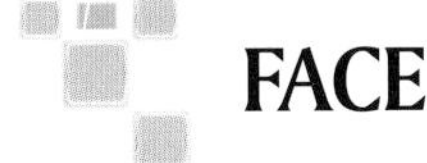

FACE

SKELETON (Fig. 7)

Identify the features on the articulated skull.

Glabella: This is the elevation in midline.

Superciliary arches: They extend out from the glabella.

Nasion: This is the depression on the bridge of the nose, where nasal bones join the frontal bone.

Cheek elevation: It is formed by zygomatic bone.

Maxilla: Forms a major part of the facial skeleton and lodges the upper teeth.

Symphysis menti: This is the part where two halfs of the mandible meet in the midline.

Angle of the mandible: This is the posterior sharp pointed end of the bone.

Orbital margin: This is formed superiorly by the frontal bone, medially by maxilla, inferiorly by maxilla and zygomatic bone and laterally by the zygomatic bone.

Nasal aperture: See that it is formed by the nasal bone and maxilla.

Infraorbital foramen: Note this below the inferior orbital margin.

Mandible: See the ramus and the body of the mandible.

Mental foramen: See this foramen on the mandible.

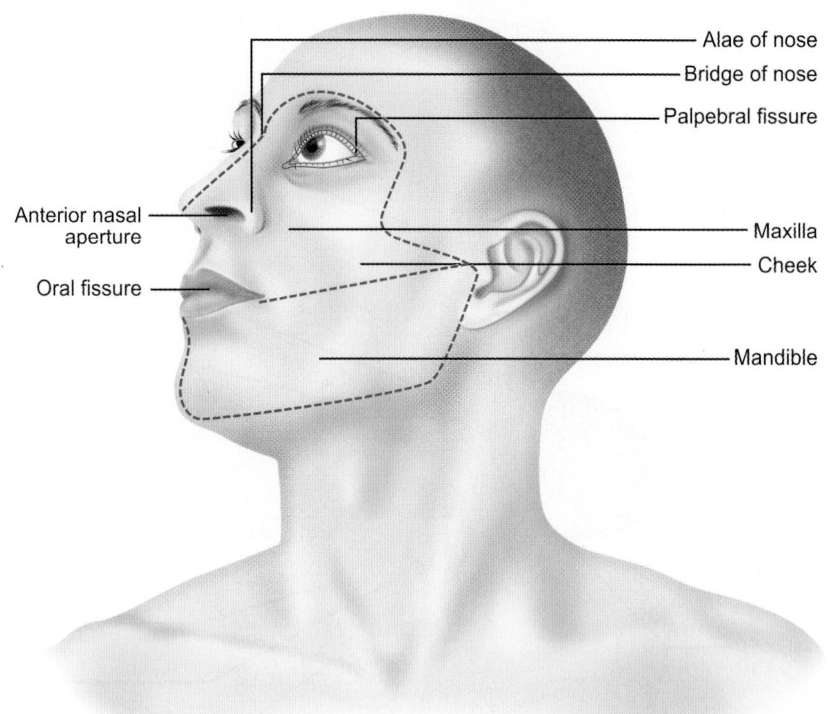

FIGURE 8 Dissection lines and surface anatomy—face

SURFACE ANATOMY (Fig. 8)

Identify the following on the living body and correlate it with the skull.

Palpebral fissure: This is the gap between the two eyelids.

External nose: This is formed by the ***bridge of the nose:*** This is the bony part of the nose, ***alae of the nose***—feel them, they are formed of cartilage and the ***anterior nasal aperture—***is the external opening of the nose.

Cheek: Feel the hard zygomatic bone beneath your cheek.

Maxilla: Feel the maxilla, note the upper jaw formed by this.

Mandible: Feel and move it in your fingers. It forms the lower jaw.

Oral fissure: This is the gap between the two lips.

Facial artery pulsations: Clench the teeth feel the masseter. Put your fingers in front of the muscle and feel the pulsations of the artery.

Superficial temporal artery pulsations: Put the fingers in front of the pinna of the ear over the zygomatic arch and feel the pulsations.

Dissection: Make a vertical incision from the nasion to the symphysis menti. Make a horizontal incision from the angle of the mouth to the ear. Make a horizontal incision from the symphysis menti to the angle of the mandible to the mastoid process. Make an incision along the margin of the eyelid. Reflect the skin and totally remove the skin. Here the skin is very thin and the muscles of facial expression are inserted into it. While reflecting the skin, constantly make sure that the muscle is not damaged.

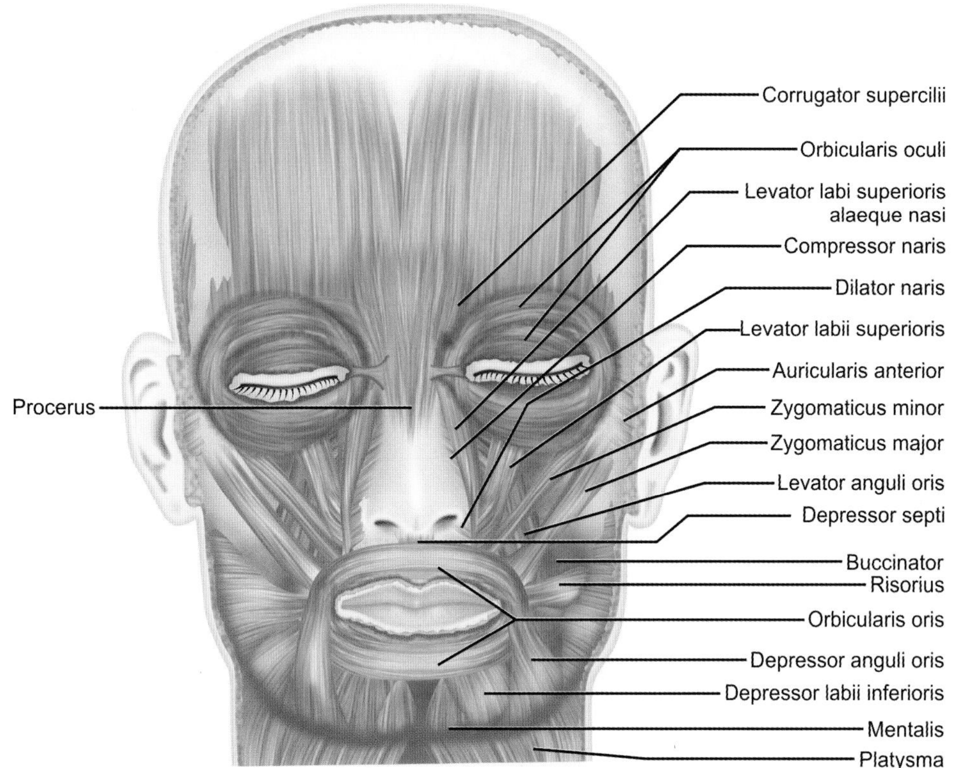

FIGURE 9 Muscles of facial expression

MUSCLES OF FACIAL EXPRESSION (Fig. 9)

The muscles of facial expression belong to the panniculus carnosus group of musculature. They control the orifices of the special senses. They have a bony origin and a cutaneous insertion, and so are capable of moving the skin of the face and scalp. Try to locate each of these muscles.

Muscle of the Eyelid

Corrugator supercilii: This extends from the bridge of the nose to the forehead. This produces vertical wrinkles of the forehead skin.

Orbicularis oculi: Identify this muscle within the eyelid. It is an elliptical muscle. It takes origin from the medial palpebral ligament. It has a ***palpebral part*** within the eyelids and this gently closes the eyelids. It has an ***orbital part*** which extends on to the adjoining orbital margin. This part screws the lids towards the medial side. It has a ***lacrimal part*** which is attached to the lacrimal sac and opens the lacrimal sac.

Muscles of the Nasal Aperture

Compressor nares: This is seen on the bridge of nose.

Dilator nares: This is inserted into the alae of the nose.

Depressor septi: This is inserted into the septum from the maxilla.

Levator *labi* superioris *alaequi* nasi: This muscle extends from medial side of orbital wall to the alae of the nose.

All the muscles of external nose are small and have a limited movement in humans. They perform the movements specified in their names.

Muscles of Oral Aperture

Orbicularis oris: This is the sphincter of the oral aperture. It is an elliptical muscle extending from the maxilla to the mandible in the midline.

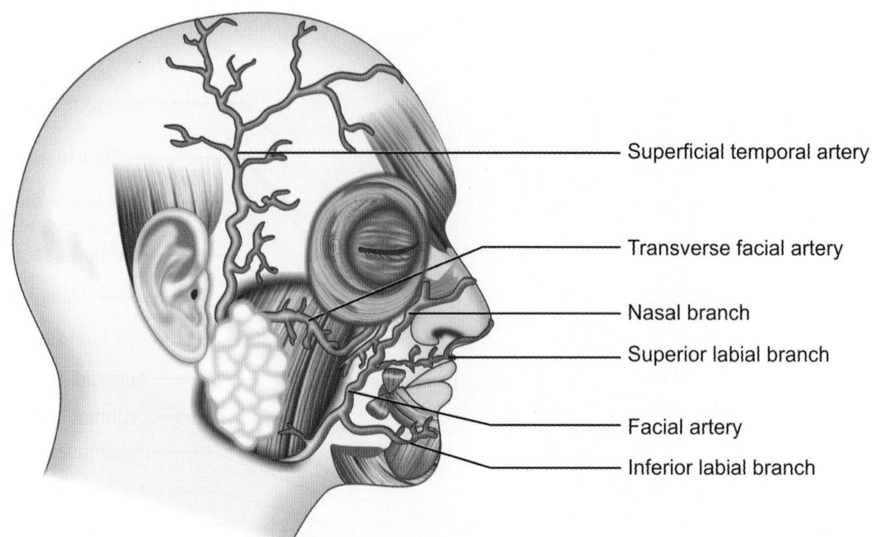

FIGURE 10 Blood vessels—face

The following muscles stretch from the neighboring bones into the lips, like the spokes of a wheel and act as dilators.

Zygomaticus major: This extends from zygomatic bone to the angle of oral aperture.

Zygomaticus minor: This extends from zygomatic bone to the angle of oral aperture. This muscle lies medial to the major.

Levator anguli oris: This extends from below the infraorbital foramen to the angle of oral aperture.

Levator labi superioris: This extends from above the infraorbital foramen to the upper lip.

Depressor anguli oris: This extends from the mandible to the angle of the oral aperture.

Depressor labi inferioris: extends from the mandible to the lower lip.

Risorius: This extends from the parotid fascia to the angle of the oral aperture. It is a smiling muscle.

Muscles of the Ear

Auricularis anterior: Lies in front of the ear.

Auricularis superior: Lies superior to the ear.

Auricularis posterior: Lies posterior to the ear.

Other Muscles

Corrugator supercilii: This extends from the bridge of the nose to the eyebrow.

Procerus: This extends from the bridge of the nose into the skin over glabella.

Mentalis: This extends from the mandible into the skin of the chin.
These small muscles act on the nearby skin.

BLOOD VESSELS (Fig. 10)

Dissection: Locate the superficial temporal artery in front of the external auditory meatus. Here it is superficial, not covered by musculature. Trace the artery and all its branches from the upper border of the parotid gland to the scalp. Similarly identify the facial artery along the lower border of the mandible in front of the masseter muscle. Again here it is superficial. From here trace it up to the angle of the eye. Trace all its branches on the way.

Superficial temporal artery: It is the terminal branch of the external carotid artery. It ascends up into the scalp and supplies the temporal area above the zygomatic arch. The ***transverse facial artery***—Locate this artery below and parallel to the zygomatic arch. It is a branch of the superficial temporal artery. It runs parallel to the zygomatic arch and above the parotid duct. It supplies the cheek region.

Facial artery: It is a branch of the external carotid artery. It reaches the face in front of the masseter muscle. It ascends up to the angle of the eye. It is tortuous in its course. This is to accommodate the artery during movements of the mouth. It gives inferior labial artery to supply the lower lip, superior labial artery to supply the upper lip and nasal artery to supply the side of the nose. Trace these arteries. The corresponding veins accompany the artery.

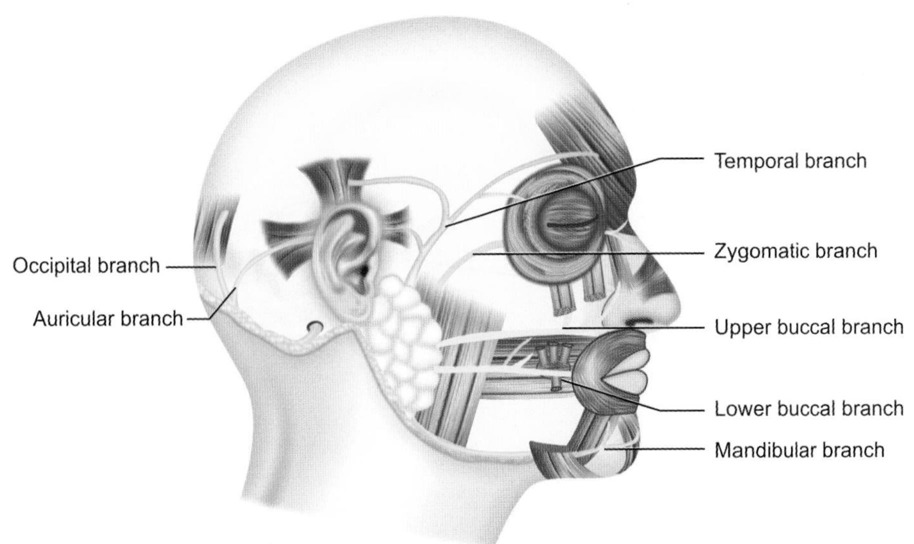

FIGURE 11 Facial nerve—face

FACIAL NERVE (Fig. 11)

The facial nerve is the 7th cranial nerve and is the motor nerve of this region. It supplies all the muscles of facial expression. Its branches are to be located around the parotid gland. They enter the face deep to the parotid gland. The branches of the nerve appear along the borders of the parotid gland, pass deep to the muscles and supply them on their deeper aspect. The distribution is highly variable. Following gives standard distribution.

Dissection: Identify the branches of the facial nerve along the borders of the parotid gland as described below and trace them to their destinations by cutting through the muscles.

Temporal branch: It is seen along the upper border of the parotid gland in front of the superficial temporal artery. This nerve runs parallel with the artery and supplies the auricularis superior, anterior frontal belly of occipitofrontalis and orbicularis oculi.

Dissection: Cut across the zygomaticus major and zygomaticus minor and lift the muscles superiorly.

Zygomatic branch: This runs parallel to the zygomatic arch, supplies the muscles zygomaticus major and zygomaticus minor arising from the zygomatic bone. It runs further to supply the muscles of nose. Trace these branches.

Upper buccal branch: This leaves the parotid gland anteriorly. Trace this nerve. It runs between the transverse facial artery and the parotid duct. Trace it forwards into the muscles of upper lip, i.e. orbicularis oris levator labi superioris and levator anguli oris.

Lower buccal nerve: Trace this nerve from the anterior border of the parotid gland, below and parallel to the parotid duct and supplies the buccinator and risorius muscle.

Dissection: Cut across the risorius, depressor anguli oris and reflect the muscles downwards.

Mandibular branch: This arises near the lower border of mandible (can be seen in the neck dissection). It enters the deep surface of depressor anguli oris and depressor labi inferioris to supply them. Trace these branches.

Cervical branch: This supplies the platysma and can be seen in neck dissection.

Occipital branch: This supplies the posterior auricular muscle.

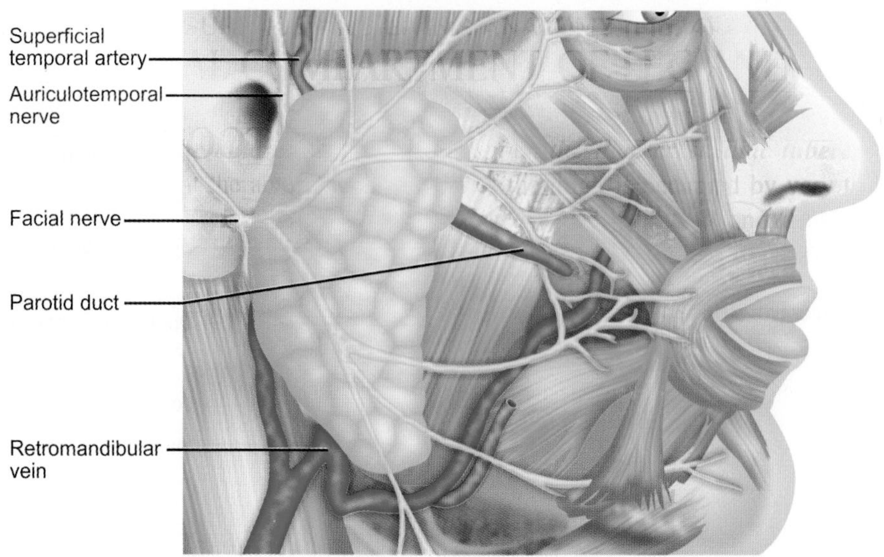

FIGURE 12 Parotid gland

PAROTID GLAND

Parotid gland (Fig. 12) is a salivary gland. It is the biggest of the salivary glands. It is enclosed in the deep fascia of the neck. It is called parotid fascia. Note the irregular shape of the gland. Superiorly it extends up to the zygomatic arch and the external auditory meatus. You have already noted the nerves and blood vessels in relation to the gland.

Parotid duct: Trace this from the middle of the anterior border of the gland. Trace it forward between the upper and lower buccal nerves. Note that it pierces the buccal pad of fat and the buccinator muscle. Its opening in the oral cavity can be seen at a later dissection.

Dissection: The parotid gland encloses the neurovascular bundle reaching the face. You try to identify them by dissecting through the gland.

Facial nerve: This is the most superficial of the structures within the gland. Dissect the branches of the nerve into the gland. Its arrangement in the gland is variable. However in general it is seen as two trunks, an upper and a lower. A small part of the gland is clasped between the two divisions. The part superficial is considered as the superficial part. Slowly remove this.

Retromandibular vein: Identify this vein running vertically within the substance of the gland. It is formed by the union of the ***superficial temporal and the maxillary veins***. It divides into an anterior and a posterior division within the substance. Locate these branches.

External carotid artery: Trace this artery in the gap between the posterior border of the mandible and the mastoid processes. Trace the superficial temporal artery and the maxillary artery which are its terminal divisions. The part of the gland that is removed to trace these vessels is the deep part of the gland.

Lymph nodes: Many a lymph nodes were removed during the dissection and these are the parotid lymph nodes.

Trigeminal nerve branches supply the skin of the face. The nerve fibres are very thin, pass through the skull before reaching the skin. Try to locate them as per their position, and it is not essential to trace all the branches.

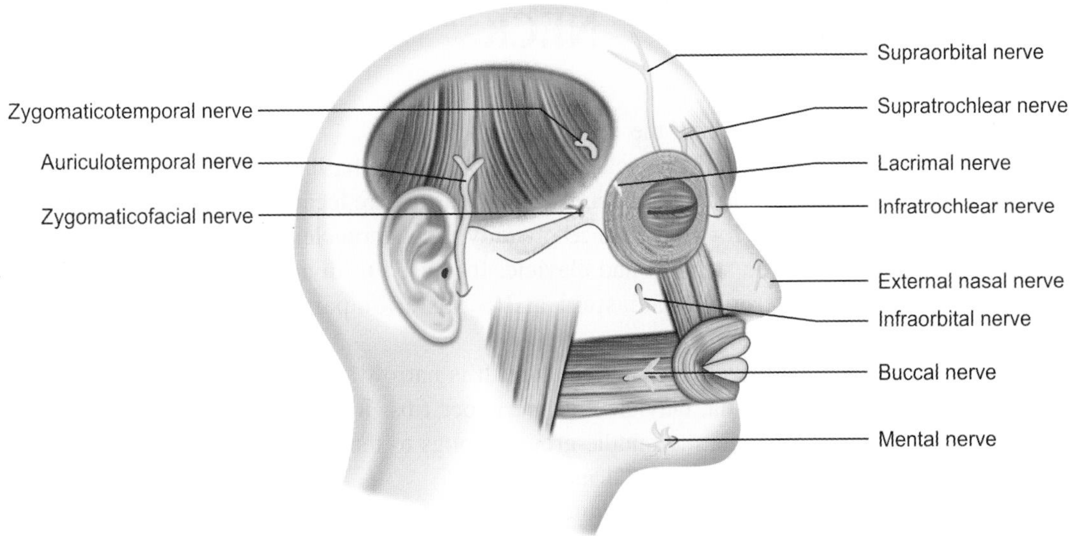

FIGURE 13 Branches of trigeminal nerve

SENSORY NERVES—BRANCHES OF TRIGEMINAL NERVE (Fig. 13)

Trigeminal nerve is the 5th cranial nerve and is sensory to the skin of the face. It has three divisions – the ophthalmic, maxillary and mandibular. The terminal branches of these divisions reach the face through the foraminae in the skull.

Dissection: Reflect the muscles and identify the deeply placed branches of the following nerves.

OPHTHALMIC DIVISION

Supratrochlear nerve and supraorbital nerve: These nerves were already identified in the dissection of the scalp. Relocate them and trace supratrochlear nerve through the orbicularis oculi to the trochlea and the supraorbital nerve to the supraorbital notch near the medial aspect of the orbit.

Lacrimal nerve: This is a very small branch piercing the upper eyelid on its lateral aspect.

Infratrochlear nerve: This is a very small branch on the bridge of the nose medial to the medial palpebral ligament.

External nasal nerve: This is a very small branch on the bridge of the nose. It pierces to the surface between the nasal bone and alae of the cartilage.

MAXILLARY DIVISION

Zygomaticotemporal nerve: It is a very small branch piercing through the temporal fascia above the zygomatic arch.

Zygomaticofacial nerve: It is a very small branch piercing through the zygomatic bone on the face. Try to see its position on a dry skull.

Infraorbital nerve: This is a thick nerve, reaches the face through the infraorbital foramen. Lift the orbicularis oculi and the levator labi superioris, feel the intraorbital foramen, and locate the thick infraorbital nerve which comes out as a bunch of nerves.

MANDIBULAR DIVISION

Auriculotemporal nerve: This was already identified in the dissection of the scalp. Relocate the nerve and trace up to the upper border of the parotid gland.

Buccal nerve: This is a deep branch. It passes through buccal pad of fat and buccinator muscle to supply the skin of the cheek. Identify this at this stage so that it can be traced in a later deeper dissection.

Mental nerve: This is a thick nerve and reaches the face through the mental foramen. Lift the depressor labi inferioris to locate this nerve.

NECK

Study the neck on a living person and observe the following:

Note that the cervical vertebrae are posteriorly located. The neck extends far higher on the posterior aspect, compared to the anterior aspect. In the midline anteriorly, the trachea and esophagus are located. These are supported by cartilages. The neck can be divided into two parts for convenience of study. The sternocleidomastoid is the key muscle here. It extends from the mastoid process to the sternum and clavicle. It is used to divide the neck into an anterior part, the anterior triangle in front of the sternocleidomastoid and a posterior part, the posterior triangle behind the sternocleidomastoid.

The ***posterior triangle*** is made up of vertebral musculature. It is narrow superiorly, but widens inferiorly and spans from the vertebral processes to the scapula, clavicle and the upper ribs. It presents a layered appearance. The most superficial group belongs to the upper limb, the middle group belongs to the erector spinae group of musculature. The deep group belongs to the rotator group of vertebral musculature.

The ***anterior triangle*** is made up of visceral structures. In its upper part it is the pharynx, the common passage of both respiratory and digestive system. Inferiorly it divides into trachea and esophagus. The thyroid and parathyroids form the prominent structures ventral to the trachea.

The ***neurovascular bundle*** lies between the two. The veins of the neck called the jugular system of veins form a superficial group and a deep group. Branches of the arch of the aorta enter the neck as brachiocephalic artery on the right side and as common carotid artery and the subclavian artery on the left side. They supply the upper limb, head and neck and the brain. The lymph nodes accompany the veins by forming a superficial and a deep group.

9th, 10th, 11th and 12th cranial nerves show their presence in the neck region. The somatic nerves form the cervical and brachial plexuses. The sympathetic chain along with three ganglia are noted here.

SKELETON (Fig. 14)

The skeleton of the neck is formed by the cervical vertebrae. Go to an articulated skeleton and identify the vertebrae. Do a detailed study of the individual vertebrae.

Atlas: This is the first cervical vertebra. It articulates with the skull. Identify its anterior arch, anterior tubercle, lateral masses, foramen transversarium, articulating surfaces on the lateral masses, posterior arch, posterior tubercle and the groove for the vertebral artery on the posterior arch.

Axis: This is the second cervical vertebra. It has an odontoid process which is the detached part of the body of the atlas. It resembles other cervical vertebrae except for this process. Identify the body, odontoid process, transverse process, pedicle, lamina and the bifid spine. This articulates superiorly with the atlas by a pivot joint.

Three to seven vertebrae: Identify the general features of these vertebrae. They present a body, pedicle, the transverse process with a foramen transversarium, anterior tubercle, costotransverse bar and a posterior tubercle, lamina and a bifid spine.

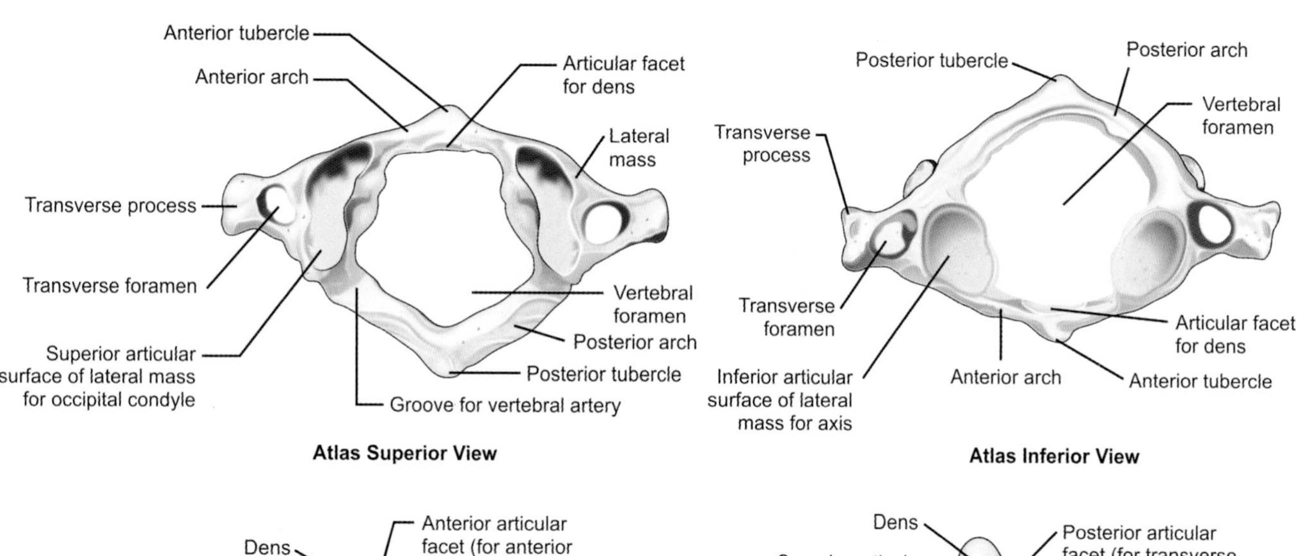

Atlas Superior View

Atlas Inferior View

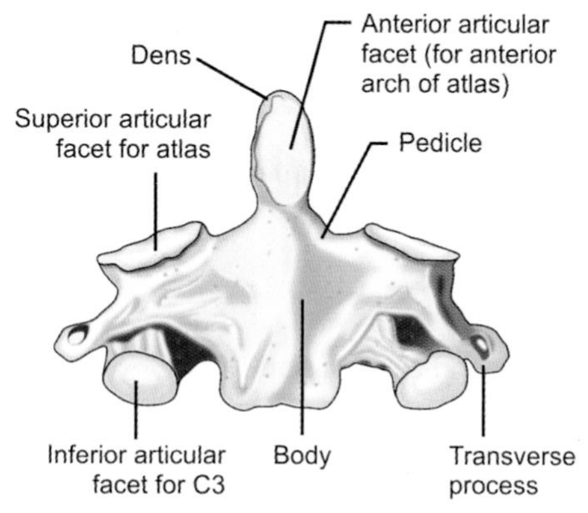

Axis Anterior View

Dens
Superior articular facet for atlas
Posterior articular facet (for transverse ligament of atlas)
Interarticular part
Transverse process
Lamina
Inferior articular process
Spinous process

Axis Posterosuperior View

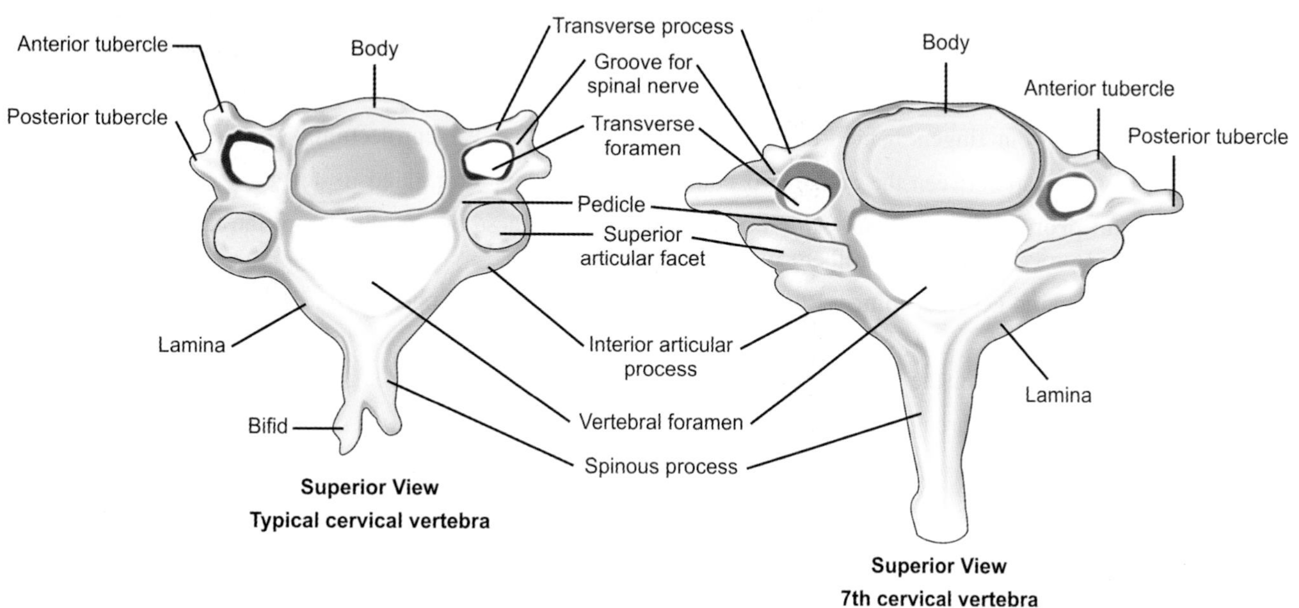

Superior View
Typical cervical vertebra

Superior View
7th cervical vertebra

FIGURE 14 Skeleton—neck

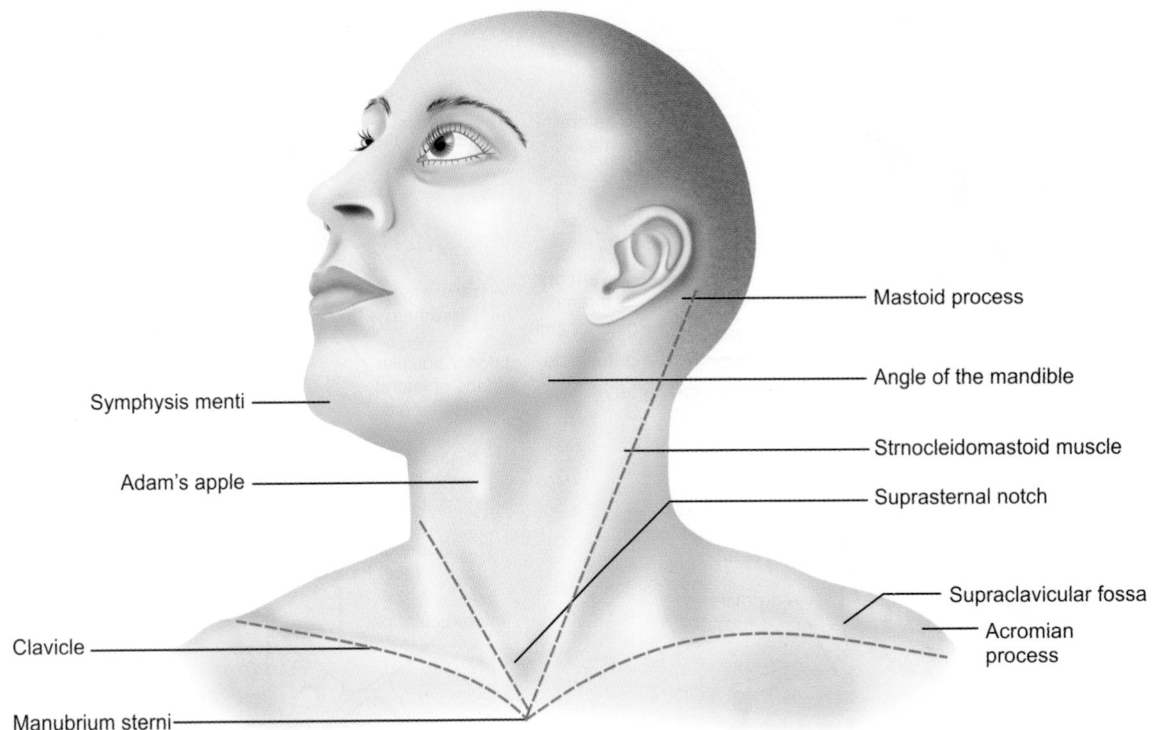

FIGURE 15 Surface anatomy of the neck and skin incision

SURFACE ANATOMY (Fig. 15)

Most of the following structures were already identified by you. As they form boundaries for this region, they are once again emphasized.

Symphysis menti: It is the lower point of the mandible in the midline.

Lower border of the mandible: Run your fingers from the symphysis menti to the angle of the mandible.

Angle of the mandible: The posteroinferior corner of the mandible at the junction of the body and ramus.

Mastoid process: Put your fingers behind the ear and feel for the downward projection.

Press and identify the gap between the above two points and note the parotid gland in it.

External occipital protuberance and **superior nuchal line:** Identify these on the skull from the midline to the lower end of the mastoid process and relocate them on the cadaver.

Ligamentum nuchae and cervical spines: Run your fingers along the midline posteriorly till you reach the 7th cervical vertebral prominence.

Acromion process: Lies under the shoulder prominence, feel this by pressing through the deltoid muscle.

Clavicle: It is subcutaneous throughout its length and can be felt all along.

Suprasternal notch: This lies at the upper border of the manubrium sterni between the two clavicles.

Hyoid bone: Run your fingers downward from the symphysis menti along the midline and clasp the bone between your two fingers. You move it by holding the greater cornu of the bone.

Thyroid cartilage: This causes a prominence more pronounced in male members called Adam's apple. Again clasp it between your fingers.

Cricoid cartilage and tracheal rings: These can be felt in the midline below the thyroid.

Supraclavicular fossa: This is a depression above the middle of the clavicle and posterior to the sternocleidomastoid muscle.

Sternocleidomastoid muscle: Turn the head to one side and identify the muscle which stands out extending from manubrium sterni to mastoid process.

External jugular vein: Identify this vein, on a well developed body.

External carotid artery: Feel the hyoid bone, and press your fingers in, to feel the carotid artery.

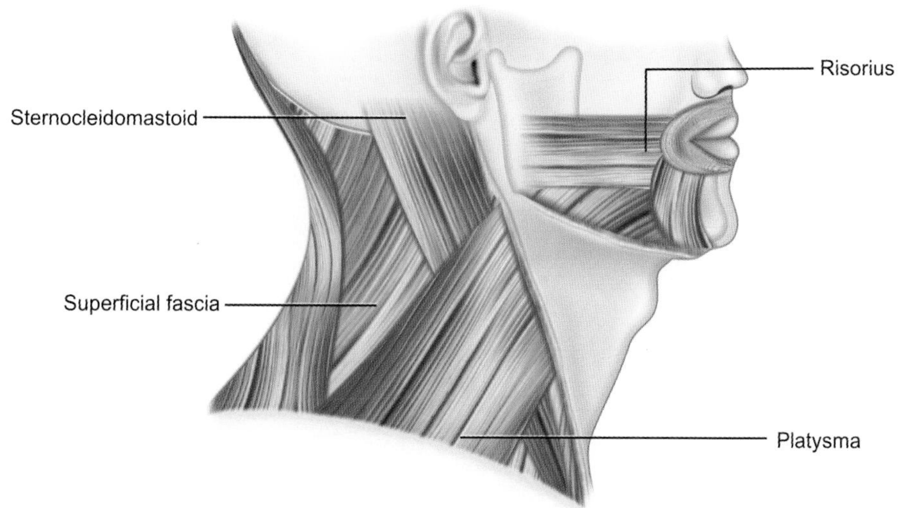

FIGURE 16 Platysma muscle—neck

POSTERIOR TRIANGLE

Posterior triangle is the area between the sternocleidomastoid and trapezius extending from the middle of the clavicle to the superior nuchal line. It is a narrow long strip of triangle. This can be divided into two subtriangles by the inferior belly of omohyoid muscle. The upper part is called the occipital triangle and the lower part is called the subclavian triangle.

BOUNDARIES

Anterior border is formed by the posterior border of sternocleidomastoid muscle; posterior border is formed by the anterior border of the trapezius muscle; roof is formed by the skin, superficial fascia with cutaneous vessels and nerves and platysma muscle; floor is formed by the prevertebral muscles—the semispinalis capitis, splenius capitis, levator scapulae and scalenus medius. Number of structures cross this area to reach their destination in the present study follow the structures as they appear in the dissection.

Dissection (Fig. 15): Support the body with a block placed near the shoulders, so that the neck hangs down stretching it. Turn the head to one side and do the skin reflection as far as you can. (1) Put an incision from the mastoid process to the midline above the manubrium sterni along the anterior border of the sternocleidomastoid muscle. (2) Put a transverse incision from the manubrium sterni to the acromian process (done). Reflect the skin, starting from the sternocleidomastoid muscle to the back. Inferiorly reflect it up to the acromian process, superiorly reflect as far as you can. Skin here is very thin. While reflecting the skin make sure you are able to see the obliquely running muscle fibres of platysma.

Platysma muscle (Fig. 16): It is a thin subcutaneous muscle stretching over the sternocleidomastoid to the clavicle. It helps in tightening the neck skin. It is supplied by the cervical branch of the facial nerve.

Dissection: Carefully lift the platysma from the clavicle and reflect it towards the sternocleidomastoid muscle, it can be reflected fully in a later dissection. Identify the cutaneous structures.

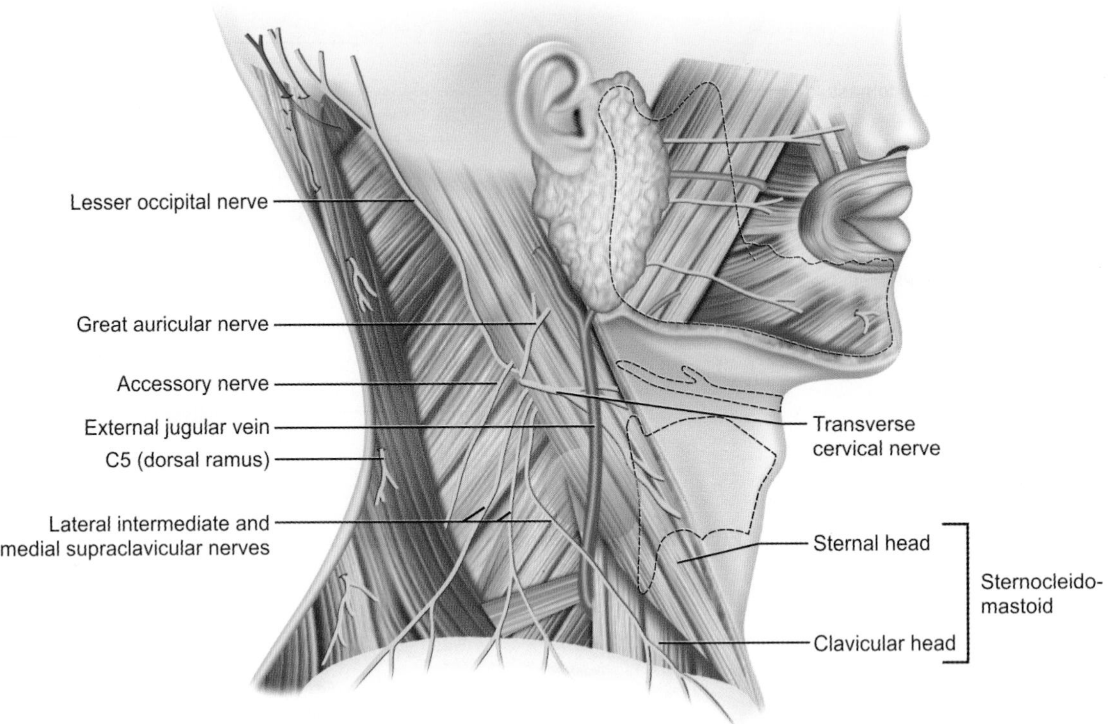

FIGURE 17 Cutaneous structures and deep fascia—neck

CUTANEOUS STRUCTURES (Fig. 17)

External jugular vein: Locate this vein on the sternocleidomastoid muscle and trace it till it pierces through the deep fascia, posterior to the sternocleidomastoid muscle. It receives suprascapular and transverse cervical veins.

Cutaneous nerves: Trace the nerves along the posterior border of the sternocleidomastoid muscle. Note that the ***supraclavicular nerves*** descend down toward the clavicle, the ***lesser occipital nerve*** towards the scalp. The ***great auricular nerve*** crosses on to the sternocleidomastoid muscle to reach the external ear. The ***transverse cervical nerve*** runs across the sternocleidomastoid muscle.

The accessory nerve, (XIth cranial nerve) passes between the two layers of the investing layer of the cervical fascia. It loops with the lesser occipital nerve. This helps in identifying this nerve. You need to clean the fascia to locate this nerve.

DEEP FASCIA—INVESTING LAYER OF CERVICAL FASCIA

The trapezius and sternocleidomastoid belong to the superficial group of musculature. Both these muscles are enclosed in the investing layer of cervical fascia. The fascia extends from the ligamentum nuchae, encloses the trapezius, then the two layers unite along its anterior border to form the roof of the posterior triangle, encloses the sternocleidomastoid muscle covers the structures of the anterior triangle to be continuous with the fascia of the opposite side.

Dissection: Clean the fascia over the sternocleidomastoid and trapezius and the fascia between the two muscles, and study the muscles. Cut the supraclavicular nerves and remove.

Sternocleidomastoid: It is the key muscle in the neck region. It has a clavicular head and a sternal head. Look for the origin of the clavicular head from the superior border and anterior surface of the medial 1/3 of the clavicle. Here it has a muscular origin. The sternal head arises from the anterior surface of the manubrium sternum. Both the origins soon join to form a thick muscle mass, which extends posteriorly to be inserted. Locate its insertion into the mastoid process along a curved line.

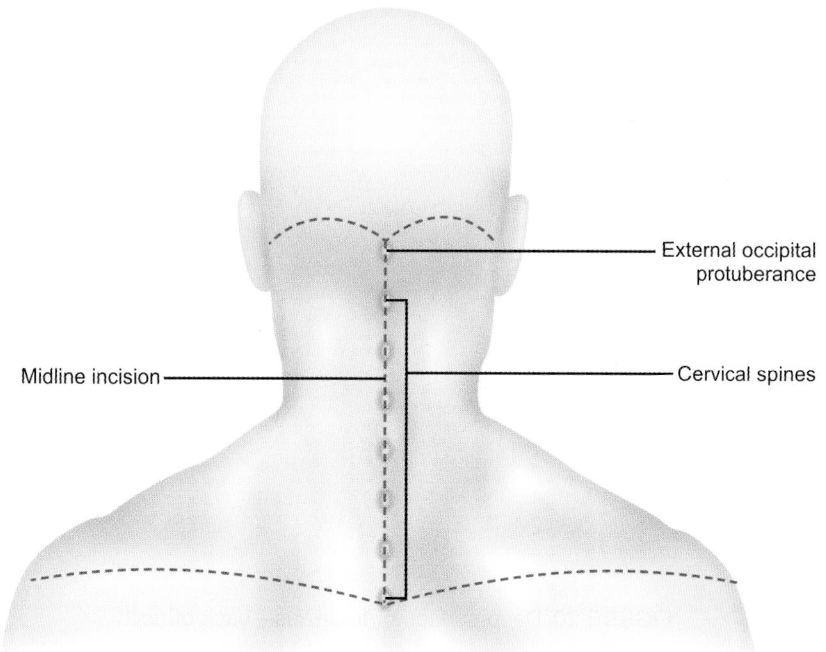

FIGURE 18 Incision lines and Surface anatomy—back of neck

Action: Look at this muscle extending from the front to the back of the neck. It pulls the mastoid processes downwards, thus results in lifting the face upwards. When muscle of one side acts it will pull the mastoid forwards thus turning the face to the opposite side.

BACK OF THE NECK SKIN INCISIONS (Fig. 18)

Dissection: Turn the body to a prone position. (1) Make a midline incision from the external occipital protuberance to the 7th cervical spine. If you are using the same body throughout for dissection, then the lower part is already dissected. Reflect the skin from the back of the neck, while doing so make sure that you are not damaging the trapezius muscle.

SUPERFICIAL FASCIA and CUTANEOUS STRUCTURES (Fig. 19)

Superficial fascia and cutaneous structures: Here superficial fascia has lot of connective tissue, so feels tough, and it is filled with fine fat.

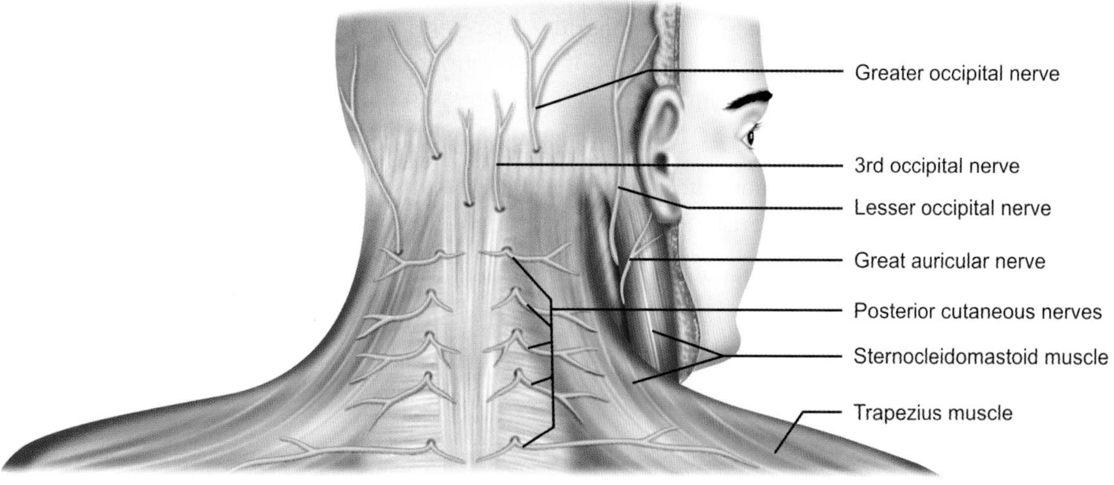

FIGURE 19 Cutaneous structures—back of neck

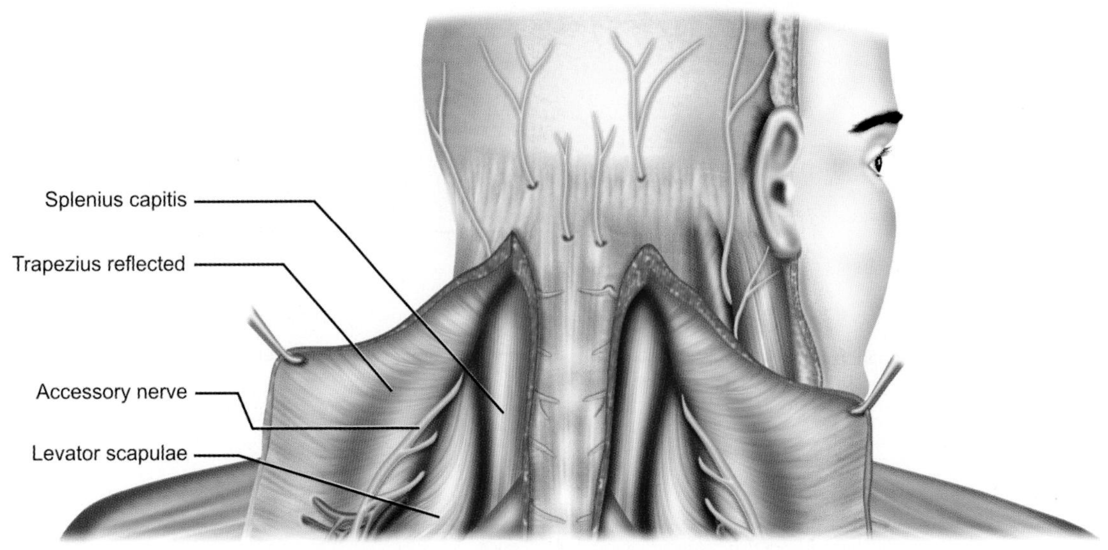

FIGURE 20 Deep surface of trapezius—back of neck

Greater occipital nerve: This nerve is already identified in the scalp region, trace it down, between the trapezius and sternocleidomastoid. Note the occipital artery accompanying this.

Third occipital nerve (C3): This nerve pierces lateral to the 3rd cervical spine. If possible locate this. The other posterior cutaneous nerves from 4th to 8th also pierce in their respective positions lateral to the midline to supply the skin on the posterior aspect. They are small and do not bother to trace all of them.

Lesser occipital nerve: Trace this nerve along the posterior border of the sternocleidomastoid muscle.

Dissection: Clean the trapezius and define its boundaries.

Trapezius: This is a muscle of the upper limb. It attaches the upper limb to the trunk bones.

Origin: It extends from the external occipital protuberance to the last thoracic spine in the midline, (the thoracic part has already been dissected) and from the medial 1/3 of the superior nuchal line. Trace this part now.

Dissection (Fig. 20): Separate the remaining part of the trapezius from its origin from the superior nuchal line and the ligamentum nuchae. Trace the accessory nerve and cervical branches entering into the undersurface of the trapezius muscle. After tracing this you may remove the muscle totally as it is partly removed.

Now identify the muscles that lie deep to the trapezius. They form the posterolateral group of musculature. They constitute two groups—The erector spinae (extensors of spine) group and the lateral rotator group.

The occipital artery and the posterior rami of the cervical nerves supply this musculature. Try to see as much as you can. Try to reflect the muscles layer by layer.

Occipital artery: It is the artery of supply to this region. It gives off a superficial and a deep branch, which goes between the muscles to supply them. Trace these branches as you are reflecting the muscles.

Motor nerves: The posterior rami of the upper cervical nerves give branches to supply the muscles of the back.

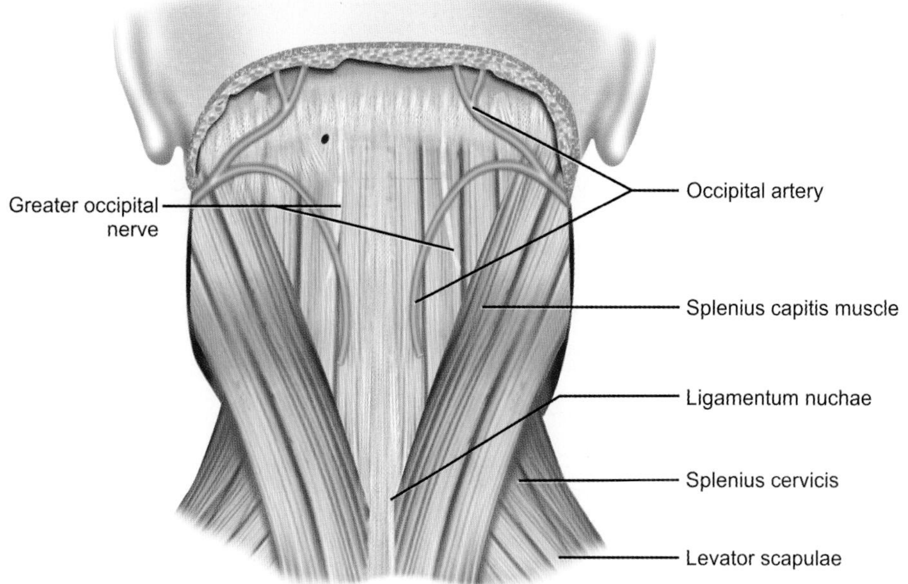

FIGURE 21 Splenius capitis and cervicis

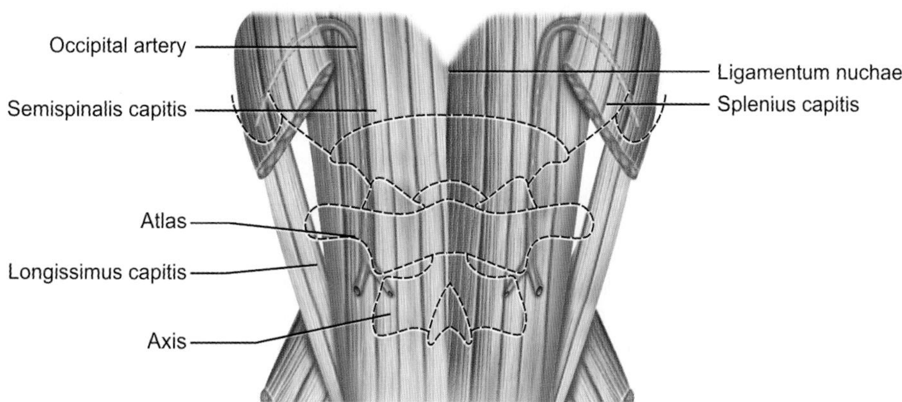

FIGURE 22 Semispinalis capitis and longissimus capitis

Splenius capitis (Fig. 21): Identify this muscle from the direction of its fibres. They extend from the midline to the lateral side.

Trace its origin from the lower part of the ligamentum nuchae and the upper six thoracic vertebral spines. Note its insertion into the superior nuchal line and mastoid process, deep to the sternocleidomastoid muscle.

Dissection: Lift the splenius capitis from its lateral side, and detach it from the skull. Reflect the muscle medially.

See the deeper ***splenius cervices*** muscle. Its origin is same as the capitis but few of these fibres get inserted into the transverse process of the upper four cervical vertebrae. This is called the splenius cervices.

Dissection: Detach this muscle from the transverse processes and reflect it medially to the midline taking care to preserve the cutaneous vessels and nerves already identified.

Semispinalis capitis (Fig. 22): This muscle fibres run opposite to the splenius capitis muscle. This muscle extends from lateral to medial side. It arises from the transverse process of upper six thoracic and lower four cervical vertebrae and is inserted into the medial aspect of the area between the superior and inferior nuchal lines.

Dissection: First trace the greater occipital nerve through the muscle and preserve it, then detach this muscle from its insertion and pull it towards the transverse processes.

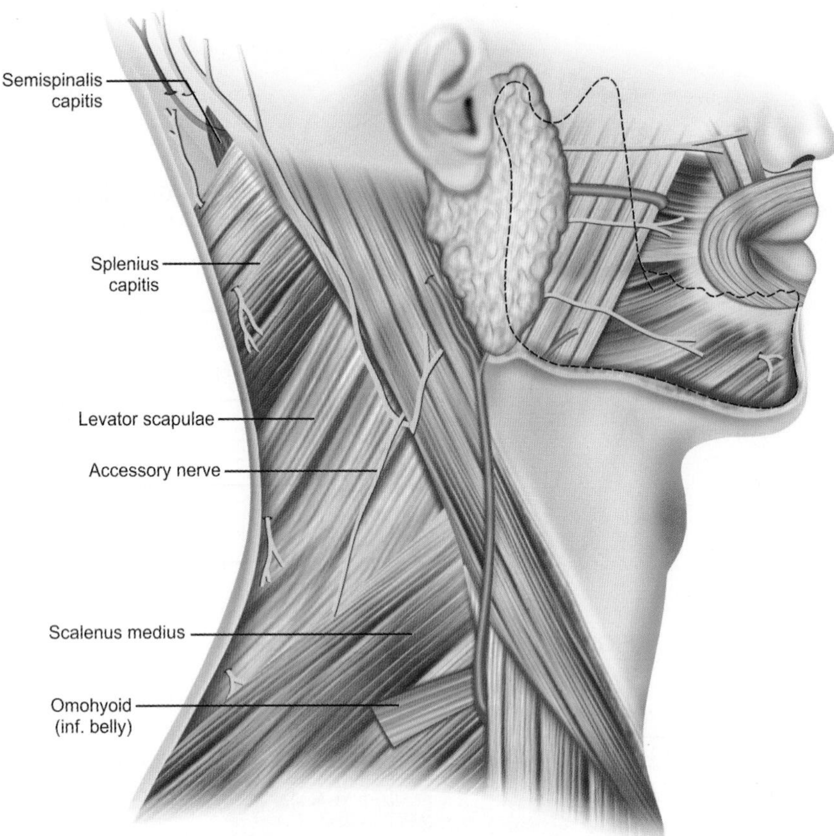

FIGURE 23 Muscles of posterior triangle floor—lateral aspect

Longissimus capitis: Identify this muscle under cover of the splenius capitis. It extends from the upper thoracic transverse processes to be inserted into the mastoid process. Detach this muscle from the mastoid process to get a clearer view of the suboccipital triangle. The fibres which get inserted into the posterior aspect of the cervical transverse processes is called the longissimus cervicis muscle. You may identify these fibres.

Action of all the above muscles belonging to the superficial group of erector spine group of muscles perform extension of the cervical part of vertebral column.

Dissection: You may cut and remove all the above muscles to get a clear view of the deeper suboccipital triangle.

Ligamentum nuchae: Identify this midline thick ligament extending from the external occipital protuberance to the 7th cervical vertebra. This is a thick ligament made up of elastic fibres. With reflexion of the posterior muscles this ligament becomes visible. Appreciate its thickness and length.

The following muscles were cut in the upper limb dissection. Trace them to their origins. They are lateral rotators of the vertebral column.

Levator scapulae (Fig. 23): Note this lateral muscle. This arises from the transverse processes of the upper four cervical vertebrae. It is inserted into the medial border of the scapula above the spine (as the upper limb is already detached, note its lower cut end and confirm its insertion on scapula).

Scalenus medius: It is another lateral muscle. It arises from the posterior tubercles of the transverse processes of cervical vertebrae. It is inserted into the external surface on the middle of the first rib (confirm its insertion as a part of the first rib is still present with the trunk).

Inferior belly of omohyoid: It is an obliquely running muscle. It arises from the upper border of the scapula medial to the suprascapular notch (as the upper limb is detached it is cut but confirm it on the bone). It is inserted into the intermediate tendon which is under cover of the sternocleidomastoid (This will be studied in the anterior triangle).

The blood vessels and nerves forming the contents can be better traced in a later dissection.

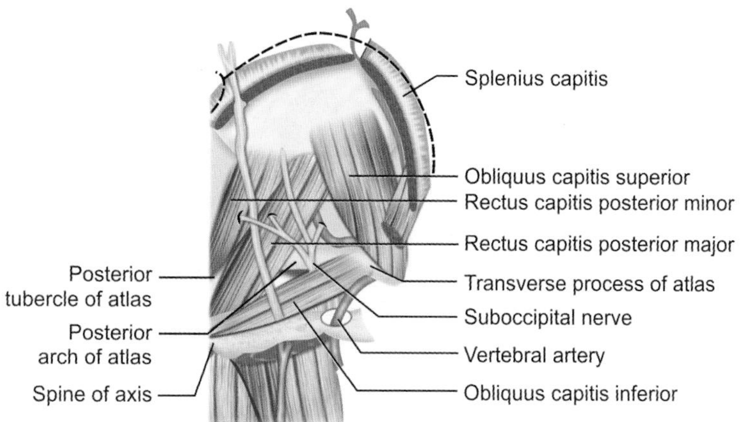

FIGURE 24 Suboccipital triangle—boundaries

SUBOCCIPITAL TRIANGLE (Fig. 24)

Suboccipital triangle is a muscular triangle made up of deep layer of erector spinae group of musculature. The ***roof*** is formed of skin, superficial fascia, trapezius muscle, splenius capitis and semispinalis capitis muscle. These are the muscles you had already seen and reflected.

Dissection: Feel the posterior tubercle of atlas and the spine of the axis in the midline. Feel the arch and the transverse process of the atlas laterally. The muscles seen in the deeper layer are covered by connective tissue. Within this connective tissue look for the neurovascular bundle entering the muscles. The nerves are branches of 1st cervical posterior ramus. The arteries come from the occipital artery. The veins drain into the suboccipital plexus of veins. The veins fill this area. Now clean this area, remove the veins and trace the nerves entering the muscles. Identify the muscles.

The ***medial boundary*** is formed by two muscles.

Identify the bigger lateral muscle, the ***rectus capitis posterior major***. It partly overlaps the medial rectus capitis posterior minor muscle. It arises from the spine of the axis and gets inserted into the area between the inferior nuchal line and the foramen magnum lateral to the rectus capitis posterior minor.

Dissection: Reflect this muscle from its insertion and identify the rectus capitis posterior minor.

Rectus capitis posterior minor: This is a small muscle on the medial side. It arises from the posterior tubercle of atlas and gets inserted into the area between the inferior nuchal line and foramen magnum.

Identify the ***superolateral boundary***. It is formed by the ***obliquus capitis superior***. It arises from the transverse process of atlas and is inserted into the area between the superior nuchal line and inferior nuchal line lateral to the insertion of semispinalis muscle.

Identify the ***obliquus capitis inferior***. This forms the inferior boundary. It arises from the spine of the axis and gets inserted into the transverse process of the axis.

Nerve supply of all the above muscles are supplied by the C1 posterior ramus—the suboccipital nerve.

Action: All the above muscles are rotators of the axis at the atlantoaxial joint. It is a pivot joint (see the bones, articulate them and perform the movements. Here the axis is the fixed part over which the atlas and the occiput rotates).

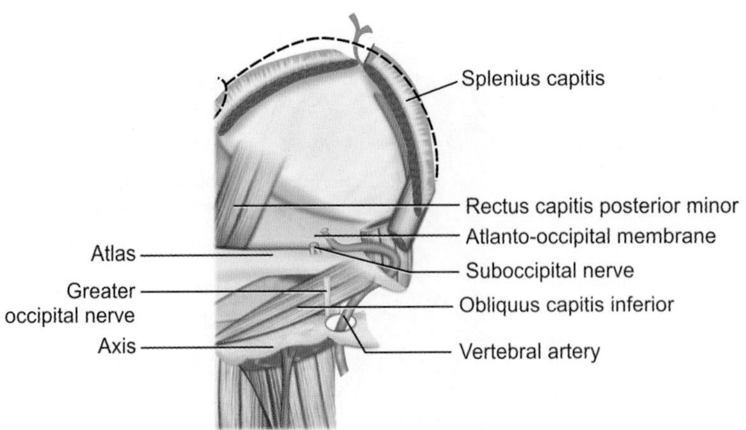

FIGURE 25 Suboccipital triangle—floor

SUBOCCIPITAL TRIANGLE—FLOOR (Fig. 25)

Dissection: Reflect the obliquus capitis superior by detaching it from the insertion, and turn it down. Clean the area between the muscles. It is full of suboccipital plexus of veins. While doing so once again look for the nerves entering into the muscles.

Greater occipital nerve: Relocate this nerve and note that it emerges below the obliquus capitis inferior, pierces the semispinalis capitis to reach the scalp.

Suboccipital nerve: It is seen immediately above the posterior arch of atlas between it and the vertebral artery. It communicates with the greater occipital nerve and supplies all the suboccipital muscles.

Identify the structures forming the floor of the suboccipital triangle.

Feel the prominent ***posterior arch of atlas***. It is the bony prominence extending from right to left.

Vertebral artery: Identify this soft bulging artery extending from the foramen transversarium of the atlas to the foramen magnum.

Posterior atlanto-occipital membrane: Locate this medial to the vertebral artery. It extends from the posterior arch of atlas to the margin of the foramen magnum. Feel it, it is a resilient structure.

ANTERIOR TRIANGLE

This is the area in front of the sternocleidomastoid to the midline. It extends superiorly from the mastoid process to the angle of the mandible, along the lower border of the mandible to the symphysis menti. Inferiorly it extends from the medial ends of the clavicle and the upper border of the manubrium sternum.

INCISION LINES (Fig. 26)

Dissection: Make a midline incision from the symphysis menti to the manubrium sterni. Reflect and remove this bit of the skin between the sternocleidomastoid and the midline. Skin here is very thin and the platysma is the subcutaneous muscle, start the reflection from the sternocleidomastoid side to the midline taking care to preserve the platysma.

PLATYSMA (Fig. 27): This is the subcutaneous muscle of the neck. It extends downwards and laterally from the lower border of the mandible, crosses over the clavicle to be inserted into the skin.

Dissection: Lift up this muscle from the lower border of the mandible.

Cervical branch of facial nerve: Look for this nerve on the undersurface of the muscle. It enters the muscle behind the angle of the mandible at the lower border of the parotid gland.

Identify the following structures in the midline.

The symphysis menti, median raphae, thyrohyoid membrane, anterior angle of thyroid cartilage (Adam's apple) cricotracheal membrane and upper tracheal rings.

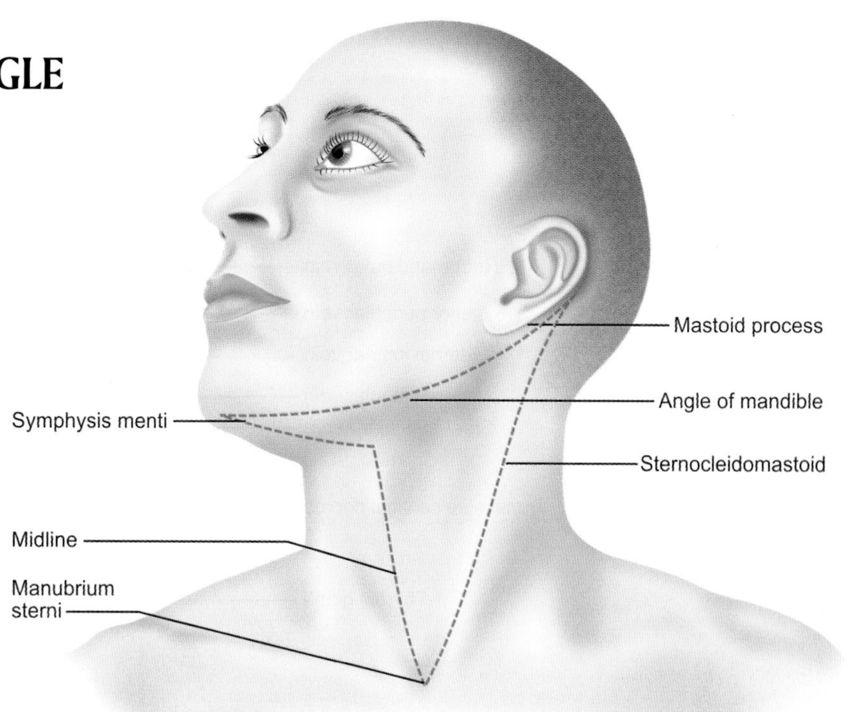

FIGURE 26 Incision lines—anterior triangle

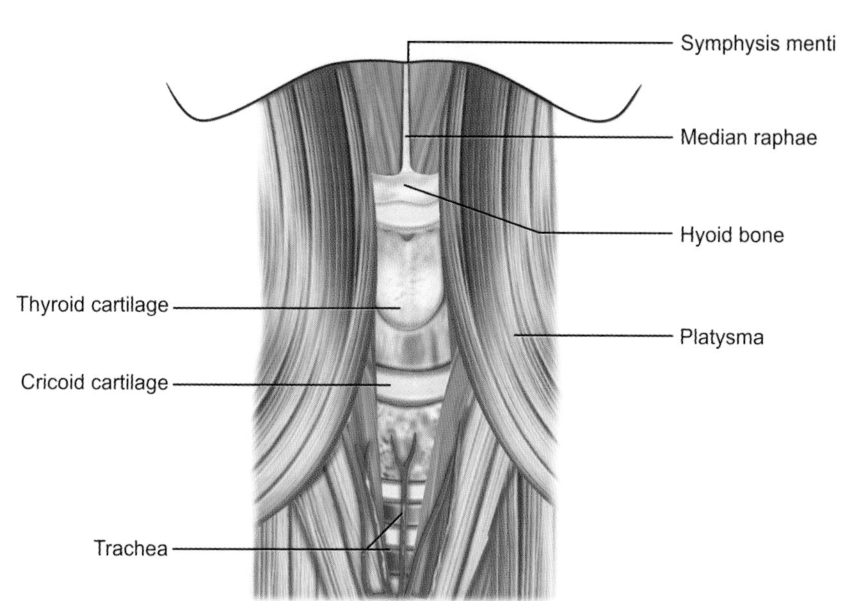

FIGURE 27 Platysma and midline structures

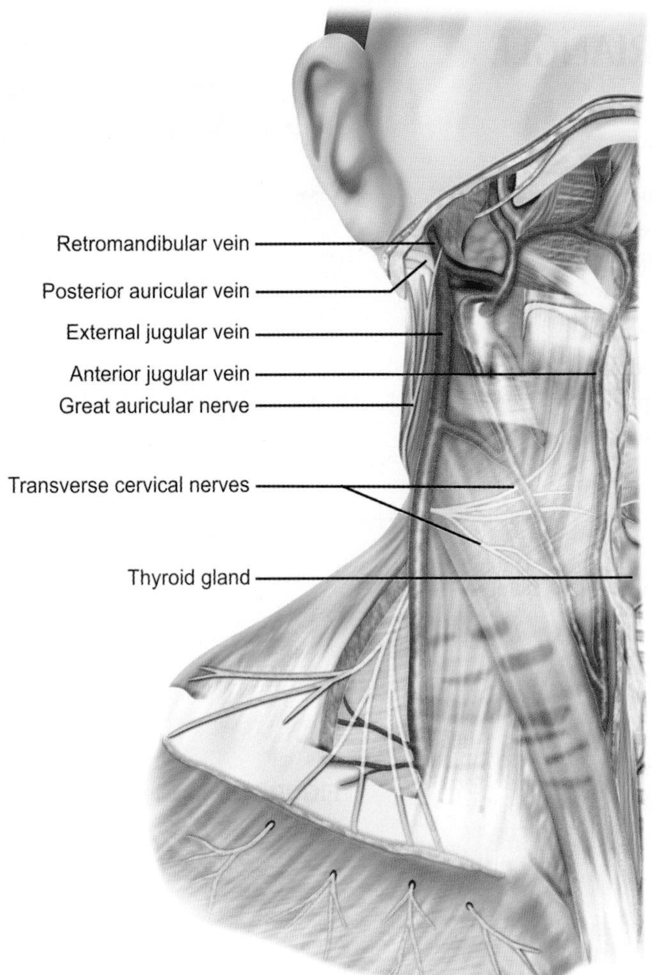

FIGURE 28 Cutaneous structures

CUTANEOUS STRUCTURES (Fig. 28)

External jugular vein: This was already identified at its lower end. Trace it up to its formation. It is formed by the union of posterior auricular vein and the posterior branch of the retromandibular vein. This is one of the superficial veins which can be easily accessed in the body.

Anterior jugular vein: Identify this thin vein lateral to the midline. It begins below and near the symphysis menti, runs down crosses laterally to enter into the external jugular vein.

Cutaneous Nerves

Great auricular nerve: Trace this nerve from the middle of the sternocleidomastoid to the ear lobule along the superficial surface of the sternocleidomastoid. It is a part of the cervical plexus and supplies the skin up to the angle of the mandible.

Transverse cervical nerve: Trace it from the middle of the sternocleidomastoid to the midline across the muscle.

Supraclavicular nerves: Trace these nerves from middle of the posterior border of the sternocleidomastoid to over the clavicle. They are generally three in number—the medial, intermediate and lateral branches. (These were already cut).

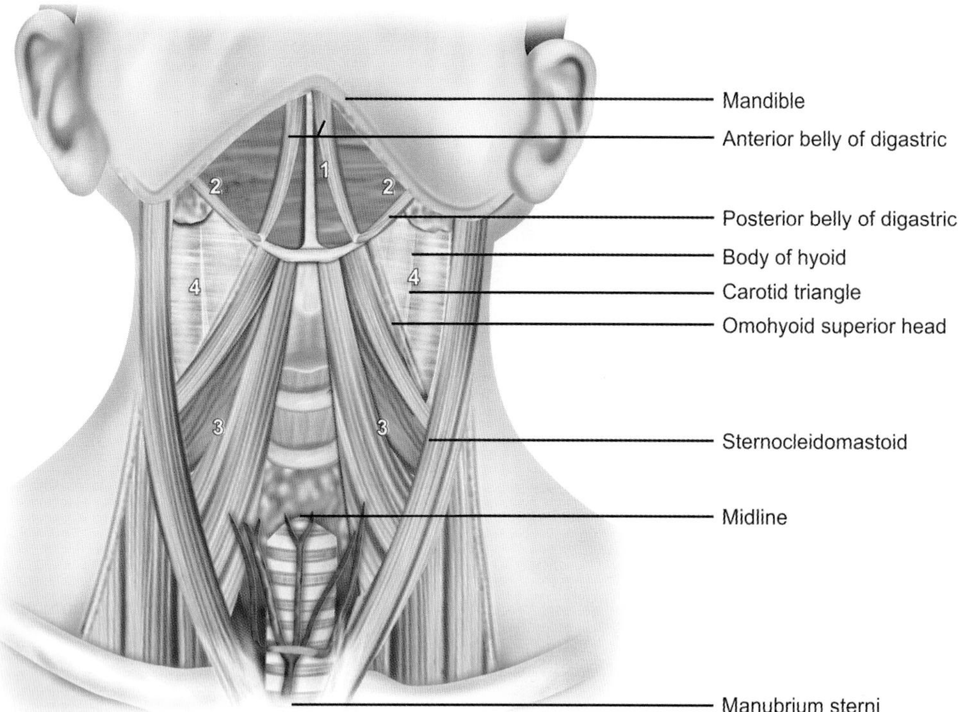

FIGURE 29 Anterior triangle—subdivisions

ANTERIOR TRIANGLE—SUBDIVISIONS (Fig. 29)

Dissection: Support the head on a block. Let the head fall back. Clean the structures in the anterior triangle and identify its subdivisions.

The anterior triangle is the triangular area from the anterior border of the sternocleidomastoid, the lower border of the mandible and the midline. In this area, identify the anterior belly of digastric, posterior belly of digastric and the superior belly of omohyoid. These muscles are used to divide the anterior triangle into four smaller triangles for convenience of description. Study them.

1. **Submental triangle:** This is a midline triangle. Identify the body of the hyoid bone. This forms its base. Look for the anterior bellies of the digastric muscles. These form the limbs of the triangle.
2. **Submandibular triangle /digastric triangle:** Feel the lower border of the mandible. This forms the base of this triangle. Identify the anterior and posterior bellies of the digastric muscle. They form the sides of the triangle. See the prominent submandibular gland in this region.
3. **Muscular triangle:** Look at the muscles on either side of the midline below the hyoid bone. It is made up of two layers. The superficial layer is split vertically. The medial muscle is sternohyoid, and the lateral muscle is the superior belly of omohyoid (the deeper muscles can be seen in a later dissection).
4. **Carotid triangle:** It is the lateral triangle. The base is formed by the anterior border of the sternocleidomastoid muscle. The limbs are formed by the posterior belly of digastric and superior belly of omohyoid. The neurovascular bundle of neck is located here.

Dissection: Cut and remove the cutaneous nerves and external jugular vein near the sternocleidomastoid muscle keeping their origins intact. Detach the muscle from the sternum and clavicle. In the upper half of the muscle look for the accessory nerve through the muscle and trace it to the point where it comes out of the carotid sheath near the angle of the mandible. You may slit the sternocleidomastoid muscle while locating the accessory nerve and remove it.

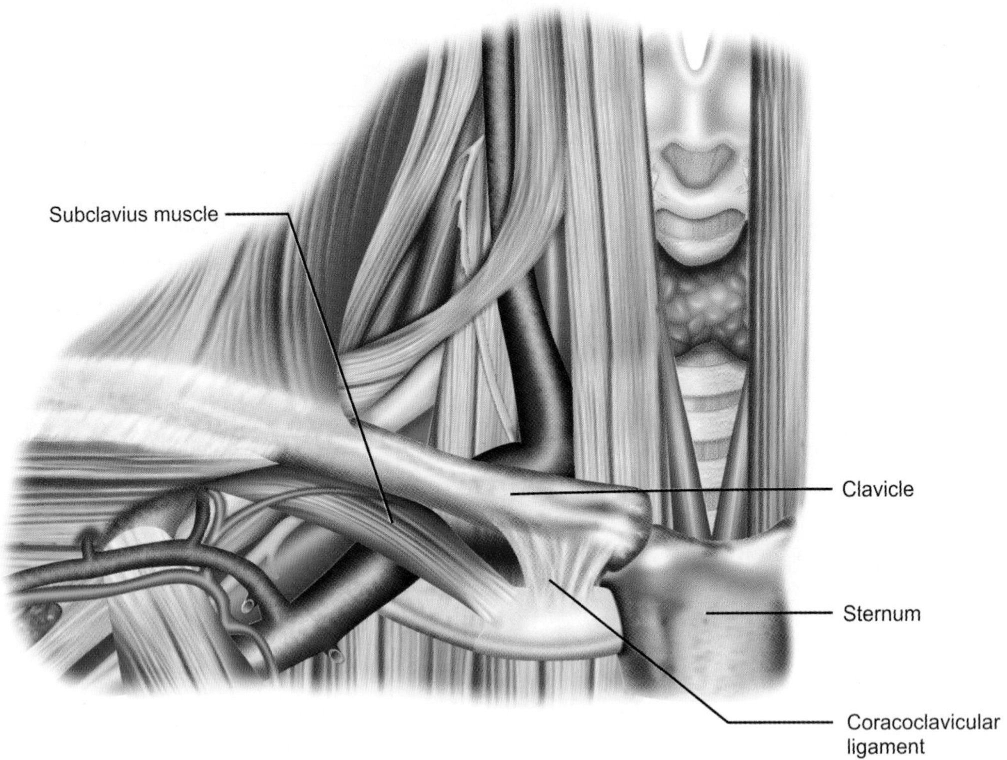

FIGURE 30 Sternoclavicular joint and subclavius muscle

STERNOCLAVICULAR JOINT–DISARTICULATION (Fig. 30)

Subclavius muscle: This was already studied while doing the upper limb dissection. Restudy this muscle. It arises from the 1st rib and costal cartilage, moves upward and laterally to be inserted into the undersurface of the clavicle in the subclavian groove.

Dissection: Detach this muscle from the undersurface of the clavicle, from the inferior side. This will preserve the nerve supply to the muscle.

Sternoclavicular Joint

It is a joint of the pectoral girdle attaching it to the trunk skeleton. It is a plane synovial joint. The medial surface of the clavicle articulates with the upper facet on the manubrium sternum. It is covered by capsule on all sides and is thicker anteriorly.

Costoclavicular ligament: Locate this ligament on the undersurface of the medial end of the clavicle and the upper surface of the 1st costal cartilage.

Dissection: Cut through the capsule anteriorly and open the joint cavity and see the intraarticular disc. It is a thick fibrocartilagenous disc. The capsule is attached to its periphery. The cartilagenous disc is inferiorly attached to the first rib. Gliding and rotatory movements are feasible at this joint. Detach the clavicle by separating it near the joint.

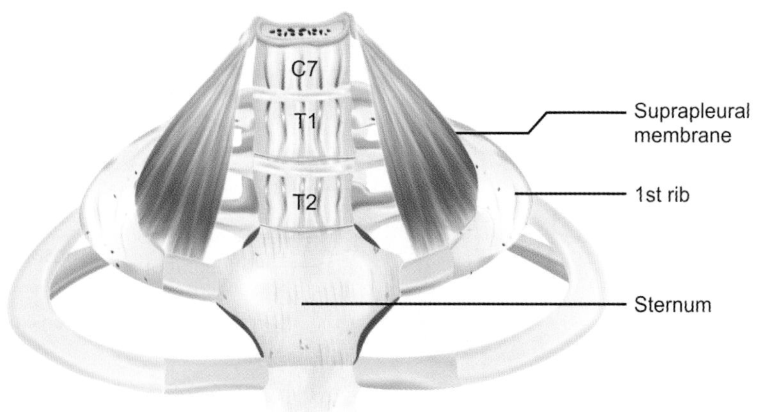

FIGURE 31 Inlet of thorax

INLET OF THORAX (Fig. 31)

The inlet of thorax is formed by the 1st thoracic vertebra, the 1st rib and the upper border of manubrium sternum. The rib is obliquely placed. The upper border of the manubrium lies at the level of the lower border of the 2nd thoracic vertebra. The inlet is closed on either side by the suprapleural membrane covering the lung and pleura. The trachea, esophagus and the neurovascular bundle passes in the midline between the two lungs. Due to the obliquity of the 1st rib all the structures passing between the thorax and the neck are exposed above the 1st rib, but they are covered by the positioning of the clavicle and subclavius muscle. The gap between the scapula, outer border of first rib and the clavicle is the apex of the axilla through which the neurovascular bundle reaches the upper limb (See the bony parts on a skeleton).

Suprapleural membrane/Sibson's fascia/scalenus minimus: This is the fascia covering the pleura. Locate its extent. This is the scalenus minimus muscle which is totally replaced by membrane. It arises from the tip of the transverse process of the 7th cervical vertebra and is inserted into the inner border of the first rib. Feel this from both thorax side and neck side. Clear this fascia to see the continuity of the structures from the thorax.

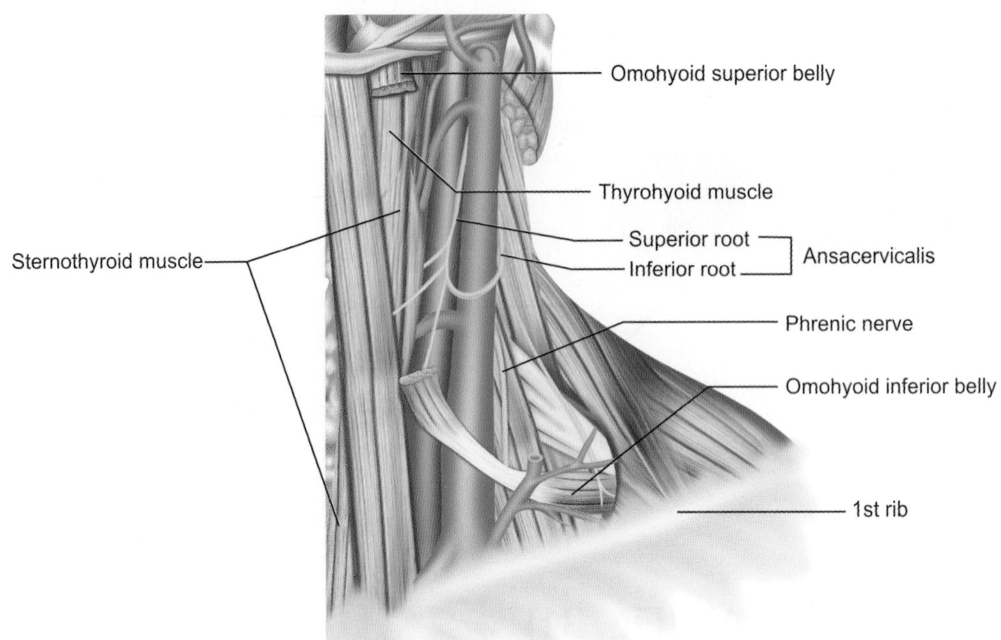

FIGURE 32 Muscular triangle and ansa cervicalis

MUSCULAR TRIANGLE

STUDY OF MUSCLES (Fig. 32)

Here the muscles are arranged in two layers—a superficial sternohyoid and omohyoid and a deeper sternothyroid and thyrohyoid muscles.

Omohyoid muscle: It arises from the body and the greater horn of the hyoid bone. Note a thick sling of connective tissue that connects the intermediate tendon to the back of the clavicle. Lift up this muscle and look for the nerve supplying the bellies on their undersurface. They are supplied by branches of the ansa cervicalis.

Sternohyoid: Note this muscle medial to the omohyoid. It arises from the back of the manubrium sternum and is inserted into the lower border of the body of the hyoid. Trace the nerve of supply from the ansa cervicalis into this muscle.

Dissection: Cut the omohyoid superior belly transversely near its origin and reflect the muscle downwards.

Sternothyroid: Identify this muscle which lies deep to the sternohyoid muscle. It arises from the back of the manubrium sternum, below the origin of the sternohyoid. It is inserted into the oblique line of thyroid cartilage. It is supplied by a branch of the ansa cervicalis.

Actions: All the strap muscles depress the larynx.

Ansa Cervicalis

It is a nerve loop over the surfaces of the carotid sheath. Its loop supplies the strap muscles—omohyoid both the bellies, sternohyoid and sternothyroid muscles.

Dissection: Identify this nerve loop now. The nerve loop lies outside the carotid sheath in its wall. Put plenty of water over the carotid sheath. The connective yields and the nerves stand out.

Superior root of ansa cervicalis: Trace this limb between the internal jugular vein and the common carotid artery. Trace it superiorly and note that it is a branch of the hypoglossal nerve.

Inferior root of ansa cervicalis: Look for two branches winding round the internal jugular vein joining together and joining the superior root of ansa.

Ansa cercivalis is a part of the cervical plexus. It is contributed by C1, 2 and 3 ventral rami. The C1 fibres reach ansa through hypoglossal nerve and the C2 and 3 fibres wind round the internal jugular vein.

The loop formation is variable in its position. Branches to the strap muscles are given off from the loop.

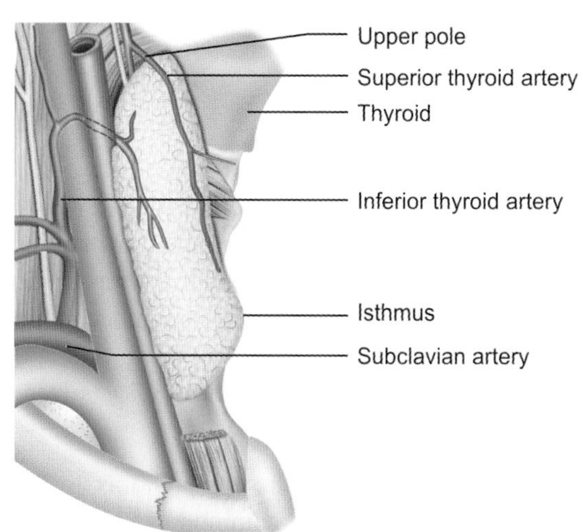

FIGURE 33 Thyroid gland

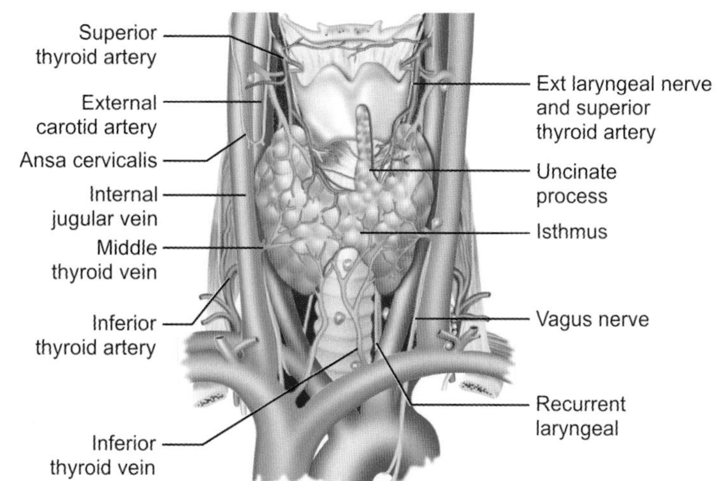

FIGURE 34 Thyroid gland—anterior view

Thyrohyoid muscle: This is also one among the muscles of muscular triangle. It arises from the oblique line on the thyroid cartilage and is inserted into the lower border of the greater cornu of the hyoid bone. It is supplied by C1 fibres through a branch of the hypoglossal nerve. It is an elevator of larynx. Trace the nerve into the muscle.

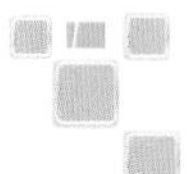

THYROID AND PARATHYROID (Figs 33 and 34)

Dissection: Cut and remove the sternohyoid and sternothyroid muscles. These form the superficial relation of the thyroid gland. The thyroid and parathyroid are connected to the trachea by pretracheal fascia. Clean the pretracheal fascia and see the thyroid and parathyroid glands. They are endocrine glands located in the midline in the lower part of neck. Identify this organ, see its parts and blood supply. The thyroid gland presents two lobes and an isthmus.

Lobes: Locate them on the sides. They are conical in shape. The upper pointed end extends up to the oblique line of thyroid cartilage. Inferiorly it is broader and extends up to the inlet of thorax. Each lobe presents a medial surface, anterior surface and a posterior surface.

Note: That the medial surface is related to the trachea and esophagus at its lower part, larynx and pharynx at its upper part. The posterior surface is related to carotid sheath. Anterior surface is overlapped by the strap muscles.

The isthmus lies over the 2, 3, and 4th tracheal rings. Levator glandulae thyroid is a small strip of the glandular tissue extends from the left side of the upper border of the isthmus to the hyoid bone. It is variable in size.

Blood Supply

Identify the superior thyroid artery at the upper pole of the gland. The ***superior thyroid artery*** divides into anterior and posterior branches, trace them as for as possible. The superior thyroid artery is accompanied by external laryngeal nerve. Trace it to the cricothyroid muscle. The ***inferior thyroid artery*** enters the lower pole of the thyroid. It arises from the 1st part of the subclavian artery. This branch supplies the inferior part of the thyroid gland. The ***thyroidea ima artery*** is a branch of the aorta and enters the lower border of the isthmus.

Veins: Generally there are three veins draining the thyroid lobes. The superior and middle thyroid veins drain into the internal jugular vein and the inferior thyroid vein drains the isthmus into the brachiocephalic vein. The ***lymphatic drainage*** accompanies the veins. Trace the recurrent laryngeal nerve which accompanies the inferior thyroid artery. The association of the nerve to the artery is to be taken care of during thyroid surgeries.

Dissection: Separate one half of the thyroid gland from the trachea take it out to see the way which is moulded to fit into the viscera. Study the posterior aspect and locate the parathyroid glands.

Parathyroid glands: Clean the connective capsule and locate the parathyroid glands. The superior parathyroid lies in the middle of the gland. The inferior parathyroid gland lies nearer to the inferior pole of the thyroid.

NEUROVASCULAR BUNDLE

The subclavian artery, its branches, the common carotid artery, the internal carotid artery, the external carotid artery and its branches form the arterial system in the neck. The anterior, external and internal jugular veins with their tributaries form the venous system. The 9th, 10th, 11th and 12th cranial nerves, the cervical and brachial plexus and the sympathetic chain form the nerves of the neck. Superficial and deep lymph nodes accompany these veins. The brachiocephalic trunk divides into common carotid artery and the subclavian artery on the right side whereas the common carotid and subclavian arteries arise independently from the arch of the aorta on the left side. Locate and trace these vessels from the thorax.

Carotid sheath: It is the thick fascial sheath which encloses the neurovascular bundle from the upper thorax to the base of the skull. It encloses the internal jugular vein and vagus nerve throughout its extent, the common carotid artery in the lower part and internal carotid artery in its upper part. It encloses the glossopharyngeal and the accessory nerve along with the vagus nerve in its upper part.

Dissection: Feel the internal jugular vein, the common carotid artery and the internal carotid artery. Clean the carotid sheath and expose the contents. Within the carotid triangle identify the internal jugular vein, internal carotid artery, the vagus nerve and the accessory nerve.

VEINS (Fig. 35)

Identify the major veins, the external jugular, subclavian, internal jugular and the brachiocephalic veins; if possible locate its tributaries.

External jugular vein: It lies superficial to the sternocleidomastoid and receives veins of the posterior region—the transverse cervical and the dorsal scapular. It receives the anterior jugular vein from the anterior aspect (already identified).

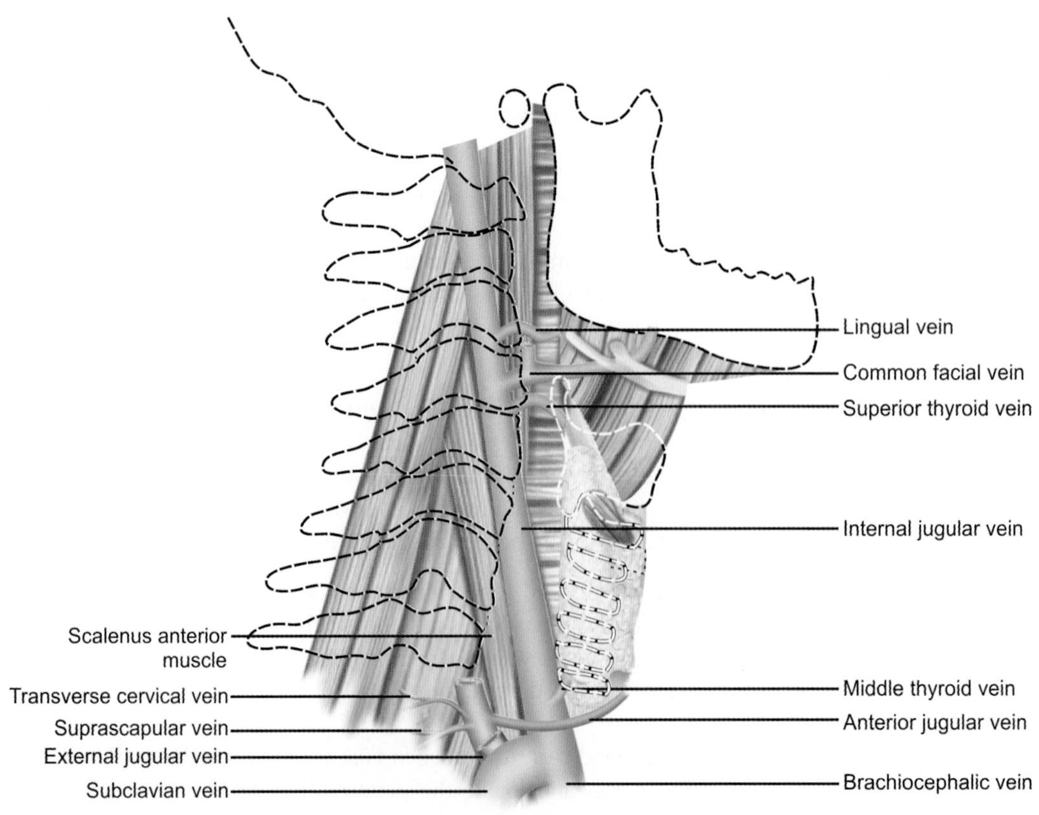

FIGURE 35 Veins of neck

The subclavian vein: It extends from the outer border of the 1st rib to the inner aspect of the sternoclavicular joint, where it joins with the internal jugular vein to form the brachiocephalic vein. It receives external jugular veins.

Brachiocephalic vein: This descends down from the sternoclavicular joint to the 1st rib. It receives the veins accompanying the branch of the subclavian artery. It receives vertebral, inferior thyroid, internal thoracic and superior intercostals veins.

Thoracic duct: Locate this lymphatic duct on the left side. It is in front of the 7th cervical vertebra, crosses the subclavian artery and suprapleural membrane to reach the left brachiocephalic vein and empties into it (the thoracic duct the big lymphatic channel has already been identified in the thorax). Trace it up, to its termination.

Right lymphatic duct is a smaller channel. It opens into the right brachiocephalic vein near its formation.

Internal jugular vein: Identify this vein by cleaning the connective tissue of the carotid sheath. It enters the neck at the level of the jugular foramen. It descends down parallel to the carotid arteries. Try to locate its tributaries—the common facial vein, lingual vein, superior thyroid vein, the middle thyroid vein, the subclavian vein and the anterior jugular vein. Except the anterior jugular vein all the other veins accompany the corresponding arteries.

Dissection: Cut the subclavian vein, external jugular vein and the internal jugular vein. Remove them leaving a part of the brachiocephalic vein in situ.

SUBCLAVIAN TRIANGLE

The area between the middle 1/3rd of clavicle, inferior belly of omohyoid and posterior border of sternocleidomastoid muscle is the subclavian triangle. This lodges the subclavian vessels, brachial plexus and other nerves.

SUBCLAVIAN ARTERY (Fig. 36)

The subclavian artery is the artery of the upper limb. It leaves the thorax, crosses over the root of the neck to reach the axilla of the upper limb at the outer border of first rib. Trace the subclavian artery. Note its relation to the scalenus anterior muscle. Conventionally it is divided into three parts—1st part from the sternoclavicular joint to the medial border of the scalenus anterior, the second part—behind the scalenus anterior and the third part between the lateral border of the scalenus anterior to the outer border of 1st rib.

Dissection: Detach the scalenus anterior from the scalene tubercle, lift it up preserve the phrenic nerve which lies on the scalenus anterior muscle. Trace the branches of subclavian artery.

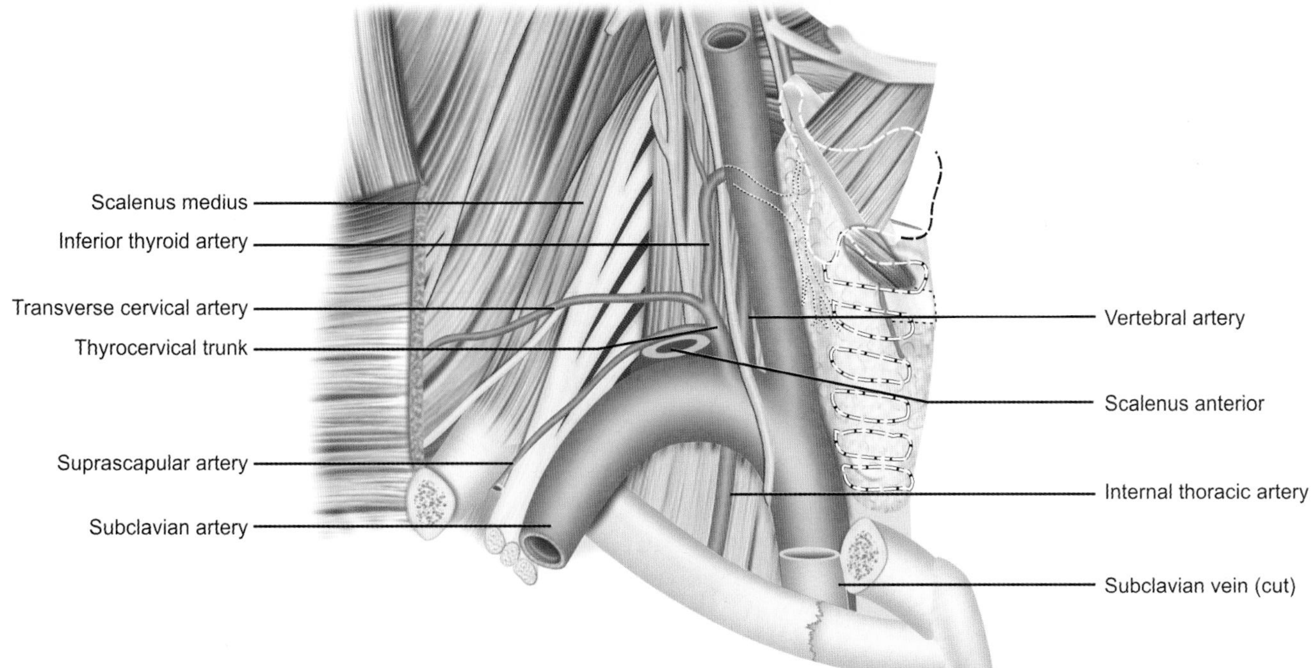

FIGURE 36 Subclavian artery

Vertebral artery: It is the first branch of the subclavian artery, arises from the anterior aspect, near the transverse process of the 7th cervical vertebra, lies between the scalenus anterior and longus coli and enters the foramen transversarium of the 6th cervical vertebrae.

Thyrocervical trunk: It is the lateral branch from the superior aspect of the subclavian artery. It generally gives off three branches. The ***inferior thyroid artery*** turns medially to enter into the posteroinferior aspect of the thyroid gland. The ***transverse cervical artery***—trace this artery across the scalenus anterior and the levator scapulae, there it divides into two branches, the superficial branch enters the deep aspect of the trapezius along with the accessory nerve and the deeper branch goes deeper to levator scapulae and rhomboidei along the medial border of the scapula. These branches were already studied in the dissection of the upper limb.

Internal thoracic artery: It arises from the inferior aspect of the subclavian artery crosses the suprapleural membrane reaches the posterior aspect of the sternoclavicular joint (its thoracic part was already dissected in thoracic).

From the second part of the subclavian artery: Locate this artery by pulling the artery forwards and look for its branches. The ***superior intercostal artery*** runs down close to the first two ribs and gives off branches into the intercostals spaces. The ***deep cervical artery*** ascends up in front of the scalenus anterior and transverse process of cervical vertebrae and gives off number of muscular branches.

The **third part of the subclavian artery** does not have any branches.

CAROTID ARTERIES (Fig. 37)

Dissection: Clean the carotid sheath and identify the artery at a superficial plane. Note that the common carotid artery divides into internal and external carotid artery opposite the upper border of thyroid cartilage.

Common carotid artery: On the right side it is a branch of the brachiocephalic trunk, on the left side it is a branch directly from the arch of the aorta. Trace it down to its origin.

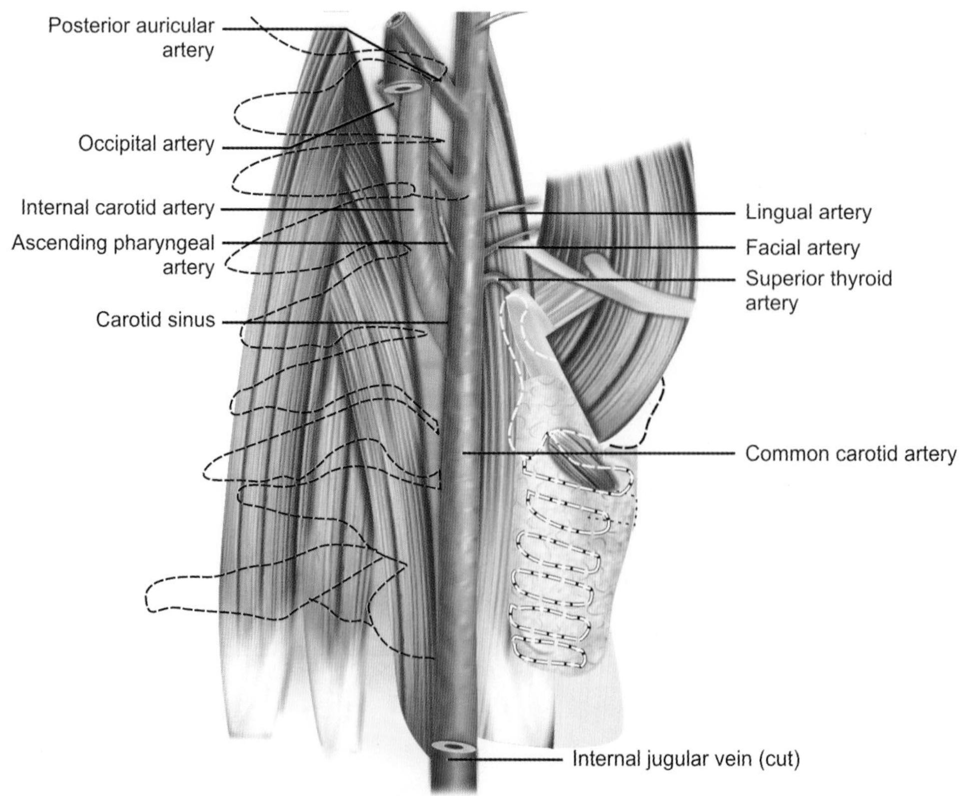

FIGURE 37 Carotid arteries

Carotid sinus: This is the enlarged upper end of the common carotid artery near its division. At this point the artery has got specialized nerve endings which act as baroreceptors.

Internal carotid artery: This is the artery which supplies brain. It ascends up to the carotid canal in the skull without giving any branche in the neck. It lies parallel and posterior to the external carotid artery. It lies within the carotid sheath throughout its extent.

External carotid artery: It is the artery of the neck and face. It gives off number of branches to supply these regions. Identify the following branches of the external carotid artery.

Dissection: Clean the connective tissue and identify the branches arising from the external carotid artery.

Superior thyroid artery: This is the first artery from the anterior surface of the *external carotid artery above the level* of superior horn of thyroid cartilage. Trace its branches—the infrahyoid branch which runs along the lower border of hyoid bone; the superior laryngeal artery which pierces the thyrohyoid membrane, the muscular branches to sternocleidomastoid and cricothyroid muscle; anterior and posterior thyroid branches near the apex of the thyroid gland.

Lingual artery: It is the next branch from the anterior aspect of the external carotid. It is given off at the level of the greater cornua of hyoid. It presents a looped appearance and disappears under cover of mylohyoid muscle. The branches of the artery can be seen at a later dissection.

Facial artery: Locate this artery immediately above the lingual artery. Trace this artery to the angle of mandible. There it gives off ascending palatine, tonsillar, glandular branches to submandibular gland and submental branch which accompanies the mylohyoid nerve to supply anterior belly of digastric and mylohyoid muscle. Try to see these branches. Beyond this the artery is already traced in the face.

Occipital artery: Note this branch which is given off from the posterior aspect of the external carotid artery near the greater cornua of hyoid, opposite to the facial artery. Trace this artery to the mastoid process along the lower border of posterior belly of digastric muscle, and into the suboccipital triangle where it is already studied. It gives off muscular branches to sternocleidomastoid muscle, and meningeal branch to pass through the jugular foramen.

Posterior auricular artery: This is another artery given off from the posterior aspect. This runs towards the back of the ear along the upper border of the posterior belly of digastric muscle.

Ascending pharyngeal artery: Pull the external carotid artery laterally and look for a small branch of this artery, the ascending pharyngeal artery. It supplies the muscles of pharynx.

Superficial temporal and the maxillary arteries are the terminal branches of the external carotid and are seen in face dissection.

Dissection: Cut and remove the veins you can cut and remove the common carotid artery. Cut the branches of the external carotid artery near their emergence and remove the external carotid artery upto the angle of mandible. This gives a clearer view to visualize the nerves.

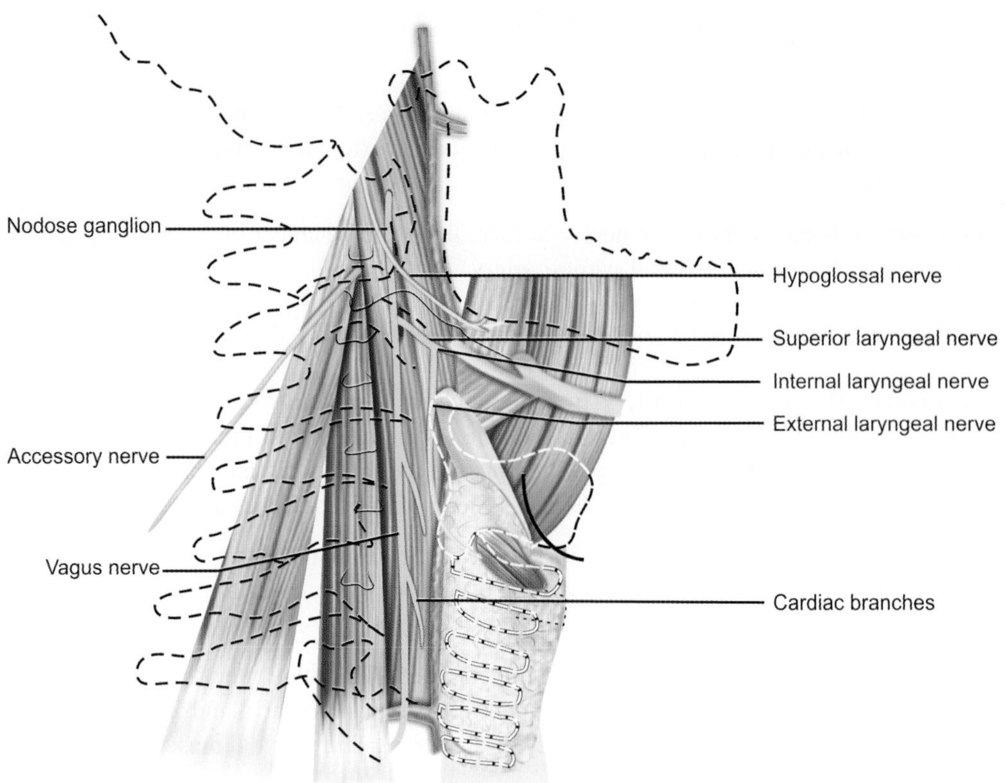

FIGURE 38 Cranial nerves

CRANIAL NERVES (Fig. 38)

9th, 10th, 11th and 12th cranial nerves, and all the cervical nerves forming the cervical and brachial plexus and sympathetic chain are located in the neck region. The cranial nerves are located in the carotid sheath along with the blood vessels. The spinal nerves lie between the scalenus anterior and scalenus medius muscles. The sympathetic chain lies in front of the transverse processes of the vertebrae. Try to locate them.

Hypoglossal nerve: It is the 12th cranial nerve. Locate this nerve between the internal jugular vein and internal carotid artery and inferior to the occipital artery. Trace it across the external carotid artery and crossing the lingual artery to enter deep to the mylohyoid muscle.

Accessory nerve: The 11th cranial nerve lies posterior and lateral to internal jugular vein. It enters the sternocleidomastoid near the posterior belly of digastric.

Vagus nerve: It is the 10th cranial nerve. Identify it in the interval between the internal jugular vein, internal and common carotid arteries. Trace it down into the thorax.

Superior laryngeal nerve is a branch of the vagus nerve. Locate this nerve deep to the carotid artery, trace it forwards. It accompanies the superior thyroid artery. The superior laryngeal nerve gives off the internal and external laryngeal nerves. Trace the internal laryngeal nerve along with the laryngeal branch of superior thyroid artery to the thyrohyoid membrane, the external laryngeal nerve runs down to supply the cricothyroid muscle.

Glossopharyngeal nerve: It is the 9th cranial nerve and will be seen at a later dissection.

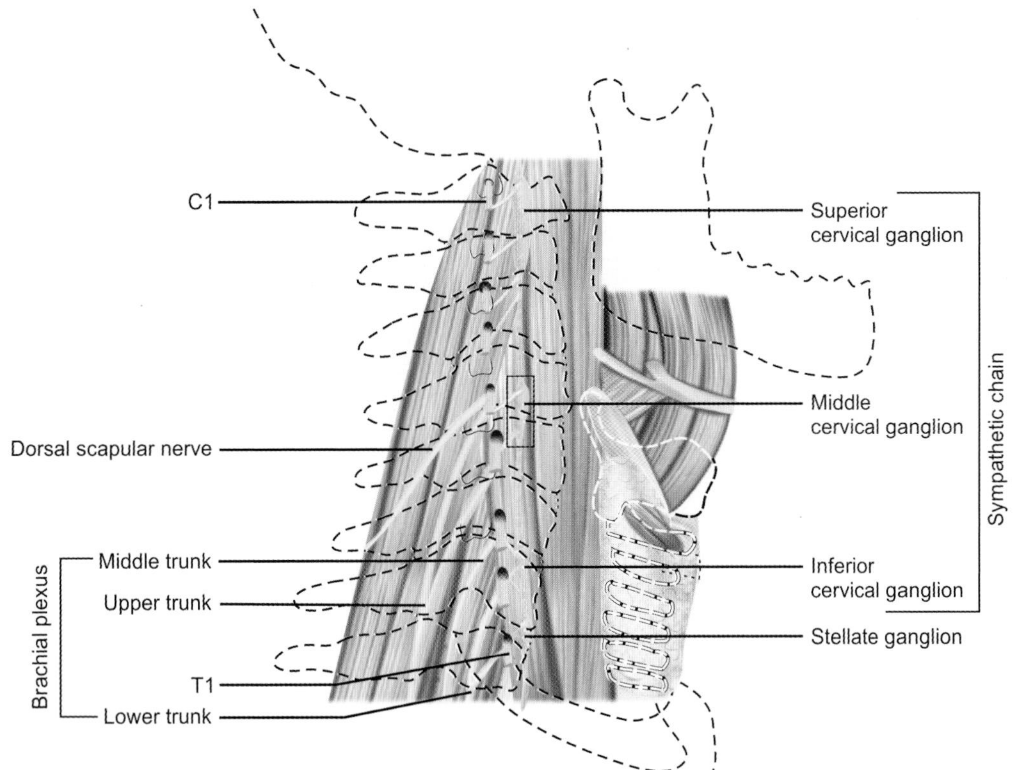

FIGURE 39 Sympathetic chain and spinal nerves

SYMPATHETIC CHAIN AND SPINAL NERVES (Fig. 39)

Sympathetic trunk: Pull the carotid vessels medially with a hook and see the sympathetic chain in front of the transverse processes of the cervical vertebrae. Trace its total length. Look for the superior cervical ganglion in front of the 2nd and 3rd cervical vertebrae, the middle cervical ganglion near the 5th cervical vertebra and the inferior cervical ganglion near the neck of the first rib. The inferior cervical ganglion joins with the 1st thoracic nerve to form the stellate ganglion.

Ansa subclavia: Trace this loop between the middle and inferior cervical ganglia in front of the subclavian artery on the right side.

Gray rami communicantes: These connect the superior cervical ganglion to upper 4 cervical nerves, middle cervical ganglion to 5th and 6th cervical nerves and the inferior cervical ganglion to 7th, 8th cervical nerves, trace as many as possible.

Visceral branches are given off to pharynx, esophagus and heart. These are medial branches, trace as many as possible.

Vascular branches: These accompany the blood vessels, trace as many as you can.

Cervical ventral rami: Trace all the cervical nerves emerging between the vertebrae. They lie on the scalenus medius muscle.

All the cutaneous nerves, the great auricular, lesser occipital transverse cervical supraclavicular were already traced. Trace them to their origin from the cervical nerves and also trace the inferior root of ansa cervicalis to the C2, 3 roots.

Muscular branches: Trace these branches entering into the sternocleidomastoid, levator scapulae, scalenus anterior medius and posterior.

Brachial plexus: Trace the cervical 5,6,7,8 and T1 roots. Note that 5 and 6 join to form upper trunk, 7 forms middle trunk and C8, T1 form lower trunk. Trace these to the first rib. Note that the lower trunk lies deeper to the subclavian artery.

Long thoracic nerve/nerve to serratus anterior, dorsal scapular nerve/nerve to rhomboids, phrenic nerve to diaphragm—trace these nerves to the roots of brachial plexus.

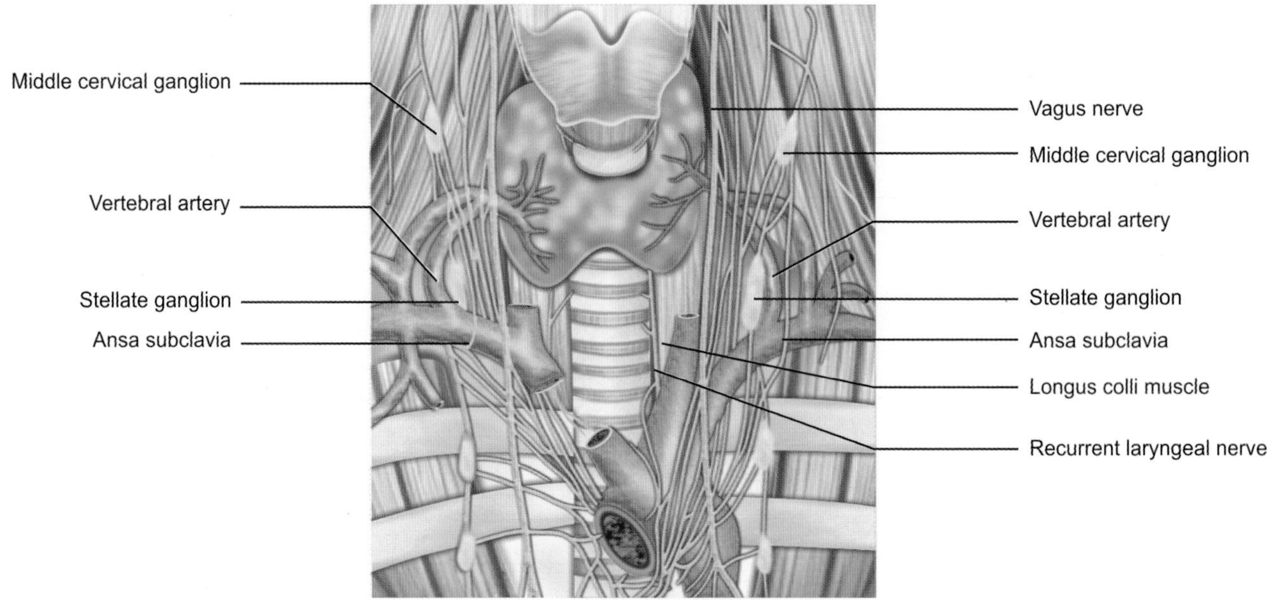

FIGURE 40 Vertebral triangle

Suprascapular nerve is given off from the upper trunk. It crosses in front of the scalenus medius deep to the omohyoid. It supplies the muscles on the posterior aspect of scapula.

Nerve to subclavius: It arises from the upper trunk. Trace it down across the subclavian artery to reach the upper surface of the subclavius muscle.

Phrenic nerve: Note this nerve on the anterior surface of the scalenus anterior muscle and trace it into thorax. This nerve supplies diaphragm and it has already been traced.

VERTEBRAL TRIANGLE (Fig. 40)

It is the area between the longus colli, 1st rib and scalenus anterior muscle.

Dissection: Cut the 1st rib near the scalenus anterior on either side and remove it with the sternum. Identify the continuations of the structures from the neck into the thorax. Trace the arch of the aorta and its branches, the brachiocephalic trunk, the left common carotid artery and the left subclavian artery. Trace the trachea and esophagus. Try to see the following nerves near the neck of the first rib.

Stellate ganglion: It is the inferior sympathetic ganglion. Identify this in front of the neck of the first rib. Note the ansa subclavian arising from here to connect this with the middle cervical sympathetic ganglion.

Vertebral artery: See this arising from the superior aspect of the first part of the vertebral artery. Trace it into the 6th foramen transversarium.

First thoracic nerve: Trace this nerve to join the 8th cervical nerve to form the lower trunk of the brachial plexus.

Recurrent laryngeal nerve: Trace this nerve from the vagus and looping around the subclavian artery on the right side. On the left side it is given at a much higher level. Trace this nerve into the groove between the trachea and esophagus.

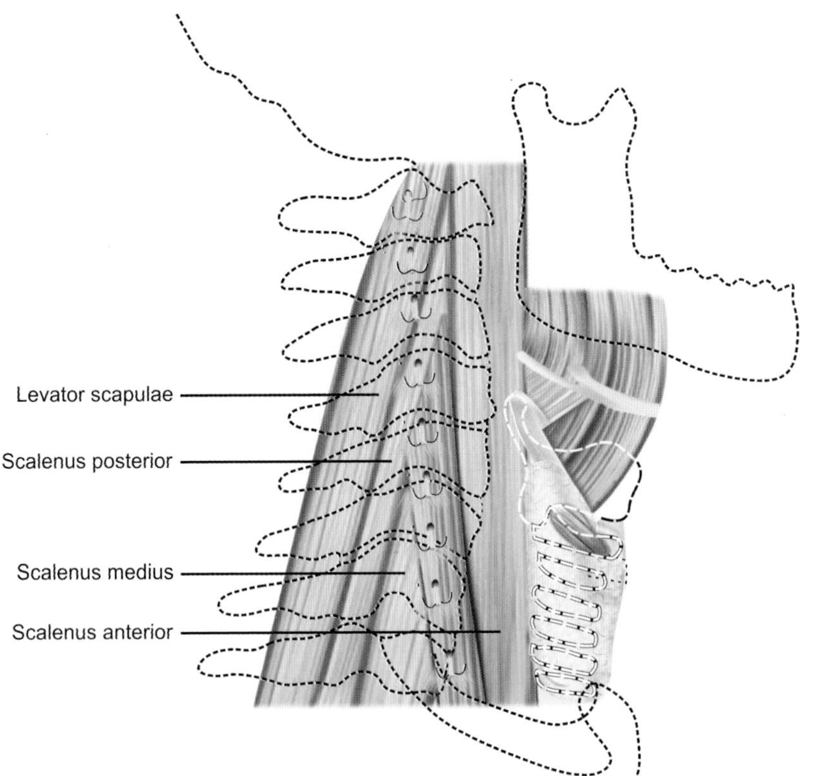

FIGURE 41 Lateral musculature

MUSCULATURE (Fig. 41)

Scalenus anterior muscle: Clean the scalenus anterior muscle. It arises from the transverse processes of 3rd to 6th cervical vertebrae. The three heads join together and descend down to reach the scalene tubercle on the inner border of the 1st rib. The muscle separates subclavian vein from the subclavian artery. Remove this muscle totally preserving the phrenic nerve. This muscle is already detached, trace it to its origin.

Scalenus medius: This muscle lies posterior to the brachial plexus. It arises from the posterior tubercles of the transverse processes of 2nd to 6th cervical vestebrae. The fibres join together to insert into the superior surface of the first rib, posterior to the groove for the subclavian artery.

Scalenus posterior: This is a small muscle arising from the 3rd to 6th posterior tubercles of the transverse processes and is inserted into the external surface of the middle of the second rib.

Ventral musculature: Try to identify the following musculature, after studying all the viscera.

Longus colli: It is the muscle on the ventral aspect of the vertebral column. Push the viscera medially and try to locate the muscle. It extends from the transverse processes to the bodies of the cervical vertebra and upper three thoracic vertebrae. Superiorly it reaches the anterior tubercle of atlas.

Nerves: These are all supplied by the segmental cervical nerves.

Action: All these muscles are flexors of the cervical vertebrae.

Rectus capitis anterior: This is a ventral muscle. Try to see this in a dissected specimen. It extends from the lateral mass of atlas, to the base of the skull in front of condyles. It is a flexor of the occiput.

Rectus capitis lateralis: It is an anterolateral muscle. It arises from the superior surface of the transverse process of atlas and gets inserted into the jugular process of the occipital bone. It is a lateral rotator. It is supplied by the ventral ramus of first cervical nerve. Trace this nerve between the above two muscle. It supplies both the muscles.

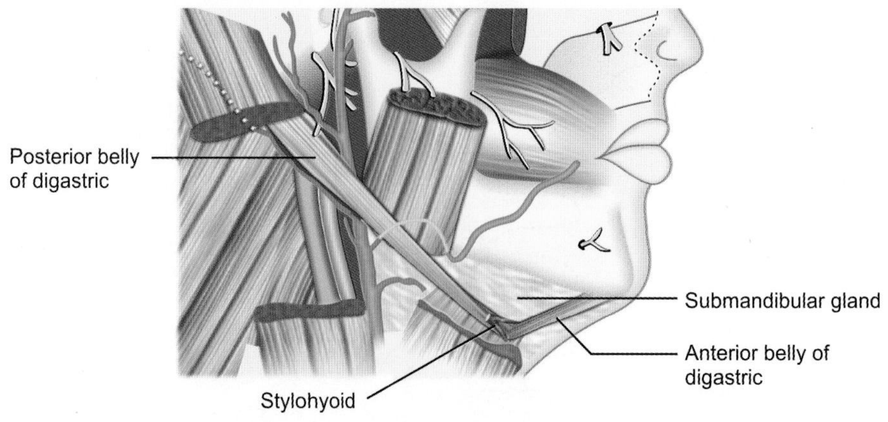

FIGURE 42 Digastric triangle

DIGASTRIC TRIANGLE (Fig. 42)

Stylohyoid muscle: Note this superficial muscle. It arises from the styloid process, lies superficial to the posterior belly of digastric, clasps the intermediate tendon of digastric to the hyoid bone. It is supplied by the facial nerve.

Dissection: Cut the tendon near the insertion, pull the muscle up, and look for its nerve supply.

Digastric muscle: It has got two bellies, it extends from mastoid process to the chin. Note the posterior belly near the angle of the mandible and trace it to its origin. It arises from a groove medial to the mastoid process. Note the anterior belly near the chin. It arises from the fossa on the undersurface of the mandible. Trace it down towards the insertion. The muscle is inserted by means of an intermediate tendon which is anchored to the greater cornu of hyoid bone by the stylohyoid tendon.

The above muscles are elevators of the hyoid bone. They help in deglutition.

Dissection: Detach the tendon from the sling and cut it. Separate the two bellies. Pull them towards their origins and look for their nerve supply entering into their undersurfaces. **Nerve to posterior belly of digastric**—pull the muscle laterally look for this nerve. It is given off from the posterior auricular branch of the facial nerve. **Nerve to the anterior belly of digastric**. Pull the muscle medially and look for the nerve near its origin. It is given off from the mylohyoid branch of the inferior alveolar nerve.

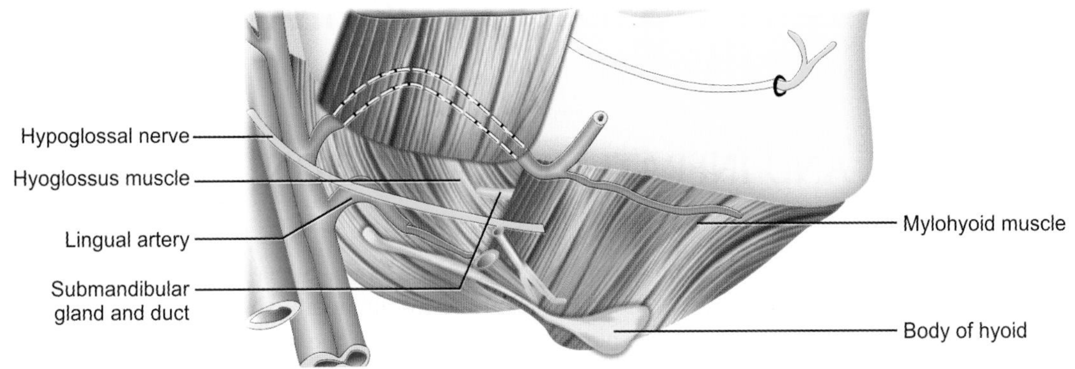

FIGURE 43 Submandibular region

SUBMANDIBULAR GLAND (Fig. 43)

Submandibular gland: It is one of the salivary glands. What is seen between the two bellies of the digastric muscle is the superficial part of the gland. Note that it is occupying the space between the mandible laterally and the mylohyoid muscle medially. Note the submandibular fossa on a mandible, which is caused by this gland.

Dissection: Separate the gland from the neighboring structures. Look for its blood supply from the facial artery. With a scissors cut the gland near its posterior margin where it turns inside to become the deep part and remove the superficial part of the gland.

Mylohyoid muscle: Identify this muscle lying deep to the submandibular salivary gland and extending up to the midline. The mylohyoid muscle arises from the mylohyoid line on the inner aspect of the body of the mandible and is inserted into the upper border of body of the hyoid bone. In the midline it joins with the muscle of the opposite side and forms a raphae. It is supplied by the mylohyoid branch of the mandibular nerve. Press the muscle and look for the nerve entering into the lateral surface of the muscle. This supplies the anterior belly of digastric also. See both the branches. It is an elevator of larynx.

Look for the free posterior border of this muscle and identify the hypoglossal nerve and the deep part of the submandibular gland and its duct disappearing behind this border.

Hyoglossus muscle: Identify this muscle lying posterior and deeper to the mylohyoid muscle. The hyoglossus muscle arises from the greater cornua of the hyoid bone. The insertion of this muscle will be seen in the tongue dissection.

Lingual artery: Note this artery passing deep to the hyoglossus muscle.

DEEP DISSECTION OF HEAD

TEMPORAL AND INFRATEMPORAL REGION

The temporal fossa is the area over the squamous part of the temporal bone. Superiorly it is limited by the superior temporal lines. Inferiorly the temporal fossa is continuous with the infratemporal fossa.

The infratemporal fossa is the area between the pterygoid plates, base of the skull and the mandible (*Identify these on the skull*).

Temporal and infratemporal region are occupied by muscles of mastication. The temporomandibular joint lies surrounded by its muscles. The neurovascular bundle to supply this region is mandibular nerve and second part of maxillary artery.

Masseter muscle (Fig. 44): It is a thick muscle on the lateral aspect of the ramus of the mandible. It arises from the inferior margin and deep surface of the zygomatic arch. It is inserted into the lateral surface of the ramus. Note the direction of its fibres, they run downwards and posteriorly.

Action: It elevates, protracts and helps in side to side movement.

Dissection: Cut through the zygomatic arch on either side of the origin of the masseter and reflect it downwards, while doing so locate the neurovascular bundle entering on its deep surface through the mandibular notch (Cut a bit of the muscle along with the neurovascular bundle for identification at a later date).

Temporal fascia: Study this thick fascia over the temporal fossa. It is attached to the superior temporal line (locate it on the skull) above and the upper border of the zygomatic arch below. Note that while removing the masseter this margin is cut, and the temporalis below this level is devoid of the fascia. The temporal fascia gives attachment to the temporalis muscle on its deeper aspect.

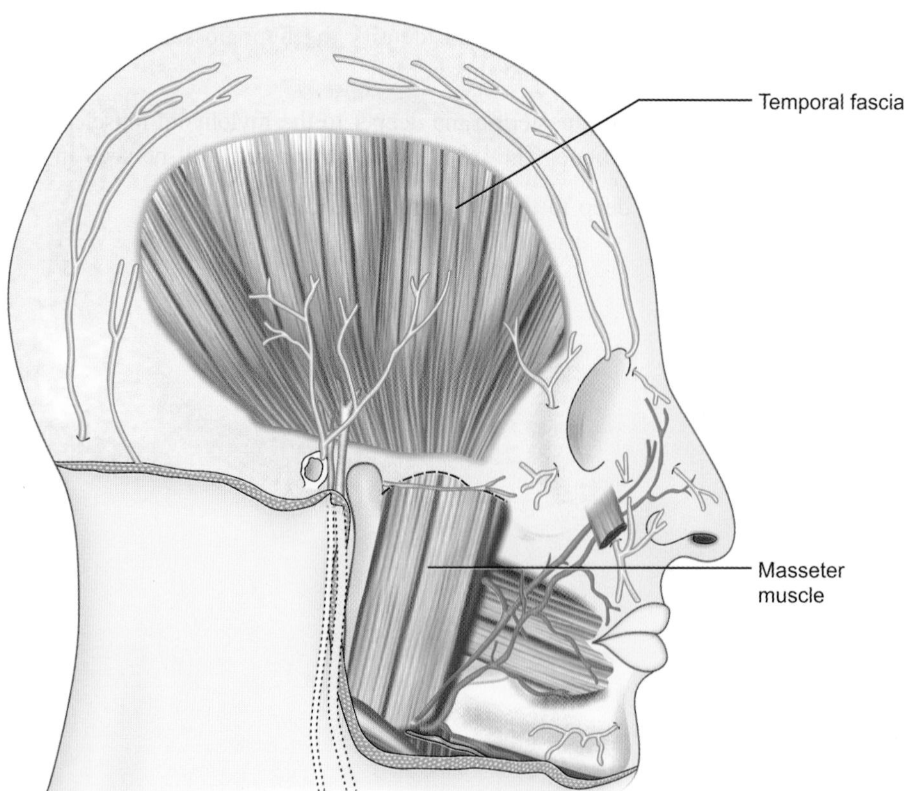

FIGURE 44 Masseter muscle and temporal fascia

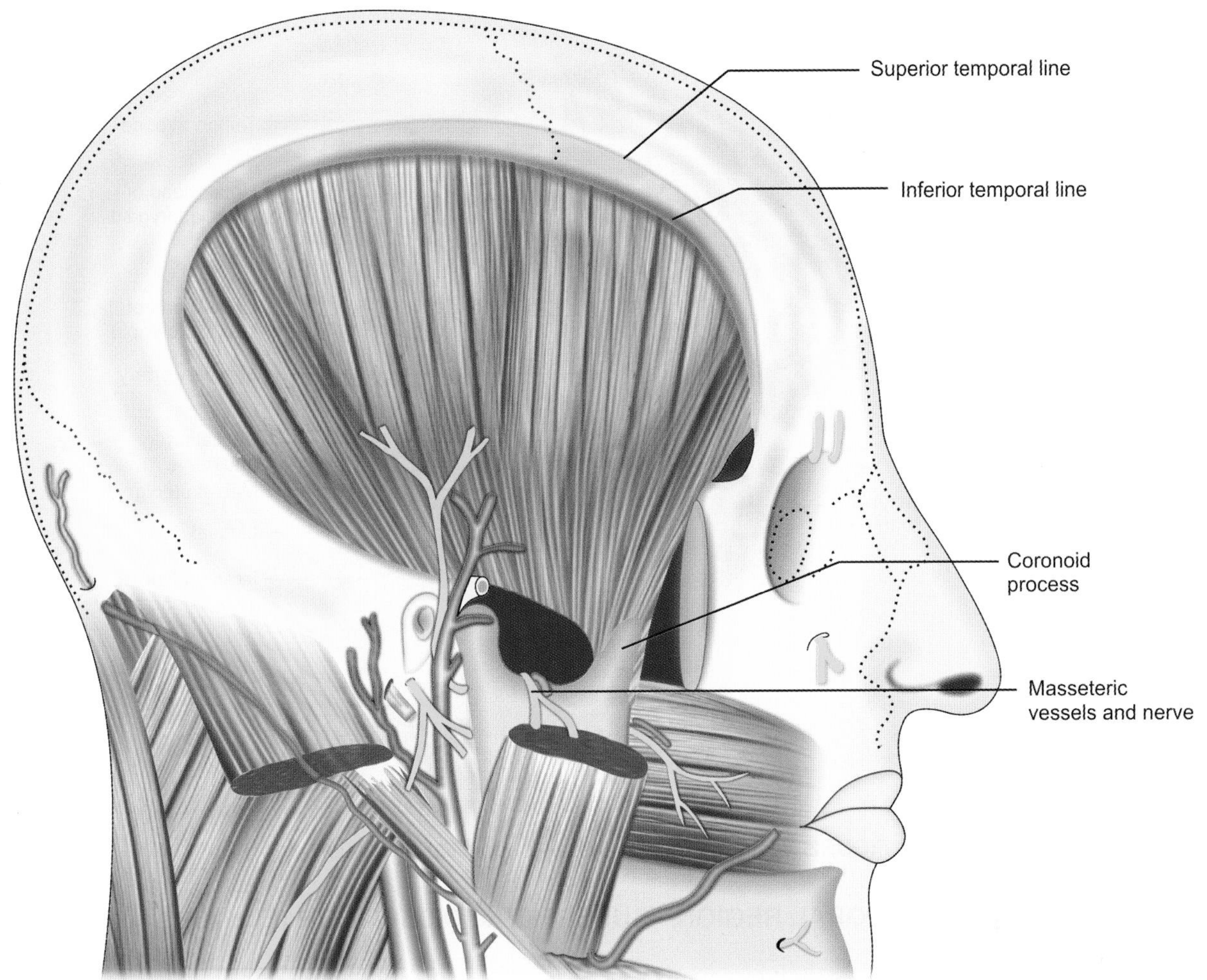

FIGURE 45 Temporalis muscle

Temporalis muscle (Fig. 45): It is a fan-shaped muscle occupying the temporal fossa. The muscle arises from the temporal fossa up to the inferior temporal line and from the temporal fascia. Note its insertion into the coronoid process, along its anterior border and inner surface. Note the direction of the fibres. The posterior fibres traverse horizontally and the anterior fibres traverse vertically. The muscle is a retractor and an elevator.

Dissection: Saw and cut the coronoid process by an oblique cut and remove the lower part of the muscle to see the neurovascular bundle on its undersurface between the muscle and temporal bone. The arteries are two in number and are called deep temporal arteries. The nerves are temporal nerves and they arise from the anterior division of the mandibular nerve.

Stylomandibular ligament: Locate the styloid process and trace this ligament to the angle of the mandible. It is the deep part of the parotid fascia, acts as a sling to suspend mandible.

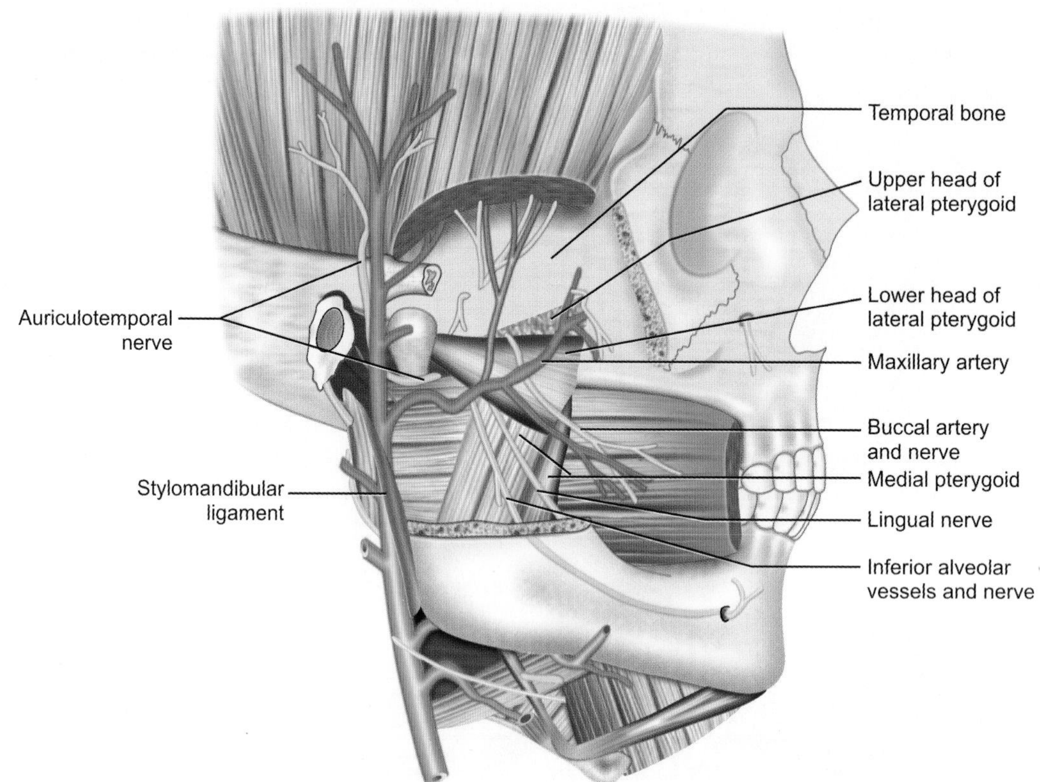

FIGURE 46 Infratemporal fossa—superficial dissection

INFRATEMPORAL REGION—SUPERFICIAL DISSECTION (Fig. 46)

Dissection: Remove the masseter totally and cut the ramus of the mandible by two cuts. The upper cut just below the neck of the mandible and a lower cut from the lower end of the anterior border of the mandible to the angle of the mandible. Remove the bone and clean and identify the structures seen in the fossa. While cutting put a forceps deep to the bone and take care of the nerves that lie deep. Let the cut go above lingula of mandible.

Maxillary artery second part: It is a superficial structure seen in here. It generally runs across the lateral pterygoid, or it goes deep, either below the inferior head or between the two heads of lateral pterygoid muscle. Locate the muscular branches to masseter, temporalis, pterygoid muscles and the buccal artery, accompanying the buccal branch of mandibular nerve.

The buccal branch of mandibular nerve is a sensory branch to supply the buccal pad of fat and the skin over the cheek. Locate this nerve passing between the two heads of lateral pterygoid to the cheek.

Lateral pterygoid muscle: This muscle occupies the upper part of the fossa. It arises by two heads, the upper head from the inferior surface of the greater wing of sphenoid, the lower head from the outer surface of the lateral pterygoid plate (confirm these parts on skull). The two bellies unite together to be inserted into the pterygoid fossa on the neck of the mandible. Note that its fibres ascend up from below, and run posteriorly from the front. It is a depressor, protractor and also helps in side to side movement. It is supplied by mandibular nerve on its deeper surface.

Medial pterygoid muscle: This occupies the lower area of the infratemporal fossa. It has a superficial and a deep head. The superficial head arises from the maxillary tuberosity and the deep head arises from the medial aspect of the lateral pterygoid plate. These two heads soon unite and get inserted into the medial aspect of the angle and ramus of the mandible (see them on the skull). Note that the fibres run downwards, posteriorly and laterally. It is an elevator, protractor and helps in side to side movement. Nerve supply is given off from the trunk of the mandibular nerve. It enters the infratemporal fossa through the foramen ovale (locate this foramen on the skull). Locate this nerve near the base of the skull.

Mandibular nerve: It is a branch of the trigeminal nerve. It leaves cranial cavity through the foramen ovale. As soon as it enters the infratemporal fossa it gives off three branches from the trunk, and then divides into an anterior division and a posterior division. ***The trunk*** gives off the nervus spinous, nerve to medial pterygoid, nerve to tensor tympani. ***The anterior division*** is predominantly a motor division except for buccal nerve which is a sensory branch. ***The posterior division*** is predominantly sensory nerve except for the motor branch to the mylohyoid muscle and the anterior belly of digastric.

The anterior division gives off the nerve to the masseter, lateral pterygoid, deep temporal nerves. Its sensory branch is the buccal branch. All these nerves are already identified. All of them were seen between the base of the skull and the lateral pterygoid muscle.

The posterior division gives off three branches, the lingual, buccal and the inferior alveolar nerves. Locate the lingual nerve which is a thick nerve and runs from the lower border of the lateral pterygoid muscle, in an anterior direction to reach the side of the tongue. Pull it forwards and locate the chorda tympani nerve joining it on its posterior side. The point of junction with the lingual nerve is variable. The lingual nerve carries general and taste sensations from the anterior 2/3rds of the tongue. Trace the ***buccal nerve*** which lies between the two heads of the lateral pterygoid to the buccal pad of fat on the buccinator muscle. Trace the ***lingual nerve*** extending from the lower border of the lateral pterygoid to the side of the tongue. Identify the ***inferior alveolar nerve*** which lies posterior to the lingual nerve. Trace this nerve to the mandibular foramen (Identify it on a dry mandible). This is the sensory nerve to the lower jaw, its terminal branch mental nerve has already been identified in face. Trace the mylohyoid nerve from the posterior aspect of the inferior alveolar nerve. It is motor to the mylohyoid and anterior belly of the digastric muscles.

Dissection: Remove the lateral pterygoid by cutting it nearer to its insertion. You may pull it out in pieces but make sure that the neurovascular bundle is not damaged. Trace the branches of mandibular nerve.

TEMPOROMANDIBULAR JOINT (Fig. 47)

This is the only synovial joint of the skull. The head of the mandible articulates with the mandibular fossa and the articular tubercle of the temporal bone. It is covered by fibrous capsule.

Lateral ligament: It extends from the articular tubercle on the zygomatic arch to the lateral aspect of the neck of the mandible.

Dissection: Cut through this ligament and look into the articular disc which separates the joint cavity into two parts. Note that the articular disc is continuous anteriorly with the tendon of the lateral pterygoid muscle. Cut the lateral ligament and see the capsule. Capsule is attached to both the proximal and distal bony parts.

Cut and remove the neck of the mandible with the articular disc.

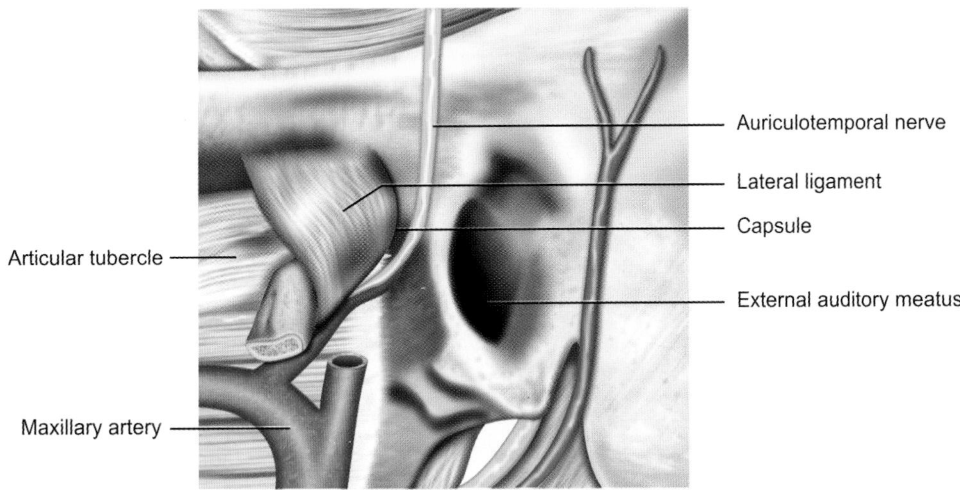

FIGURE 47 Temporomandibular joint—ligaments

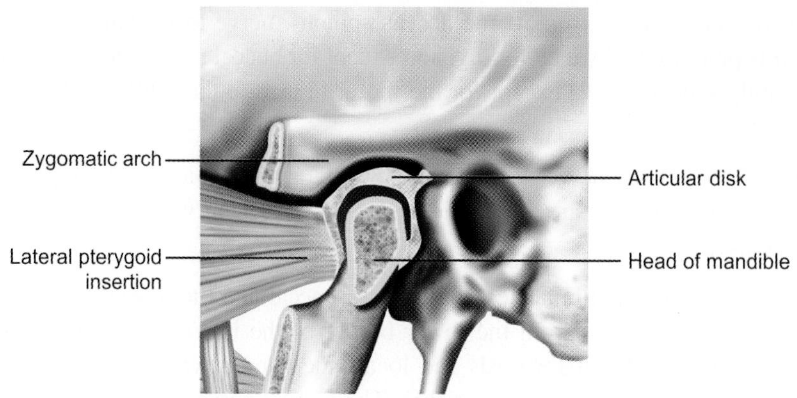

FIGURE 48 Temporomandibular joint—anterior

The articular disc (Fig. 48) is a fibrocartilaginous structure. Look that its superior surface is concavo-convex and its inferior surface is convex.

Movements: Though it is uniaxial type of joint, it performs more movements because of the presence of articular disc. Protraction, retraction, elevation, depression and side to side movements are performed here.

Study the details from a Textbook.

INFRATEMPORAL FOSSA–DEEP DISSECTION (Fig. 49)

Dissection: Cut the superficial temporal artery and remove it. Study and identify the structures seen here.

First part of the maxillary artery: Trace this artery from the external carotid artery. It is related to the neck of the mandible. It gives off five branches—auricular, anterior tympanic, accessory meningeal are fine branches. The middle meningeal artery is a bigger branch. Trace it up to the foramen spinosum. It is accompanied by the meningeal branch of the mandibular nerve. The inferior alveolar artery is another big branch. It descends down to the mandibular foramen. It enters the foramen along with the inferior alveolar nerve.

Sphenomandibular ligament: This is a thin sheet of connective tissue extending from the spine of the sphenoid (see it on the bone) to the lingula on the mandible.

Auriculotemporal nerve: It is given off from the posterior part of the posterior division of the mandibular nerve very near the skull. It generally splits into two, encloses the middle meningeal artery. It ascends posteriorly behind the neck of the mandible to supply the skin on the lateral aspect of the scalp (this has already been identified).

Otic ganglion is a parasympathetic ganglion connected to the mandibular nerve. Pull the posterior division forwards and locate this tiny ganglion with its spider like connections. It is at a deeper plane between the nerve to medial pterygoid and the tensor veli palatini.

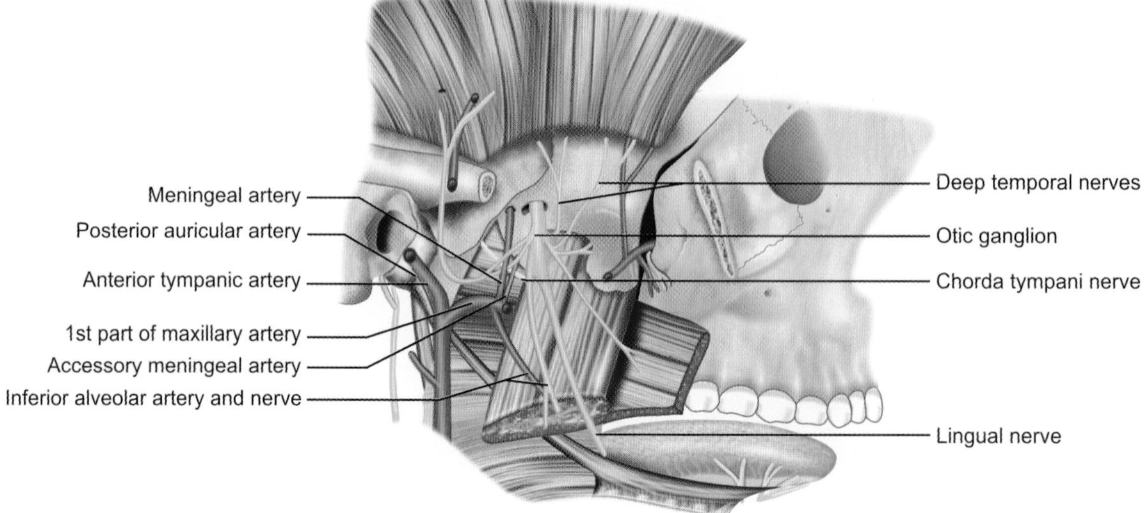

FIGURE 49 Infratemporal fossa—deep dissection

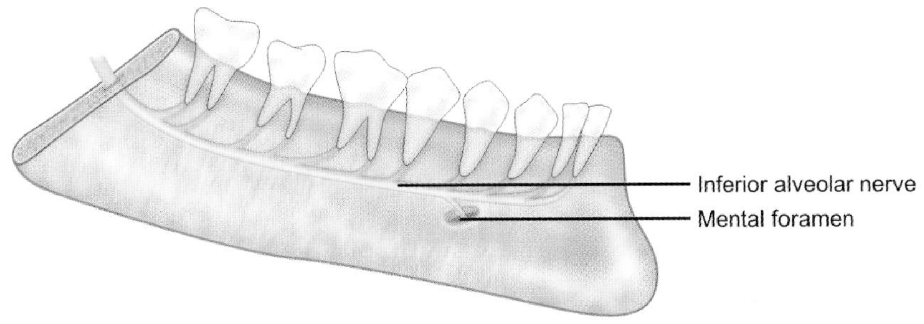

FIGURE 50 Inferior alveolar nerve

Chorda tympani nerve: Identify this nerve joining the posterior aspect of the lingual nerve. It leaves the skull through the petrotympanic fissure (identify this on the skull) and its point of joining the lingual nerve is variable in position. The chorda tympani nerve is a branch of the facial nerve and it carries the secretomotor fibres to the submandibular and sublingual salivary glands and taste sensations from the anterior two thirds of the tongue.

Dissection (Fig. 50): Chisel and chip the body of the mandible up to the point of the mental foramen. While doing this, separate the two tables of mandible, identify the inferior alveolar nerve. Remove the outer table up to the mental foramen. After seeing the inferior alveolar nerve, cut the mandible in the midline, cut the nerve near the mandibular foramen and remove the mandible. Detach the mylohyoid muscle from its origin from the mylohyoid line of the mandible. Reidentify the nerve supply from inferior alveolar nerve.

STYLOID APPARATUS (Fig. 51)

Dissection: Feel the styloid process lateral to the superior constrictor and identify the following.

Styloglossus muscle: Trace this muscle forwards and downwards to the area between the hyoglossus and mylohyoid muscle. This is one of the extrinsic muscles of the tongue. It arises from the anterior surface of the styloid process and is inserted into the lateral side of the tongue. It is a retractor of tongue.

Stylohyoid muscle: Trace this muscle from the posterior aspect of the styloid process to the hyoid bone. It arises from the posterior surface of the styloid process and at its insertion it splits into two parts clasps the intermediate tendon of the digastric to the greater cornu of hyoid bone. It is an elevator of the hyoid bone. It is supplied by the posterior branch of the facial nerve (this muscle was already cut in the digastric triangle dissection).

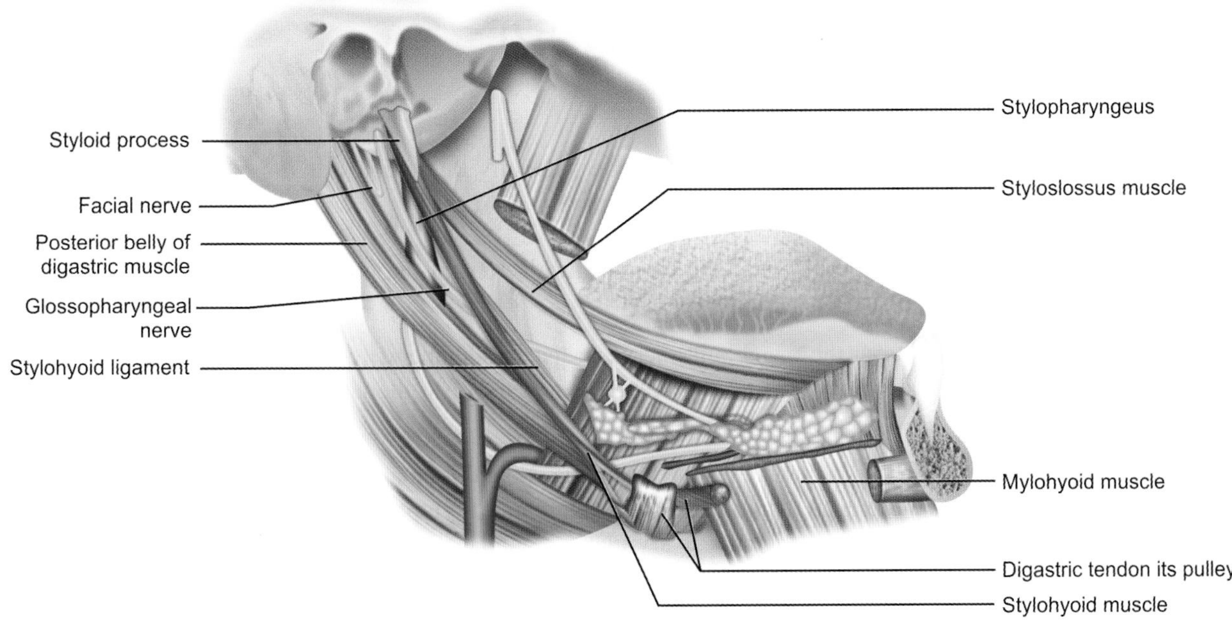

FIGURE 51 Styloid apparatus

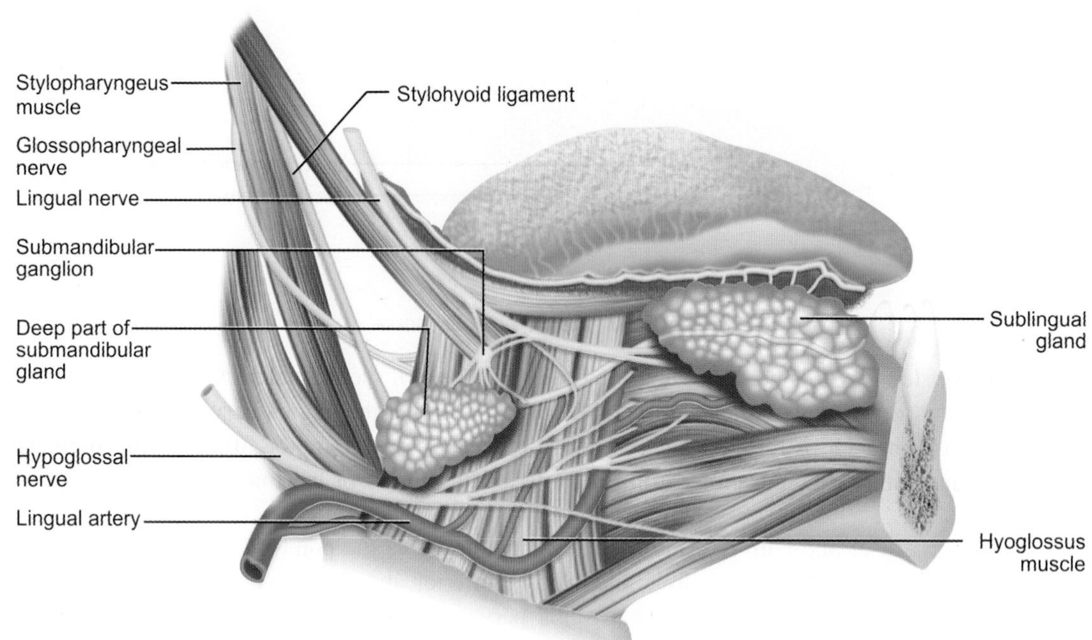

FIGURE 52 Submandibular region

Stylopharyngeus muscle: This is a muscle on the medial side of the styloid process. It arises from the medial surface of the styloid process and is inserted into the posterior border of the thyroid cartilage. It is another longitudinal muscle of the pharynx. It enters the pharynx between the superior and middle constrictor of pharynx.

Glossopharyngeal nerve: Locate this nerve winding round the stylopharyngeus muscle. This supplies the stylopharyngeus muscle. After it enters into the pharynx it is sensory to pharynx and posterior 1/3rd of tongue.

Stylohyoid ligament: Locate this thin ligament extending from the tip of the styloid process to the lesser cornua of the hyoid bone. It is internal to the stylohyoid muscle.

Facial nerge: Note the cut part of this nerve at stylomastoid foramen.

SUBMANDIBULAR REGION (Fig. 52)

Dissection: Cut the mylohyoid muscle near the hyoid bone. Identify the hyoglossus muscle and the structures on the hyoglossus muscle.

Hyoglossus muscle: It is an extrinsic muscle of the tongue. It arises from the greater horn and body of the hyoid bone. It is inserted into the lateral side of the tongue.

Lingual nerve: Trace this nerve from the mandibular nerve in the intratemporal fossa. It runs across the hyoglossus muscle near its upper border. Trace it forward to the tongue. It is sensory to the anterior 2/3rds of tongue. It carries both general and taste sensations.

Submandibular ganglion: It is one of the parasympathetic ganglia. Note this small ganglion suspended from the lingual nerve by two roots. It receives the preganglionic fibres from the chorda tympani nerve. The fibres after relay in the ganglion supply the submandibular and sublingual salivary glands. See the fine branches arising from the ganglion and entering the deep part of the submandibular gland. The secretomotor fibres to the sublingual gland reach in, through lingual nerve.

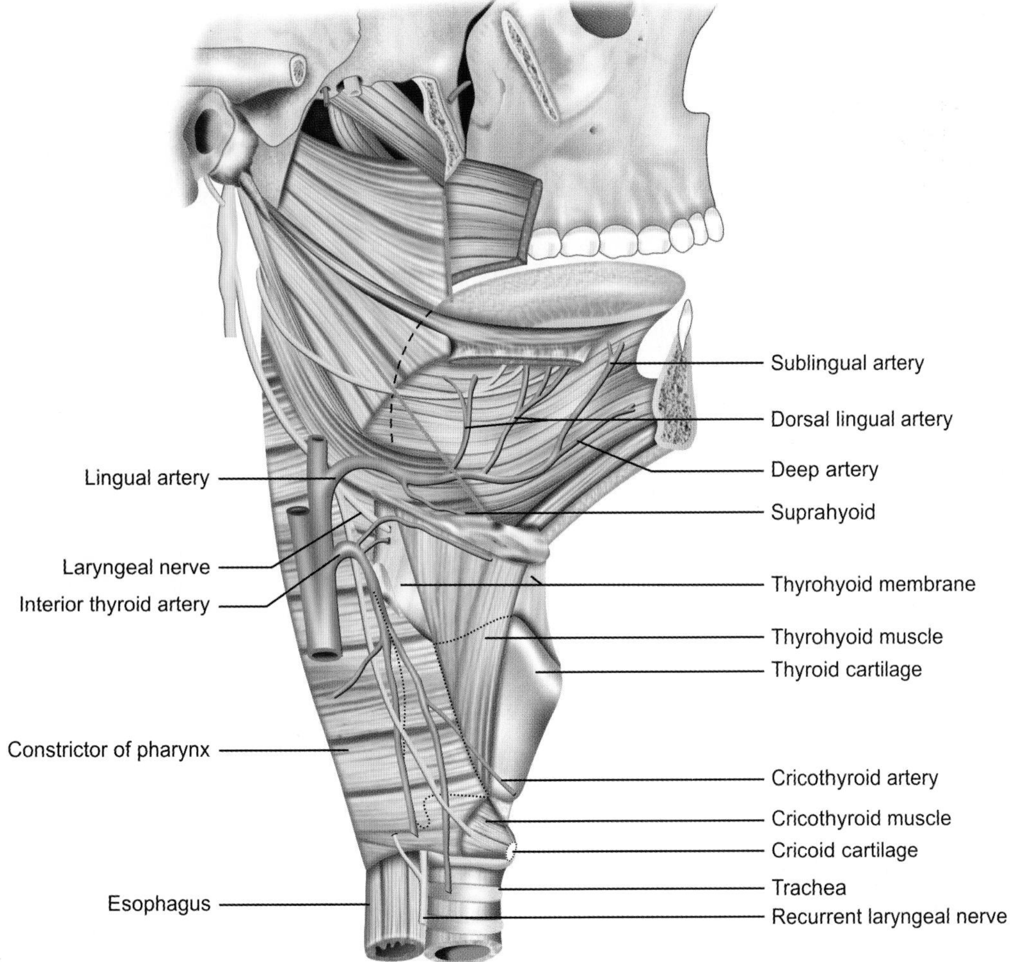

FIGURE 53 Lingual artery

Deep part of the submandibular salivary gland: Note this small part deep to the mylohyoid and on the hyoglossus muscle. Trace its thick duct to the undersurface of the tongue near the midline. Observe its opening.

Sublingual salivary gland: Note this gland distal to the hyoglossus muscle on the lateral aspect of the genioglossus muscle.

Hypoglossal nerve: This is the 12th cranial nerve. Trace its origin into the carotid sheath. It runs across the hyoglossus muscle along its lower aspect. Note its communication to the lingual nerve. It is a motor nerve to supply the thyrohyoid (already studied), the styloglossus, hyoglossus, genioglossus, geniohyoid and the intrinsic muscles of tongue.

Lingual Artery (Fig. 53)

Locate this artery opposite to the greater horn of the hyoid bone, arising from the external carotid artery. Locate its first branch, the ***suprahyoid branch***. It passes along the upper border of the hyoid bone. ***Now detach the hyoglossus muscle from the hyoid bone, lift it up, and trace the lingual artery.*** Note the two ascending branches. These are the ***dorsal lingual branches.*** These branches supply the tongue up to the mucous membrane. Identify the fine branch that supplies the sublingual gland, the ***sublingual artery.*** Beyond this the continuation of the artery is called as the ***deep artery*** of the tongue.

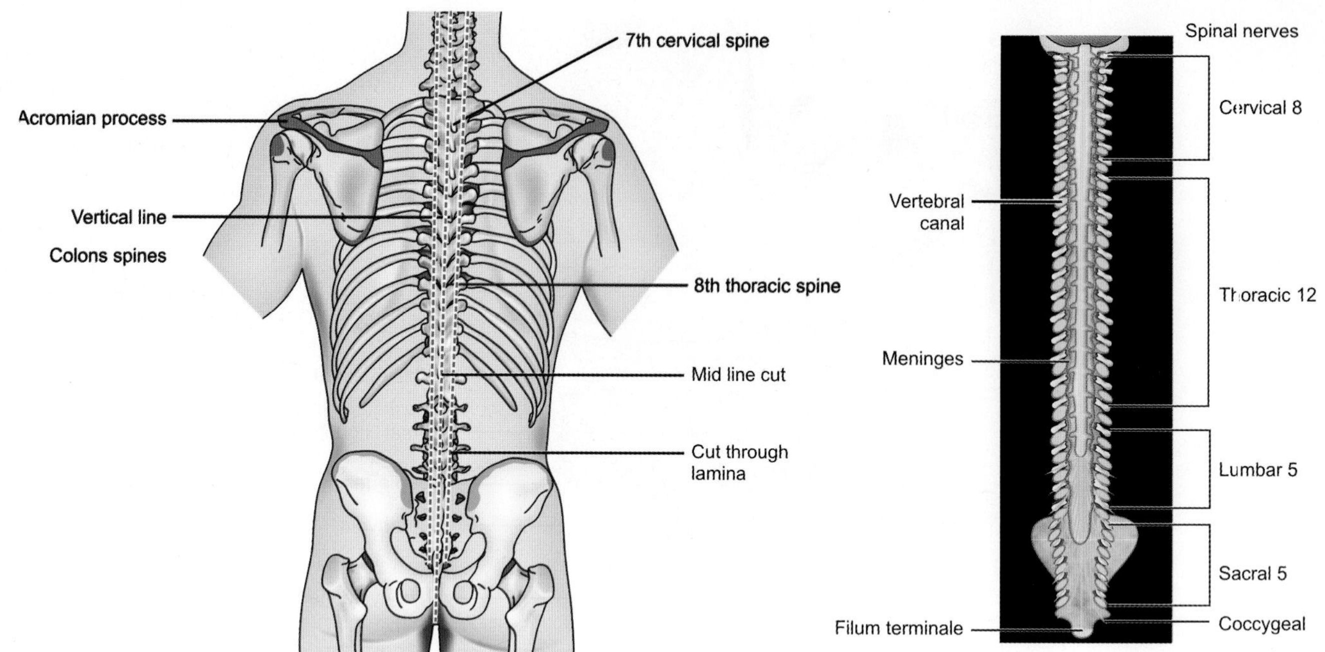

FIGURE 54 Removal of the spinal cord

REMOVAL OF SPINAL CORD

By this time you have dissected all the postvertebral muscles. Confirm once more that the postvertebral muscles are grouped as the erector spinae group of musculature, signifying their action as an extensor of the vertebral column.

It extends from the sacrum to the external occipital protuberance. In the lumbar region it lies between the middle and posterior layers of the thoracolumbar fascia. In the thoracic region it extends from the spines of the vertebrae to the angles of the ribs. In the neck region it is best developed and well separated. It extends between the spines of the vertebrae to the posterior tubercles of the cervical vertebrae. Inferiorly they extend on to the upper two ribs, superiorly they occupy the space between the external occipital protuberance and the superior nuchal line to the foramen magnum **(Fig. 54)**.

Dissection: Put the body in a raised prone position, with the neck supported and the head pulled down. Cut and remove all the erector spinae group of muscles from the sacral region to the external occipital protuberance. Expose the vertebrae between the spines and the transverse processes. Use chisel and a saw to cut through the lamina of the vertebrae from the sacrum to the atlas. Slowly chip and remove the total posterior part of the vertebral column from the sacrum to the atlas. Note that the laminae are united by the ligamentum flava. Now you are in the epidural space.

Epidural space: It is the area between the vertebral column and the dura mater. It is filled with ***vertebral plexus** of veins*. They drain the venous blood from the vertebrae and the spinal cord.

The vertebral plexus of veins are devoid of valves. They communicate with the segmental veins. It is easy for pelvic infections to pass through this route to secondarily infect the vertebrae and brain.

Dissection: Clean the vertebral venous plexus seen in here. The covering that is seen is the dura mater.

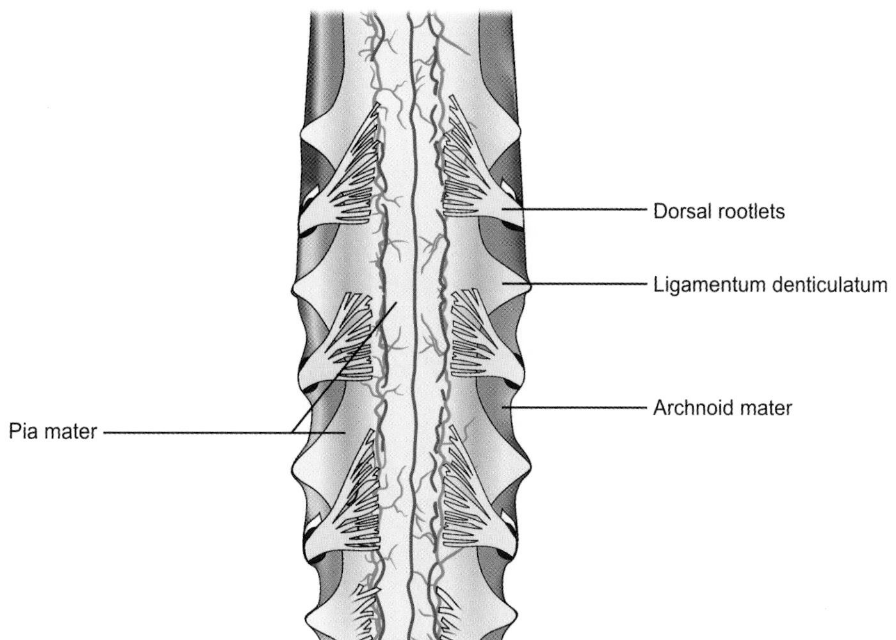

FIGURE 55 Dura mater (spinal cord)

Dura mater (Fig. 55): It is the outermost layer of the meninges. It is a tough sheet. Try to mobilize the spinal cord and see. Note that the spinal nerves leave the vertebral canal through the intervertebral foraminae. They are covered by the meninges. The dura mater extends from the foramen magnum to the second sacral vertebra, beyond that identify the thin filum terminale extending up to the coccyx.

Dissection: Remove the spinal cord along with the meninges by gradually cutting the spinal nerves and lifting it from the vertebral canal. Remove the spinal cord from the cervical level to the sacral level. As you are lifting note that the spinal cord extends up to the lower border of the first lumbar vertebra, beyond that it is made up of bunch of nerves. As you are lifting note the lower end of the dura mater closing at the level of the second sacral vertebra and the meninges continue as the filum terminale to the coccygeal vertebra.

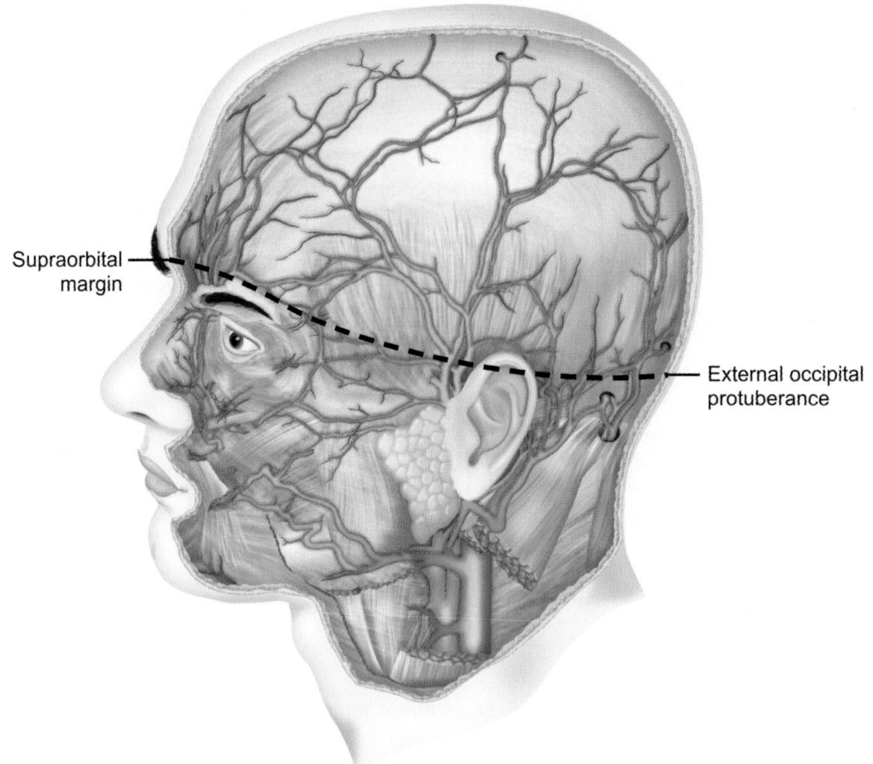

FIGURE 56 Removal of the skull cap

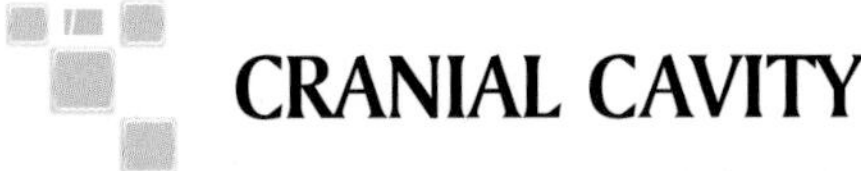

CRANIAL CAVITY

The cranial cavity is occupied by the brain. It is covered by three meninges—the pia mater, the arachnoid mater and the dura mater in that order from inside out. The dura mater is very thick. It is made up of two layers, the endosteal and the meningeal layers. The meningeal layer sends in sheets to separate different parts of the brain. The venous sinuses lie at the point of their separation. All the cranial nerves leave the cranial cavity through the foraminae in the skull.

In this study you remove the brain from the cranial cavity along with the pia and arachnoid mater. While removing the brain you will be cutting the cranial nerves arising from it. You will study the dura mater and the venous sinuses as you try to remove the brain.

Dissection (Fig. 56): Removal of skull cap—clean all the muscles from the scalp, back, suboccipital muscles and temporalis.

Take a wet chalk piece and make a mark from (1) Just below the supraorbital margin anteriorly (2) along the upper border of the attachment of auricle, (3) to a point below the external occipital protuberance. Cut it with a saw and remove the skull cap making sure that you retain the dura mater *in situ*. Use hand or edge of the scalpel to ease the dura mater from the skull. In general near the midline there can be erosion of the skull cap by the arachnoid granulations. Take more care in this area.

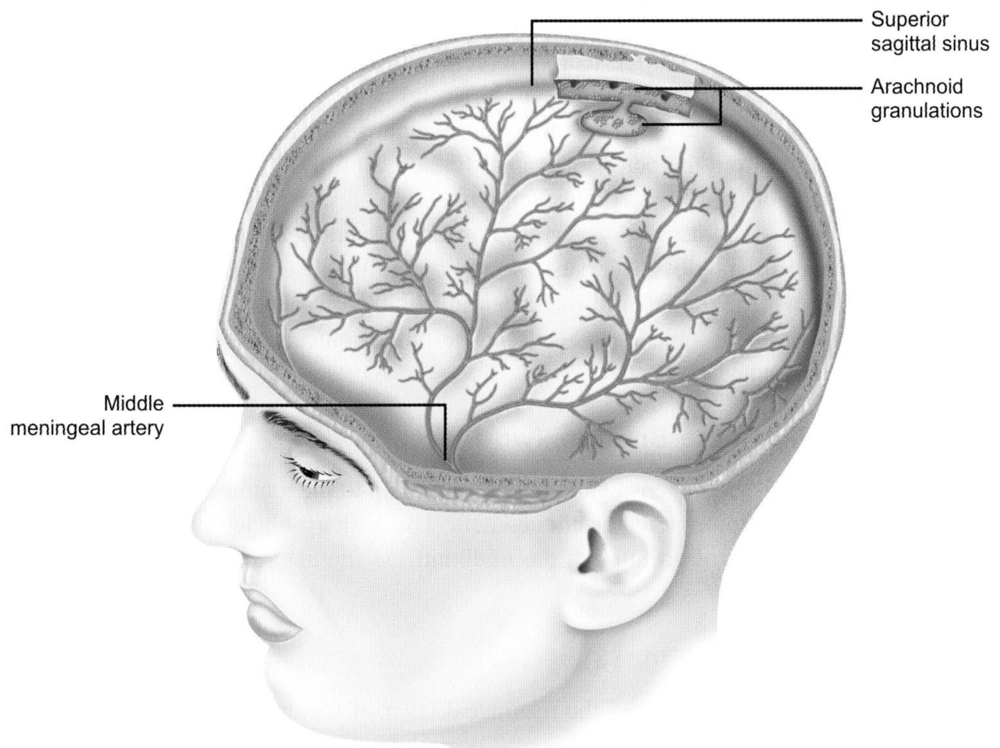

FIGURE 57 Dura matter (Brain)

Dura Matter (Fig. 57)

It is the thick white glistening meninges that is exposed now. Note the prominent ***middle meningeal artery*** on the superolateral aspect of the dura mater. This reaches the dura through the foramen spinosum. This is a branch of the first part of the maxillary artery. This is the major artery of supply to the dura mater.

VENOUS SINUSES

The veins of the cranial cavity present a nonvalvular sinus pattern. The venous sinuses lie between the endosteal and meningeal layer of the dura mater. The superior sagittal sinus, the inferior sagittal sinus and the straight sinus lie in the midline. The sphenoparietal sinus, the cavernous sinus, the intercavernous sinuses, the superior and inferior petrosal sinuses are paired sinuses and lie on either side of the midline.

Superior sagittal sinus: This lies in the midline from the foramen cecum to the level of external occipital protuberance. Slit the dura matter in the midline and see its interior. Put fine probes and identify the veins opening into it. These veins drain the cerebrum.

Arachnoid granulations: These are fine grape like structures projecting into the venous lacunae by the side of the superior sagittal sinus. These are projections of the arachnoid mater. The cerebrospinal fluid located in the subarachnoid space is poured into the venous sinus here.

Dissection: Make two parallel cuts on either side of the superior sagittal sinus. Make a coronal cut from one ear to the other ear through the dura mater reflect the four flaps towards the side of the skull. Leave the falx cerebri in position. Study the forebrain. Look at the frontal lobe, parietal lobe, occipital and temporal lobes of the cerebrum. Lift them up from the anterior, middle cranial fossae. Lift up the frontal lobes, and see in the midline. You can see the optic nerves, optic chiasma, internal carotid arteries and infundibular stalk. With fine scissors cut them, continue to cut the oculomotor nerve, trochlear which are located at a slightly posterior plane.

Turn the body to a prone position. Lift the occipital lobes and see the tentorium cerebelli. Locate its attached margin. It extends from the internal occipital protuberance, along the occipital bone to the superior border of the petrous part of the temporal bone.

Identify the transverse sinus along the occipital bone.

Falx cerebri: Identify this from the crista galli to the level of external occipital protuberance. Cut it near the crista galli and pull it up to the tentorium cerebelli. Cut the tentorium cerebelli inner to the attached margin (Central part of the tentorium lies between the cerebrum and cerebellum). Ease the cerebellum from the posterior cranial fossa and feel the foramen magnum and medulla oblongata. Nearer to foramen magnum pull the falx cerebelli posteriorly and lift the cerebellum and medulla oblongata from the posterior cranial fossa. Carefully lift the temporal and occipital lobes. Put a scissors along the inner surface of the petrous part of temporal bone and cut the facial, vestibulocochlear, trigeminal, glossopharyngeal, abducent, vagus and accessory nerves. Put the scissors near the foramen magnum along its sides and cut the vertebral arteries and hypoglossal nerves. Slowly carefully lift up the whole brain. In this removal the whole brain is removed along with the arachnoid mater and all blood vessels and nerves. Along with the brain the central part of the tentorium cerebelli comes off. So it can be pulled out after the removal, and put it back in the anatomical position and can be studied.

Alternative Method to Remove the Brain in Two Pieces

Dissection: Cut the falx cerebri near the cristagalli and pull it up, up to the tentorium cerebelli. Lift the temporal, occipital lobes of the cerebrum from the tentorium cerebelli. Use a sharp blade, make a transverse cut through the brain in the midline. The cut will go through the midbrain. As the anterior structures were already cut the forebrain can be lifted up easily.

Study of the Tentorium Cerebelli (Fig. 58)

Look for the glistening dura mater. It is a fold of the meningeal layer of the dura mater. It has got an attached margin along the inner side of the occipital bone from the internal occipital protuberance to the petrous part of the temporal bone, along the superior border of the petrous part of the temporal bone to the posterior clinoid process. Free margin of tentorium cerebelli is a 'U' shaped margin and anteriorly it is attached to the anterior clinoid process.

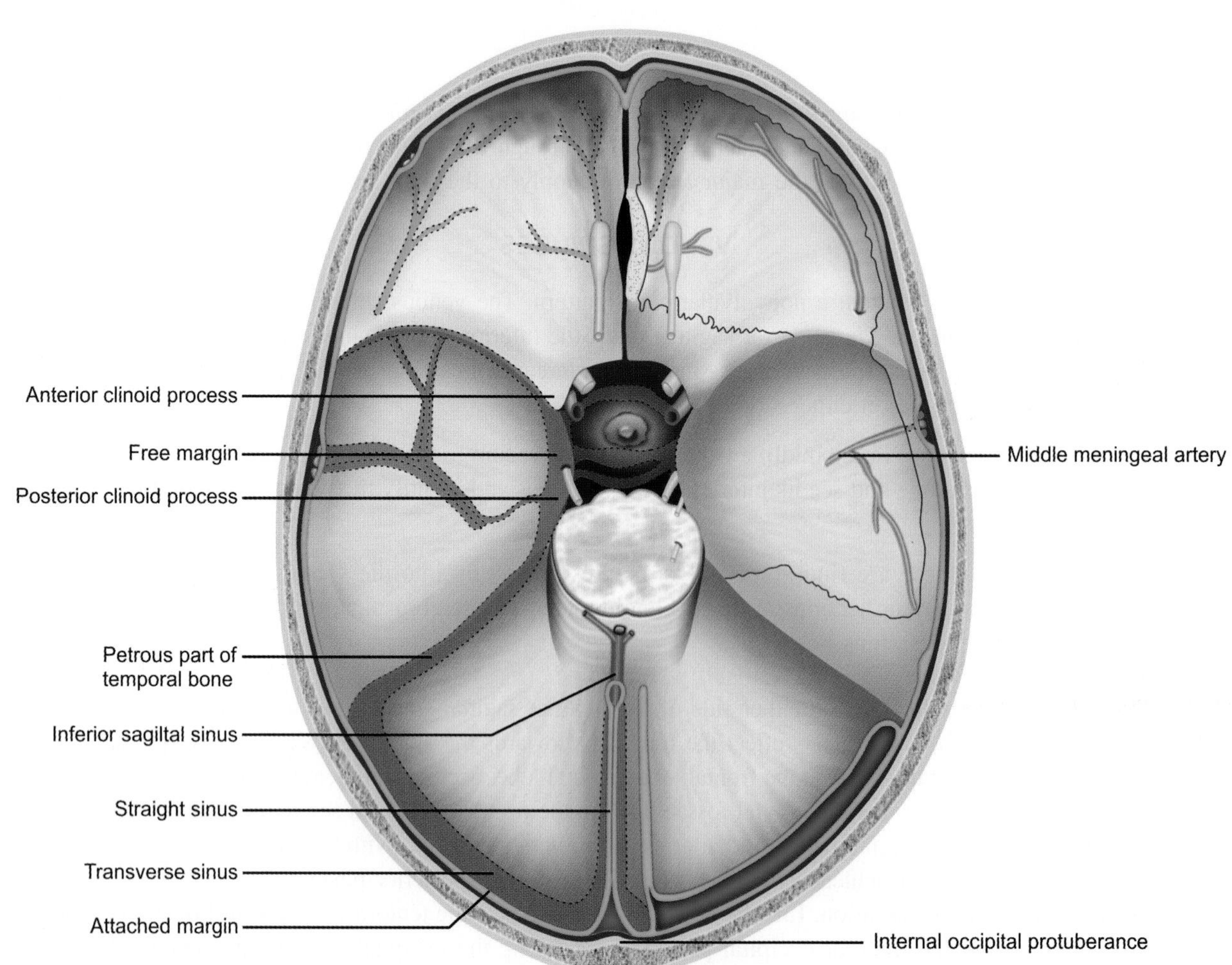

FIGURE 58 Tentorium cerebelli

Straight sinus: Locate this at the junction of superior sagittal sinus with the tentorium cerebelli.

Transverse sinus: Slit the tentorium cerebelli along the attached margin of the tentorium cerebelli with the occipital bone. Observe the transverse sinus.

Inferior sagittal sinus: See this in the free margin of the falx cerebri and identify the formation of straight sinus by the union of inferior sagittal sinus and great cerebral vein of Galen.

Dissection: Cut through the attached margin of the tentorium cerebelli and remove it. Note the trochlear nerve located between the free and attached margins of the tentorium cerebelli.

Observe the hindbrain. See the cerebellum in the posterior cranial fossa. Note the midbrain, pons and medulla oblongata anterior to the cerebellum. Push the brainstem posteriorly. Note the oculomotor, trochlear, trigeminal, facial and vestibulocochlear nerves. Cut them nearer to the bone. Push the medulla oblongata further and cut the 6, 9,10,11,12 cranial nerves and the vertebral artery nearer to the foramen magnum and jugular foramen.

Push the brainstem and cerebellum forwards, pull the falx cerebelli backwards and cut the medulla oblongata near the foramen magnum and lift the hindbrain. This will remove the hindbrain along with all the cranial nerves from 3rd to 12th and the vertebral artery along with pia and arachnoid mater.

Middle meningeal artery: Note this bulging artery within the lateral aspect of the dura mater. Note its branches supplying the dura mater. Trace it down to its emergence from the foramen spinosum.

INTERIOR OF SKULL (Fig. 59)

After removing the brain, the interior of the skull which now is still covered by the dura mater, the arteries, dural venous sinuses and cranial nerves can be studied.

ARTERIES

Vertebral artery: This enters the cranial cavity through the foramen magnum. Note the cut end of this artery within the foramen magnum.

VENOUS SINUSES

Internal carotid artery: Note this artery lateral to the optic chiasma. This artery enters the cranial cavity through the carotid canal, passes through the cavernous sinus (will be dissected soon) and enters the brain lateral to the optic chiasma.

Sphenoparietal sinus: This sinus lies along the lesser wing of sphenoid. This drains into cavernous sinus.

Cavernous sinus: This sinus lies lateral to the pituitary gland. The oculomotor, trochlear, ophthalmic and mandibular division of trigeminal nerve lie in the lateral wall of the cavernous sinus.

Dissection: Peel the dura mater off the lateral wall and identify these nerves.

Internal carotid artery and abducent nerve lie within the cavernous sinus. Locate them. Anterior, posterior and intercavernous sinuses connect the cavernous sinuses of either side.

Superior petrosal sinus: Slit the attached margin of the tentorium cerebelli along the petrous part of the temporal bone and note that it connects the cavernous sinus to the transverse sinus.

Inferior petrosal sinus: Locate this sinus from the cavernous sinus to the jugular foramen. It can be seen as a blue line. Slit it open and see the sinus.

Basilar plexus of veins: Locate these through the dura mater over the basilar part of the occipital bone.

Occipital sinus: Locate this within the attached margin of falx cerebelli.

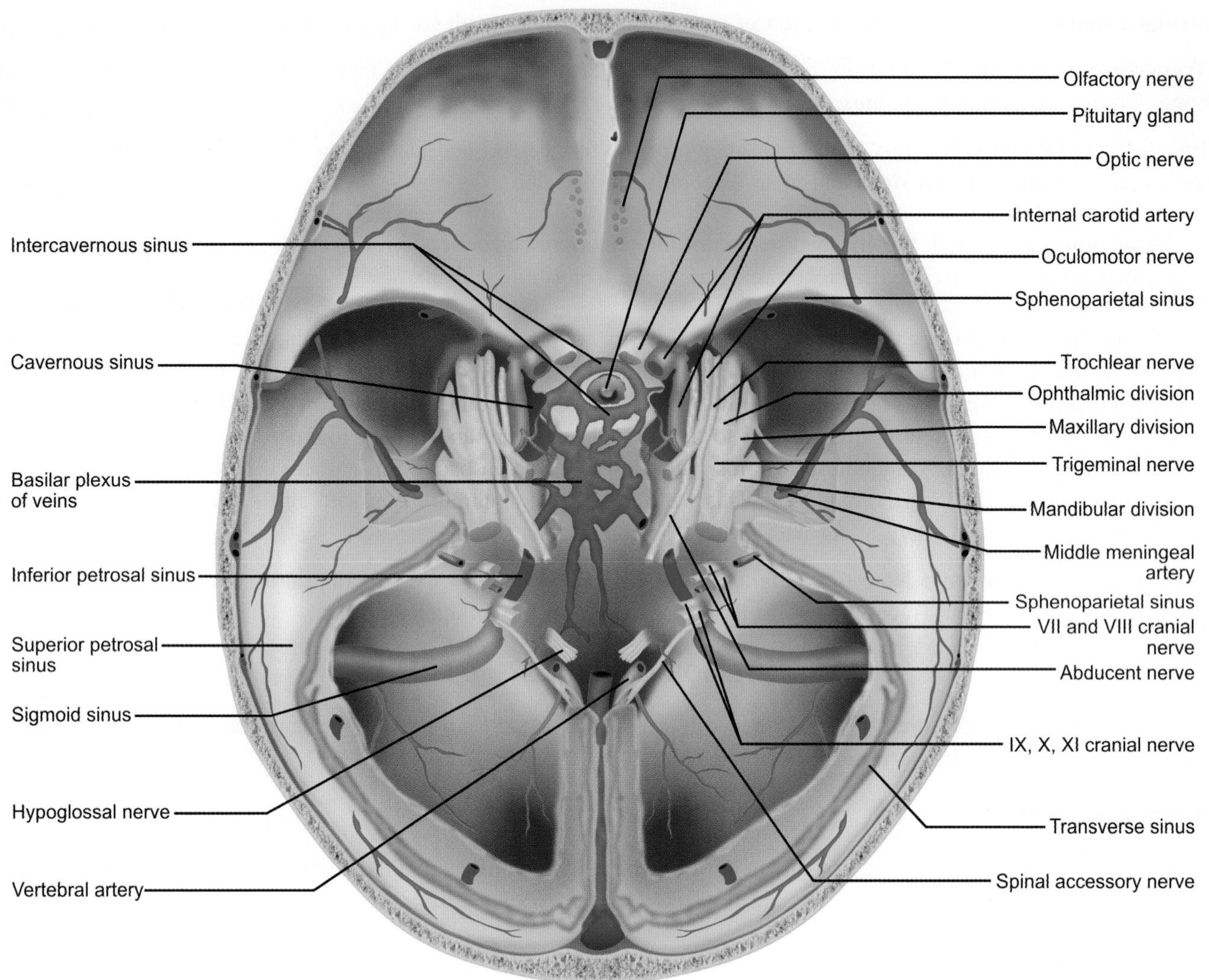

FIGURE 59 Cranial nerves and venous sinuses—base of skull

CRANIAL NERVES

I. Olfactory nerve: This enters the skull as 20 rootlets through the cribriform plate of ethmoid bone. Note these openings in the ethmoid bone. It carries olfactory sensations.

II. Optic nerve: Trace it in the optic canal. It carries visual sensations.

III. Oculomotor nerve: This is a thick nerve passing through the free margin of the tentorium, into the lateral wall of the cavernous sinus to the superior orbital fissure. It is a motor nerve. It supplies the muscles of eyeball.

IV. Trochlear nerve: This is a thin nerve. Locate it between the free and attached margins of the tentorium cerebelli passes along the lateral wall of the cavernous sinus to the superior orbital fissure. It is motor to superior oblique muscle of eyeball.

V. Trigeminal nerve: It is a thick nerve, locate it in the posterior cranial fossa. It pushes the dura mater into the middle cranial fossa forming a covering to itself called the cavum trigeminal. Slit the dura mater and locate the ganglion and its branches.

Ophthalmic division is the most superior of the divisions. It passes along the lateral wall of the cavernous sinus to the superior orbital fissure. It is a sensory nerve to the face.

Maxillary division is the middle branch of the trigeminal nerve. It runs along the lateral wall of the cavernous sinus. It is sensory to the maxilla.

Mandibular nerve leaves the cranial cavity through the mandibular foramen. It is a mixed nerve. Locate the deeper motor part of this nerve. It supplies muscles of mastication and is sensory to the face and mandible.

VI. Abducent nerve: Locate this thin nerve piercing dura mater of posterior cranial fossa. It passes through the cavernous sinus along with the internal carotid artery. Trace it to the superior orbital fissure.

VII and VIII. Facial and vestibulocochlear nerve: These nerves enter the internal auditory meatus in the petrous part of the temporal bone. Locate the fine labyrinthine artery in the posterior cranial fossa which accompanies these nerves.

IX,X and XI. Glossopharyngeal, vagus and accessory nerves: They enter the jugular foramen. Locate the spinal part of the accessory which ascends up through the foramen magnum to join the cranial part of the accessory nerve.

XII. Hypoglossal nerve: Locate this nerve passing through the hypoglossal canal just above the foramen magnum.

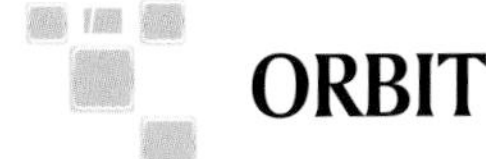

ORBIT

BONY ORBIT (Fig. 60)

Study the bony orbit on the dry skull. Note that it is a pyramidal shaped area. Its medial walls are parallel to each other whereas its lateral walls diverge laterally. Locate the followings:

Optic canal is formed by the two roots of the lesser wing of the sphenoid and the body of the sphenoid.

Superior orbital fissure is formed by the lesser wing and greater wing of sphenoid.

Inferior orbital fissure formed by the greater wing of sphenoid, maxilla and the zygomatic bone.

Anterior, posterior ethmoid canals are fine canals between the ethmoid and the frontal bone.

Internal orifice in the zygomatic bone is a fine foramen in the zygomatic bone.

Trochlea is a rough part on the medial part of the roof.

Supraorbital foramen or notch can be felt in the supraorbital margin.

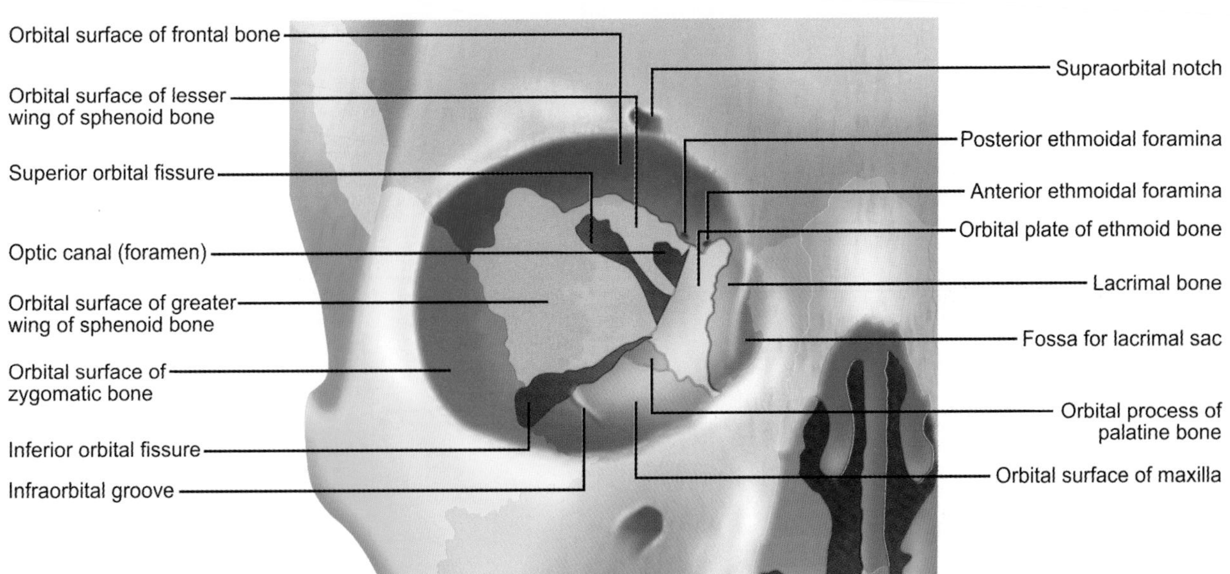

FIGURE 60 Bony orbit

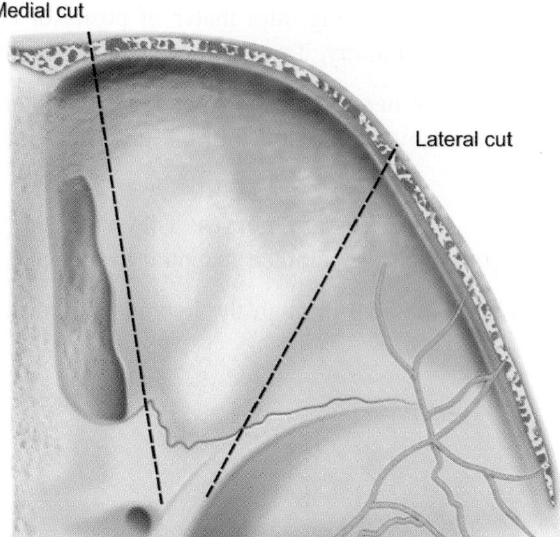

FIGURE 61 Dissection of orbit

Dissection (Fig. 61): Make two saw cuts along the medial and lateral ends of the superior orbital margin to the superior orbital fissure. Remove the roof and lateral wall of the orbit taking care not to damage the deeply located orbital periosteum.

SUPERFICIAL STRUCTURES OF THE ORBIT

Orbital periosteum envelops the contents of the orbit. The orbit has the lacrimal gland, eyeball with the optic nerve, muscles to move the eyeball, sensory nerves to supply the internal structures and skin, autonomic fibres to supply the interior of eyeball and the ophthalmic artery with its accompanying veins. You will identify all these structures as and when they appear in dissection **(Fig. 62)**.

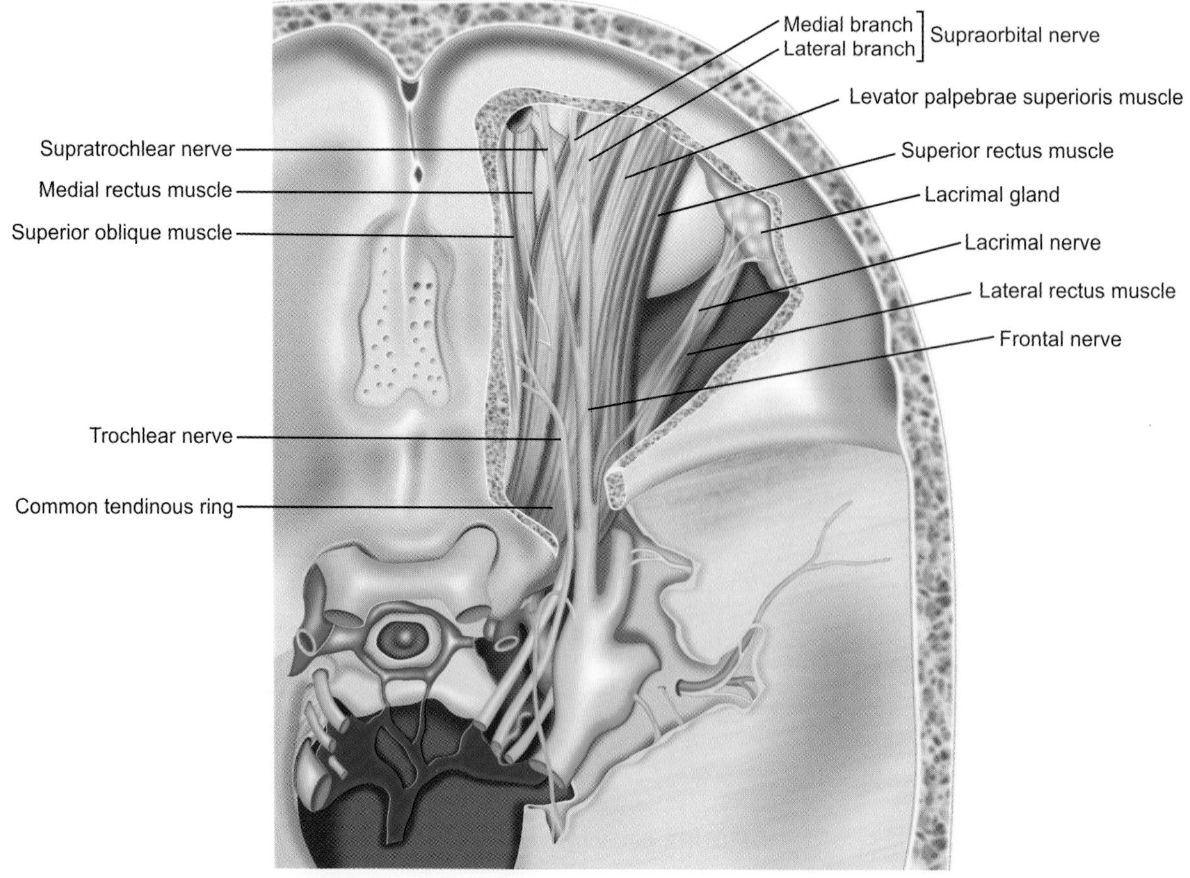

FIGURE 62 Superficial structures of the orbit – superior aspect

Dissection: Cut and remove the thick glistening orbital periosteum from the roof. Identify the three nerves extending from the middle cranial fossa to the orbit.

Trochlear nerve: Trace this most medial nerve into the superior margin of the superior oblique muscle nearer to its origin. Trace this nerve back to the lateral wall of the cavernous sinus. It supplies the superior oblique muscle.

Frontal nerve: This is the thick nerve seen right in the middle. Trace it back to the ophthalmic division of trigeminal nerve. Note that it immediately divides into two branches, the medial supratrochlear branch and thick lateral supraorbital nerve. Trace the nerves forwards along the superior orbital margin to the scalp. It is sensory to scalp.

Lacrimal nerve: It is a thin lateral branch along the superiolateral margin. Trace it back to the ophthalmic division and trace it forward to the lacrimal gland. Trace a fine zygomatic branch joining this nerve. The zygomatic branch brings in secretomotor fibres from the maxillary nerve to the lacrimal gland.

Lacrimal gland: It secretes tears. It is a light yellow color gland located on the anterolateral aspect of the orbit. It is divided into a superficial and a deeper part by the aponeurosis of the levator palpebrae superioris muscle. Locate this gland and identify its parts.

Dissection: Detach the nerves and reflect them towards the middle cranial fossa.

MUSCULATURE OF THE ORBIT

Orbit lodges the four recti, two oblique which act on the eyeball and a palpebral muscle which elevates the upper lid. The significant feature here is that the recti arise from a common tendinous ring located proximally near the superior orbital fissure. They all insert into the anterior half of the eyeball. Note that they move anterolaterally to reach their insertion. The oblique are inserted into the posterior half of the eyeball and they run anteroposteriorly.

Superior oblique muscle: Locate this muscle along the superomedial margin of the orbit. It arises from the common tendinous ring. Trace it to the trochlea at the anterior end and feel it. It is inserted into the superolateral surface of the eyeball posterior to the equator (you will see the insertion after reflecting the other muscles). Locate its nerve supply from the trochlear nerve.

Dissection: Cut the muscle between the origin and trochlea

Levator palpebrae superioris: Identify this muscle which occupies the whole central area. It arises from the under surface of the orbital plate of the frontal bone and is inserted into the upper eyelid. Note the deeper fibres inserted into the conjunctiva. The muscle fibres spread out as they move forwards. Note that it elevates the upper eyelid by pulling it.

Dissection: Cut it in the centre reflect the proximal part towards its origin and the distal part towards its insertion.

Superior rectus: Note this muscle immediately deep to the levator palpebrae superioris. It arises from the tendinous ring. Note the margin from where it arises. Trace its insertion into the superior part of the eyeball in front of the equator. It is an elevator of the cornea.

Medial rectus muscle: Locate this muscle along the medial side of the orbit. It arises from the tendinous ring and gets inserted into the medial side of the eyeball. It is an adductor of the eyeball.

All the three muscles are supplied by upper division of the oculomotor nerve. The nerve enters into the muscles on their deeper aspect.

Dissection: Cut the muscle in the center and reflect the proximal part towards the origin and the distal part towards the insertion. Cut through the tendinous ring between the origin of the superior rectus and lateral rectus. Locate the oculomotor nerve entering into the orbit through the superior orbital fissure. Trace it backwards to its location in the cavernous sinus. Trace its branches entering into the levator palpebrae superioris, superior rectus and medial rectus.

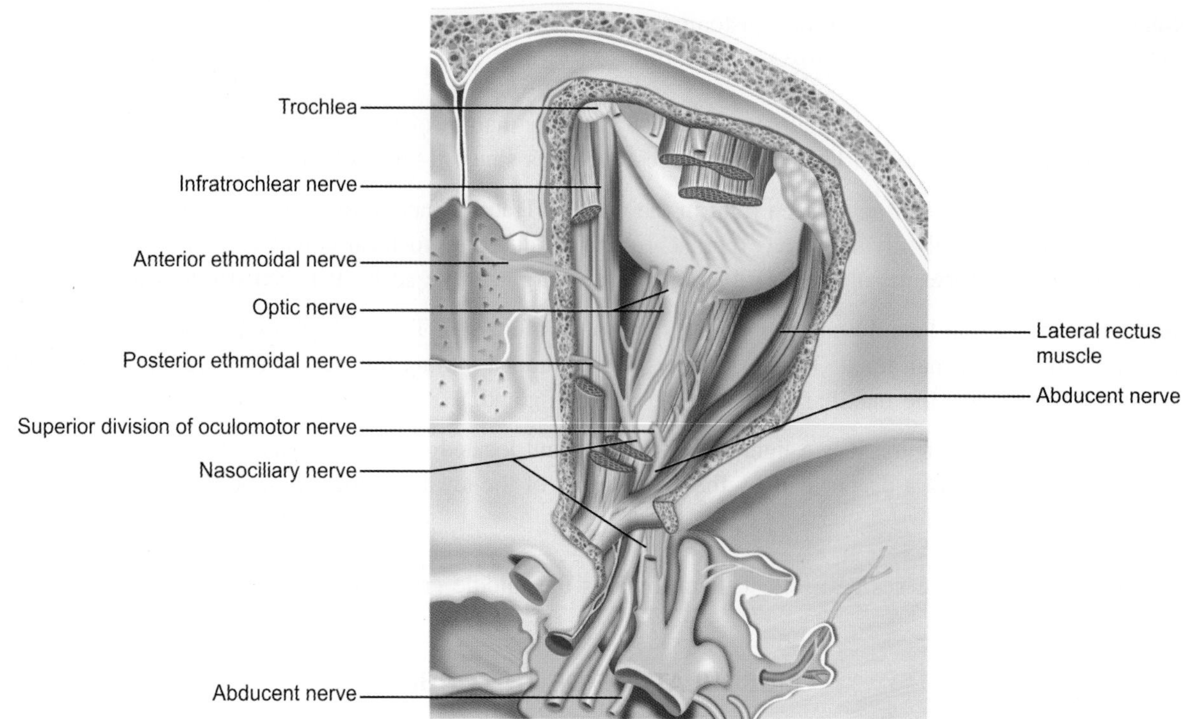

FIGURE 63 Deep structures in the orbit

DEEP STRUCTURES OF ORBIT (Fig. 63)

Insertion of superior oblique: Trace this muscle from the level of the trochlea. Note that the muscle becomes aponeurotic and spreads out. It is inserted into the superolateral surface of the eyeball posterior to the equator. Clean the orbital fat and trace the insertion. Note that this muscle pulls the posterior part of the eye all upwards and medially and produces downward and lateral movement of the cornea

Nasociliary nerve: Clear the fat in the orbit and locate the nasociliary nerve crossing the optic nerve from lateral to medial. Trace it back to the ophthalmic division and forwards to the ethmoid between medial rectus and superior oblique muscles. This is the sensory nerve to the orbital structures and the ethmoidal air sinuses. It gives off fine ***anterior and posterior ethmoidal nerves*** which pass through the canals in the ethmoid bone. The anterior ethmoidal nerve after supplying the ethmoidal air sinus enters the nasal cavity to supply the mucous membrane of nose. The nasociliary reaches the face as the ***infratrochlear nerve*** and supplies the skin of the face.

Lateral rectus muscle: Locate this muscle along the lateral side of the orbit. It arises from the tendinous ring and is inserted into the lateral aspect of the eyeball. It is an abductor and is supplied by the abducent nerve.

Abducent nerve: Locate this nerve into the inner aspect of the muscle. Trace it backwards to the superior orbital fissure and the cavernous sinus.

Optic nerve: Locate this thick nerve entering into the orbit through the optic canal. It is the sensory nerve to carry the visual sensations.

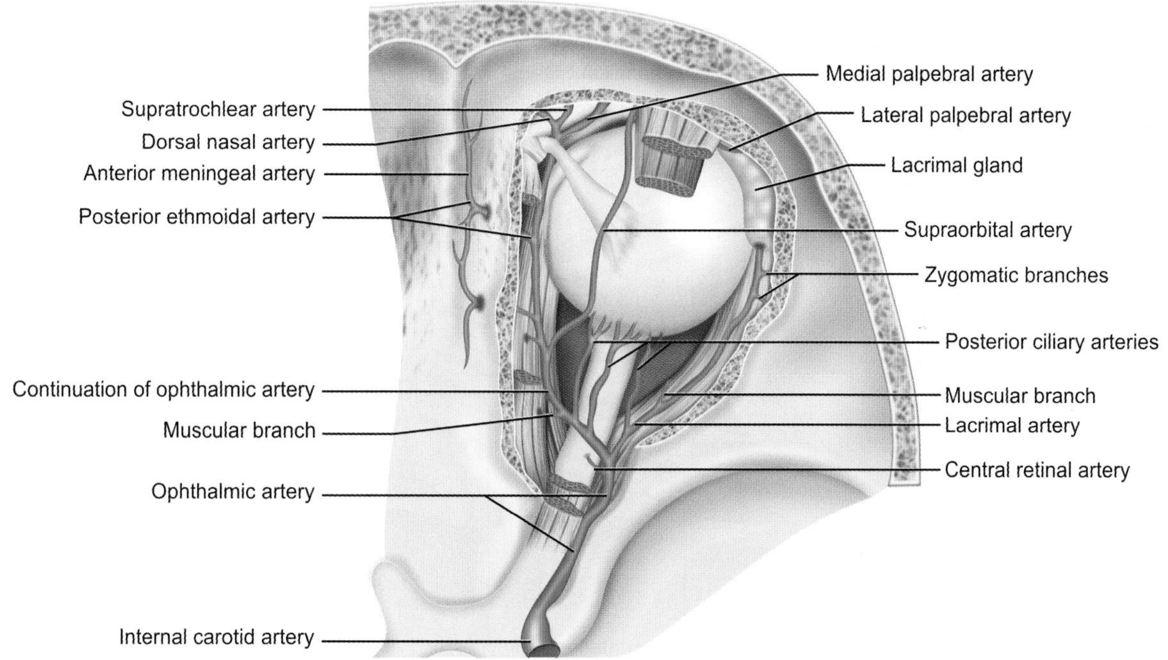

FIGURE 64 Ophthalmic artery

OPHTHALMIC ARTERY

Ophthalmic Artery (Fig. 64)

Locate this artery inferior to the optic nerve in the optic canal. Trace it forwards and see all its fine branches. It divides into a ***lacrimal branch*** which moves forwards and into the eyelid after supplying the lacrimal gland. The medial branch crosses the optic nerve either superficial or deep to the nerve. As it crosses the nerve it gives off ***ciliary branches*** to supply the eyeball. The ***central artery of retina*** enters the optic nerve while the ophthalmic artery lies deep to the optic nerve. It is an end artery and supplies the retina. The ophthalmic artery further runs medially and parallel to the medial wall of the orbit. Here it gives off the ***ethmoidal branches*** to enter the ethmoidal canals. They supply the ethmoidal air sinuses. The ***supraorbital*** is an independent branch. The ophthalmic artery gives the ***medial palpebral artery,*** to the lids, ***supratrochlear artery*** to the scalp and ***dorsal nasal*** to the nose. Throughout its course it gives off branches to supply the orbital structures.

Veins in the orbit exhibit a plexiform arrangement and leave the orbit as superior and inferior ophthalmic veins. The ***superior ophthalmic vein*** accompanies most of the branches of the artery and leaves through the superior orbital fissure and drains into cavernous sinus. The ***inferior ophthalmic vein*** drains the inferior structures and leaves it through the inferior orbital fissure. This drains into the pterygoid plexus of veins.

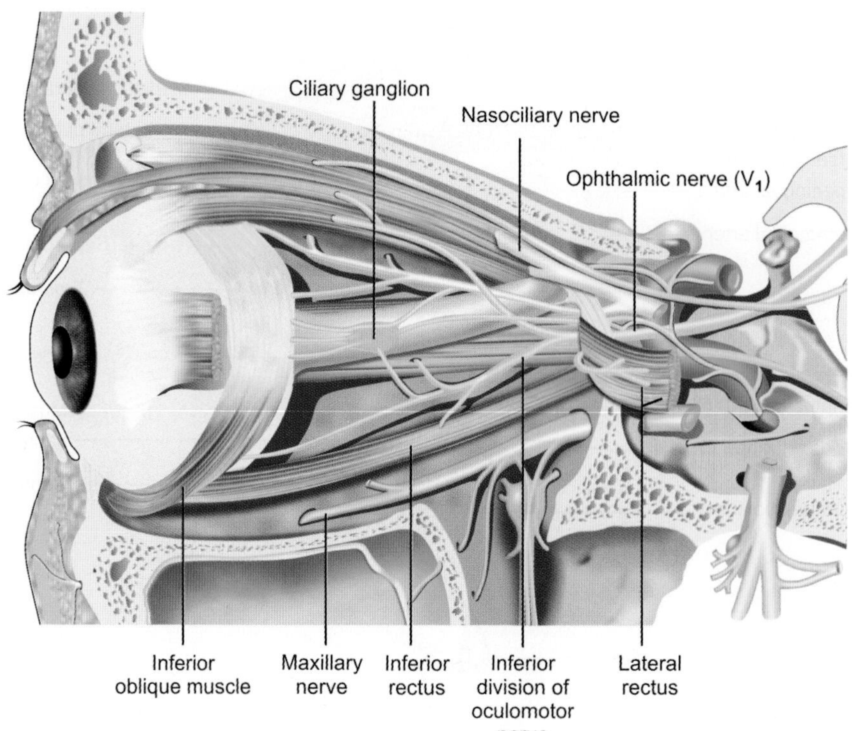

FIGURE 65 Lateral exposure of orbit

Dissection: Try to chip the lateral wall of the orbit up to the superior orbital fissure. This gives more space here to trace the important structures. Cut the lateral rectus muscle in its center and reflect it. See the following structures **(Fig. 65).**

Ciliary ganglion is a parasympathetic ganglion. Pull the optic nerve medially and locate this small ganglion between it and the lateral rectus. Very near the apex of the orbit. You can see it suspended by the nasociliary and inferior division of oculomotor nerve. Locate the ***short*** and ***long ciliary nerves*** arising from the ganglion and from the nasociliary nerve. Trace them reaching the back of the eyeball. These carry the autonomic and sensory fibres to the muscles within the eyeball.

Inferior oblique muscle: Locate this muscle in the floor extending from medial to lateral side. It arises from the medial aspect of the floor of the orbit. It is inserted into the inferolateral surface of the eyeball, posterior to the equator. It pulls the posterior aspect of the eyeball downwards and medially thus resulting in the upward and lateral movement of the cornea.

Inferior rectus muscle: Depress the inferior oblique muscle and pull the eyeball up and locate this muscle in the undersurface of the eyeball. It arises from the fibrous tendinous ring on its inferior aspect. It is inserted into the eyeball on its inferior surface ***anterior to the equator***.

Inferior division of oculomotor nerve: Locate this nerve lateral to the optic nerve. It enters into the orbit through the superior orbital fissure. Trace it back to the oculomotor nerve. Trace its branches entering into the inferior rectus and inferior oblique muscles on their internal surfaces.

Maxillary nerve: Trace this nerve from the middle cranial fossa through the foramen rotundum to the floor of the orbit. Trace it into the infraorbital groove/canal.

Facial sheath of the eyeball: Pull the eyeball upwards and locate the connective tissue sheath from below the eyeball to the medial and lateral bony walls. They are called medial and lateral palpebral ligaments. All the muscles of the eyeball get inserted into the eyeball through this facial sheath.

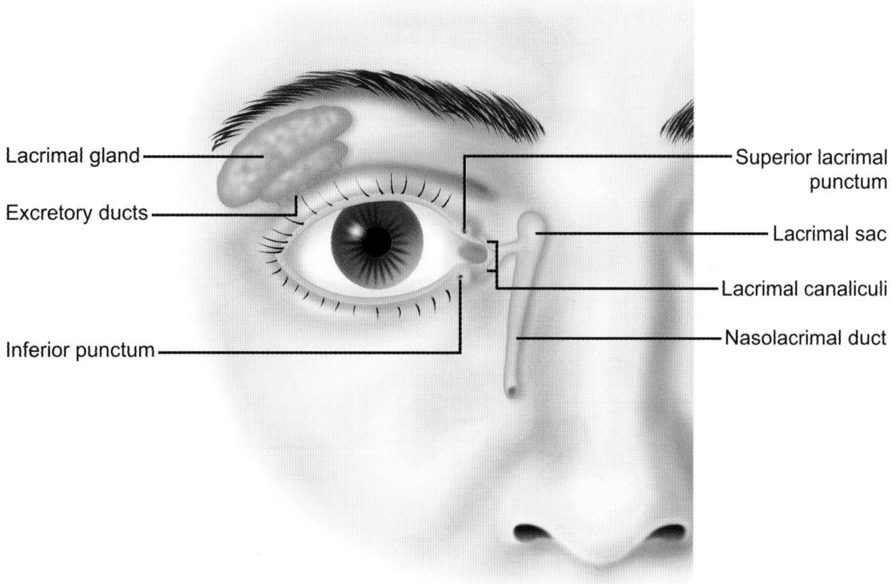

FIGURE 66 Lacrimal apparatus

LACRIMAL APPARATUS (Fig. 66)

The lacrimal apparatus manufactures tears, pours it on to the eyeball to moisten the eyeball. The excess tears are drained to the nasal cavity.

Lacrimal apparatus consists of ***lacrimal gland*** with its ***excretory ducts***—this lies within the orbit, ***conjunctival sac***—this is the space between the two eyelids and the eyeball, ***lacrimal papillae and puncta***—these lie within the medial ends of the eyelid, the ***lacrimal canaliculi***—these run from the puncta to the lacrimal sac, the lacrimal sac—this lies deeper to the medial palpebral ligament, the ***nasolacrimal duct***—this drains the lacrimal sac to the ***inferior nasal meatus***.

Many of these structures are small and deeply placed and are difficult to identify. The structures are described at the appropriate place.

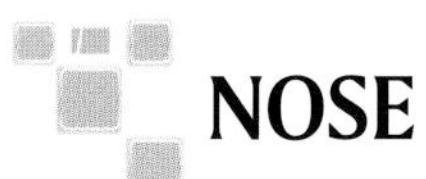

NOSE

The part of the nose that is seen externally is ***external nose***. Feel it and note that it is both bony and cartilaginous. But when it is cut in the midline the total area extending from the anterior nasal aperture to the posterior choanae is considered as the nasal cavity.

Nasal cavity is a respiratory passage. It is divided into two parts by a septum. The surface area of the nasal cavity is increased by bony projections. The bones surrounding the nasal cavity are pneumatic bones, filled with air. They help in the resonance of the voice. The part seen externally is called the external nose. It is made up of both bone and cartilage. All the bones and cartilages of the nasal cavity are covered by the mucoperiosteum. The function of the cavernous tissue is to control the temperature of the passing air. It warms in cold climate and cools in warm climates. The roof of the nasal cavity is olfactory in nature and is supplied by the olfactory nerves.

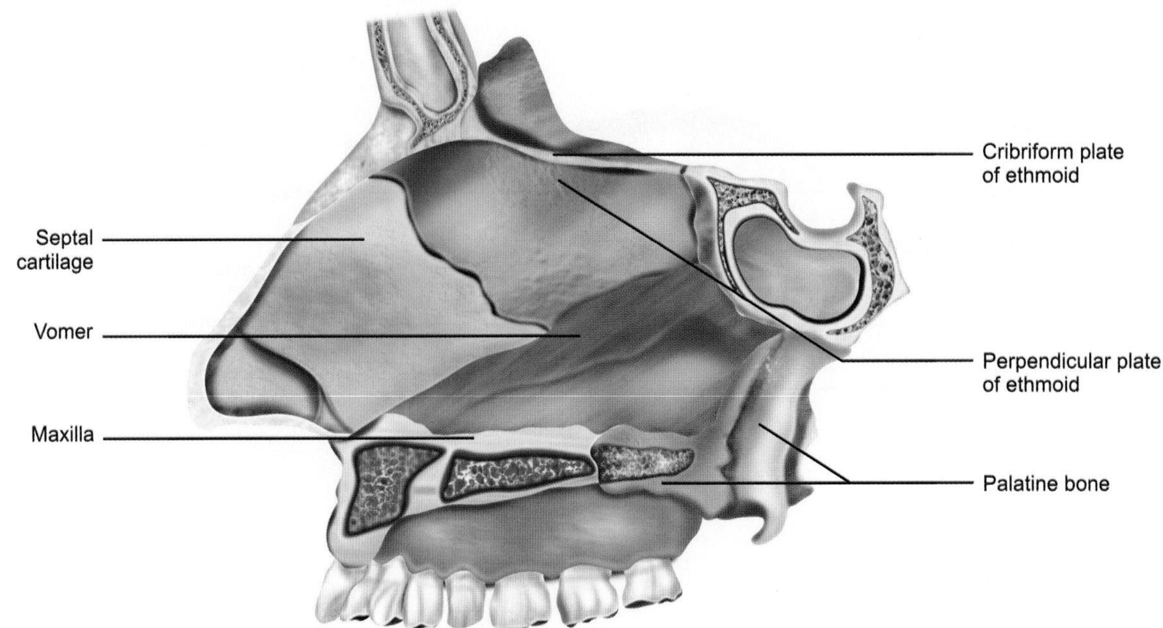

FIGURE 67 Nasal septum

BOUNDARIES OF THE NASAL CAVITY (Figs 67 to 69)

It is divided into two halves by the median nasal septum. Note that it is made up of bone as well as cartilage. Identify the ethmoid, vomer and the space for the septal cartilage.

Observe that the lateral wall exhibits projections called conchae. Note that the wall is made up of maxilla, lacrimal, ethmoid, palatine, sphenoid and inferior nasal concha. Note the sphenopalatine foramen in the vertical plate of the palatine bone between its two roots. Note the area for cartilage.

Dissection: Use a band saw and detach the neck at the level of 7th cervical vertebra and make a sagittal section in the midline and separate it into two halves.

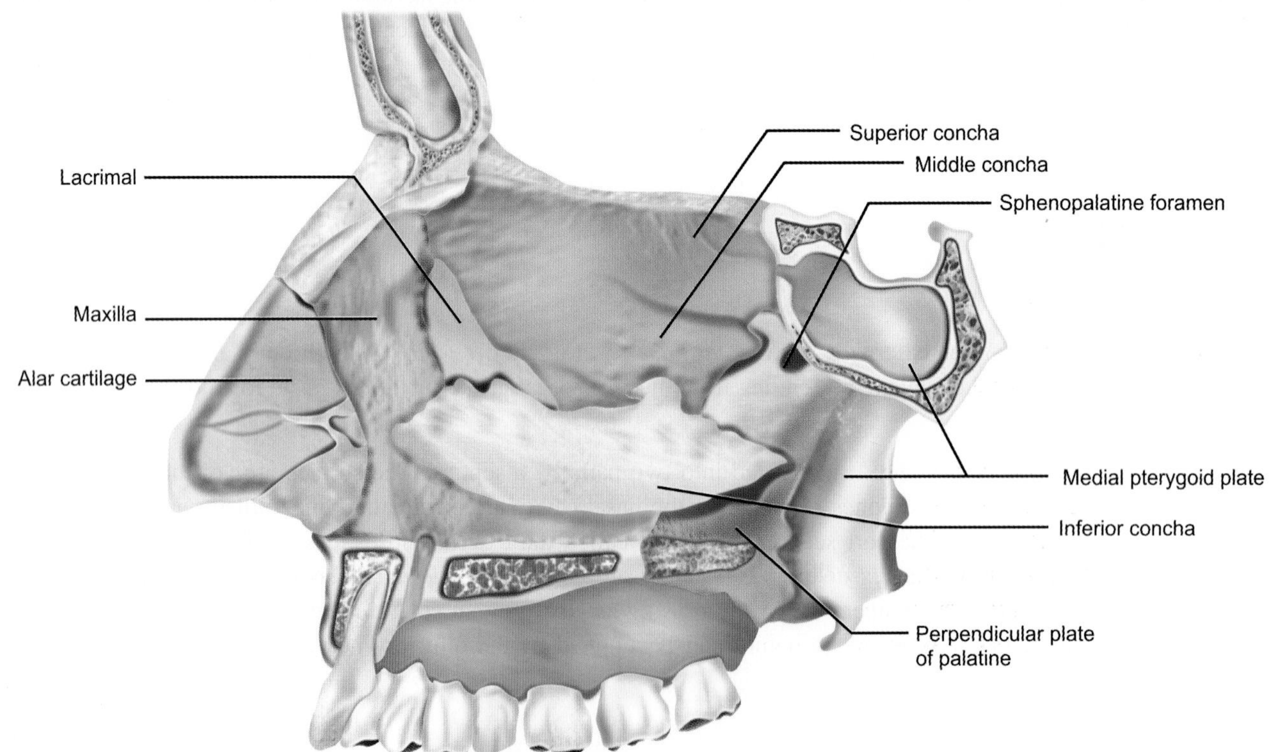

FIGURE 68 Lateral wall of nose

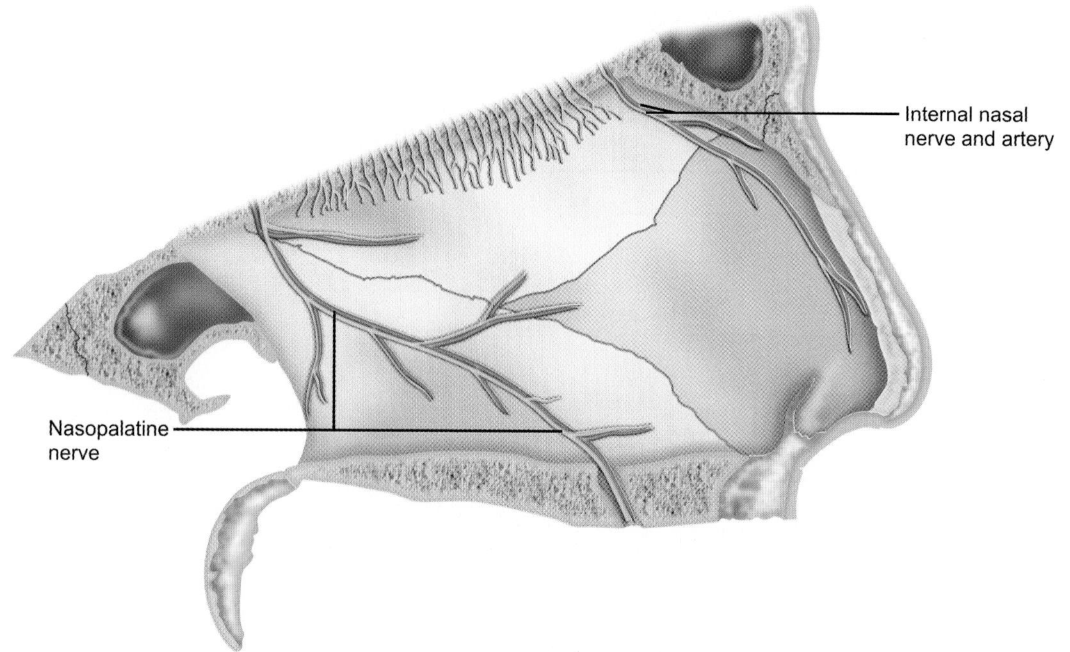

FIGURE 69 Vessels and nerves of nasal septum

See the *median septum* in the section and feel that it is covered by mucoperiosteum.

Dissection: Strip the mucoperiosteum and try to locate the thin nasopalatine nerve and artery posteriorly and identify the internal nasal nerve and artery (branches of nasociliary) anteriorly.

Identify the **roof** that is sloping both anteriorly as well as posteriorly.

Floor: The floor of the nasal cavity is same as the roof of the oral cavity. It is formed by the palate (It will be studied at a later stage of dissection).

Choanae is the posterior margin of the nasal cavity where it is continuous with the nasopharynx. It is bounded by the roof, lateral wall, septum and floor of the nasal cavity.

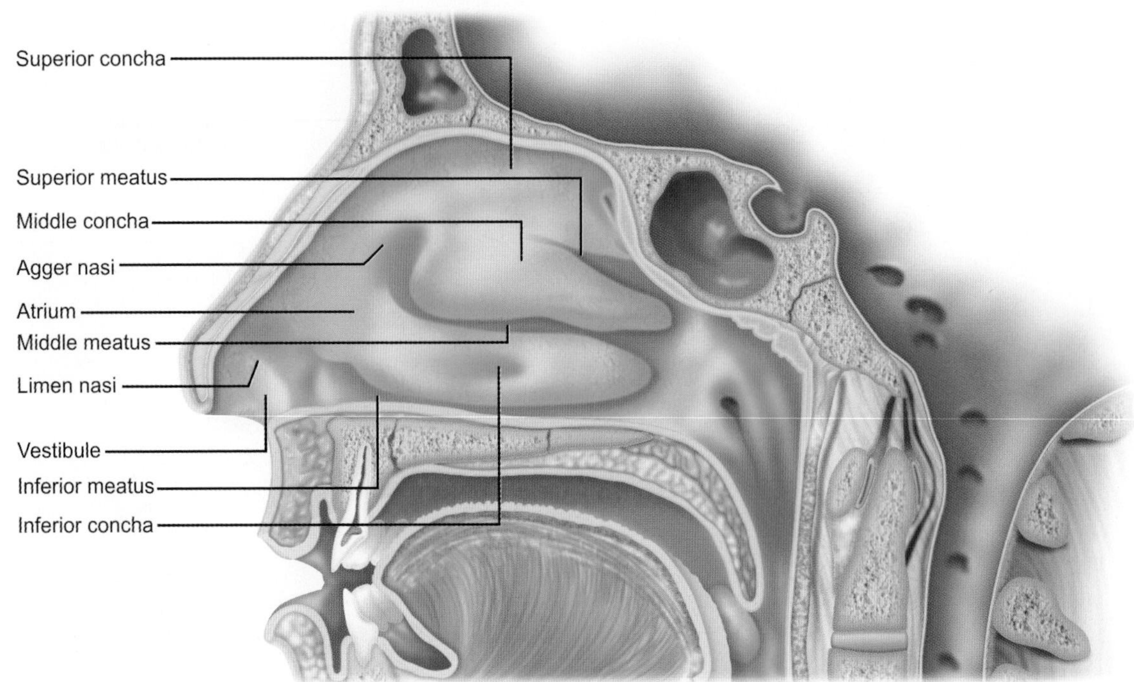

FIGURE 70 Lateral wall of nose

LATERAL WALL OF NOSE (Fig. 70)

Vestibule: It is the depressed area immediately internal to the anterior nasal aperture. Note the small thick hairs called vibrissae. The vestibule is bounded superiorly by the ***limen nasi***. The area above the limen is the ***atrium***. It is limited superiorly by ***agger nasi*** an elevation. The atrium lies continuous with the middle meatus.

Conchae: These are the bony elevations seen in the lateral wall. They are generally three in number—the ***superior, middle*** and ***inferior conchae.*** The superior and middle are projections of the ethmoid bone and the inferior is an individual bone. Put a fine forceps and identify the gaps, the meatuses. The nasal cavity is surrounded by air sinuses, superiorly, posteriorly and laterally. These sinuses open into the meatuses. Feel the thick membrane covering the conchae. These are cavernous in nature, i.e. they are filled with capillary plexus.

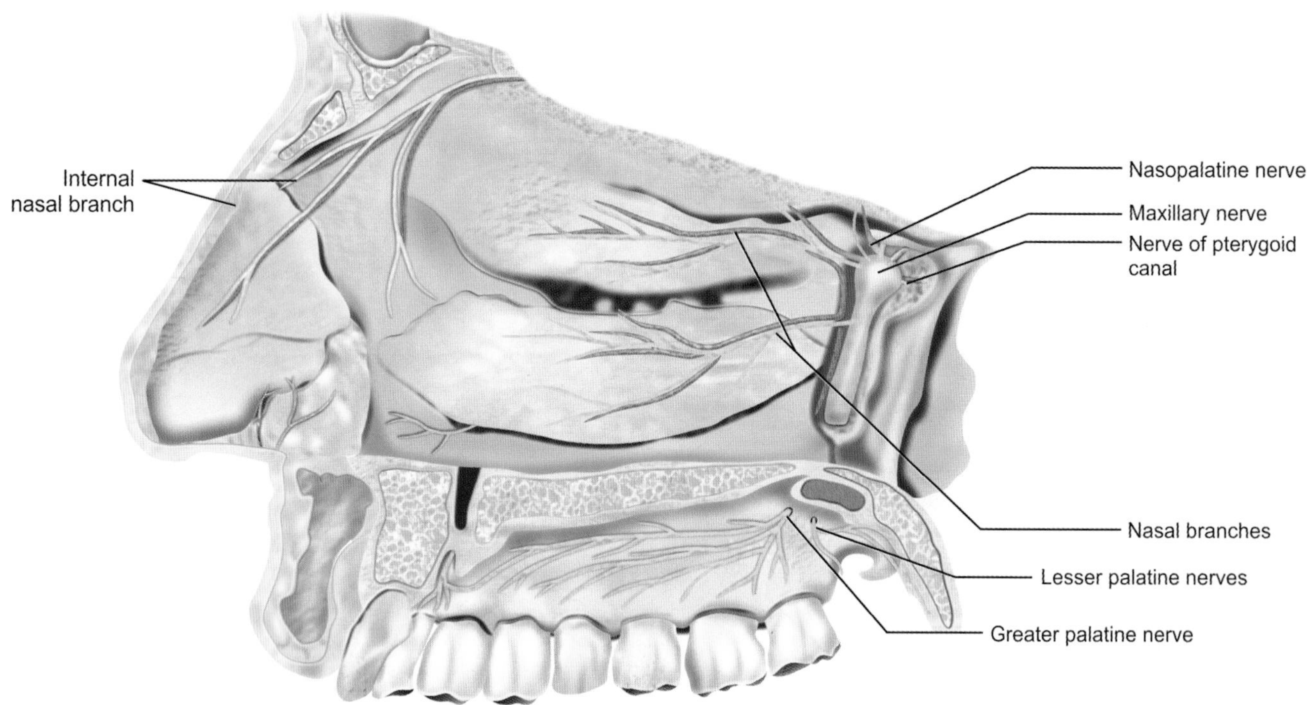

FIGURE 71 Pterygopalatine ganglion

PTERYGOPALATINE GANGLION (Fig. 71)

Dissection: Strip the mucoperiosteum behind the conchae and locate the pterygopalatine fossa. Locate the thick maxillary nerve and study the pterygopalatine ganglion.

Pterygopalatine ganglion is a parasympathetic ganglion. It is connected to the maxillary nerve by two roots. It carries both general sensory fibres and secretomotor fibres. See the two roots and the pterygopalatine ganglion hanging down from the ***maxillary nerve***. Trace the ***nerve of the pterygoid canal*** entering into the ganglion. These carry the preganglionic secretomotor fibres. Trace the branches arising from the pterygopalatine ganglion. The ***greater and lesser palatine*** nerves descend down and reach the roof of the palate. The ***pharyngeal branch*** goes posteriorly, the ***nasal branches*** traverse forward and ***nasopalatine*** *nerve* crosses and reaches the septum.

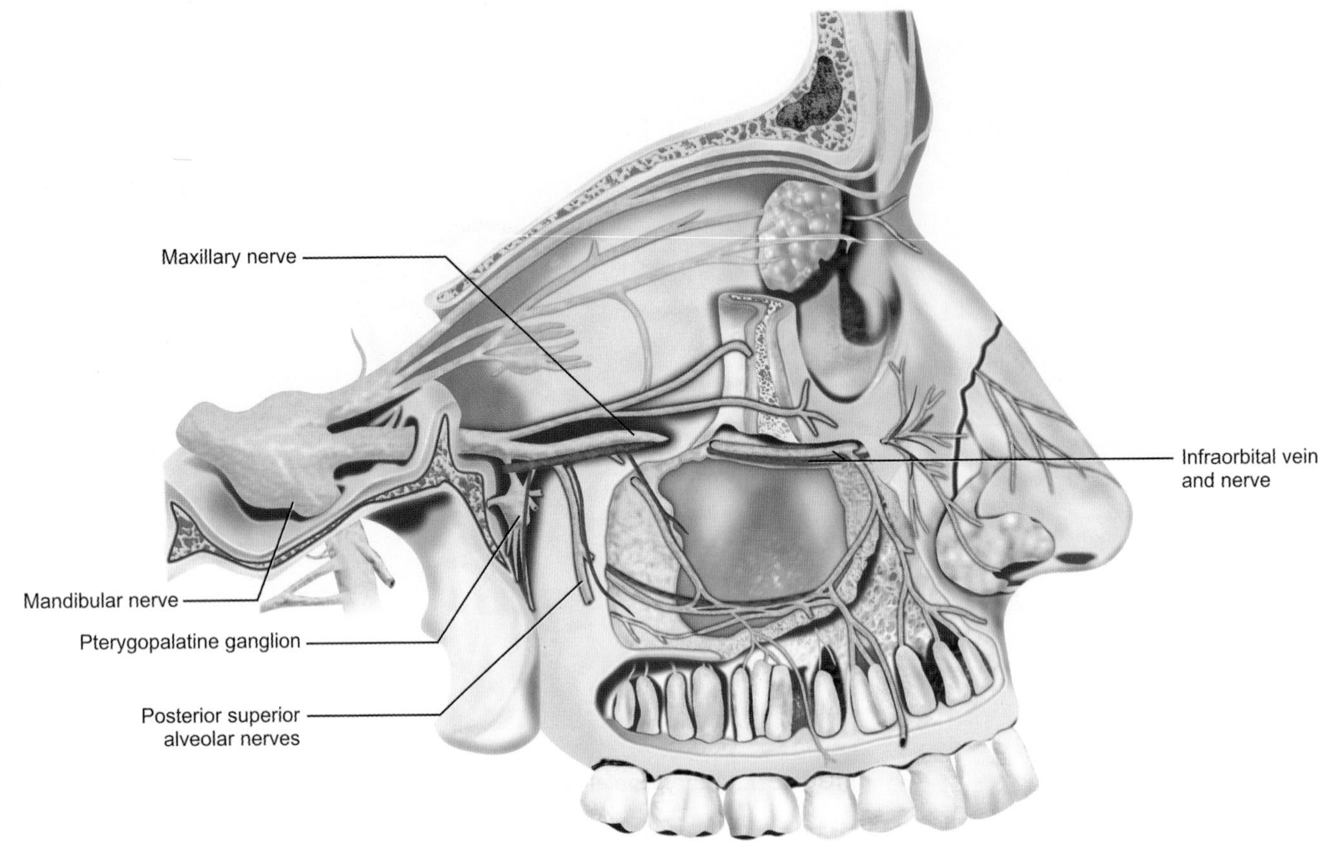

FIGURE 72 Maxillary nerve

MAXILLARY NERVE (Fig. 72)

Dissection: Turn the part to the outer side, and break the bone of the middle cranial fossa with a bone forceps. Identify the maxillary nerve in the middle cranial fossa near the cavernous sinus.

The ***maxillary nerve*** reaches the pterygopalatine fossa through the foramen rotundum. It moves forward into the floor of the orbit. See the ***posterior superior alveolar nerves*** that it gives off before reaching the orbit. They supply the maxillary teeth and the maxillary air sinus.

Arterial supply is by ***maxillary artery***. The third part of the maxillary artery reaches the pterygopalatine fossa after passing through the infratemporal fossa. It accompanies the maxillary nerve in the pterygopalatine fossa. It continues as the infraorbital artery in the floor of the orbit. Locate this artery and its branches in the pterygopalatine fossa. It gives off ***posterior superior alveolar, greater palatine, lesser palatine, nasopalatine, pharyngeal and artery accompanying the nerve of the pterygoid canal. Study of air sinuses and meatuses.***

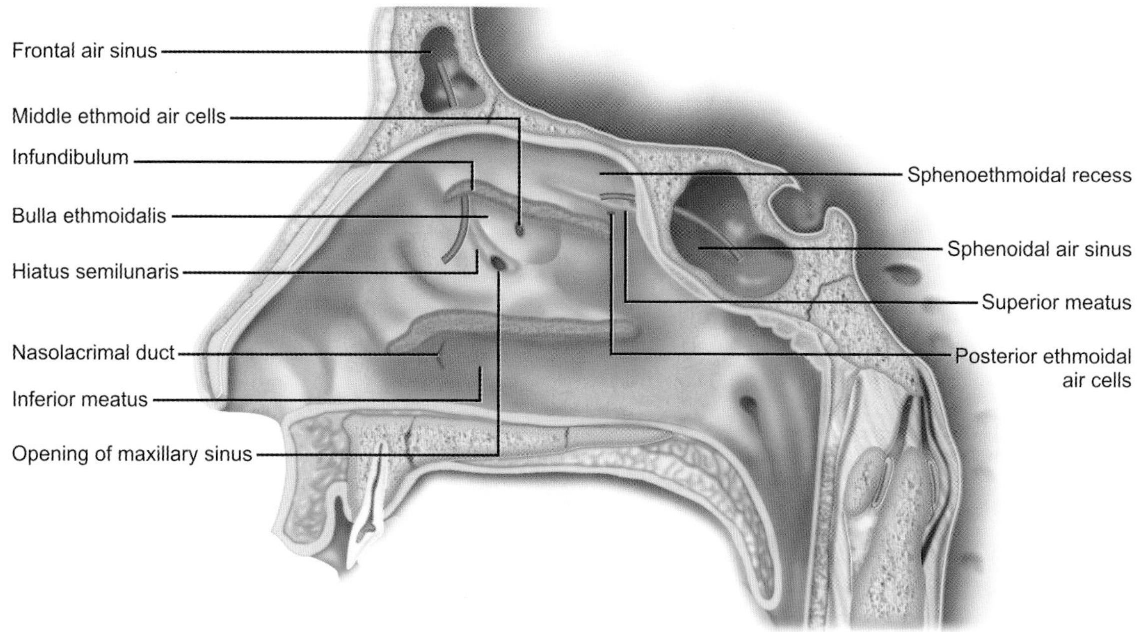

FIGURE 73 Meatuses and air sinuses

STUDY OF AIR SINUSES AND MEATUSES (Fig. 73)

Dissection: Cut the conchae with a scissors near their attachment.

Sphenoethmoidal recess: This is the space above and posterior to the superior concha. The ***sphenoidal air sinus*** opens into this. Locate this in the body of the sphenoid bone. It is divided into two halves by and unequal septum. Pass a probe from the sinus to the sphenoethmoidal recess.

Superior meatus: Identify this deep to the superior concha. The ***posterior ethmoidal air cells*** open into this. Cut the superior concha with a scissors. Note that two to three air cells open into it. Put a probe into them and note that they belong to posterior group of ethmoidal air cells. There are around 8 to 10 cells on the ethmoid bone. They are grouped into posterior middle and anterior group.

Middle meatus: It is the space deeper to the middle concha. Cut the middle concha with a scissors very near its attachment. Note the ***bulla ethmoidalis.*** It is a bulge in the center of the meatus. Note 2 to 3 air cells opening into it. Put a probe through them and note they are in the center of the ethmoid bone. These are ***middle ethmoidal air cells.*** Identify the groove below the bulla ethmoidalis. This is the ***hiatus semilunaris.*** It receives ***frontal, ethmoidal*** and ***maxillary air sinuses.***

Put a probe into the anterior end of the hiatus and push it up and note that they are continuous with the air cells in the anterior part of the ethmoid through a small infundibulum. These are the ***anterior ethmoidal air cells.***

Frontal air sinus: Put another probe through the cut frontal air sinus into the anterior end of the hiatus semilunaris through the infundibulum.

Maxillary air sinus: It occupies the whole maxilla (identify this on a dry skull. Identify its opening in the floor of the hiatus semilunaris. Pass a probe downwards and note its depth. Note that the rear premolars and molars project into it). Realize the mechanical disadvantage of this sinus, as its opening is above the base, due to this, the maxillary air sinus gets often infected.

Inferior meatus: Note that it is widest of all meatuses. It receives the ***nasolacrimal duct.*** It is nearer to the anterior end of the meatus. Pass a fine probe into the nasolacrimal duct. It passes through the bony wall to reach the lacrimal sac in the medial end of the orbit. Feel the lacrimal sac.

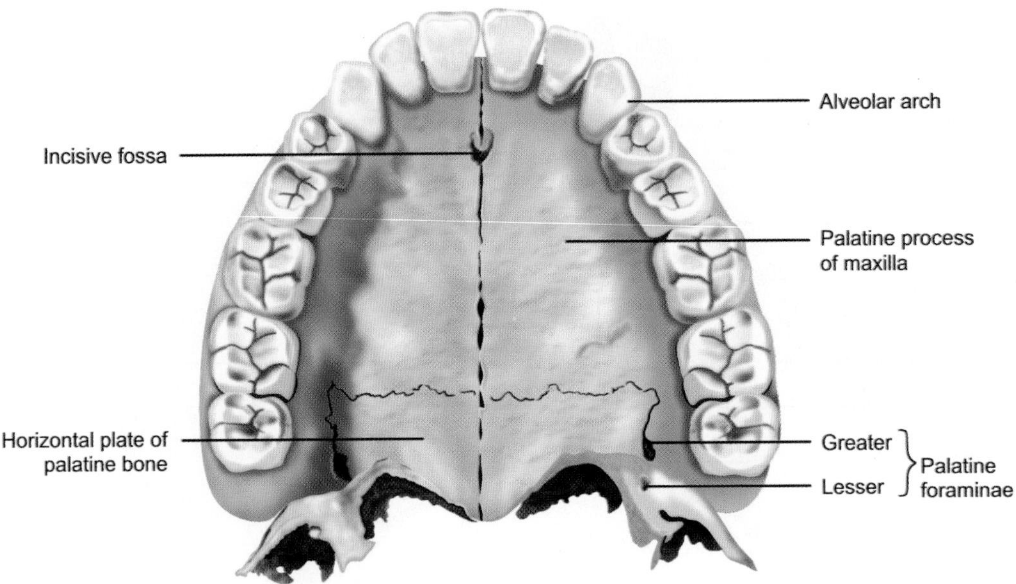

FIGURE 74 Bony hard palate

Neurovascular bundle of the nasal cavity: Nasal cavity is supplied by the branches of the maxillary nerve and maxillary artery. They reach the nasal cavity through the pterygopalatine fossa.

PALATE (Figs 74 and 75)

The palate is made up of hard palate and soft palate. The hard palate separates the nasal cavity from the oral cavity. The soft palate separates the nasopharynx from the oropharynx. The midline posterior projection from the soft palate is called the uvula.

Hard palate: It is made up of bones. Identify the bones forming the hard palate on a dry skull. They are maxilla and the palatine bone.

Dissection: Strip the mucus membrane from the hard palate and identify the greater and lesser palatine vessels and nerves reaching here through the foraminae of the same name. They are branches of the maxillary nerve through the pterygopalatine ganglion. They are both sensory as well as secretomotor to the hard palate.

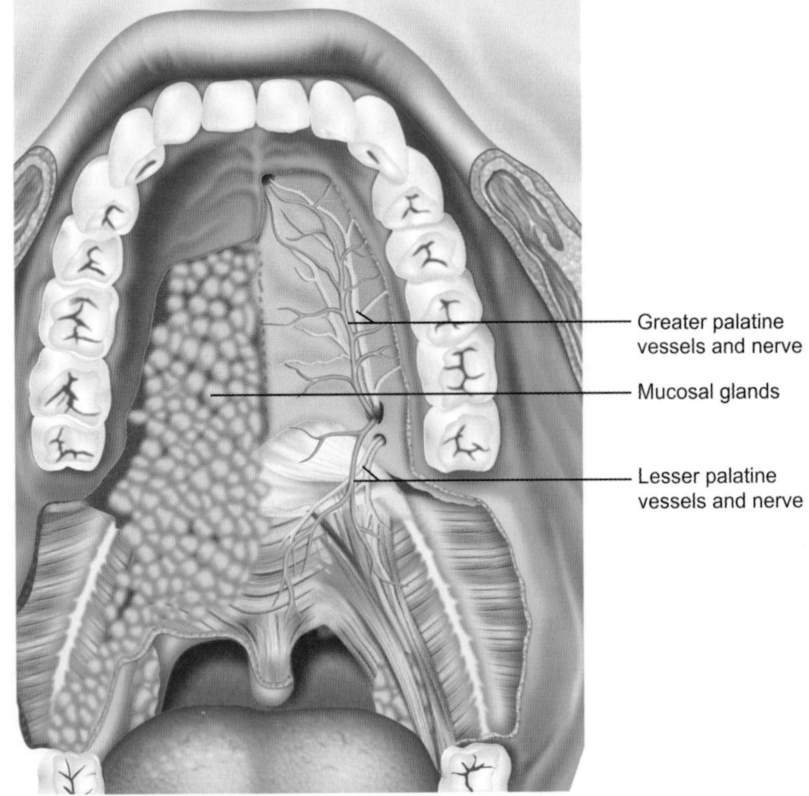

FIGURE 75 Hard palate

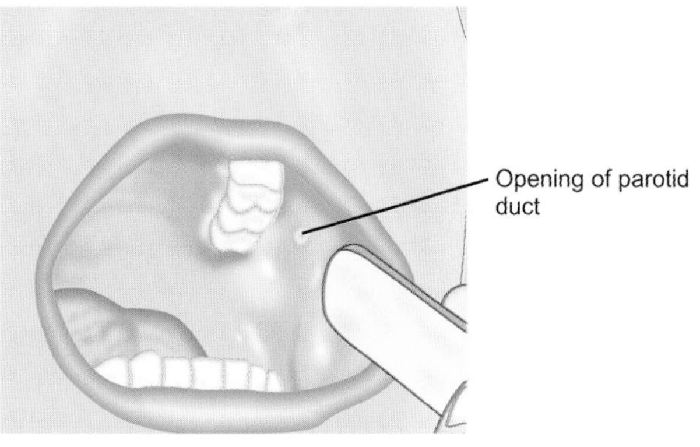

FIGURE 76 Vestibule

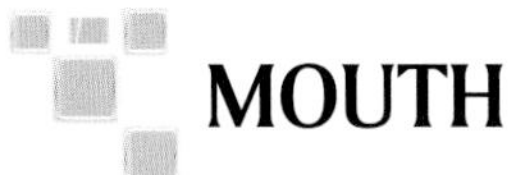

MOUTH

The mouth has two parts—the vestibule and the oral cavity. The vestibule lies external to the teeth and the oral cavity lies between the maxilla and mandible. The partition between the nasal cavity and oral cavity is formed by the hard palate. The oral cavity lodges the tongue.

Vestibule (Fig. 76): This is the area between the cheeks laterally and maxilla and mandible medially. The parotid duct opens into it opposite to the upper second molar tooth. If possible try to locate its end (this can be seen well in a living subject).

TONGUE (Figs 77 and 78)

Dorsum of the tongue is the superior surface facing the hard palate (See all the parts in a living person also). Note the ***sulcus terminalis*** near the posterior part. It is a V shaped sulcus which separates the anterior 2/3rd from posterior 1/3rd. In the anterior 2/3 note the fine ***filiform papillae.*** See the rounded ***fungiform papillae*** between the filiform papillae. Locate the ***circumvallate papillae*** behind the sulcus. In the remaining part of the posterior 1/3—note the grooves. These grooves receive the openings of the deeply placed glands. The elevations between the grooves is due to the lymphoid tissue.

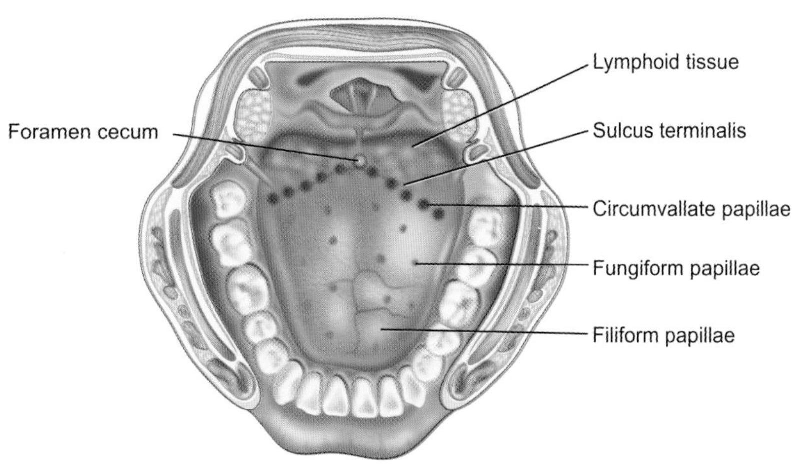

FIGURE 77 Dorsum of tongue

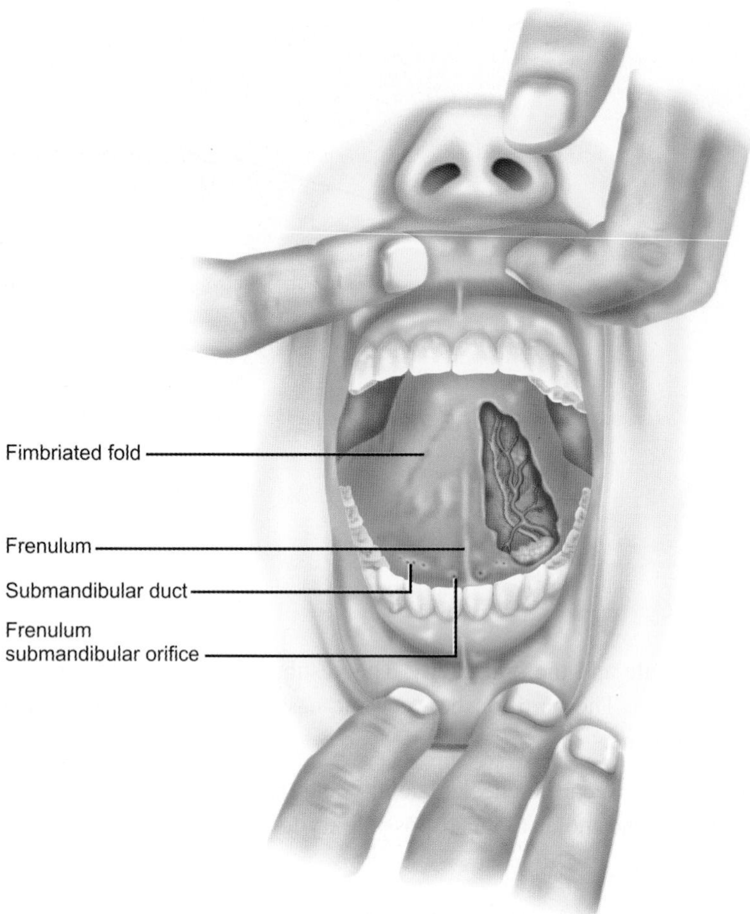

FIGURE 78 Ventral surface of tongue

Ventral surface of tongue*:** Lift the tongue up and note the ***frenulum* in the midline,** ***fimbriated fold laterally and ***sublingual fold*** and ***orifice of the submandibular duct*** in the floor (see these in a living person).

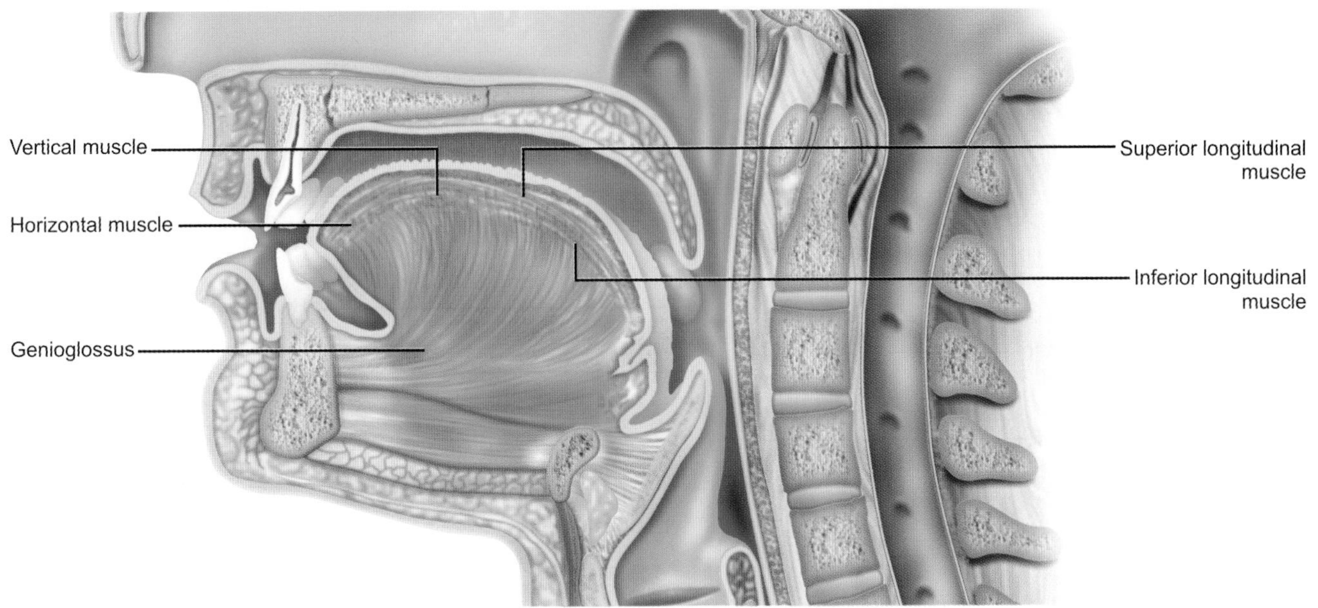

FIGURE 79 Intrinsic musculature of tongue

MUSCLES OF TONGUE (Fig. 79)

Muscles of tongue can be divided into intrinsic and extrinsic muscles. The muscles are bilateral and are separated by a central fibrous septum. The intrinsic muscles have no bony attachment.

In a paramedian section of the tongue the intrinsic muscles can be identified. They are arranged as: ***Superior longitudinal layer*** lies immediately beneath the dorsum of the tongue. ***Vertical muscle fibres*** run down vertically. ***Horizontal fibres*** intermingle with the vertical fibres. ***Inferior longitudinal fibres*** lie below these above muscles.

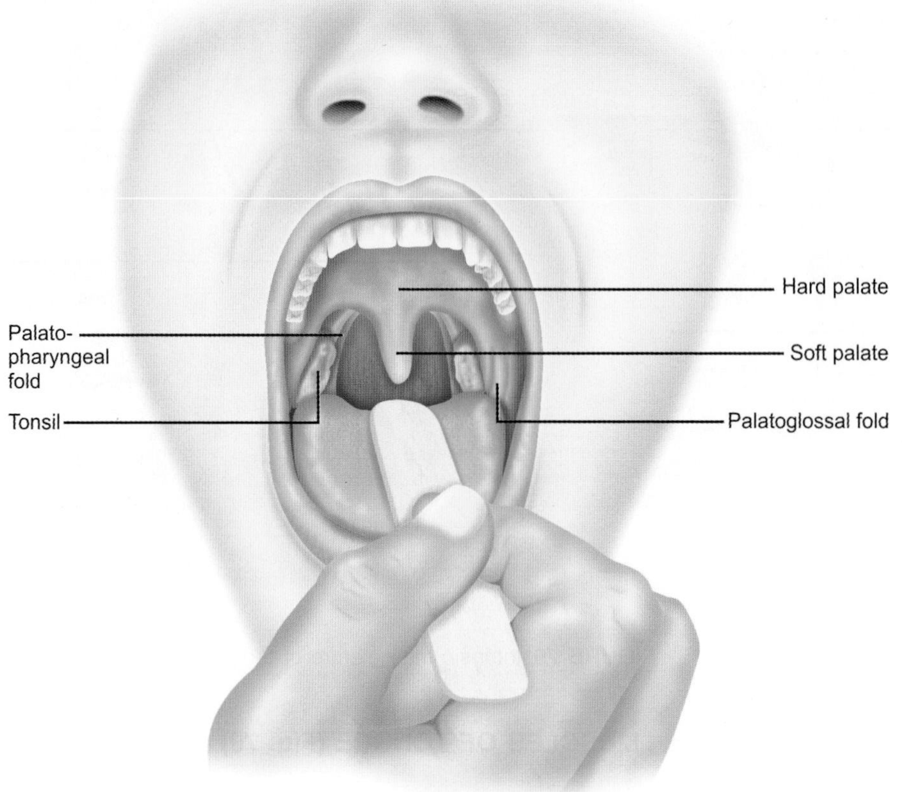

FIGURE 80 Fauces

Genioglossus: This is the extrinsic muscle from the superior genial tubercle lies between the inferior longitudinal fibres and genial tubercles. This is a fan-shaped muscle. It is a depressor of the tongue (other extrinsic muscles will be seen in a later dissection).

Fauces (Fig. 80): It is the junction between the oral cavity and the oropharynx. It is formed by two pillars—the anterior palatoglossal fold and posterior palatopharyngeal fold. Between the two pillars the palatine tonsil is located.

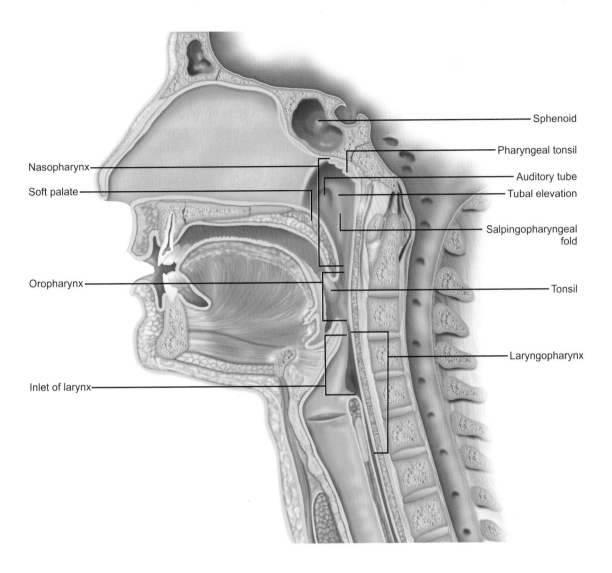

Sphenoid
Pharyngeal tonsil
Nasopharynx
Auditory tube
Soft palate
Tubal elevation
Salpingopharyngeal fold
Oropharynx
Tonsil
Laryngopharynx
Inlet of larynx

FIGURE 81 Interior of pharynx

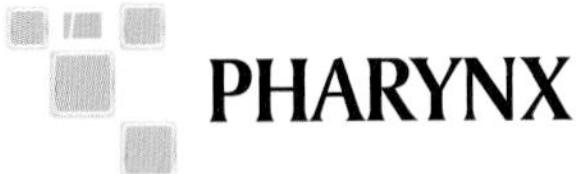

PHARYNX

The pharynx is a funnel shaped fibromuscular tube extending from the base of the skull to the 6th cervical vertebra. It is divided into three parts—the nasopharynx, oropharynx and laryngopharynx **(Fig. 81)**.

Boundaries: The roof of ***nasopharynx*** is formed by the sphenoid bone. It is continuous with the nasal cavity anteriorly. The junction is called the choanae. The lateral wall shows the auditory opening. Inferiorly and anteriorly it is separated from the oral cavity by the soft palate. Posteriorly and inferiorly it is continuous with the oropharynx. The roof of the ***oropharynx*** is same as the floor of the nasopharynx. Oropharynx is continuous with the oral cavity anteriorly and superiorly. Anteriorly and inferiorly the sloping posterior 1/3rd of tongue forms the boundary. The junction between the oropharynx and oral cavity is called the oropharyngeal isthmus. It is formed by the palatoglossal fold. The lateral wall forms fauces and lodges tonsil. The ***laryngopharynx*** is continuous with the larynx anteriorly. The opening into the larynx is called inlet of the larynx. The laryngopharynx lies behind and parallel with the larynx. It continues below as the esophagus.

It is the common passage for air and food. Its interior is covered by mucous membrane. Structurally, the pharynx has four layers. Innermost mucosal layer, followed by submucosal layer, the external muscular layer, covered by adventitial layer.

Dissection: In this study from the interior you will see the mucous membrane, the submucosal lymphoid tissue and the inner longitudinal layer of the musculature. You will identify the lymphoid tissue as bulges. You need to strip the mucous membrane to identify the musculature.

Nasopharynx: See the position of the ***pharyngeal tonsil.*** It is the collection of lymphoid tissue in the roof of the pharynx. It can easily be identified deeper to the mucous membrane. Identify the ***opening of the auditory tube*** in the lateral wall. It is a longitudinal slit with anterior and posterior walls. The posterior wall is more prominent and is called ***tubal elevation.*** It is due to tubal tonsil, the aggregation of the lymphoid tissue here. A mucosal fold continues down from the tubal elevation and is called the ***salpingopharyngeal fold.*** The fold is raised by the salpingopharyngeal muscle.

SOFT PALATE (Fig. 82)

Soft palate is the posterior part of the palate and it is muscular. It is made up of five muscles. Two muscles can be seen from above and two muscles from below and one muscle posteriorly.

Dissection: Strip the nasopharynx mucous membrane.

Tensor veli palatine: Identify this muscle lateral and anterior to the auditory tube. It runs vertically on the external side of the auditory tube. It arises from the scaphoid fossa lateral side of auditory tube and spine of the sphenoid (identify them on the dry skull). It hooks round the pterygoid hamulus and gets inserted in the form of an aponeurosis which forms the core for the soft palate. It is a tensor of the soft palate. Nerve supply. It is supplied by the mandibular near trunk just below the foramen ovale (this was identified in the infratemporal fossa dissection).

Dissection: Pass a probe through the auditory tube. The muscle in front of it is the tensor veli palatine and the muscle behind it is the levator veli palatine.

Levator veli palatine: It arises from the undersurface of the petrous part of the temporal bone and the medial surface of the cartilage of the auditory tube. It is inserted into the superior surface of the palatine aponeurosis. It is an elevator of the palate.

Musculus uvulae: Strip the mucous membrane over the uvula and locate this centrally located muscle. It arises from the spine and gets into the mucous membrane.

Salpingopharyngeus: This muscle is the longitudinal muscle of the pharynx. It arises from the lower part of the auditory tube and is inserted into the posterior border of thyroid cartilage. Pull the muscle up and feel the insertion and its action as an elevator of larynx.

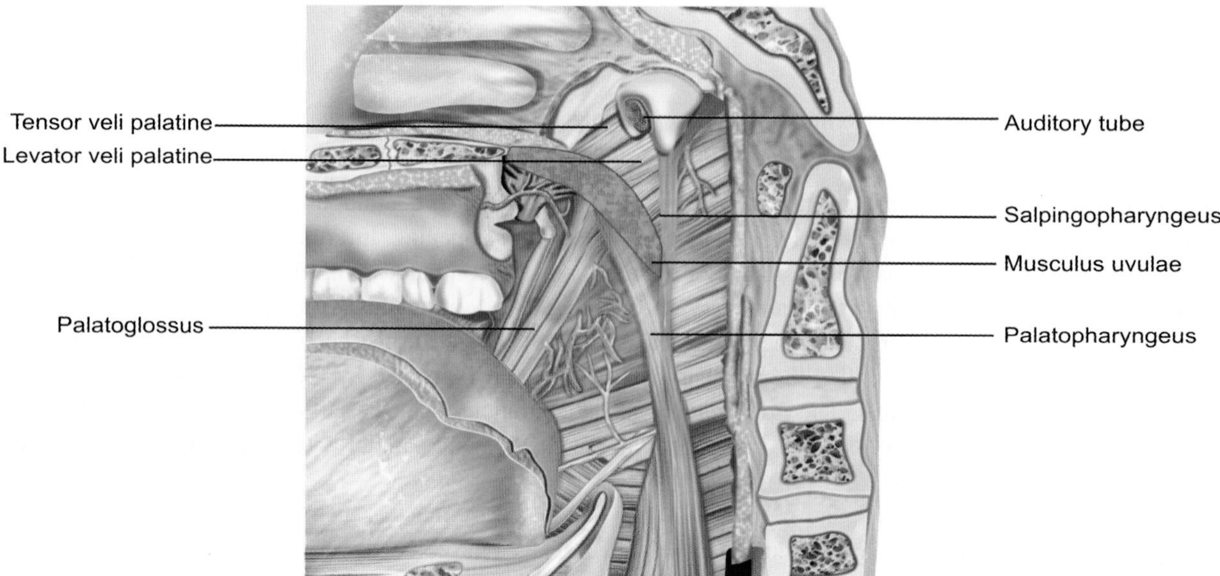

FIGURE 82 Soft palate

Dissection: Strip the mucous membrane of the oropharynx and see the musculature.

Palatoglossus muscle: This muslce forms the anterior pillar of the fauces. This is an extrinsic muscle of the tongue arising from the soft palate. It arises from the undersurface of the palatine aponeurosis. It is inserted into the side of the tongue.

Palatopharyngeus muscle. This muscle forms the posterior pillar of the fauces. It arises from the posterior border of the hard palate and the palatine aponeurosis. It runs downwards and is inserted into posterior border of the thyroid cartilage. This is also an elevator of the larynx.

Passavant's muscle: Few of the fibres of the palatopharyngeus muscle run straight back to the midline raising an elevation in the lateral wall. It acts like a sphincter between nasal and oral pharynx, along with the soft palate.

Nerve supply: All the muscles of the pharynx and the soft palate are supplied by the cranial accessory nerve through the pharyngeal plexus located in the pharyngeal wall except the tensor veli palatine which is supplied by the mandibular nerve.

Tonsil: Note this lymphoid tissue between the palatoglossal and palatopharyngeal fold. It shows pitted appearance.

OROPHARYNX (Fig. 83)

Anteroinferior wall of the oropharynx: This is formed by the posterior part of tongue. Note the following structures by pushing the tongue forwards.

Median glossoepiglottic fold: It is a raised mucosal fold in the midline extending from the back of the tongue to the center of the epiglottis.

Lateral glossoepiglottic folds: These are two lateral mucosal folds to the right and left of the median fold.

Vallecula: It is the central depression between the median and lateral glossoepiglottic folds.

Laryngopharynx It coexists with the larynx, in other words, the larynx forms the anterior wall to this part of the pharynx (this will be studied with larynx).

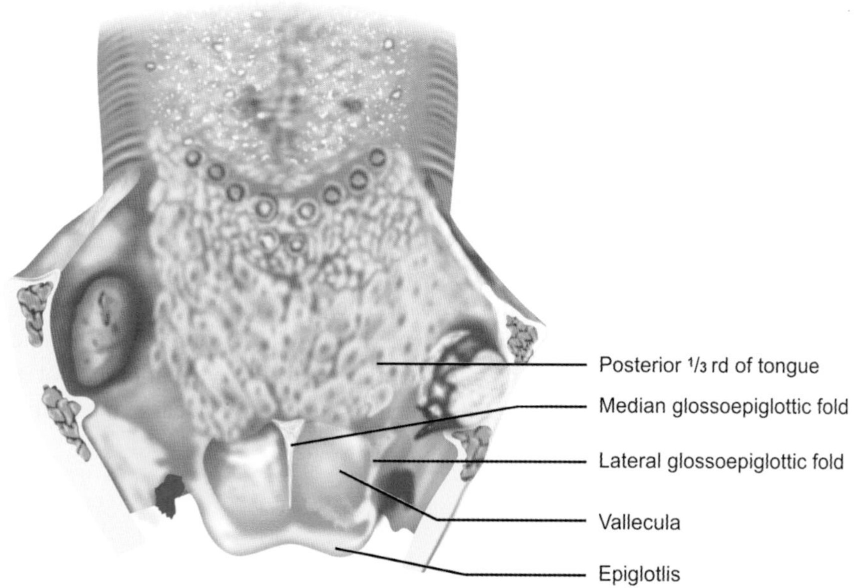

FIGURE 83 Anterioinferior wall of oropharynx

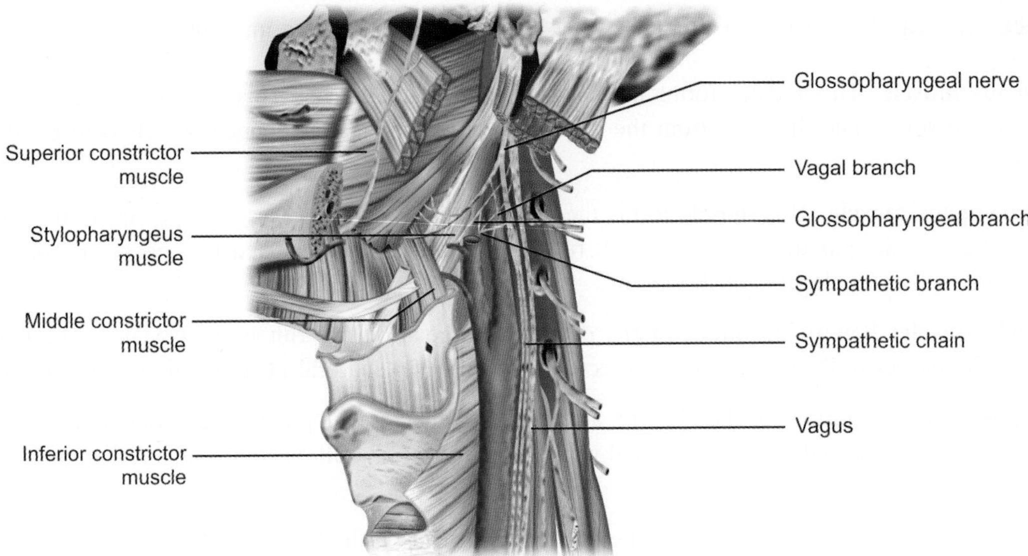

FIGURE 84 Structures from the lateral aspect

STUDY OF THE STRUCTURES FROM THE LATERAL ASPECT (Fig. 84)

The pharynx extends from the basiocciput to the 6th cervical vertebra. It is covered by adventitial layer. Clean this connective tissue and try to identify the following structures from above downwards on the lateral aspect. This is the external circular muscular layer. It is made up of three muscles one fitting into the other, like buckets.

Superior constrictor muscle: It is the upper circular muscle of the pharynx. Identify the muscle. It arises from the medial pterygoid plate, pterygomandibular raphae and mandible behind the third molar tooth. At its upper border identifies the anterior tensor veli palatini and posterior levator veli palatini with the auditor tube in between.

Middle constrictor muscle: Locate this muscle lying deeper to the hyoglossus. It arises from greater, lesser cornu of the hyoid bone and the lower part of the stylohyoid ligament. The fibres span out posteriorly to reach the midline.

Inferior constrictor muscle: Note this muscle below and external to the middle constrictor. It arises from the oblique line of thyroid cartilage and from the lateral side of the cricoid cartilage. It is Inserted into the midline raphae located posteriorly.

All the three constrictors of pharynx insert into a median raphae posteriorly. They are supplied by cranial accessory nerve through the pharyngeal plexus.

Dissection: Peel the connective tissue from the posterior aspect of the pharyngeal musculature. Try to identify as many nerve branches as possible.

Pharyngeal plexus: It is a plexus of nerves deep to the pharyngeal fascia. It is formed by the (i) pharyngeal branch of the vagus, but it carries the cranial accessory fibres. Thus it receives through a communication near the jugular foramen. These fibres supply the muscles of pharynx and soft palate. (ii) Pharyngeal branch of glossopharyngeal nerve. It is sensory to the mucous membrane. (iii) pharyngeal branch of superior cervical sympathetic ganglion. This carries vasomotor fibres to the blood vessels of the pharynx.

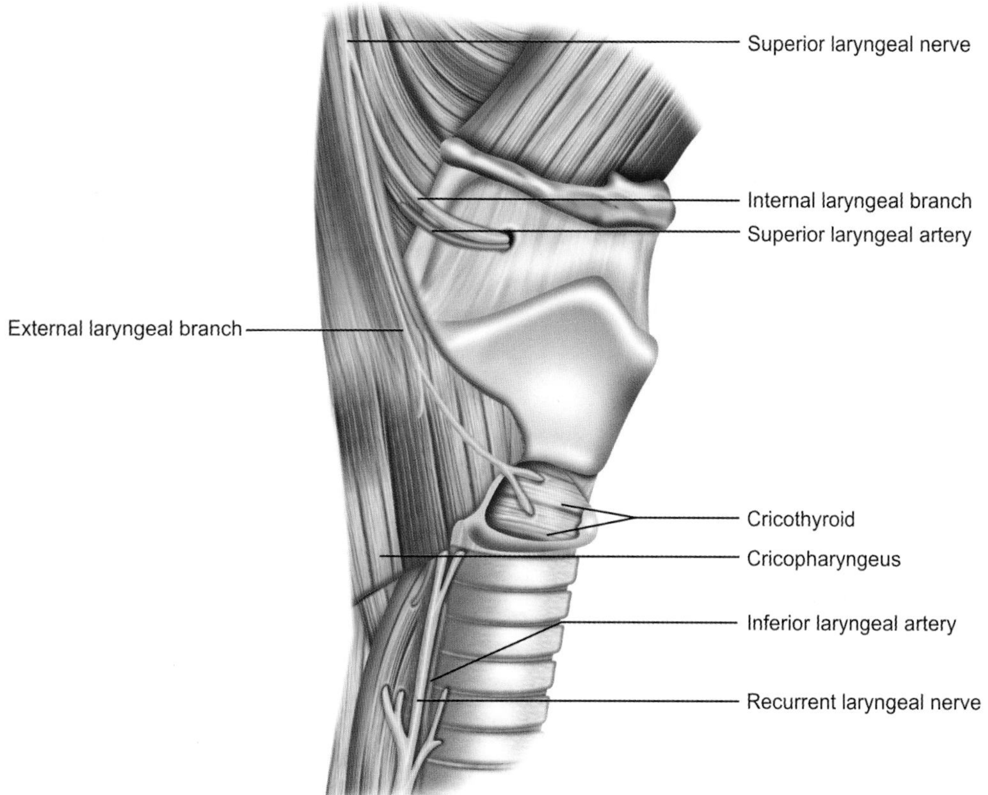

FIGURE 85 Larynx—neurovascular bundle

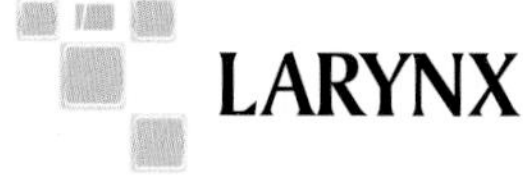

LARYNX

Larynx is an organ of voice production. It extends from the 4th to 6th cervical vertebrae. It is around 5 cm long, 4 cm in width and 3.5 cm in anterior posterior diameter. It is a fibrocartilaginous structure. It has an obliquely placed inlet of the larynx. It opens into the pharynx.

NEUROVASCULAR BUNDLE (Fig. 85)

Dissection: Reidentify the neurovascular bundle entering into the larynx before taking it out of the body.

Internal laryngeal nerve and superior laryngeal vessels: These enter the larynx through the thyrohyoid membrane. Superior laryngeal artery is a branch of superior thyroid and nerve is a branch of superior laryngeal nerve. This nerve is sensory above the rima glottidis. External laryngeal nerve is a branch of the superior laryngeal, branch of the vagus nerve.

Inferior laryngeal artery and the recurrent laryngeal nerve: Trace these two structures entering into the larynx between trachea and esophagus below the inferior constrictor muscle. The recurrent laryngeal nerve is a motor nerve to muscles of larynx and sensory to mucous membrane below the rima glottidis.

Dissection: Remove the larynx from the body (where it is not bisected in a sagittal plane) by cutting it above the hyoid bone, and the sides of the pharyngeal wall and clean the fascia. Inferiorly cut it near the 3rd tracheal ring. Feel the following cartilages, bones and membranes.

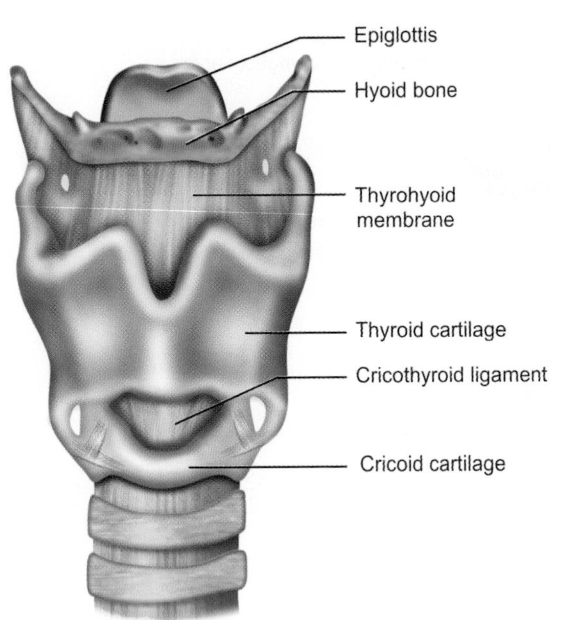

FIGURE 86 Skeleton of larynx—anterior view

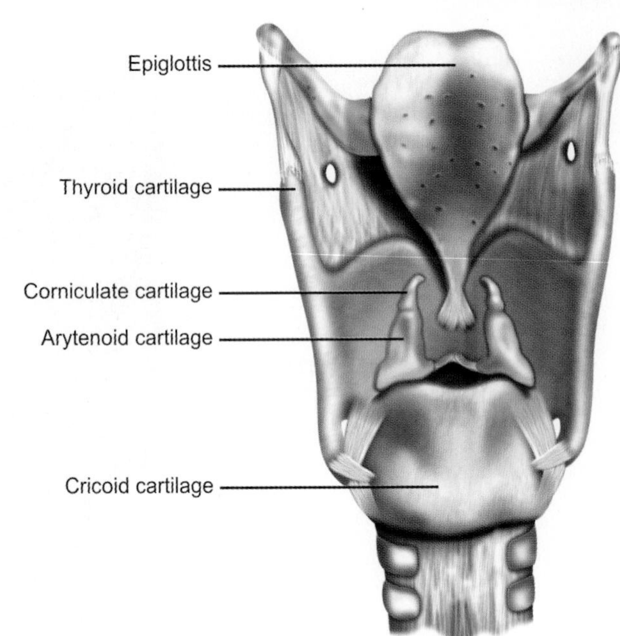

FIGURE 87 Skeleton of larynx—posterior view

SKELETON OF LARYNX (Figs 86 and 87)

Hyoid bone: This forms the superior boundary of the larynx. It has got a wide body in the center, greater cornua extending laterally and lesser cornua at the junction of body and greater cornua.

Thyrohyoid membrane: Identify this membrane extending between the upper border of hyoid bone to the upper border of thyroid cartilage. It shows two thickenings medial (in the midline) and lateral (towards the ends) thyrohyoid ligaments.

Thyroid cartilage: This cartilage has two laminae. They unite anteriorly in the midline to form an angle. This is called Adams apple or laryngeal prominence. It is around 90° degrees in males and 120° in females. It has two horns, the superior and inferior horns. The inferior horn articulates with the cricoid cartilage.

Cricothyroid ligament: Feel this ligament between the thyroid and cricoid cartilage on the anterolateral aspect. Push the back of the forceps and note that it is attached to the inner aspect of the thyroid cartilage near its middle.

Cricoid cartilage: Feel the broad posterior lamina of the cricoid cartilage and the anterior arch shaped part. Totally it resembles a signet ring.

Arytenoid cartilages: Feel these pyramidal shaped cartilages on the superior surface of the cricoid cartilages. Feel its three surfaces, the medial, lateral and the base. It has three angles, the superior (articulating with corniculate cartilage), the anterior is called vocal process and lateral is called muscular process.

Corniculate cartilage: It is a comma shaped cartilage articulating with the superior angle of arytenoid.

Cuneiform cartilage: Feel it. It is a nodule in the aryepiglottic fold.

Epiglottis: Identify this leaf shaped cartilage on the posterior aspect of the hyoid and thyroid cartilages. It can easily be bent forwards and backwards. It is connected to the hyoid by hyoepiglottic ligament and to the thyroid by thyroepiglottic ligament.

Quadrangular membrane: You clasp this membrane between your fingers. It extends from the anterior border of the arytenoid cartilage to the side of the epiglottis. As the name signifies it is quadrangular in shape. It has a superior border called aryepiglottic ligament. This forms part of inlet of larynx. Its inferior free border forms the vestibular ligament. The quadrangular membrane separates the vestibule of the larynx from the piriform fossa, the space between the larynx and the thyroid cartilage.

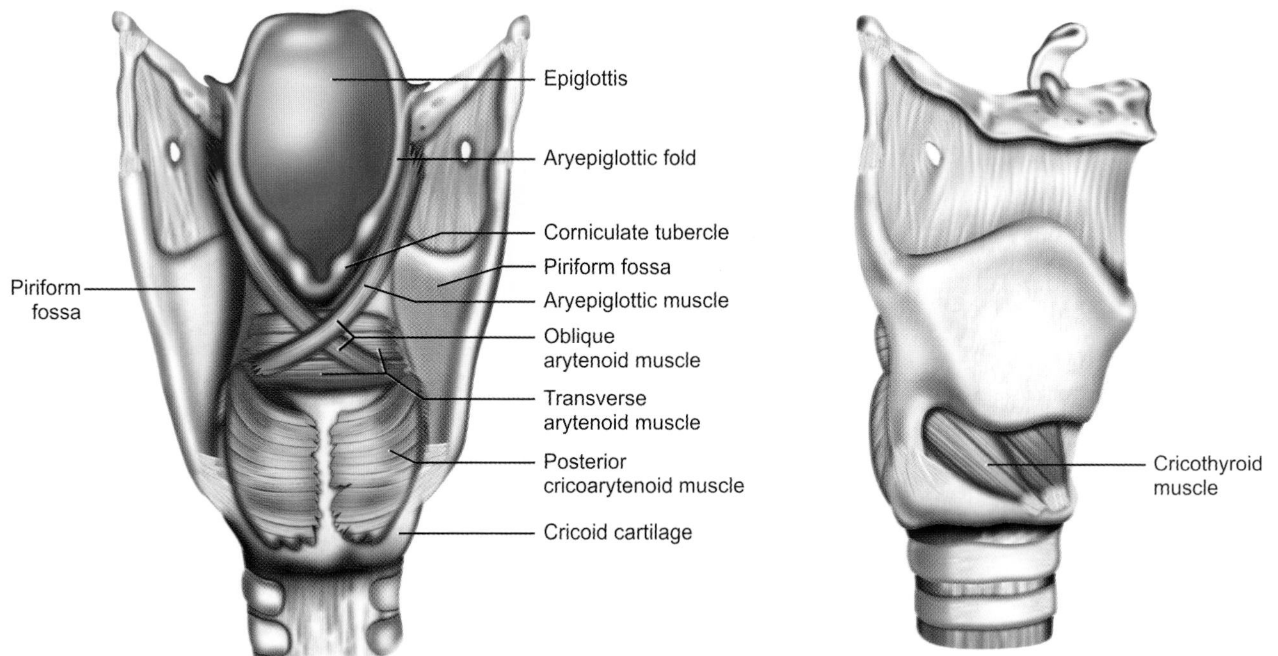

FIGURE 88 Muscles of larynx

INLET OF LARYNX

Turn the larynx to its posterior aspect and observe and feel the inlet of the larynx. It is formed by the upper border of the epiglottis, aryepiglottic folds, arytenoids cartilages and interarytenoid mucous membrane.

Dissection: Peel the adventitial layer from the outer surface of the larynx and identify the muscles.

MUSCLES (Fig. 88)

Posterior cricoarytenoid: Identify this muscle on the posterior aspect of the lamina of cricoid cartilage. It arises from the same and is inserted into the muscular process of the arytenoids cartilage. Note that the fibres are transverse in the upper part, these act as lateral rotators, and the lower fibres slope up, and these would pull the arytenoid downward thus producing abduction.

Oblique arytenoid: See it between the two arytenoids. It arises from the posterior aspect of one arytenoid and is inserted into the apex of the other arytenoid. Note that the fibres of both sides cross each other like an x. It acts along with aryepiglottis muscle to close the inlet of the larynx.

Transverse arytenoid: This muscle is deeper to the oblique arytenoid. It extends from one arytenoids to the other arytenoid. This muscle acts as an adductor.

Aryepiglottic muscle: Trace this muscle in the free margin of aryepiglottic fold. It arises from the apex of the arytenoids to be inserted into the side of the epiglottis. The aryepiglottis along with the oblique arytenoid acts like a scissors and closes the inlet of the larynx.

Cricothyroid: See this on the lateral aspect. It arises from the lateral aspect of the cricoid cartilage and is inserted into the lower border of the thyroid cartilage. It is a tensor of the vocal cords. It is supplied by the external laryngeal nerve.

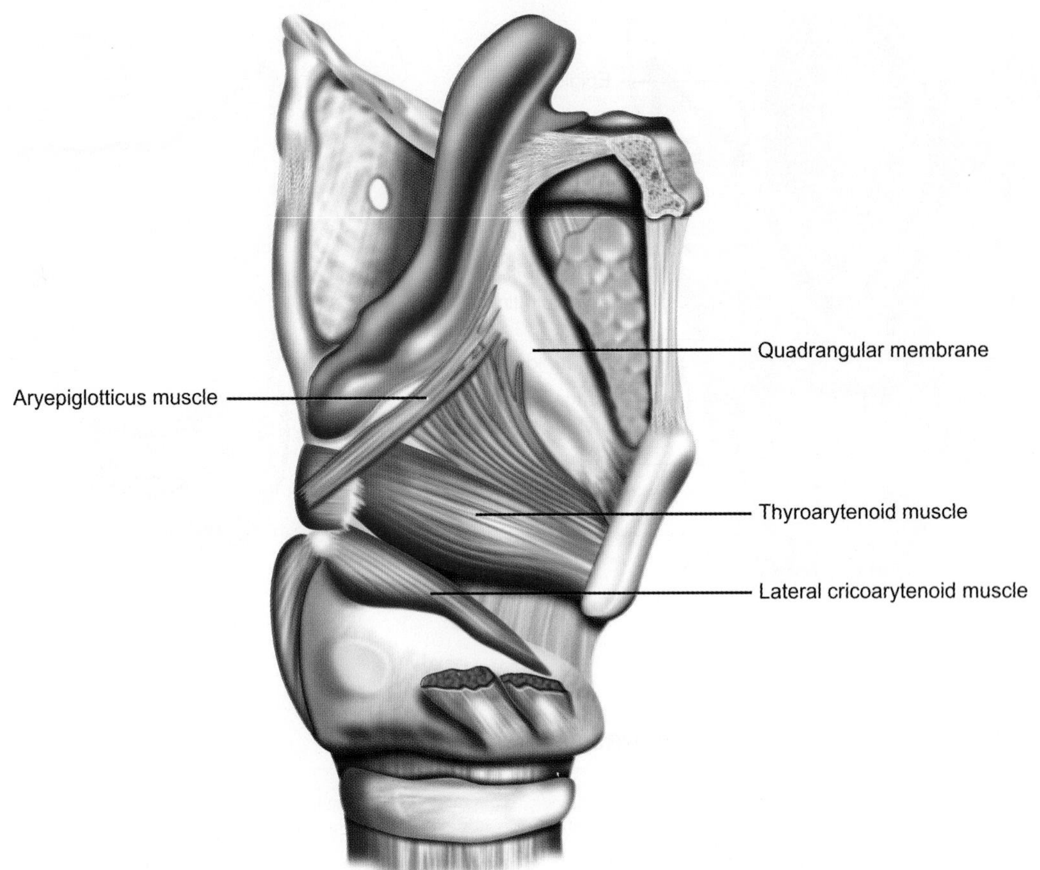

FIGURE 89 Deep muscles of larynx

Lateral cricoarytenoid muscle (Fig. 89): Trace this deeper muscle. It arises from the upper border of the cricoid cartilage. It is inserted into the muscular process. It is an abductor of vocal cords.

Dissection: Cut the posterior wall of larynx in the midline and open it. See the interior.

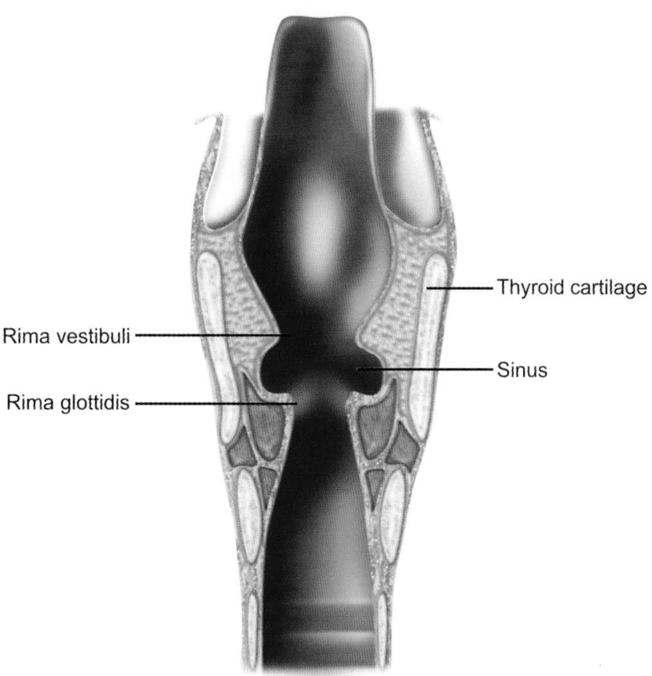

FIGURE 90 Interior of larynx

INTERIOR OF LARYNX (Fig. 90)

Rima vestibuli: It is the lower border of the quadrangular membrane. It is thickened at its lower part and is called vestibular ligament. It is covered by mucous membrane called vestibular folds. The gap between the two vestibular folds is called the rima vestibuli.

Rima glottidis: It is the gap between the two vocal ligaments. The thickened upper end of the cricothyroid membrane is called the vocal ligament. The mucous membrane covering it forms the vocal fold. The gap extending from the back of the thyroid cartilage to the posterior wall is called the rima glottidis. It has got an anterior intermembranous part and posterior intercartilaginous part between the two arytenoid cartilages.

Sinus: It is the gap between the rima vestibuli and rima glottidis.

Saccule: Put a probe through the sinus and extend it upwards. This is an extension of the sinus lateral to the quadrangular membrane. In birds it is very much well developed.

Vestibule: It is the part of the larynx, above the rima vestibuli to the inlet of the larynx. See its anterior wall, is far higher and formed by the epiglottis.

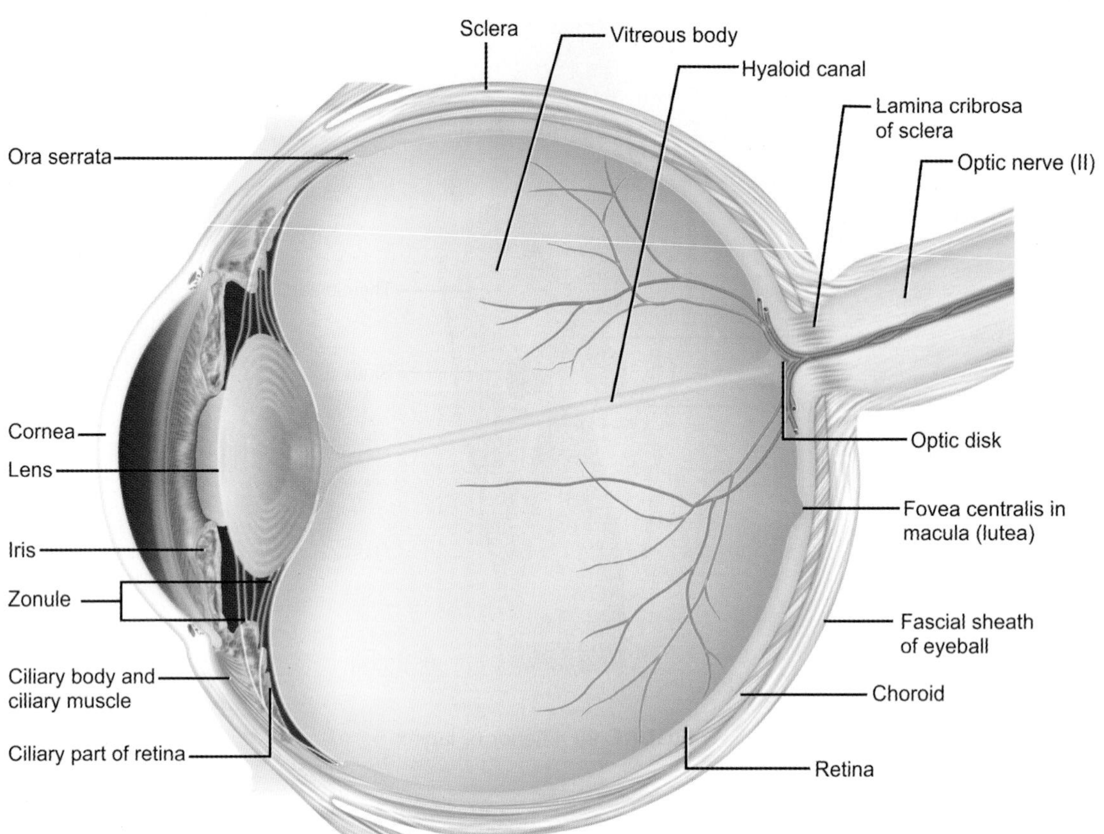

FIGURE 91 Sagittal section of eyeball

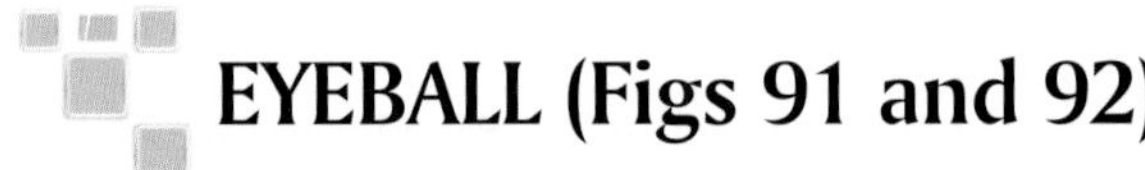

EYEBALL (Figs 91 and 92)

Dissection: It is easy to study bull's eye as they are big in size and well developed. Clean the muscles on the external surface. Take two eyeballs cut one along the equator in a coronal section dividing it into anterior and posterior halves, the other anteroposteriorly into two halves. See the following.

Cornea: Cornea is the outer protective coat. It forms the anterior 1/6th of the outer coat of the eyeball. It is transparent.

Sclera: It forms the posterior 5/6th of the outer coat of the eyeball. It is the opaque thick fibrous layer.

Vitreous body: This is the innermost jelly like body. It is enclosed by a thin capsule. It generally gets cut and falls off when the eyeball is cut.

Retina: This is the nervous layer of the eye. It looks whitish in the cut eyeball. It easily gets peeled off from the deeper choroid layer. It becomes very thin anteriorly.

Vascular layer: It is the intermediate layer. Peel the retinal layer and look at his layer. It is black in color. ***Iris*** is its anterior part and this lies in front of the lens. ***Ciliary body*—**this is the part lateral to the lens. ***Choroid***—this is the part behind the ora serrata. ***Ora serrata***—is the serrated junction between the ciliary body and choroid. This can easily be identified.

Zonule: Note this suspending fibrous structure extending from the ciliary body to the lens.

Lens: This is the biconvex structure suspended by the zonular fibres.

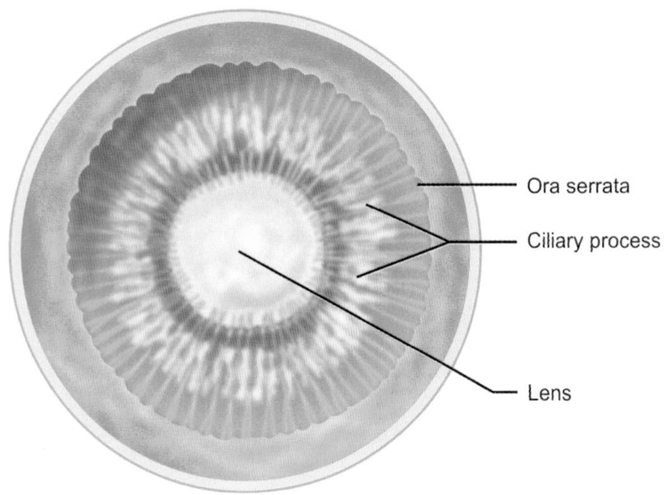

FIGURE 92 Coronal section of eyeball

MUSCLES OF THE EYEBALL

Ciliary muscle: Locate this muscle within the ciliary body.

The sphincter and dilator pupilae: These are the muscles present within the iris. You can see these muscles in the cut parts of the ciliary body and iris. These muscles are supplied by the autonomic nervous system, through the ciliary ganglion.

Optic disc and optic nerve: Identify these structures at the posterior medial part of the eyeball.

Anterior ciliary arteries: These arteries enter the sclera near the sclerocorneal junction. The posterior ciliary arteries pierce the sclera around the optic nerve. All the arteries are branches of the ophthalmic artery.

Venae vorticose: These are the veins draining the eyeball. They pierce the eyeball near the equator and drain into ophthalmic veins.

CHAPTER 8

CENTRAL NERVOUS SYSTEM

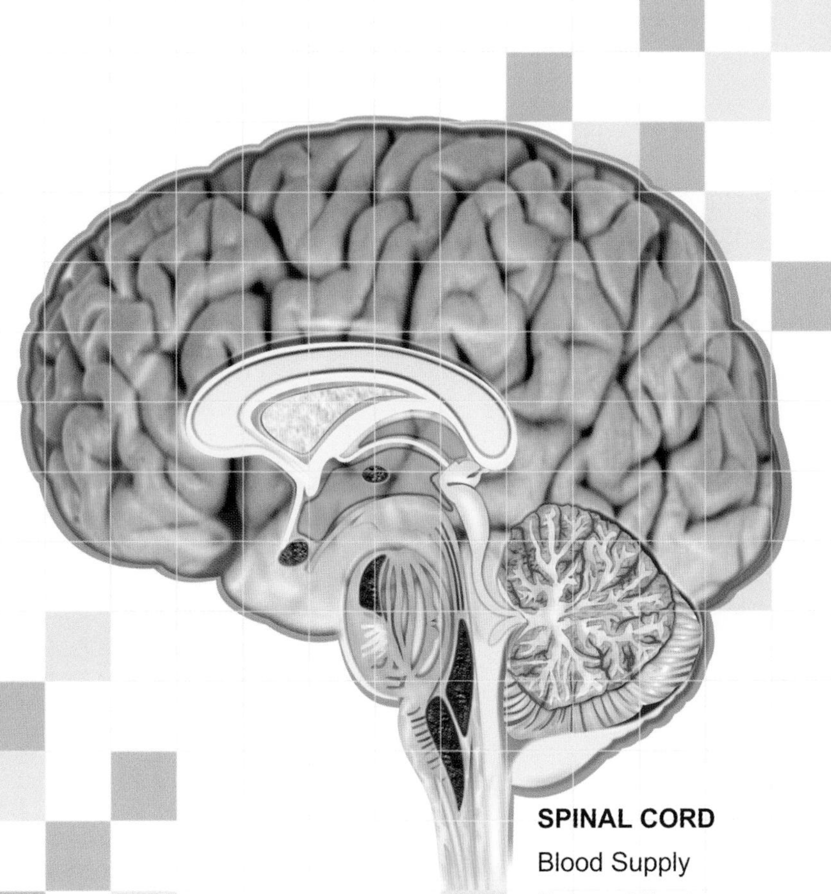

SPINAL CORD

You removed the spinal cord from the vertebral canal along with the meninges. Take out the detached preserved spinal cord and lay it on the table with the ventral surface facing you. The spinal cord is covered by meninges.

MENINGES: The spinal cord is covered by the thick outer ***dura mater.*** The ***arachnoid mater*** is thinner and lies inner to the dura mater. The dura and arachnoid are almost adherent in the cadaver. The space between them is a capillary subdural space.

Dissection: Slit through the dura, arachnoid by a longitudinal cut in the midline both from anterior as well as from the posterior part from the cervical level to the sacral level. Pull and see the arachnoid mater on the inner aspect of the dura mater.

BLOOD SUPPLY OF SPINAL CORD (Figs 1A and B)

The space between the arachnoid and pia mater is the subarachnoid space. It is filled with cerebrospinal fluid in the living. It lodges the blood vessels.

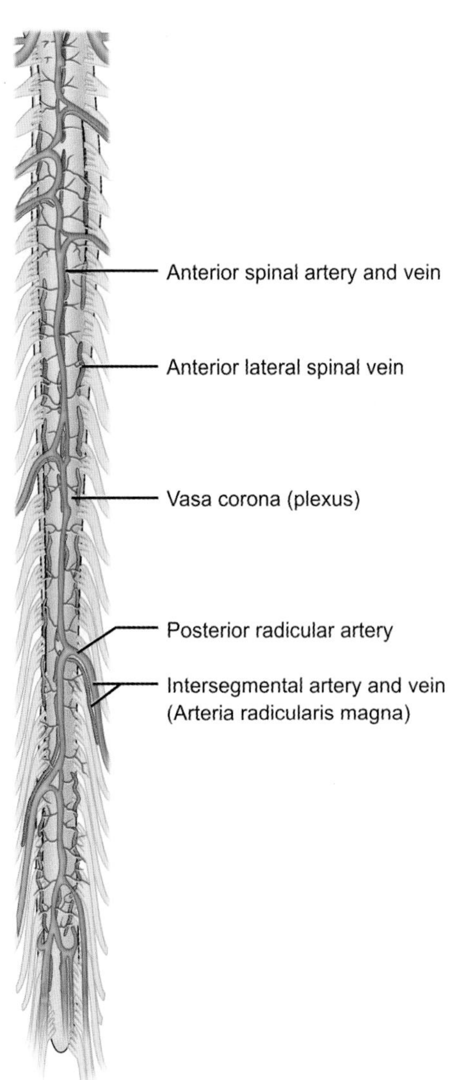

FIGURE 1A Blood supply of spinal cord—anterior aspect

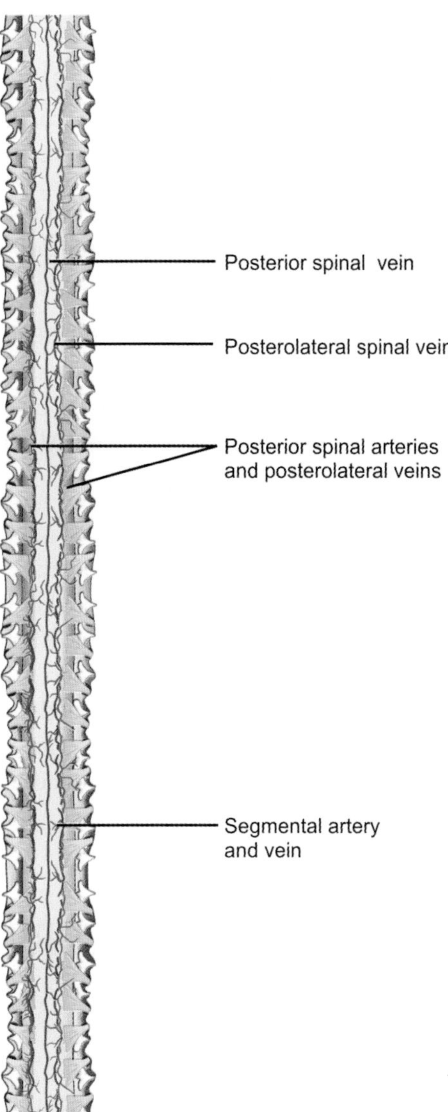

FIGURE 1B Blood supply of spinal cord—posterior aspect

The spinal cord is supplied by vertebral arteries and intersegmental arteries. They lie in the subarachnoid space, anastomose and penetrate the pia mater to enter the substance of the spinal cord. Once they penetrate the nervous tissue they are end arteries. Accompanying veins drain into vertebral plexus of veins.

Dissection: Clean and identify the blood vessels. Note the anterior spinal artery ventrally in the midline. See the posterior spinal arteries near the dorsal roots. Identify six longitudinal venous channels, one each in the midline anteriorly and posteriorly, and four along the dorsal and ventral nerve roots.

Anterior spinal artery: It is formed by the union of medial branches of vertebral artery in the cranial cavity. This runs in the anterior median fissure. Here it gives off small branches which enter the white matter. In the lower levels it is supported by segmental arteries.

Posterior spinal arteries: These are two in number. These are lateral branches of vertebral arteries or inferior cerebellar arteries. They are given off in the cranial cavity. They run down from there along the dorsal nerve roots.

Segmental arteries: Identify them along with the nerves. They enter the vertebral canal through the intervertebral foramina. Trace them along the ventral and dorsal nerve rootlets. They divide and run transversely over the spinal cord and are called anterior and posterior radicular arteries. The segmental arteries are variable in number. Identify at least few of the arteries.

Vasa corona: These are fine circularly placed branches from the radicular arteries which form an interconnecting plexus.

Arteria radicularis magna: It is bigger in caliber and supplies the lower segments of the spinal cord. This varies in position. It may arise either from one of the lower thoracic segmental or upper lumbar segmental arteries.

The anterior spinal, posterior spinal and the vasa corona send central perpendicular branches to supply the substance. Once they enter the cord they are end arteries. Pull the arteries and identify these branches. Thrombosis in any of these vessels leads to insufficiency of blood and results in ischemia.

Veins of the spinal cord: They stand out because of their black coloration. They appear tortuous, and anastomose freely. Normally six longitudinal channels are easily identifiable. They are along the anterior median fissure, posterior median sulcus and along the four groups of nerve rootlets. They accompany the nerve roots and drain into the segmental veins.

Pia mater: This lies deeper and is adherent with the spinal cord. It is loose over the rootlets of the nerves and forms the ligamentum denticulata between the spinal nerves. They are generally 21 in number. They are tooth like processes and are attached to arachnoid and dura mater. The pia mater penetrates into the anterior median fissure of the spinal cord and is called the linea splendens. All the three meningeal layers continue on the outgoing spinal nerves and form a sheath over them.

Dissection: Clean the blood vessels and identify pia mater by pulling it on the surface of the spinal cord. Identify its extensions, the ligamenta denticulata. Put the pointed ends of the forceps near the points where the nerves are leaving the meninges and note that they are covered by the pia, arachnoid and dura mater. They gradually become continuous with the epineurium of the nerves. Trace the spinal nerves, pick them up nearer to the formation of the spinal nerve, trace it backwards to the spinal cord. Note that each spinal nerve enters the spinal cord as dorsal and ventral rootlets. Trace the spinal nerves down to the lower end. Note that these nerves are much longer in the lower part. This is due to the shortening of the spinal cord. At the lower end identify the aggregation of the spinal nerves, the cauda equina. Remove the pia mater and study the external features of the spinal cord.

EXTERNAL FEATURES (Figs 2 and 3)

The **spinal cord** is approximately 42-45 cm long. It is flattened anteroposteriorly.

It presents wide ***enlargements*** in the ***cervical*** and ***lumbar*** regions. This is due to the formation of nerve plexuses in these regions viz cervical, brachial and lumbosacral plexuses.

Conus medullaris: It is the cone like lower part of the spinal cord.

Filum terminale: This is the continuation of the pia and coccygeal nerve fibres. Identify this in the midline at the lower end of conus medullaris.

Cauda equina: Note this bunch of nerves extending from the lower part of the spinal cord to the lumbar, sacral, coccygeal intervertebral foraminae.

Anterior median fissure: It is a longitudinal ventral midline fissure which lodges the anterior spinal artery.

Anterolateral sulcus: Trace the ventral rootlets of the spinal nerves traversing this groove. Each spinal nerve has 6 to 8 rootlets leaving from here.

Posterolateral sulcus: Turn the cord posteriorly and identify this sulcus into which the posterior rootlets enter the spinal cord from the dorsal root ganglia. They may be 6 to 8 in number.

Posterior median sulcus: It is in the midline on the posterior aspect. The posterior spinal vein lies here.

SPINAL SEGMENT

Though spinal cord is continuous, looking at the attachment of the rootlets of the spinal nerve, a spinal segment can be determined. Note that the segments are longer in the cervical and thoracic level, whereas they are very short in lumbar and sacral segments. This is due to the shortening of the spinal cord due to its slower growth in comparison to the growth of the vertebral column. There are ***32 spinal segments***. Each segment of the spinal cord supplies a body segment.

Each spinal segment functionally has two parts. The ***sensory part***—receives sensations from the external and internal environment through the dorsal nerve roots. Once they enter the spinal cord the fibres are separated according to the sensations that they carry. They relay in different nuclei within the spinal cord. The second order neurons in this sensory pathway are sent to thalamus. The ***motor part***—ventral roots carry the motor neurons. They reach the muscle of a particular segment and supply them. These motor fibres are controlled by the higher centers in the cerebral cortex.

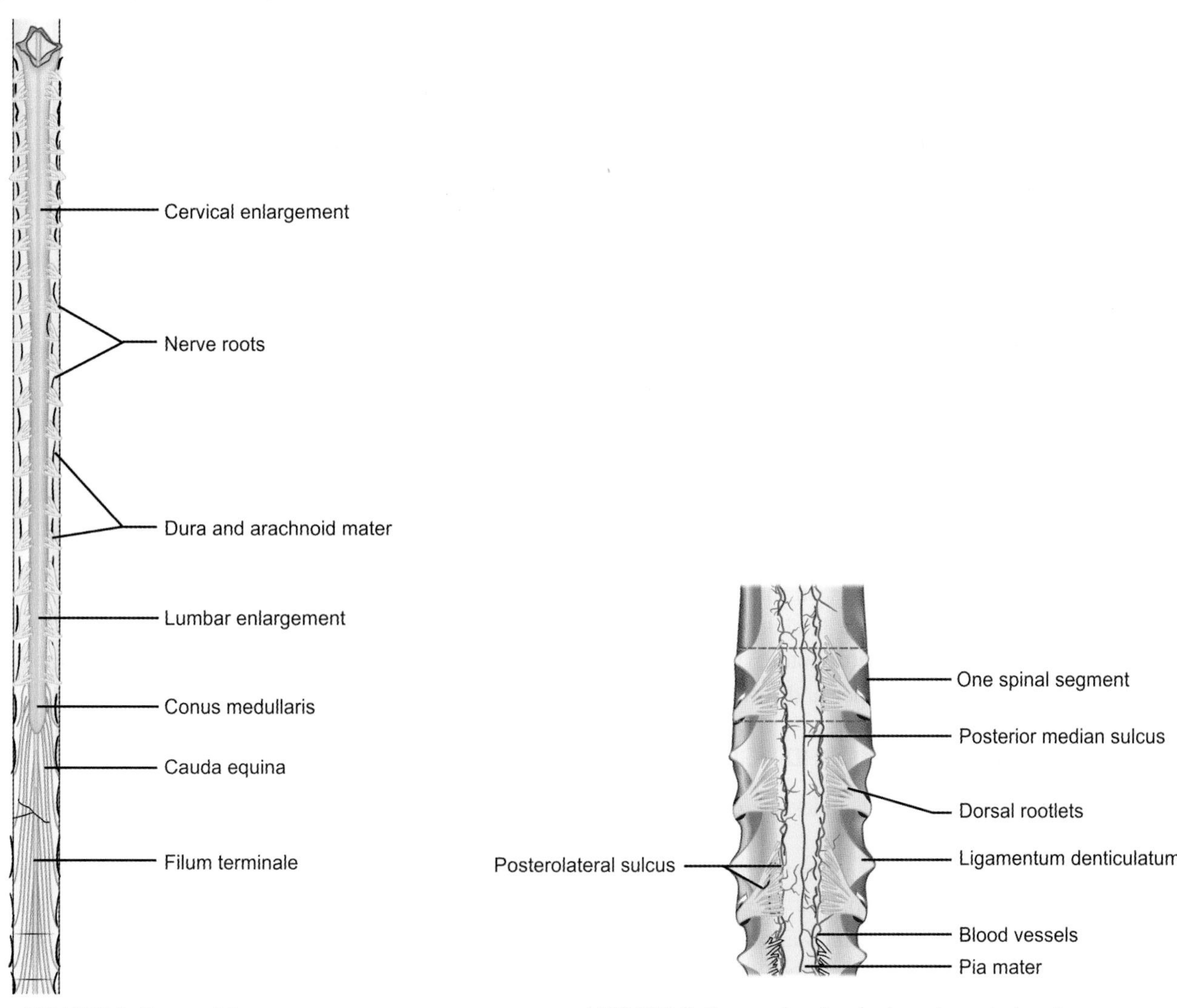

FIGURE 2 External features

FIGURE 3 Segments of spinal cord–posterior view

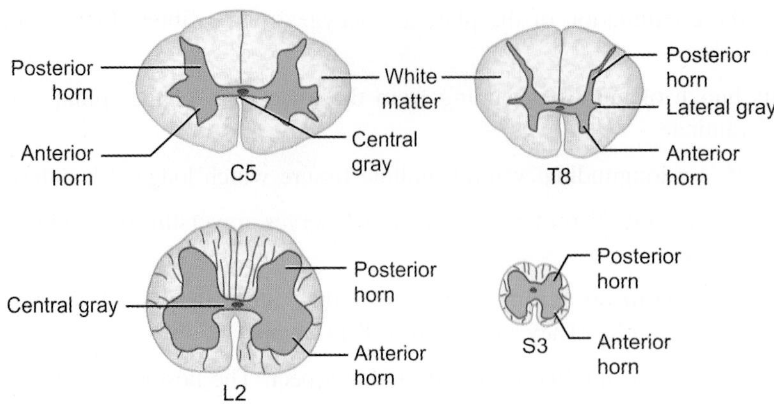

FIGURE 4 Structure of spinal cord. The sections show proportion of gray and white mater at different segmental levels

INTERNAL STRUCTURE (Fig. 4)

The spinal cord structurally exhibits two parts, the ***gray matter*** and the ***white matter***. The fibres which enter and leave the cord form the white matter. Group of fibres which perform a particular function occupy a particular position and are called tracts. They occupy a peripheral position and appear white in fresh specimens as they are myelinated. The gray matter lies internally and is made up of aggregation of cell bodies. The cells connected with a particular function, group together and are called nuclei. The glial cells constitute the connective tissue of the CNS. They are astrocytes and oligodendrocytes. They occupy both the gray and white matter.

To study the structure of the central nervous system in dissection hall Mulligan stain used. This stains thin CNS sections (See Appendix). This shows the gray matter deep purple and white matter white in color.

Dissection: Make 1 cm thin slices of spinal cord of midcervical, thoracic, lumbar and sacral levels. (Simultaneously observing the hematoxylin and eosin stained histological sections under dissection microscope at the same levels will be of great help in understanding the structure).

In freshly cut sections, the white matter appears dull white and the gray matter appears creamish in color.

Put the sections of different levels across and note the proportion of gray and white matter in these sections. Note that the white matter increases in quantity as we ascend up from coccygeal level to the cervical level. The fibres of the last coccygeal segment is the first one to enter the spinal cord. As we ascend up fibres of the other segments get added, by the time we reach the cervical level all the coccygeal, sacral, thoracic, and cervical level fibres get added, so the white matter is more in quantum in the cervical spinal cord when compared to the lower levels.

The gray matter size depends on the area of supply of that particular segment. The thoracic cord has the least amount of gray matter with thin H shaped area. It even shows a small lateral horn. This lodges preganglionic cell bodies of the sympathetic system motor pathway. The cervical and lumbar gray matter shows a wide anterior horn as it gives motor fibres to the upper and lower limb musculature.

SECTION OF THE SPINAL CORD—GRAY AND WHITE MATTER (Fig. 5)

CENTRAL CANAL: This occupies the center of the spinal cord. It is the persistent cavity of the neural tube.

GRAY MATTER: Gray matter is made up of cell bodies and is located in the central part of the spinal cord in the form of columns but in sections it appears like horns, so they are named as posterior horn, lateral horn, anterior horn and central gray. It presents a H shaped appearance.

Posterior horn: The cell bodies of the posterior horn form the second order neurons in the sensory pathway. They receive the axons of the neurons in the dorsal root, synapse and send the second order neurons to the thalamus and

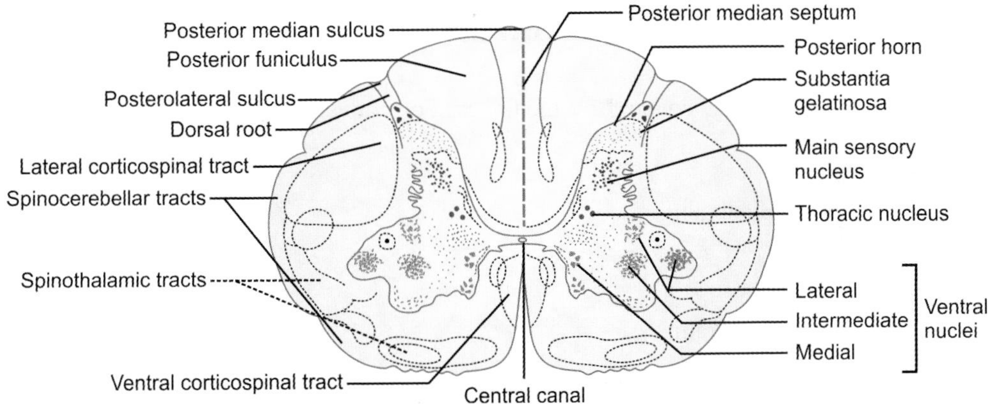

FIGURE 5 Section of spinal cord. This shows the nuclei and tracts

cerebellum. The cell bodies accumulate into groups according to the function they are related with. ***Substantial gelatinosa*** receives pain and temperature fibres and send them to thalamus. ***Main sensory nucleus*** receives touch and pressure fibres and sends them to thalamus. ***Thoracic nucleus*** (C8-L3) receives proprioceptive fibres and sends them to cerebellum.

Lateral horn nuclei (T1 to L2) lodge the cell bodies of preganglionic neurons of motor pathway of the sympathetic nervous system. They receive corticospinal fibres and send to the smooth muscles of internal organs through the sympathetic chain.

Anterior horn: Cell bodies are second order neurons in the motor pathway. They receive the motor neurons through the pyramidal tract or corticospinal tract and send its axons to the skeletal muscles through the ventral nerve roots. They can be identified as three rows of nuclei. The ***medial group*** supplies the trunk musculature. The ***intermediate group*** supplies the diaphragm. The ***lateral group*** supplies the limb musculature. The ventral horn is accordingly variable in its size.

Central gray: It is the horizontal bar of gray matter on either side of the central canal. It has the cell bodies of the autonomic neurons.

WHITE MATTER: This lies peripheral to the gray matter. It is made up of both ascending and descending fibres. They are described as posterior funiculus and anterolateral funiculus (In gross sections the fibres cannot be identified. The diagram shows the position of the fibres).

Posterior median septum is a glial septum which extends from the posterior median sulcus to the posterior aspect of the central gray. ***Posterior funiculus*** lies between the posterior median septum and posterolateral sulcus. It has first order neurons in the proprioceptive sensory pathway. These fibres pass through the dorsal root enter the spinal cord segmentally, ascend up to relay in the medulla oblongata. ***Septomarginal bundle*** is a short intersegmental pathway along the medial margin of the posterior funiculus. It is difficult to locate this in gross anatomical specimen.

Dorsal root: These fibres enter through the posterolateral sulcus. These are the axons of the cell bodies located in the dorsal root ganglion. Most of them relay in the posterior horn nuclei.

Anterolateral funiculus extends between the dorsal root and the anterior median fissure. It has both ascending and descending tracts. The ascending tracts occupy a more superficial position, whereas the descending fibres occupy a deeper position. ***Anterior and posterior spinocerebellar tracts*** are most superficial in position. They carry proprioceptive fibres from the thoracic nucleus to the cerebellum. ***Anterior*** and ***lateral spinothalamic tracts*** are second order neurons. They carry general sensations from the spinal cord to the thalamus. ***Tecto, reticulo, olivospinal tracts and spino olivary, reticular, tectal tracts*** form the tracts connecting reciprocally.

Observe the spinal cord sections at different levels. Study the arrangement, nature of crossing, function and the result of damage caused to all these tracts.

BRAIN

The brain lies within the cranial cavity, covered by meninges. For convenience of description it is divided into the following parts.

Medulla oblongata.
Pons
Cerebellum
} Hindbrain

Mid brain

Cerebral hemispheres
Diencephalon
} Forebrain

Medulla oblongata, pons and midbrain are called brainstem. They are continuous with spinal cord and have a similar structure.

To study the brain it is convenient to have a full brain as well as a midsagittal section. The full brain can be used for dissection and the section is to be used for reference.

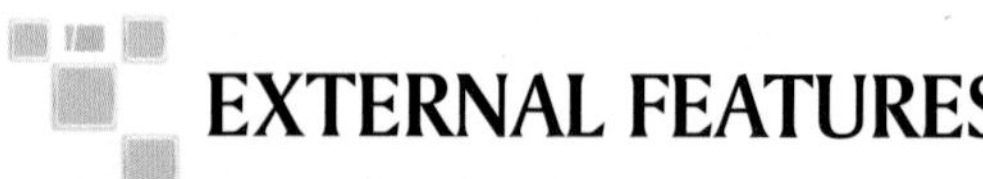

EXTERNAL FEATURES

MENINGES

When we take the stored brain out for study, it has the arachnoid and pia mater. The dura mater remains in the cranial cavity as it is firmly adherent to it.

Arachnoid mater (Fig. 6): It covers the brain on all aspects and is continuous with the spinal arachnoid mater at the foramen magnum. It crosses over all the depressions. It is thicker than pia mater, so it does not penetrate into the gaps between the parts of the brain. As a result big spaces are created between the arachnoid and pia., and these spaces are filled by CSF. These areas are called cisterns. Apart from the CSF the blood vessels lie between the arachnoid and pia.

Dissection: Peel the arachnoid mater from the ventral surface of the brain and observe the following—subarachnoid cisterns, attachment of cranial nerves and blood vessels **(Figs 6 and 7).**

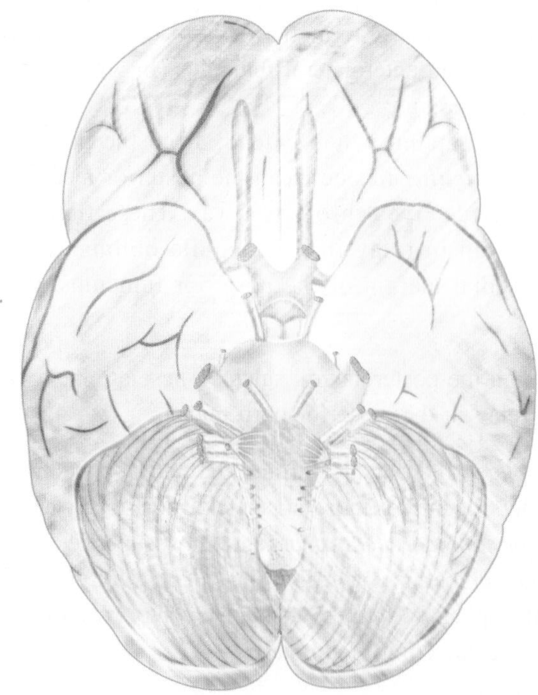

FIGURE 6 Arachnoid mater. Note that it is a thin sheet covering the blood vessels. Nerves and parts of the brain

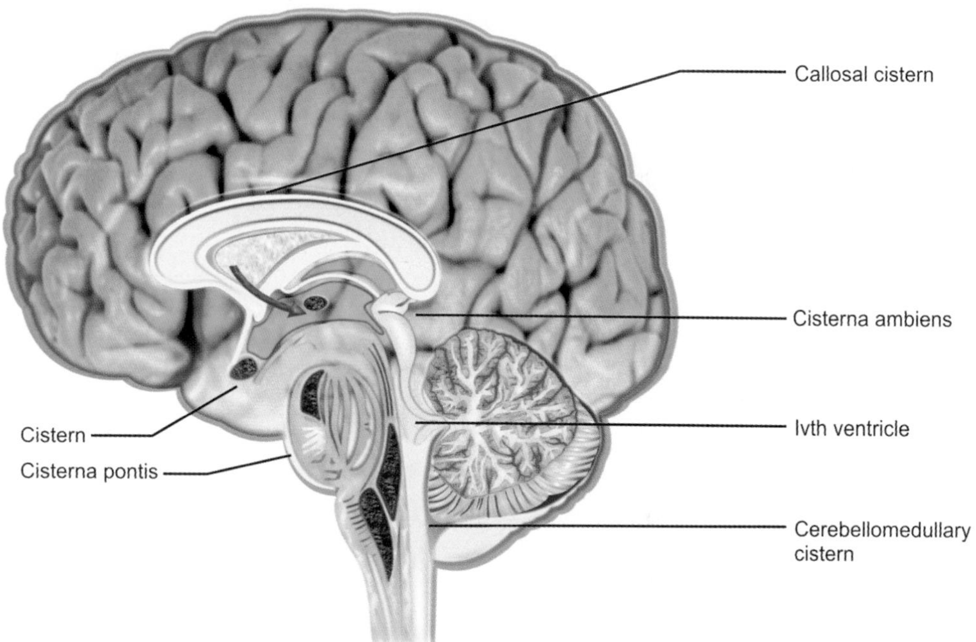

FIGURE 7 Midsagittal section showing subarachnoid cisterns

SUBARACHNOID CISTERNS

Cerebellomedullary cistern/Cisterna magna: It is present laterally and posteriorly between the pons, medulla oblongata and the cerebellum. This communicates with the fourth ventricle through the foramen of Magendie in the midline and foraminae of Luschka laterally.

Cisterna pontis: This lies anterior to the pons and lodges the basilar artery and its branches.

Interpeduncular cistern: It is seen on the ventral aspect bounded by the pons inferiorly, the temporal lobes laterally and optic chiasma anteriorly. This lodges the circle of Willis and its branches.

Callosal cistern: It is seen in midsagittal section around the corpus callosum.

Cisterna ambiens: It is seen in the midsagittal section between the splenium of the corpus callosum and the superior colliculi. It lodges the great cerebral vein.

(Study the formation, composition and circulation of CSF)

STUDY OF BLOOD VESSELS (Fig. 8)

The blood vessels are located in the subarachnoid space. The arteries come from ***vertebral artery and the internal carotid artery.*** They anastomose on the ventral aspect of the brain and from there give off branches to supply the different parts of the brain. The veins accompany the arteries, lie superficially and drain into the neighboring venous sinuses. The venous sinuses were already studied while dissecting the dura mater.

Dissection: Identify the following arteries and trace their branches. Pull them out and see the fine vessels (end arteries) penetrating into the substance of brain.

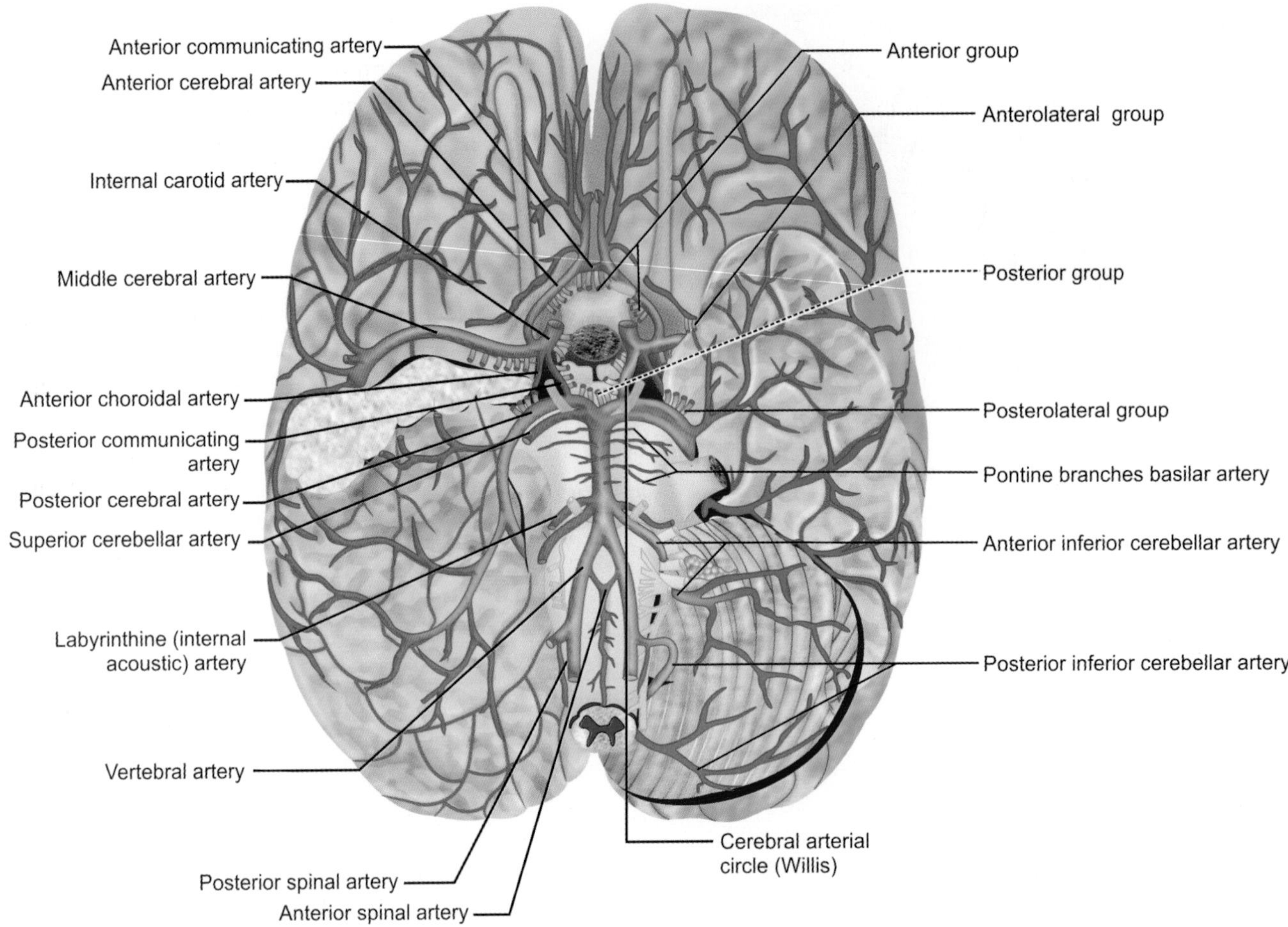

FIGURE 8 Base of the brain: showing arachnoid cisterns and arteries

VERTEBRAL ARTERIES: These arteries enter the cranial cavity through the foramen magnum along the lateral side. The right and left arteries join up together to form the basilar artery at the junction of pons and medulla oblongata.

Branches: The ***posterior spinal artery*** is first branch given off from the lateral aspect. It runs down along the dorsal rootlets of the spinal nerves. It supplies the lateral aspect of the medulla oblongata and spinal cord. ***Posterior inferior cerebellar artery*** is given off while the vertebral artery lies along the lateral side of the medulla oblongata. Generally it gives off the posterior spinal artery, or may arise as a common trunk. It passes in a tortuous course between the rootlets of the glossopharyngeal, vagus and hypoglossal nerves, where it supplies the nerves and the part of the medulla oblongata. It reaches the junction of the medulla oblongata and cerebellum where it gives off the choroidal branch to the 4th ventricle. Further when it reaches the cerebellum it supplies the posterior part of the inferior aspect of the cerebellar hemispheres. *Trace this artery and its branches.* ***Anterior spinal artery*** are two small arteries one from each vertebral artery given near their termination. They join up together to form a single spinal artery which runs in the anterior median fissure. This artery supplies the anterior and medial aspect of the medulla oblongata.

BASILAR ARTERY: It lies in the midline in front of the pons. It causes a depression along the midline of ventral aspect of pons. It divides into two posterior cerebral arteries at the upper end of pons.

Branches: ***Anterior inferior cerebellar artery*** is the 1st branch from the basilar artery. It runs a tortuous course to supply the anterior part of the inferior aspect of the cerebellum. *Trace it to the cerebellum.* ***Pontine branches*** are many small branches, they penetrate the pons and supply it. *Pull the basilar artery and identify them.* ***Labyrinthine artery*** is a branch that runs horizontally beyond the pons. It accompanies vestibulocochlear and facial nerve into the internal auditory meatus to supply the internal ear in the petrous part of the temporal bone. ***Superior cerebellar artery*** is a big branch given off from the distal part of the basilar artery. This runs round the pons to reach the superior aspect of the cerebellum and supplies it. See its ramification on the superior aspect of the cerebellum.

CIRCLE OF WILLIS

It is an arterial circle seen in the interpeduncular fossa. Note its hexagonal shaped formation.

The two ***posterior cerebral arteries*** form the inferior boundary. These are the terminal divisions of the basilar artery. *Locate these.* The ***internal carotid artery*** has entered the cranial cavity through the carotid canal. (Identify it on the skull). It reaches the brain after passing through the cavernous sinus. *Identify its three branches.* The ***posterior communicating artery*** runs downward to anatomose with the posterior cerebral artery. This forms the lateral boundary. Locate this thin branch.

Middle cerebral artery is a branch of the internal carotid. *Locate this artery in the lateral sulcus.*

Anterior cerebral artery is the terminal division of the internal carotid artery. *Locate it as it runs forward and medially to reach the cerebral fissure*, between the two cerebral hemispheres. This forms the anteriomedial boundary.

Anterior communicating artery is a small branch connecting the two anterior cerebral arteries. It forms the anterior boundary. *Pull the two cerebral hemispheres* separate and locate this artery.

CENTRAL BRANCHES: Six sets of central branches arise from the circle of Willis and penetrate the brain substance to supply deep central nuclei. These are all end arteries.

Anterior group arises from the anterior cerebral artery and anterior communicating artery. *Pull the artery forward* and note their branches penetrating the anterior part of the lateral ventricle. This group supplies the caudate nucleus, putamen and anterior aspect of internal capsule. ***Anterolateral group*** arises from the middle cerebral artery and penetrate the area between the olfactory stria and is called the anterior perforated substance. *Locate this area by gently pushing the optic chiasma medially. Pull the middle cerebral artery forwards and locate* the small branches penetrating this area. It supplies thalamus, deep nuclei and internal capsule. One of its bigger branches of great clinical importance is called arteries of cerebral hemorrhage, as this is the artery which often gets blocked. ***Anterior choroidal artery*** is another identifiable branch of the middle cerebral artery. This is given off as it passes through the lateral sulcus. *Pull the middle cerebral artery medially and locate* this artery lateral to the posterior communicating artery. It enters the choroidal fissure of the inferior horn of the lateral ventricle and forms the choroidal plexus. **Posterolateral group** arises from the posterior cerebral artery beyond the communication with the posterior communicating artery. *Locate it as it runs round the midbrain* to supply the meta thalamus and internal capsule. ***Posterior group*** arises from the posterior cerebral arteries near the midline. *Gently pull the posterior cerebral arteries towards you and locate* the group of arteries entering into the brain substance in the midline to supply the hypothalamus. This area is called the posterior perforated substance. ***Posterior choroidal artery*** is given off when posterior cerebral artery reaches the back near the splenium of the corpus callosum. Here it enters the choroidal fissure of the lateral and third ventricles and forms the choroids plexus. *Locate this artery* in the sagittal section.

CORTICAL BRANCHES: They arise from the anterior, middle and posterior cerebral arteries, the distribution can be studied at a later stage.

Dissection: Carefully remove the main arteries from the ventral aspect and identify the cranial nerves.

ATTACHMENT OF CRANIAL NERVES (Fig. 9)

Except for the trochlear nerve which is attached to the dorsal aspect, all the other eleven cranial nerves are attached to the ventral surface of the brain.

Olfactory nerve I: It has many rootlets. They pierce through the cribriform bone of the ethmoid and enter the olfactory bulb. It has got cell bodies of the second order neurons in the pathway of smell. *These nerves are too fine and they get cut while removing the brain.* They end in the olfactory bulb.

Optic nerve II: Note the thick flat nerves and the optic chiasma forming the anterior boundary of the interpeduncular fossa. It is a sensory nerve for vision.

Oculomotor nerve III: Locate this nerve between the posterior cerebral artery and the superior cerebellar artery on the medial side of the cerebral peduncles. This is a thick nerve which supplies the muscles of eyeball.

Trochlear nerve IV: Press the cerebellum gently forwards and locate this nerve below the inferior colliculi. *Trace it along the sides of the cerebral peduncles.* It supplies the superior oblique muscle.

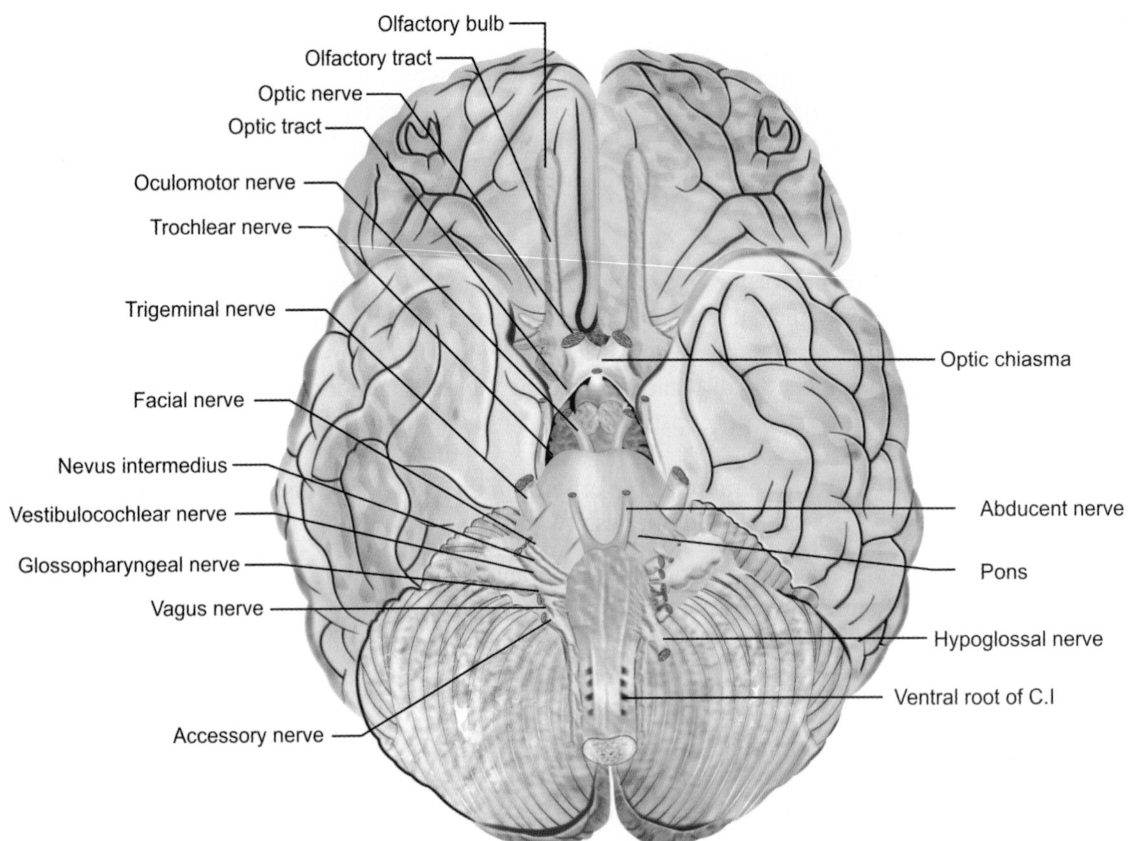

FIGURE 9 Attachment of cranial nerves

Trigeminal nerve V: It is a thick nerve attached to the ventral aspect of the pons, between the pons and middle cerebellar peduncle. You can easily make out two roots at its attachment on pons—the smaller motor root – supplies the muscles of mastication. The bigger sensory root, carries sensations from the facial skin. This separates the pons from the middle cerebellar peduncle.

Abducent nerve VI: It is thin nerve between the pons and the pyramids of medulla oblongata. It supplies the lateral rectus of the eyeball.

Facial nerve VII, nervus intermedius and vestibulocochlear nerve VIII: Locate these three thick nerves seen between the pons, medulla oblongata and the cerebellum. Facial nerve supplies muscles of facial expression, nervus intermedius carries taste sensations, vestibular nerve controls equilibrium and cochlear nerve carries auditory sensations.

Glossopharyngeal IX, vagus X and accessory XI nerves: These are attached along the posterolateral sulcus between the olive and inferior cerebellar peduncle, by number of rootlets. They supply the pharynx, larynx and GI tract. *Locate these rootlets.* They are mixed nerves. They have motor fibres to supply the muscles of branchiomeric origin and glands, carry taste and general sensations from the internal organs.

Hypoglossal nerve XII: This nerve leaves the medulla oblongata along the anterolateral sulcus between the pyramid and olive by number of rootlets. This nerve supplies the musculature of the tongue.

(Study the functional components of all these nerves)

STUDY OF MIDSAGITTAL SECTION (Fig. 10)

The prominent feature in the midsagittal section is the cavity of the brain. The central canal which is a narrow tube in the spinal cord expands in the brain to form ventricles.

VENTRICLES: The ***IV ventricle*** is the cavity of the hindbrain. Note this cavity between pons and upper medulla anteriorly and cerebellum posteriorly. ***Third ventricle*** is the cavity of the thalamic complex. It is irregular in outline and is a single cavity in the midline. Note the cerebral aqueduct connecting the third and fourth ventricles. The cavity of the cerebrum is the ***lateral ventricle.*** They are two in number one in each cerebral hemisphere. Identify the septum pellucidum which separates the two lateral ventricles.

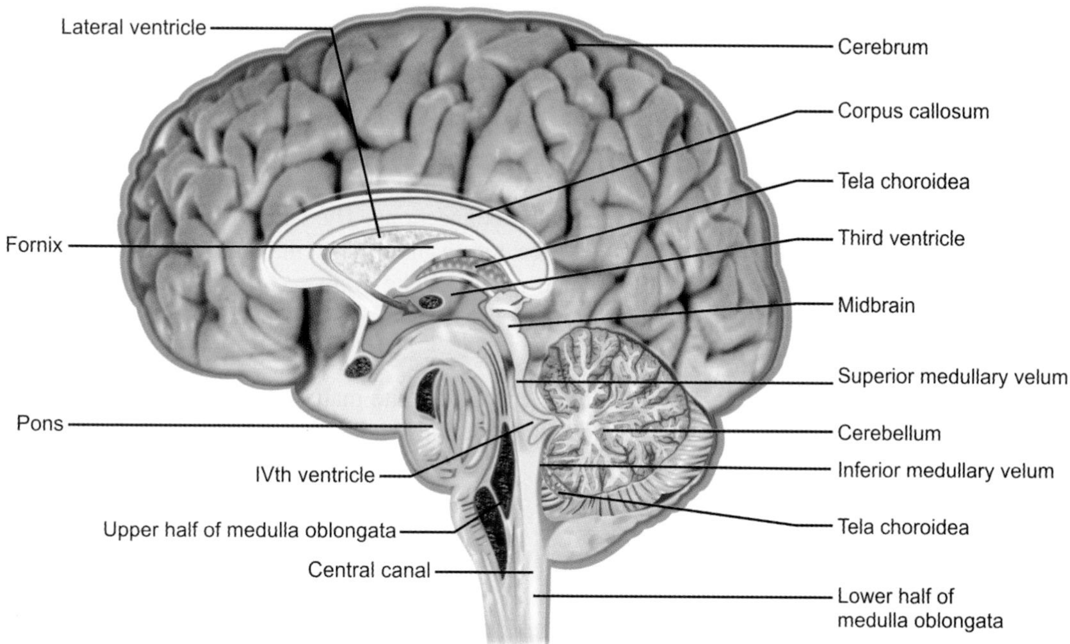

FIGURE 10 Midsagittal section

The brain substance around the ventricles is described as follows:

Lower half of medulla oblongata: Note that it is a tubular structure with the central canal more towards the posterior aspect.

Upper half of medulla oblongata: Anteriorly is more bulky, due to the accumulation of the nuclear matter. Posteriorly it is deficient. Here the central canal communicates into the cerebromedullary cistern.

Pons: This is the prominent anterior bulging part. It is clearly separated from the medulla oblongata below and the midbrain above.

Cerebellum: This occupies the area behind the upper part of the medulla oblongata and the pons. Identify the central recess forming the roof of the IVth ventricle.

Superior medullary velum: Note this thin sheet of white matter connecting the cerebellum to the midbrain in the midline. It is lined by the ependyma.

Inferior medullary velum: Note this thin white matter covered by the ependyma in the lower sloping surface of the cerebellum.

Tela choroidae: This is the blood vessels covered by the pia mater. Note this between the inferior medullary velum and the lower half of the cerebellum.

Midbrain: This part is located above the pons and cerebellum. It is relatively shorter anteriorly compared to the posterior part. The posterior part is formed by the colliculi. The cavity of the midbrain is the narrow cerebral aqueduct of Sylvius.

Thalamic complex: It is the part that lies around the third ventricle. It is made up of thalamus, hypothalamus, epithalamus and metathalamus.

Cerebrum: This is the most expanded part of the forebrain. In a sagittal section the commissural fibres which connect both sides get cut. The corpus callosum forms the prominent structure here. Identify this curved structure. Fornix is the other prominent commissure. *Note the septum pellucidum* connecting these two commissures. The part of the cerebrum seen on this surface is called the medial side.

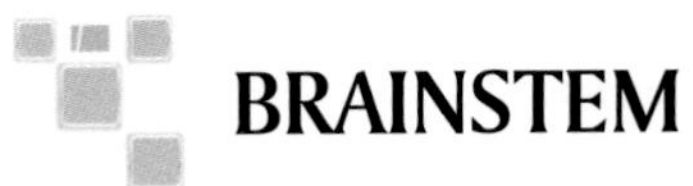

BRAINSTEM

The brainstem is made up of medulla oblongata, pons and midbrain in that order from the spinal cord to the forebrain. It is related to the basiocciput and basisphenoid anteriorly. Architecturally, it is similar to the spinal cord. The gray matter of the brain is occupied by the cranial nerves and their connections. The extrapyramidal system which produces a coordinated muscular movement has number of nuclei located in the brainstem. The fibre tracts which connect the different parts of the CNS lie external and form the white matter of the brain.

MEDULLA OBLONGATA

It is very much similar to the spinal cord in arrangement of gray and white matter. The upper half of medulla oblongata opens up posteriorly to form the IVth ventricle. Identify the external features.

Anterior Aspect (Fig. 11)

Anterior median fissure: *Locate this in the midline*. This is a continuation of the anterior median fissure of the spinal cord. Not the crossing of the fibres in the lower part. The fissure is obliterated at the lower part of the medulla oblongata and the crossing of the fibres is called the ***pyramidal decussation***. ***Foramen cecum*** is the upper expended end of the ***anterior median fissure***. *Locate this* at the junction of the pons and medulla oblongata.

Pyramids: These are elevations on either side of the anterior median fissure. Note that pyramids are prominent structures in the upper part of medulla oblongata but narrow down in the lower part. They are constituted by the corticospinal tracts. As the name signifies they are the descending fibres beginning at the cerebral cortex and reach the spinal cord. Many of the pyramidal fibres cross and form lateral corticospinal tracts and the uncrossed fibres continue as the anterior corticospinal tract. The crossing of these fibres is the pyramidal decussation.

Anterolateral sulcus: This lies between the pyramids and olive. Identify the rootlets of the hypoglossal nerve in this sulcus. This sulcus is continuous with the anterolateral sulcus of the spinal cord through which the ventral, motor roots of the spinal cord emerge. The hypoglossal nerve supplies the musculature of the tongue.

Olive: It is the raised oval elevation caused by the deeply lying olivary nucleus. It is a part of the extrapyramidal system. It receives afferents from the cortex and spinal cord and sends efferents to the cerebellum.

Posterolateral sulcus: Locate this sulcus between olive and inferior cerebellar peduncle. See the rootlets of glossopharyngeal, vagus and accessory nerves in that order from above downwards. This sulcus is continuous inferiorly with the dorsilateral sulcus through which the dorsal rootlets of the spinal nerves enter.

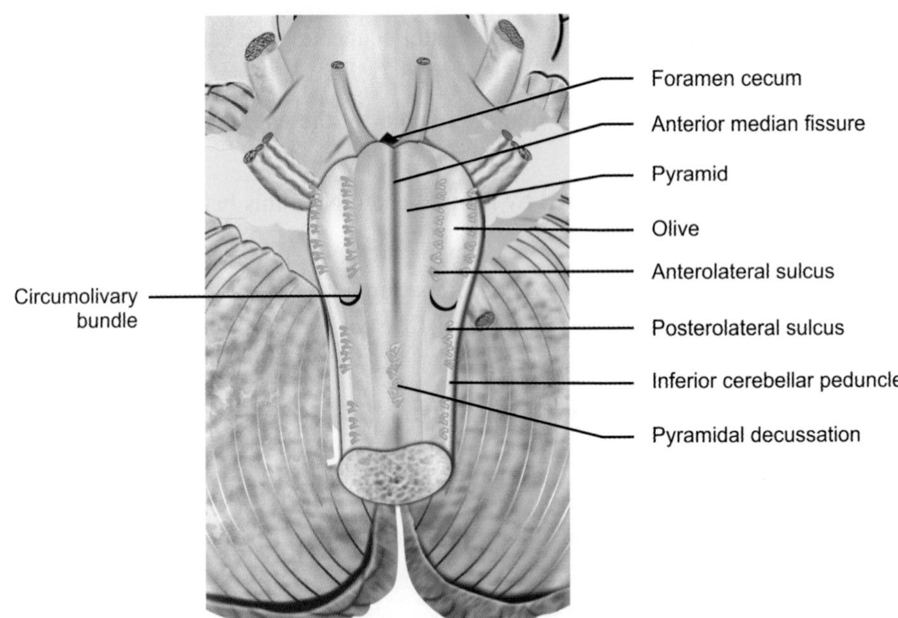

FIGURE 11 Medulla oblongata—Anterior aspect

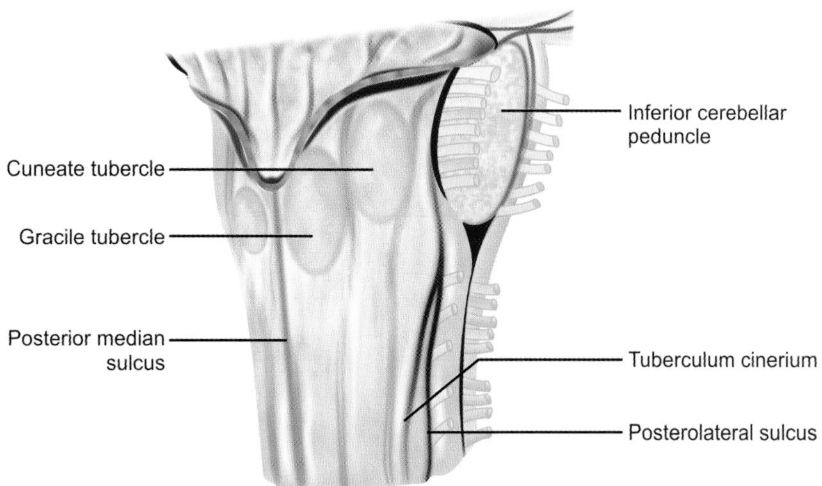

FIGURE 12 Medulla oblongata—posterior aspect

Circumolivary bundle: Locate this semicircular bundle below the olive. This begins from the displaced arcuate nuclei located on the pyramids. The fibres wind round the olive to reach the cerebellum through the inferior cerebellar peduncle. These are displaced parts of coticocerebellar fibres.

Inferior cerebellar peduncle: Locate this stem like structure lateral to the olive. It reaches deep to the middle cerebellar peduncle (will be discussed with cerebellum).

POSTERIOR ASPECT (Fig. 12)

Dissection: Turn the part posteriorly, push the medulla oblongata forwards and identify the following **(Fig. 12).**

Posterior median sulcus: Locate this midline depression on the posterior aspect of the spinal cord and it opens up in the upper part of the medulla oblongata. It is continuous with the posterior median sulcus of the spinal cord. Note that this sulcus opens up in the upper part of medulla oblongata.

Gracile tubercle: This is the elevation lateral to the widening part of the posterior median sulcus. The gracile nucleus underlies this tubercle. This nucleus receives proprioceptive fibres of the lower half of the body.

Cuneate tubercle: Locate this tubercle lying superior lateral to the gracile tubercle. It is due to the underlying cuneate nucleus. This receives proprioceptive fibres of the upper half of the body.

The second order neurons from gracile and cuneate nuclei form the internal arcuate fibres and ascend up as the medial lemniscus.

Tuberculum cinereum: Identify this elevation between the cuneate fasciculus and the posterolateral sulcus. This is caused due to the underlying spinal tract of trigeminal nerve.

Inferior cerebellar peduncle: This is a big bundle lies between the cuneate tubercle olivary nucleus.

PONS (Fig. 13)

Pons is the expanded part of the brainstem. It has a ventral part which is visible in the anterior aspect. The posterior part forms the floor of IV ventricle and is totally overlapped by the cerebellum.

Note: The ventral depression caused due to the presence of the basilar artery.

On either side of the artery the pons shows bulges. This is due to the underlying pontine nuclei. The ventral part is called the basilar part of pons. The dorsal part is called tegmentum and has cranial nerve nuclei.

Trigeminal nerve V: The fibres of trigeminal nerve are attached to the pons at the junction of pons and middle cerebellar peduncle.

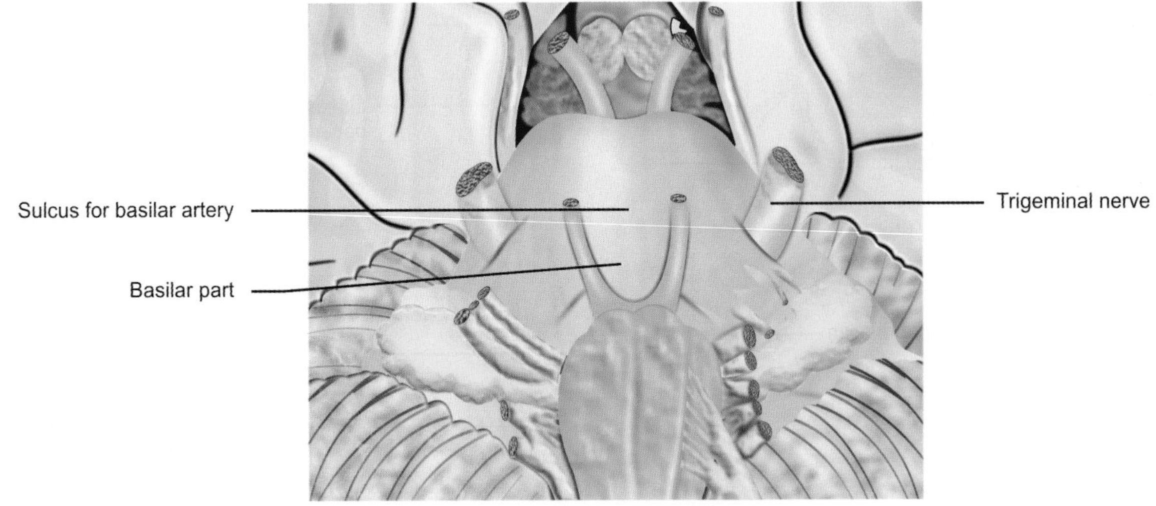

FIGURE 13 Pons—anterior aspect

MIDBRAIN

Midbrain is the upper part of the brainstem. It is a tubular structure. The cavity of midbrain is called aqueduct of Sylvius. The part anterior to the aqueduct is called the cerebral peduncle, the part posterior is called the tectum. It is made up of two pairs of colliculi and is also called as corpora quadrigemina.

ANTERIOR ASPECT (Fig. 14)

Crus cerebri: Identify this anterior most part of the cerebral peduncle. This is made up of the corticospinal and corticopontine fibres. These are the diverging fibre bundles extending from the upper border of the pons to the forebrain.

Hypothalamic structures: These parts of hypothalamus push themselves to lie between the crura. The ***tuber cinereum*** is an elevation in the midline. It is connected to the pituitary gland through infundibulum. ***Mammillary bodies*** are below the tuber cinereum and are one on either side of the midline. ***Optic chiasma*** and ***optic tract*** limit the anterior and anterolateral aspect.

Dissection: Turn the brain posteriorly, press the cerebellum downwards and identify the posterior aspect of midbrain.

POSTERIOR ASPECT (Fig. 15)

Tectum/corpora quadrigemina: The *superior* ***Colliculi*** are the upper bodies of the corpora. They are reflex centers in the visual pathway. The ***inferior colliculi*** are the lower bodies of the corpora. They are reflex centers in the auditory pathway. ***Frenulum veli*** separates the right side from the left side.

Trochlear nerve IV: This leaves below the inferior colliculi on either side of the midline. The nerve winds round the crus cerebri to reach the ventral aspect. It supplies the superior oblique muscle of the eyeball.

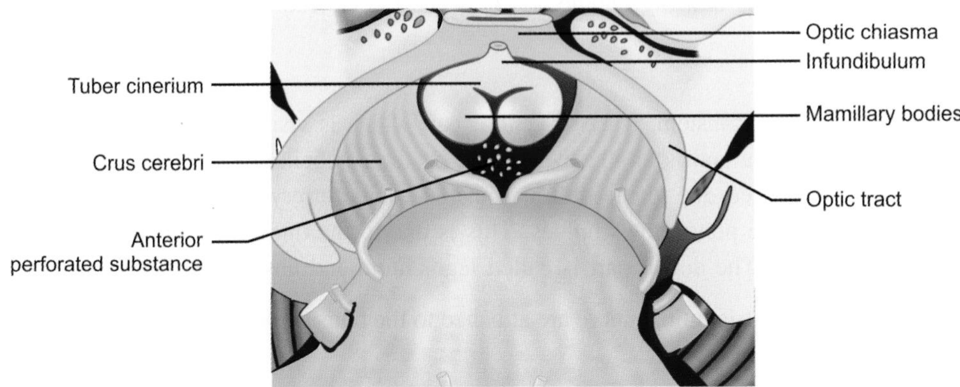

FIGURE 14 Midbrain—anterior aspect

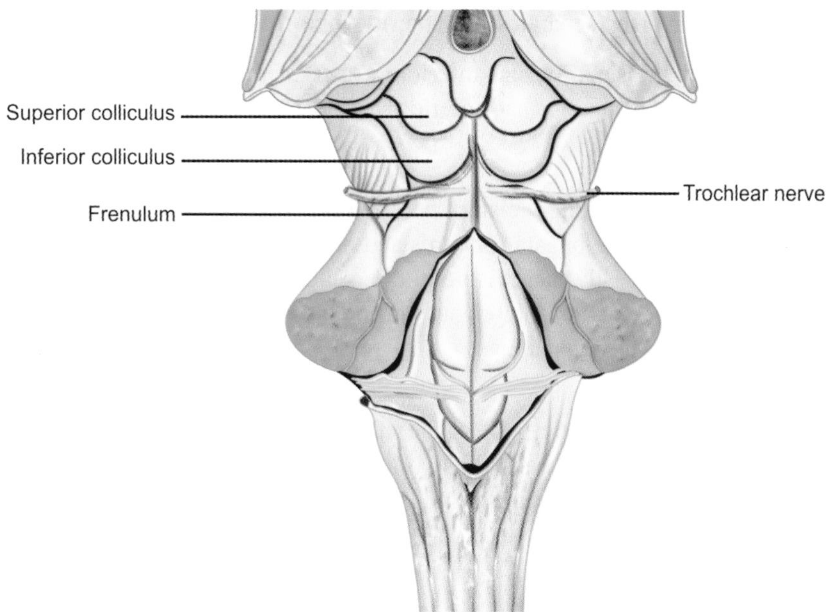

FIGURE 15 Midbrain—posterior aspect

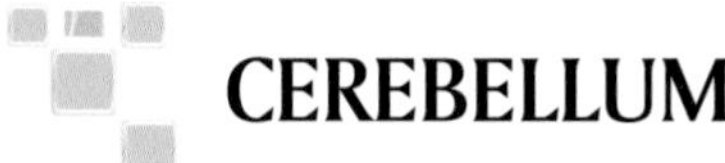

CEREBELLUM

Dissection: Sever the brainstem from the forebrain. The cut should pass anteriorly near the upper part of the crus cerebri and posteriorly through the superior colliculus. Take the part in hand and study the surfaces of cerebellum.

The cerebellum is located posterior to the pons and medulla oblongata. It is an integrating center for the muscular coordination. It receives sensory impulses particularly the proprioceptive fibres from different parts of the body. It also receives the outgoing 1st order motor neurons from the cerebral cortex. It received so many array of fibres, the cerebellum has developed an outer gray matter to receive and integrate these fibres. The incoming and outgoing fibres constitute the white matter. Fibres arising from the gray matter form internuncial neurons and end on the cerebellar nuclei. The outgoing fibres of the cerebellum arise from these internal nuclei. So its structure is very much similar to the cerebral cortex with an outer folded gray matter and a inner white matter with a internally located nuclear matter.

The cerebellum presents a superior surface, inferior surface, an anterior notch and a posterior notch.

Superior surface (Fig. 16): It is separated from the cerebrum by the tentorium cerebelli. It looks uniform with raised central elevation called the superior vermis and on either side are the cerebellar hemispheres. The vermis and hemispheres are continuous with each other.

Inferior surface: This surface also presents a central vermis and two lateral cerebellar hemispheres. The central vermis is separated from the hemispheres by the vallecular depression. Pull the cerebellum slightly and identify the inferior surface.

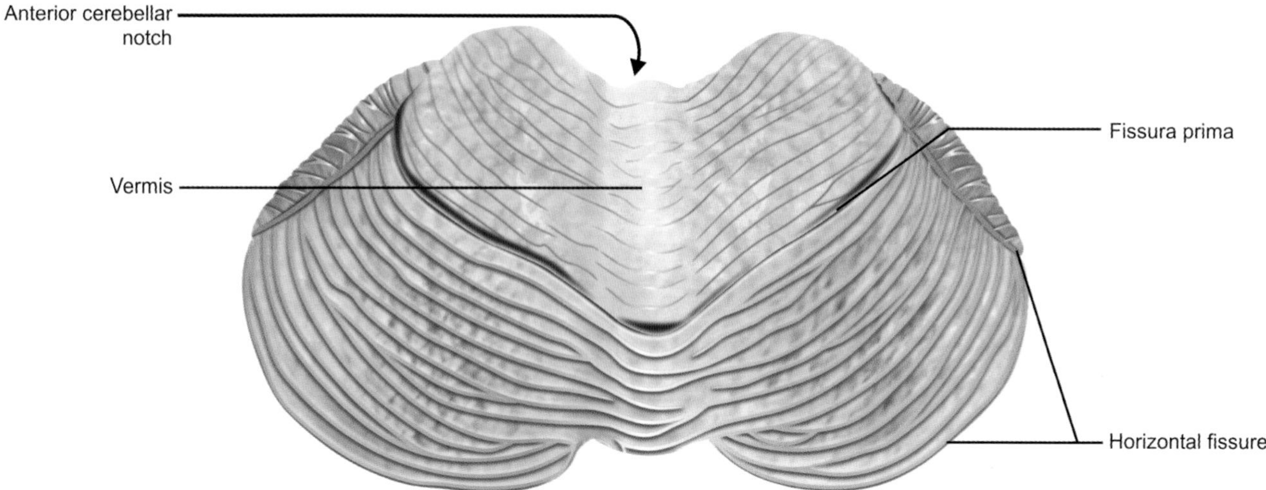

FIGURE 16 Cerebellum—superior aspect

Fissura prima: *Identify this fissure*. This separates the anterior lobe from the posterior lobe.

Horizontal fissure: This separates the superior and inferior surface of the cerebellum *Locate this* at the junction of the cerebellum with the pons where the superior and inferior surface come closer. Trace it round the cerebellum to the posterior aspect of it.

Dissection: Reidentify the cerebellomedullary cistern between the medulla oblongata and the inferior surface of cerebellum. Slightly pull the medulla oblongata forwards and note the pia mater extending between the two. The prominent foramen of Magendie is easily identifiable in the center. Trace the pia mater laterally to the junction between the cerebellum, pons and medulla oblongata, and identify the lateral foramen of Luschka. Note the projecting choroids plexus in both these openings.

Choroid plexus: It is the capillary plexus in the roof of the 4th ventricle. A branch of the posterior inferior cerebellar artery contributes to its formation. It enters between the two layers of the pia mater. It is shaped like a T when arteries of both sides meet. The blood vessels form a capillary plexus. It pushes the pia and the ependyma and is seen as a grape like structure and CSF is formed thereby filtration.

ANTERIOR CEREBELLAR NOTCH (Fig. 17)

Dissection: Cut the cerebellum from the hindbrain near the peduncles. Take the cerebellum in hand and study its features.

Look at the anterior aspect of the cut part of the cerebellum. Right in the midline a tent like depression is seen. This is the roof of the fourth ventricle in the center of the vermis, it is called ***superior recess***. *Put a blunt edge of the scalpel and see its depth*. It slops superiorly to form superior medullary velum and inferiorly to form inferior medullary velum. All these parts are lined by the ependyma.

Superior medullary velum: This is a thin sheet of white matter covered by pia mater. It ascends up to the midbrain between the two superior cerebellar peduncles.

Inferior medullary velum: Look at the inferior surface and note the thin inferior medullary velum in the midline. It forms the roof of the inferior half of the 4th ventricle. The choroid plexus of the fourth ventricle is located here.

Choroid plexus and tela choroidea: Choroid plexus is the capillary plexus located in the ventricles. The capillary plexus is covered by the pia mater and it is called tela choroidea. In the IV ventricle it is T shaped.

The cerebellum is connected to the brainstem by three cerebellar peduncles. The superior cerebellar peduncle connects it to the midbrain. The middle cerebellar peduncle connects it to the pons and the inferior cerebellar peduncles connect it to the medulla oblongata. Locate their position on the cerebellum.

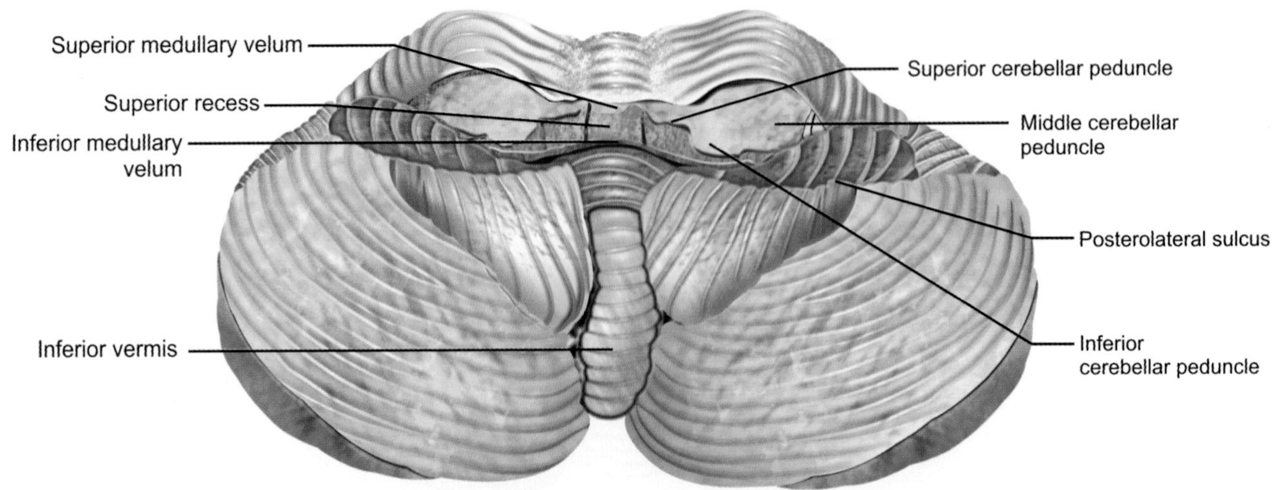

FIGURE 17 Cerebellum—inferior aspect

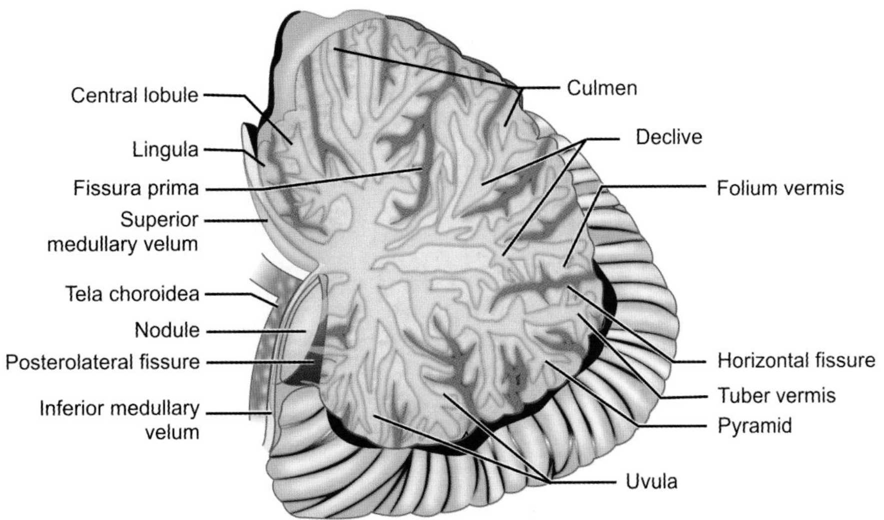

FIGURE 18 Cerebellum—vermis

VERMIS (Fig. 18)

Dissection: Cut the cerebellum in the midline and divide it into two halves.

Observe the cut parts. The vermis presents a central white core covered by gray matter. The appearance of gray and white matter looks like branches of a tree. So the arrangement is called arbor vitae arrangement.

Note that the central vermal parts extend laterally into the cerebellar hemispheres. Deep fissures separate the parts of vermis. Lot of work was done on cerebellum and is classified based on different factors.

Following is the most accepted old classification.

Cerebellum is divided into ***anterior, middle and posterior lobes.*** Each lobe has a central vermal and a lateral hemisphere part. *Identify the following parts and the prominent fissures to identify the lobes.*

Identify ***lingula*** small part sticking to the superior medullary velum. ***Culmen and declive***—identify these big vermal parts and the ***fissure prima***. The fissure separates the anterior lobe from the middle lobe. The lingual culmen declive with the lateral extensions form the ***anterior lobe. Folium vermis***—is a thin single folium below the declive. The fissure below it is the ***horizontal fissure.*** This separates the superior side from the inferior side. Trace it laterally. ***Tuber vermis, pyramid, uvula***—are shaped like a bulge, pyramid and a tongue. Identify them in that order. See their lateral extensions. The lateral extension of the uvula is the ***tonsil.*** It is a prominent part and identify this. Identify the ***posterolateral fissure***. This fissure lies between the nodule and uvula. It separates the middle lobe from the posterior lobe. ***Nodule*** is the small most anterior part of the inferior vermis. ***Flocculus and paraflocculus*** are the parts of cerebellar hemisphere extensions from the nodule. They can be easily identified projecting into the lateral recess of the fourth ventricle, the ***foramen of Lushka.*** Remove the tonsil to get a better view of the connection between the flocculus and paraflocculus.

Practice the names of all these parts of vermis and cerebellar hemisphere.

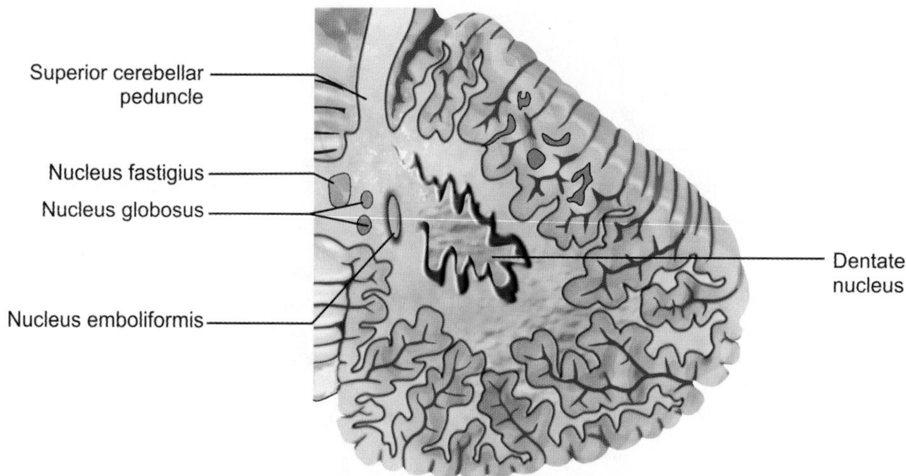

FIGURE 19 Deep cerebellar nuclei

DEEP CEREBELLAR NUCLEI (Fig. 19)

Dissection: Make a horizontal cut through the middle of the cerebellum. Note the gray matter within the white matter of the cerebellum.

Dentate nucleus: *Identify this crenated nucleus occupying the major part of the white matter.* The mouth of this nucleus faces towards the midline. It receives internuncial neurons from the gray matter. It sends efferent fibres through the superior cerebellar peduncle. They are the dentatorubral and dentatothalamic fibres. ***Nucleus globose, emboliformis and fastiggi***—these are smaller nuclear matter between the dentate nucleus and the midline. The nucleus fastigial shows reciprocal vestibular connections. Nucleus globosus and emboliform have reciprocal spinal connections.

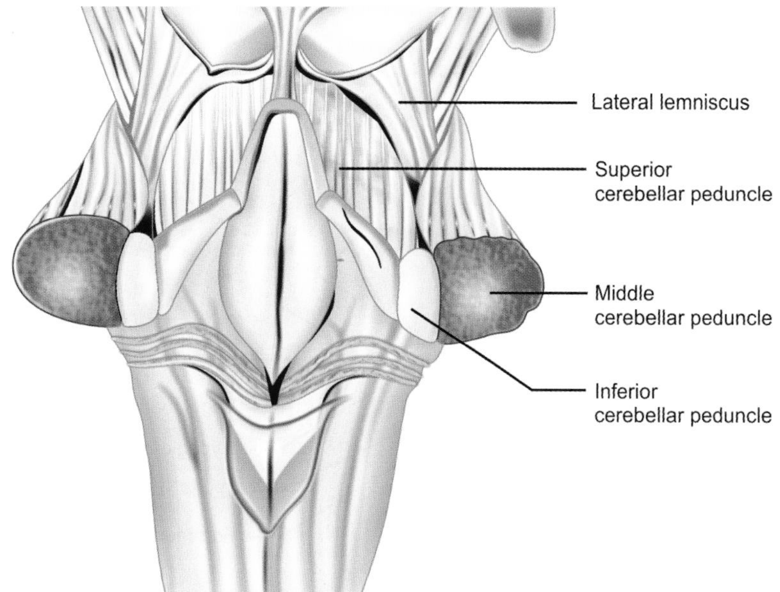

FIGURE 20 Cerebellum—peduncles

PEDUNCLES OF CEREBELLUM (Fig. 20)

The cerebellum is connected to the brainstem through cerebellar peduncles. *Identify them on the brainstem now.* They all can be seen on the posterior aspect.

Superior cerebellar peduncle: It forms the upper part of the roof of the IV ventricle. It is seen on the posterior aspect of the brainstem. It is a thick fibre bundle connecting the cerebellum to the midbrain. You can see it as a prominent bundle extending from the cerebellum to the undersurface of the superior colliculus. It is predominantly made up of efferent or outgoing fibres of cerebellum. These start in the deep nuclei of cerebellum and reach the red nucleus and thalamus. It has only one descending tract—the anterior spinocerebellar tract.

Lateral lemniscus: Identify this bundle lateral to the superior cerebellar peduncle. These are the second order neurons in the auditory pathway. They begin in the auditory nuclei located at the junction of the pons and medulla oblongata. (Though it is not a cerebellar connection, it is shown here due to visibility of this structure here).

Middle cerebellar peduncle: It is seen as a thick lateral bundle of fibres. It connects the cerebellum to the pons. It is made up of corticocerebellar fibres. The corticocerebellar fibres relay in the pontine nuclei and the second order neurons cross to the opposite side and reach the cerebellum as the inferior cerebellar fibres. It is located on the lateral side of the brainstem.

Inferior cerebellar peduncle: *Locate this bundle between the superior and middle cerebellar peduncles.* It connects the cerebellum to the medulla oblongata. It has both afferent and efferent fibres. The afferents to the cerebellum come from the olivary nuclear complex through different tracts. Olivary nucleus is a part of extrapyramidal system. It modifies the motor functions initiated by the cerebral cortex. It also receives proprioceptive fibres from the lower part of the body through spinocerebellar fibres. The vestibular fibres come from vestibular nuclei. It also has efferent fibres to vestibular nuclei and spinal cord. It is on the posterolateral side of medulla oblongata.

Study the tracts in each peduncle from a Textbook.

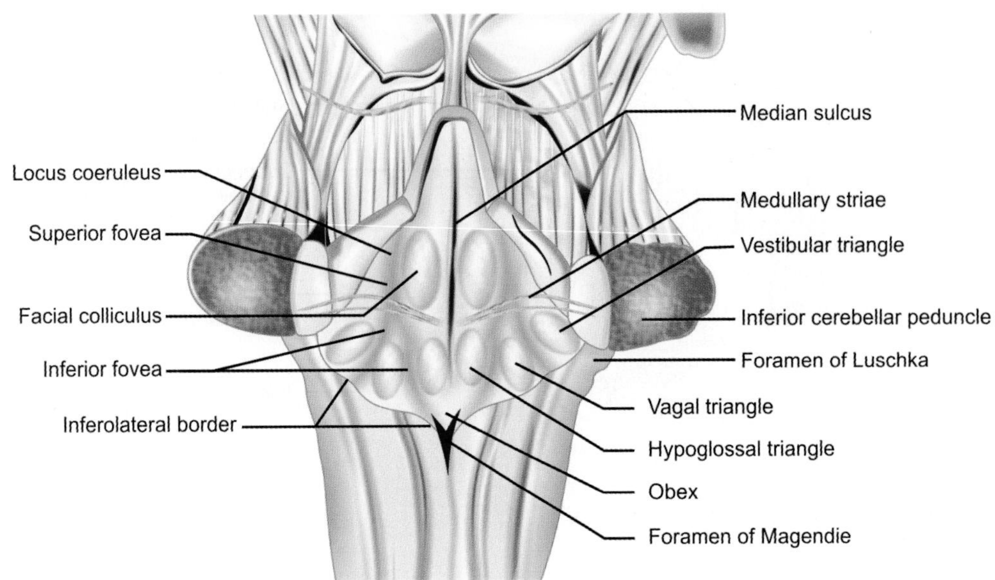

FIGURE 21 Fourth ventricle

FOURTH VENTRICLE (Fig. 21)

Fourth ventricle is the cavity of the hindbrain. It is a diamond shaped space. The floor of 4th ventricle is formed by the posterior aspect of the pons and upper half of medulla oblongata. The roof is formed by the cerebellum, and the superior and inferior medullary vela. It is tent like structure. The roof and floor meet at the curved lateral margin of the medulla oblongata except at the foramen of Magendie and foraminae of Luschka. Superiorly the 4th ventricle narrows up to form the aqueduct of the midbrain. Inferiorly it is continuous with the central canal.

Dissection: Note the following features on the posterior aspect of the brainstem.

Inferolateral border: It is formed by the obex, gracile tubercle, cuneate tubercle and the inferior cerebellar peduncle. The inferior medullary velum is attached along this margin.

Relocate the position of foramen of Magendie and the foramen of Luschka.

Median sulcus: It is the midline separation seen in the floor dividing it into right and left halves.

Medial eminence: See this elevation on either side of the sulcus in the pontine part of the fourth ventricle. This is caused by the underlying motor cranial nerve, the abducent nerve nucleus. The facial nerve fibres wind round the abducent nerve nucleus, so it is called ***facial colliculus***.

Superior fovea: Note this depression lateral to the facial colliculus. The ***locus coeruleus*** is dark area just above the superior fovea. This is due to the pigmented cells present here.

Medullary striae: Note these horizontally running fibres at the junction of the medulla oblongata and pons. These fibres arise from the displaced pontine nuclei called arcuate nuclei. They begin on the anterior aspect of the pyramids sweep backwards through the center to reach the floor of the 4th ventricle. From the center of the median sulcus they run horizontally to reach the cerebellum.

Inferior fovea: Note this inverted Y shaped depression which separates the medullary part of the medial eminence into three triangular elevations.

The hypoglossal triangle: Note this next to the median sulcus. It is caused by the hypoglossal nerve nucleus.

The vagal triangle: It is the elevation between the two limbs of the inferior fovea, caused by the vagal nerve nucleus. Funiculus separans is a thin fibrous elevation. It separates the vagal triangle from the area postrema which lies below the funiculus separans.

Vestibular triangle: Lateral to the inferior fovea and is caused by the vestibular nerve nuclei.

 Obex: This is the point where the two gracile tubercles meet.

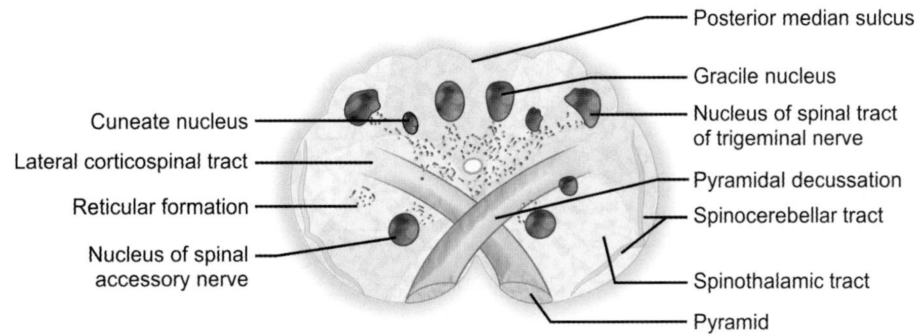

FIGURE 22: Section through the pyramidal decussation

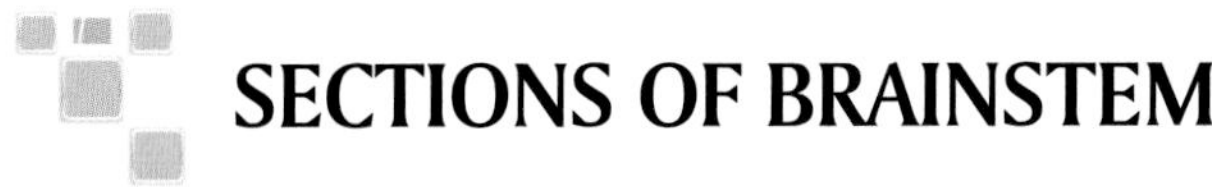

SECTIONS OF BRAINSTEM

Dissection: Make serial sections at the following levels, stain with Mulligan stain and try to identify the nuclear matter. The brainstem lodges the ascending fibres, descending fibres, cranial nerve nuclei and nuclei connected with extrapyramidal system.

SECTION THROUGH THE PYRAMIDAL DECUSSATION (Fig. 22)

The prominent feature at this level is the formation of the ***pyramidal decussation***. Note this in the midline. Note that the anterior fissure is obliterated by the crossing pyramidal fibres. These are the *descending corticospinal fibres* or 1st order neurons in the motor pathway. Ninety percent of these fibres cross at this level. These fibres cross to the opposite lateral funiculus and form the *lateral corticospinal tract*. These crossing fibres separate the anterior horn from the central gray. Below the pyramidal decussation the pyramid is very much diminished in size. It carries only 10% of the remaining corticospinal fibres and is called anterior corticospinal tract.

Gray matter: It has the same features as the spinal cord. The anterior horn has the nucleus of the ***spinal accessory nerve***. The substantia gelatinosa of the spinal cord is replaced by the ***nucleus of the spinal tract of trigeminal nerve***. This nucleus receives the pain and temperature fibres of the face. The gracile and cuneate nuclei make their appearance in the respective fasciculi.

White matter: Note the ***gracile and cuneate fasciculi*** in the posterior funiculus. These carry proprioceptive fibres. Note the anterolateral funiculus. It is occupied by the ***anterior and posterior spinocerebellar tracts.*** These are the second order neurons in the proprioceptive pathway to the cerebellum. They occupy the area nearer to the surface. ***The anterior and lateral spinothalamic tracts*** lie deep to the spinocerebellar tracts. They are crossed second order sensory fibres to the thalamus.

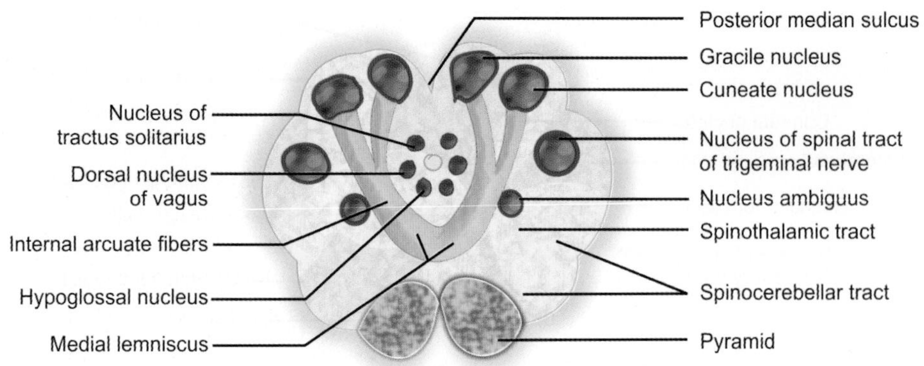

FIGURE 23: Section of the sensory decussation

SECTION OF SENSORY DECUSSATION (Fig. 23)

The prominent feature at the level is the formation of ***gracile and cuneate nuclei*** and the sensory decussation. Note these sweeping fibres from the gracile and cuneate nuclei in the posterior funiculus to the anterior funiculus round the central gray. The second order neurons beginning from here sweep the central gray, reach the area behind the pyramidal decussation. The sweeping fibres are called the ***internal arcuate fibres***. The fibres from here ascend up as the ***medial lemniscus fibres***. They carry second order neurons in the proprioceptive pathway to the thalamus.

Gray matter: The dorsal horn is represented by the ***spinal tract of trigeminal*** nerve and it lies laterally in the position of substantia gelatinosa. ***Nucleus of tractus solitarius*** lies in the central gray. The nucleus of tractus solitarius occupies a dorsal position. It is a relay center for the taste sensations. The second order neurons from here ascend up to the thalamus. ***Vagus nerve nucleus*** lies lateral in position. It is occupied by the dorsal nucleus of vagus. It has both motor and sensory components of autonomic nervous system. ***Hypoglossal nerve nucleus*** lies in the ventral gray near the midline. It is occupied by the hypoglossal nerve nucleus. It is motor to the muscles of tongue. ***Nucleus ambiguus*** is located in the position of the ventral horn. It is motor to the muscles derived from the branchial arches. ***Reticular formation*** is the fine dispersed nuclei present in the white matter present throughout the spinal cord and the brainstem.

White matter: This shows prominent pyramids lateral to the midline. The spinocerebellar and spinothalamic tracts and tracts belonging to the extrapyramidal system, all remain in their respective positions. Medial lemniscus is the newer bundle added between the central gray and pyramids. They are second order neurons in the proprioceptive pathway.

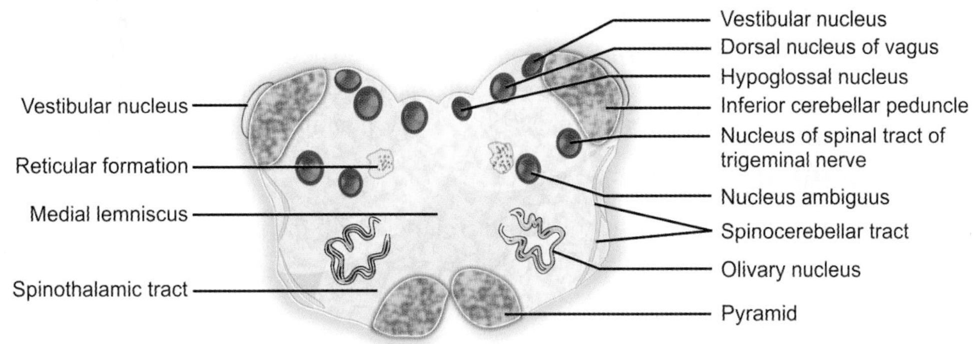

FIGURE 24: Section through the olivary nucleus

SECTION THROUGH THE OLIVARY NUCLEUS (Fig. 24)

The presence of the ***olivary nucleus*** lateral to the pyramid is the prominent feature in this section. Olivary nucleus is relay station in the cerebellar pathway. It receives fibres from the cortex and spinal cord and projects it to the cerebellum. It is a prominent indented nucleus at this level.

The central canal opens up to form the 4th ventricle.

The ***hypoglossal, vagal and vestibular nuclei*** lie in their respective triangles. Identify them based upon the triangles. ***Nucleus of tractus solitarius*** (pain sensations from face), ***nucleus ambiguus*** (branchial motor), ***nucleus of spinal tract of trigeminal*** nerve lie deep in the gray. The ***vestibular nerve nuclei*** lie on either side of the inferior cerebellar nuclei.

White matter: The ***pyramids*** anteriorly and ***inferior cerebellar peduncle*** laterally are the prominent features of the white matter. The ***spinocerebellar tracts*** occupy the peripheral position. The ***spinothalamic tract*** lies in front of the olivary nucleus. The ***medial lemniscus*** occupies the area dorsal to the pyramid. The fibres from the ***extrapyramidal system*** occupy the area between the medial longitudinal bundle and the central gray.

PONS THROUGH THE FACIAL COLLICULUS (Fig. 25)

Here pons forms the floor of the 4th ventricle. Pons exhibits dorsal tegmentum and ventral basilar part.

Tegmentum: This shows the cranial nerve nuclei in the central gray. The parts which are continuous with the medulla oblongata and midbrain occupy the area peripheral to the central gray. ***Abducent nerve nucleus*** lies deep to facial colliculus. *See the facial colliculus and identify the abducent nerve nucleus.* Note the fibres of the abducent nerve nucleus sweeping through the tegmentum. ***Facial nerve nucleus*** lies deep in the tegmentum. ***Nucleus of spinal tract of trigeminal nerve*** and ***vestibulocochlear nerve nuclei*** lie laterally.

Medial lemniscus, spinal lemniscus take a horizontal position inner to the basilar part.

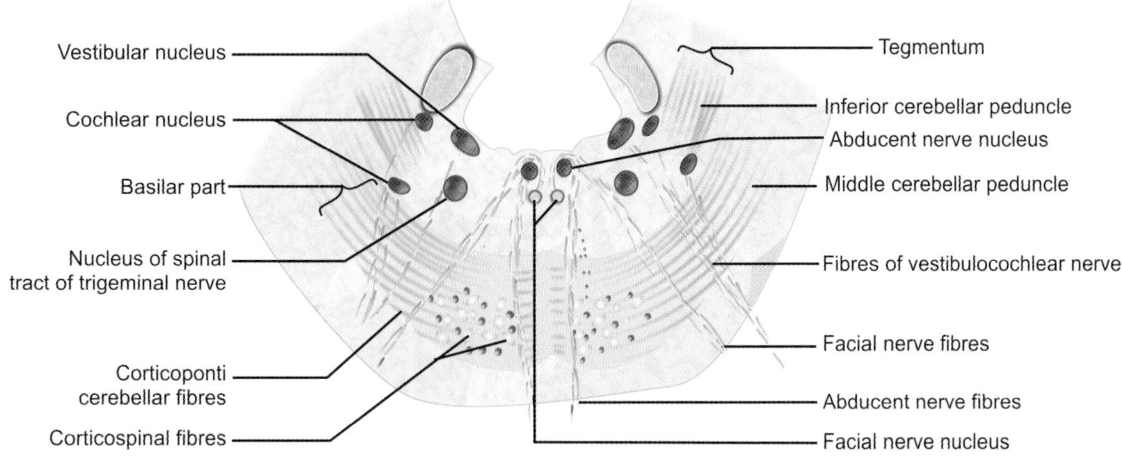

FIGURE 25: Pons through facial colliculus

Basilar part of pons: Basilar part of the pons has both cell bodies and fibres. The ***pontine nuclei*** are mixed with the fibres. The basilar part is dominated by the ***corticoponti nuclear fibres***. These fibres come from cerebral cortex relay in pontine nuclei and reach cerebellum through middle cerebellar peduncle. Identify these horizontally running fibres. Note the transversely cut vertically running corticospinal fibres. Fine pontine nuclei are seen within the basilar part.

PONS THROUGH TRIGEMINAL NERVE (Fig. 26)

Pons when cut carefully shows the enlarged cavity of the 4th ventricle with the roof formed by the superior medullary velum. Superolaterally look for the superior cerebellar peduncle.

Tegmentum

The **trigeminal nerve nuclei:** They form the major part here in the gray matter. This lies laterally, inner to the middle cerebellar peduncle. Locate the attachment of the trigeminal nerve on the pons. Trace the trigeminal nerve nucleus inner to this. Note the ***middle cerebellar peduncle*** forming and lateral aspect in this section. ***Trapezoid body*** is the horizontally running second order neurons in the auditory sensory pathway. They begin in auditory nuclei and ascend up as lateral lemniscus. This lies between the tegmentum and the basilar part of pons. The ***medial lemniscus*** from gracile and cuneate nuclei, the ***trigeminal lemniscus*** from the trigeminal nerve nucleus, the ***spinal lemniscus*** from the nuclei of spinal cord in the posterior horn, occupy the space between the trapezoid body and the basilar part of pons.

Basilar part of pons: This shows the horizontally running ***corticoponti nuclear fibres,*** vertically running corticopontine fibres and pontine nuclei. Identify them fibres to cerebellum.

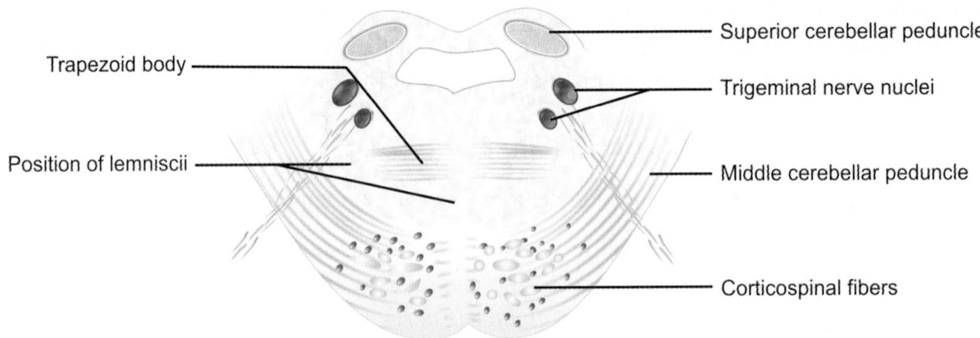

FIGURE 26: Pons through trigeminal nerve

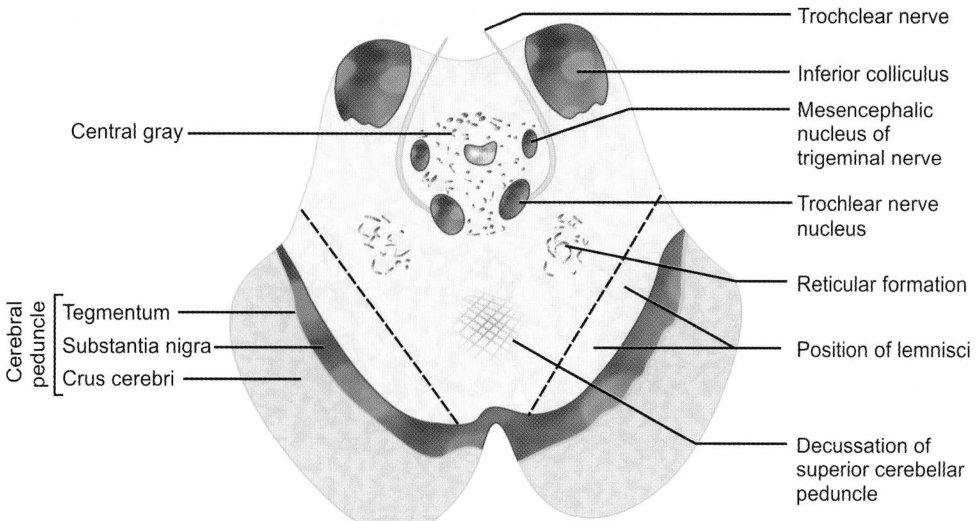

FIGURE 27: Midbrain at inferior colliculus

MIDBRAIN AT INFERIOR COLLICULUS (Fig. 27)

The midbrain is divided into two parts, tectum posterior to the central canal and cerebral peduncles in front of the central canal.

Tectum: At this level the tectum is formed by the nuclear matter of ***inferior colliculus.*** Note this nucleus. It is a reflex center in the auditory pathway. The fibres of the lateral lemniscus enters here.

Cerebral peduncle is made up of three parts—tegmentum, substantia nigra and crus cerebri.

Tegmentum: The central gray shows the ***mesencephalic nucleus of trigeminal nerve and trochlear nerve nucleus.*** The trochlear nerve nucleus occupies a position lateral to the midline whereas the mesencephalic nucleus occupies a lateral position. Decussation of ***superior cerebellar peduncle*** in the midline ventral to central gray. These are the fibres from the deep cerebellar nuclei to the thalamus. They decussate before they reach the cerebrum. **Lemnisci**—lateral, spinal, trigeminal and medial—in that order from inferior colliculus to the cerebellar decussation. Though actual separation of these fibres cannot be identified in these sections, their position can be identified.

Substantia nigra: It is the nuclear matter with melanin pigment in their cells. So the area appears black in color. It lies between tegmentum and crus cerebri. It is a part of the extrapyramidal system.

Crus cerebri: It is made of descending white fibres both corticospinal, corticonuclear and corticopontine fibres.

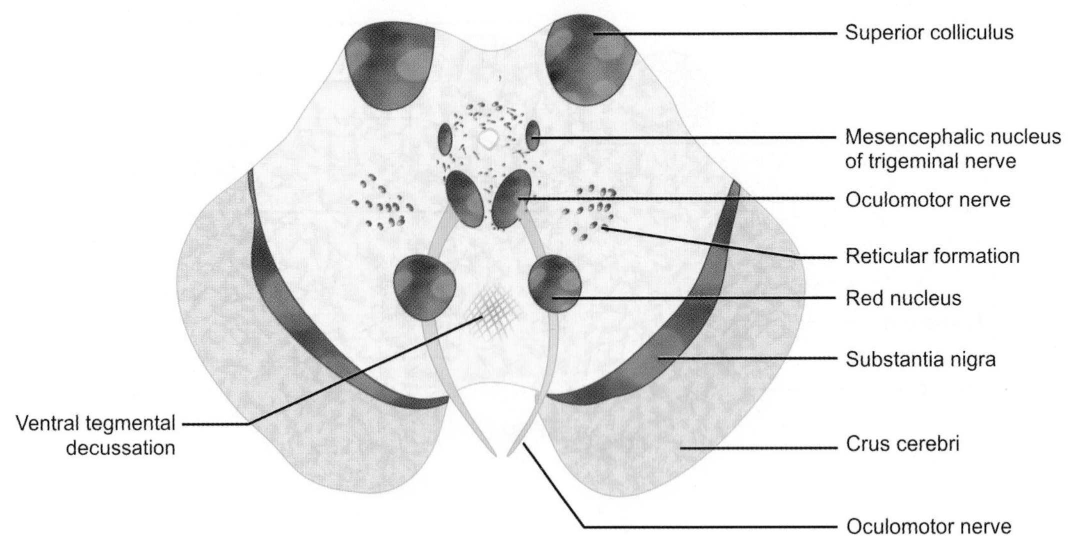

FIGURE 28: Midbrain at superior colliculus

Midbrain at Superior Collicular Level (Fig. 28)

Tectum: It shows superior colliculus. It is a nuclear matter. Note the thin white matter around it. This is due to the fibres entering into the nucleus. The superior colliculus is a reflex center for visual sensations.

Central gray: This shows ***oculomotor nerve nucleus*** on either side of the midline in the ventral gray. The ***mesencephalic nucleus of trigeminal nerve*** lies dorsal to the oculomotor nerve nucleus.

Cerebral Peduncle

Tegmentum: This shows red nucleus. This is a nuclear matter of extrapyramidal system. This is a very prominent feature at this level. The **lemnisci** show spinal, trigeminal and medial in that order from lateral to medial side, as lateral lemniscus has already entered into the inferior colliculus. Ventral tegmental decussation in the midline is caused by the rubrospinal fibres.

The substantia nigra: Note this pigmented gray matter. It is a part of the extrapyramidal system.
Crus cerebri shows the same descending fibres.

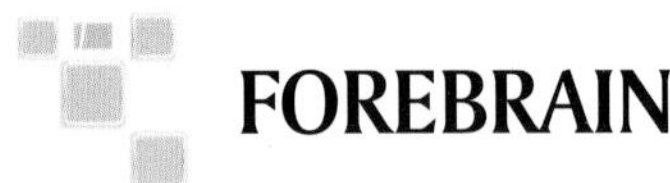

FOREBRAIN

The forebrain is made up of cerebrum and thalamic complex. The cerebrum is the well developed part of the human development. It has got outer gray matter, inner white matter and basal ganglia within the white matter. The cavity of the forebrain is the lateral ventricle. The thalamic complex is made up of thalamus, metathalamus, epithalamus, hypothalamus and subthalamus. The cavity of the thalamic complex is the third ventricle. The cerebrum and thalamic complex merge with each other and it is convenient to study them together.

The cerebrum lodges the highest sensory and motor centers of the body. Multitude of the fibres inter connect these centers with different parts of the CNS.

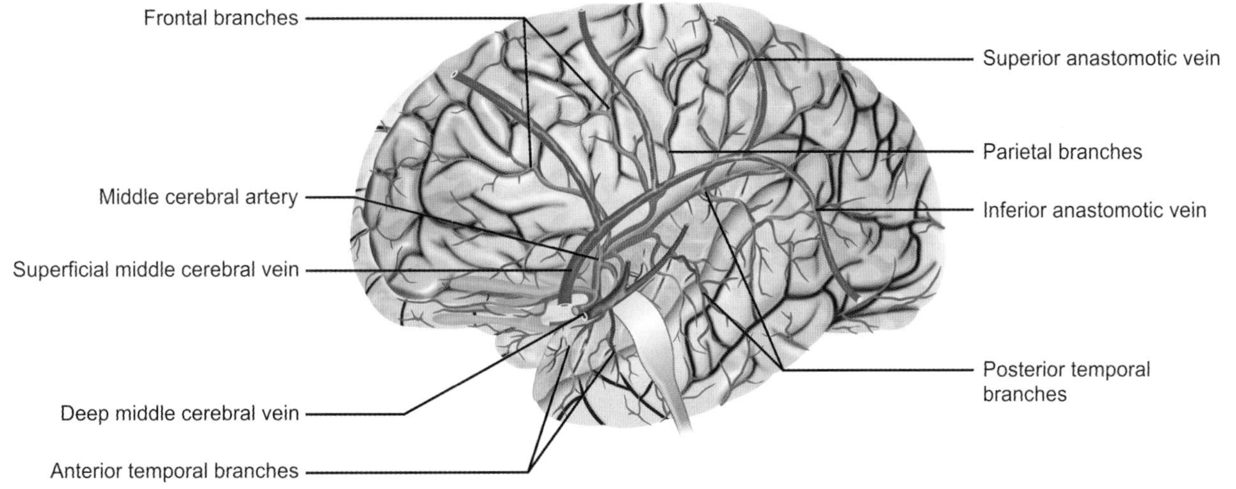

FIGURE 29: Cerebrum—blood supply of lateral surface

BLOOD SUPPLY OF FOREBRAIN

Lateral Surface (Fig. 29)

Dissection: Carefully remove the arachnoid matter from the sulci on the superolateral surface of the brain and identify the veins draining this region.

Superior cerebral veins: These are number of longitudinally running channels opening into the superior sagittal sinus.

Superficial middle cerebral vein: This drains into the cavernous sinus.

Inferior cerebral veins: These drain the temporal lobe and drain into the transverse sinus.

Superior anastomotic vein: This connects the superior sagittal sinus to the superficial middle cerebral vein. This is a slightly enlarged vein of the superior cerebral veins.

Inferior anastomotic vein: This connects middle cerebral vein to the transverse sinus. This is a slightly enlarged vein of the inferior cerebral veins.

Deep middle cerebral vein: This lies in the depth of the limen insulae. This vein drains the insula and the neighboring gyri. It drains into the basal vein which winds the external surface of the cerebral peduncle.

Dissection: Remove these veins and look for the middle cerebral artery and its branches.

Middle cerebral artery: It is a branch of the internal carotid artery at the circle of Willis. Trace it into the lateral sulcus. Identify frontal, parietal and temporal group of branches of the artery. Note the area of supply.

Dissection: With a brain knife separate the two cerebral hemispheres by a midline cut through the corpus callosum, septum pellucidum, Third ventricle to the midbrain.

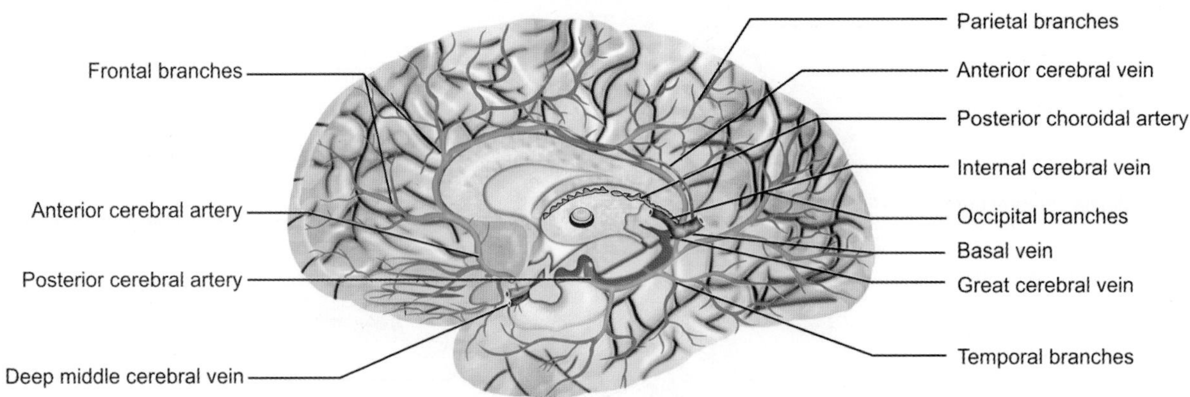

FIGURE 30: Cerebrum—blood supply medial and inferior surface

The Medial and the Inferior Surface (Fig. 30)

Anterior cerebral artery: This arises from the circle of Willis. Trace it to the parietal lobe along the superior border of the corpus callosum. This artery supplies orbital 'surface' and medial surface up to the parietooccipital sulcus.

Great cerebral vein of Galen: This lies below the splenium of the corpus callosum. Trace its two tributaries—the internal cerebral vein—this runs along the roof of the third ventricle, the basal vein along the side of the midbrain. These veins drain blood from the interior part of the forebrain.

Posterior cerebral artery: Identify this artery near the temporal lobe. Identify its temporal and occipital group of branches and note its area of supply.

Anterior choroidal artery: This lies in the gap between the temporal lobe and frontal lobe by lightly separating there. This artery arises from the middle cerebral artery. *Trace the artery into the interior of the lateral ventricle through the choroid fissure.*

Posterior choroidal artery: This arises from the posterior cerebral artery near the splenium of the corpus callosum. It enters the cerebrum below the splenium to form the choroids plexus of both third and lateral ventricle.

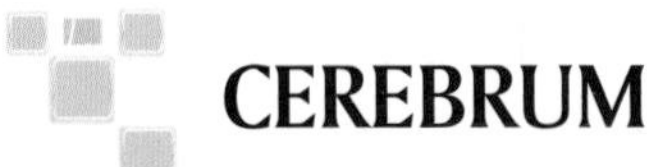

CEREBRUM

Dissection: Remove the pia matter and the blood vessels on the surface of the cerebral hemisphere leaving the central branches including the choroidal branches *in situ*.

Cerebrum moulds itself according the shape of the cranial cavity above the tentorium cerebelli. It exhibits the following general features in a hardened specimen. Customarily it is divided into four lobes based on its relations to the bones related to the surface.

GENERAL FEATURES (Fig. 31)

Frontal pole: It is the most anterior projection, occupies the anterior cranial fossa.

Temporal pole: It is the middle projection and occupies the middle cranial fossa.

Occipital pole: It is the posterior projection, lies above the tentorium cerebelli and is related to the occipital bone above the groove for transverse sinus.

Superomedial border: This extends from frontal pole to the occipital pole.

Inferolateral border: This extends from the temporal pole to occipital pole.

Medial border: It is more blunt extends from the frontal pole to the occipital pole on the medial side. It can be described as orbital, hippocampal and occipital parts.

Superolateral surface: The area between the superomedial to inferior lateral border on the lateral aspect.

Medial surface: This extends between the superomedial border to the medial border, on the medial aspect. The two medial surfaces are separated by the falx cerebri. The diencephalon is seen below the medial surface.

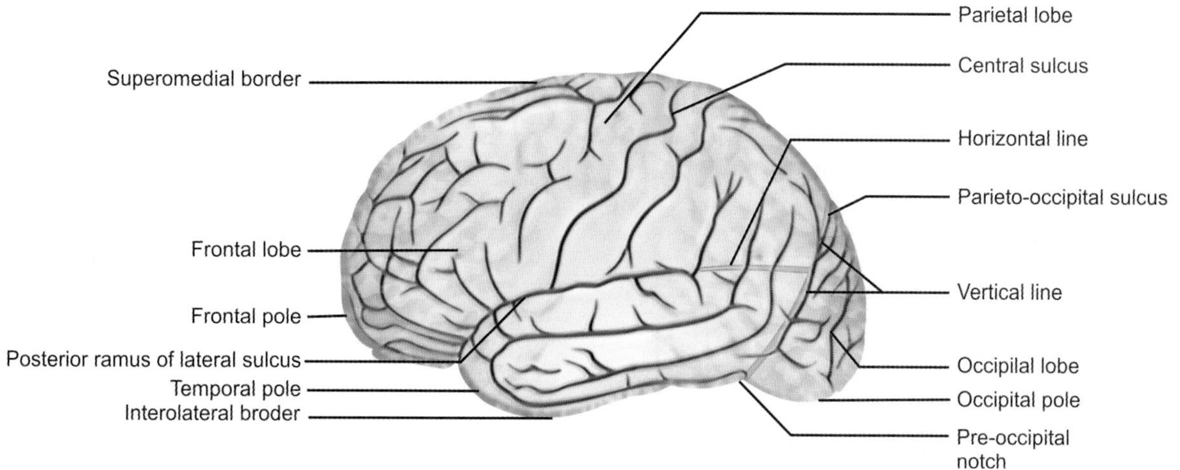

FIGURE 31: General features and lobes of cerebrum

Inferior surface: This can be divided into two parts ***orbital surface,*** the part of the frontal lobe related to the orbital plate in the anterior cranial fossa and the ***tentorial surface*** which includes the inferior surface of both temporal and occipital lobes and is related to the tentorium cerebelli and the middle cranial fossa.

LOBES OF CEREBRUM (Fig. 31)

Cerebrum can be divided for descriptive purposes into frontal, parietal, occipital and temporal lobes. To do this, identify the central sulcus, lateral sulcus, vertical imaginary line, horizontal imaginary line, temporo-occipital notch and parieto-occipital sulcus.

Occipital notch is a depression located between the temporal and occipital lobes.

Imaginary vertical line, look for the small parieto-occipital sulcus on the superolateral surface and draw a line form here to the occipital notch. Imaginary horizontal line—draw this line from the posterior limb of the lateral sulcus to the imaginary vertical line.

The part of the cerebrum in relation to the frontal bone, the area between the frontal pole, central sulcus and above the lateral sulcus is the ***frontal lobe***. It is seen on the superolateral surface as well as the medial surface. The ***parietal lobe*** is the area behind the central sulcus and between the two imaginary lines drawn earlier in this area. We can see the extensions of the temporal sulci into this area. The parietal lobe extends on to the medial surface. This area is in relation to the parietal bone. The ***temporal lobe*** is the area between these imaginary lines, lateral sulcus and inferior lateral border. It includes the temporal pole and also extends on to the medial side. This part is in relation to the middle cranial fossa. The ***occipital lobe*** is the area behind the vertical imaginary line on the superolateral aspect. It includes the occipital pole and extends on to the medial side. This part lies above the tentorium cerebelli and in relation to the occipital bone.

GYRI AND SULCI ON THE CEREBRUM

The enormous expansion of the cerebral hemisphere in humans results in folding of the cerebrum, resulting in the formation of gyri and sulci. The following, describes the basic identifiable sulci, but there can be far more sulci in individual brains. The elevated area between the sulci are the gyri. **Boardman** has assigned numbers to the areas which have a common function.

Identify the following sulci and gyri on this area and study the functional areas and their numbers.

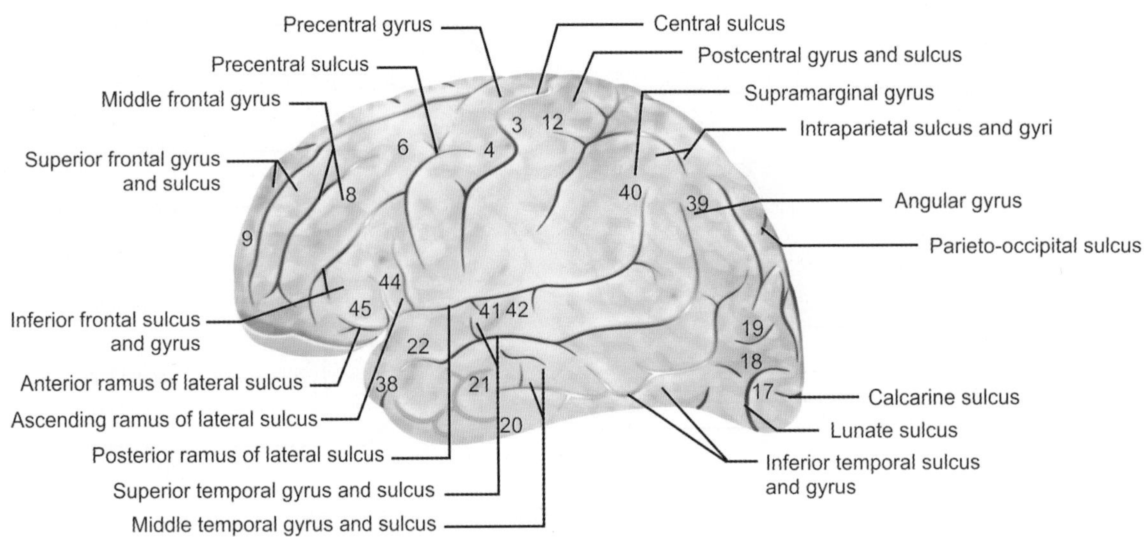

FIGURE 32: Cerebrum—superolateral surface

SUPEROLATERAL SURFACE (Fig. 32)

FRONTAL LOBE is the area in front of the central sulcus and above the lateral sulcus. This is primarily a motor area.

Lateral sulcus: It is a gap where the frontal, parietal and temporal lobes meet. Put your fingers in this sulcus and feel the frontal, parietal and temporal operculas, lightly separate them and see the submerged insula. Generally this sulcus is described as having a stem, anterior, ascending, and posterior rami. The anterior and ascending rami cut into the inferior frontal gyrus.

Central sulcus: This lies on the superomedial border. It starts midway between the frontal and occipital poles. It runs obliquely downwards and forwards to reach just above the lateral sulcus. It separates the frontal lobe from the parietal lobe. It is a complete sulcus, it separates two functional areas, the sensory and the motor area.

Precentral sulcus: It is the sulcus parallel and in front of the central sulcus.

Superior and inferior frontal sulci: These sulci run horizontally in the area in front of the precentral sulcus. Generally they are full sulci but many a times these are broken into smaller bits or there can be more than two horizontal sulci.

Precentral gyrus: It is the area between central and precentral sulcus. This is a primary motor area (area 4). The fibres starting from here control the movements of the body. They form the pyramidal tracts and relay on the motor cranial and spinal nuclei. Here the body is represented upside down. It has a big representation of the head and neck and hand as these regions perform intricate movements like speech and hand movements. ***Superior and inferior frontal gyri (area, 6.8.9.)***: They lie in front of the precentral sulcus and between the sulci of the same. These areas in the middle frontal gyrus are given a common name, the frontal eye field. This brings about consolidated movements of the both eyeballs.

Broca's area of speech (area 44, 45): It is located in the inferior frontal gyrus. Two sulci called horizontal vertical parts of the lateral sulcus project into the inferior frontal gyrus. The area between these two and the area in front of the precentral sulcus constitutes the Broca's speech area. This brings about the coordinated movements of the muscles of larynx, mouth and face to bring about speech.

PARIETAL LOBE

Postcentral sulcus: It is the sulcus parallel and posterior to the central sulcus.

Postcentral gyrus: It is the area between the central and post central sulcus area. It perceives the general sensations like pain, touch pressure from different parts of the body in area 3. Area 1, 2 are integrating centers for the general sensations.

Intraparietal sulcus: This is an irregular horizontal sulcus within this area. The part of the lateral sulcus which projects up into the parietal lobe is called the posterior ramus of lateral sulcus.

Supramarginal gyrus (area 40): It is around the posterior limb of the lateral sulcus.

Angular gyrus (area 39): It is around the superior temporal gyrus. Wernicke's area is the area of 40, 39 including the supramarginal and angular gyri. This is an integrating center in understanding written and spoken words.

Intraparietal gyri: These are superior and inferior gyri above and below the intraparietal sulcus. This area is called parietal eye field and center for stereognosis. This area is located between general, auditory and visual sensations. In this area integration of all these impulses takes place and their correlation with past experience, e.g. identification of a forceps in the hand even though we are not looking at it.

TEMPORAL LOBE

Superior and inferior temporal sulci: These run horizontally between the lateral sulcus and inferolateral border. Both the sulci curve superiorly into the parietal lobe.

Superior, middle and inferior temporal gyri: These lie between the sulci. Temporal lobe lodges the auditory area.

Primary auditory area (area 41, 42): This occupies the area opposite to the central sulcus on the superior temporal gyrus. This is called transverse temporal gyrus. *Lower the superior temporal gyrus to identify this.* It occupies the superior surface of this. The sounds we hear are interpreted here.

Secondary auditory area (area 21, 22): This occupies the remaining area of the temporal lobe. This area is the integrating area with our part experience and makes us understand what we heard, for example, the bell ringing sound is that of the ringing of a Church bell.

OCCIPITAL LOBE

Note this area behind the imaginary vertical line.

Lunate sulcus: It is a curved sulcus very near the pole. The area between the lunate sulcus and the imaginary line is occupied by the para and peristriate areas (area 18 and 19).

MEDIAL SURFACE (Fig. 33)

Turn the cerebral hemisphere on to the medial side and study the gyri and sulci.

Corpus callosum: This is the thick fibre bundle which connects both the hemispheres. The details will be studied with the commissures.

Callosal sulcus: It is the sulcus immediately above and around the corpus callosum.

Cingulate sulcus: This is parallel to the callosal sulcus between the superior medial border and the corpus callosum.

Medial frontal gyrus: This lies between the superior medial border and the cingulate sulcus up to the central sulcus. This area has the same 4.6.8.9.10 areas that are seen on the lateral surface.

Paracentral lobule: It is the area around the central sulcus on the medial side. It has sensory as well motor areas of perineum and lower limb.

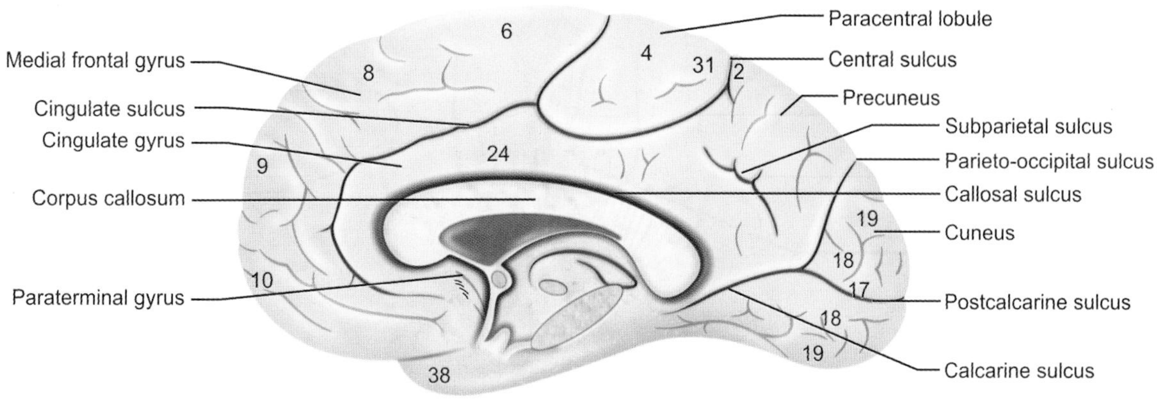

FIGURE 33: Cerebrum—medial surface

Cingulate gyrus: It is the gyrus between the cingulate and callosal sulci. This is a part of limbic lobe and in concerned with the control of internal organs.

Precuneus: It is the area between the paracentral lobule and parieto-occipital sulcus. This is the medial aspect of the parietal lobe. No particular area is assigned here. It is an integrating center.

Paraterminal gyrus: This lies in front of the lamina terminalis. This is a part of the limbic system.

OCCIPITAL LOBE

Calcarine, post-calcarine and parieto-occipital sulci form a Y shaped sulci.

Cuneus: It is the area within the Y.

Visual area (area 17): This occupies the depth and lips of the post-calcarine sulcus. This is the visuosensory area to be able to see the color and light. ***Visiopsychic area*** (area 18 and 19) extend on either side of the area 17. Posteriorly all the three areas are limited by the lunate sulcus. Area 18 and 19 are visual association areas where the objects are perceived by past experience.

INFERIOR SURFACE

Orbital Surface (Fig. 34)

Olfactory sulcus: Locate this longitudinal sulcus parallel to the medial border. The olfactory bulb and tract are located here. Gyrus rectus lies medial to the olfactory sulcus (area 11).

Orbital sulcus: It is H shaped sulcus. It occupies the remaining part of the orbital surface. Anterior, posterior, medial and lateral orbital gyri can be identified on the sides of the orbital sulci. This area is a integration center for olfactory sensations (area 10).

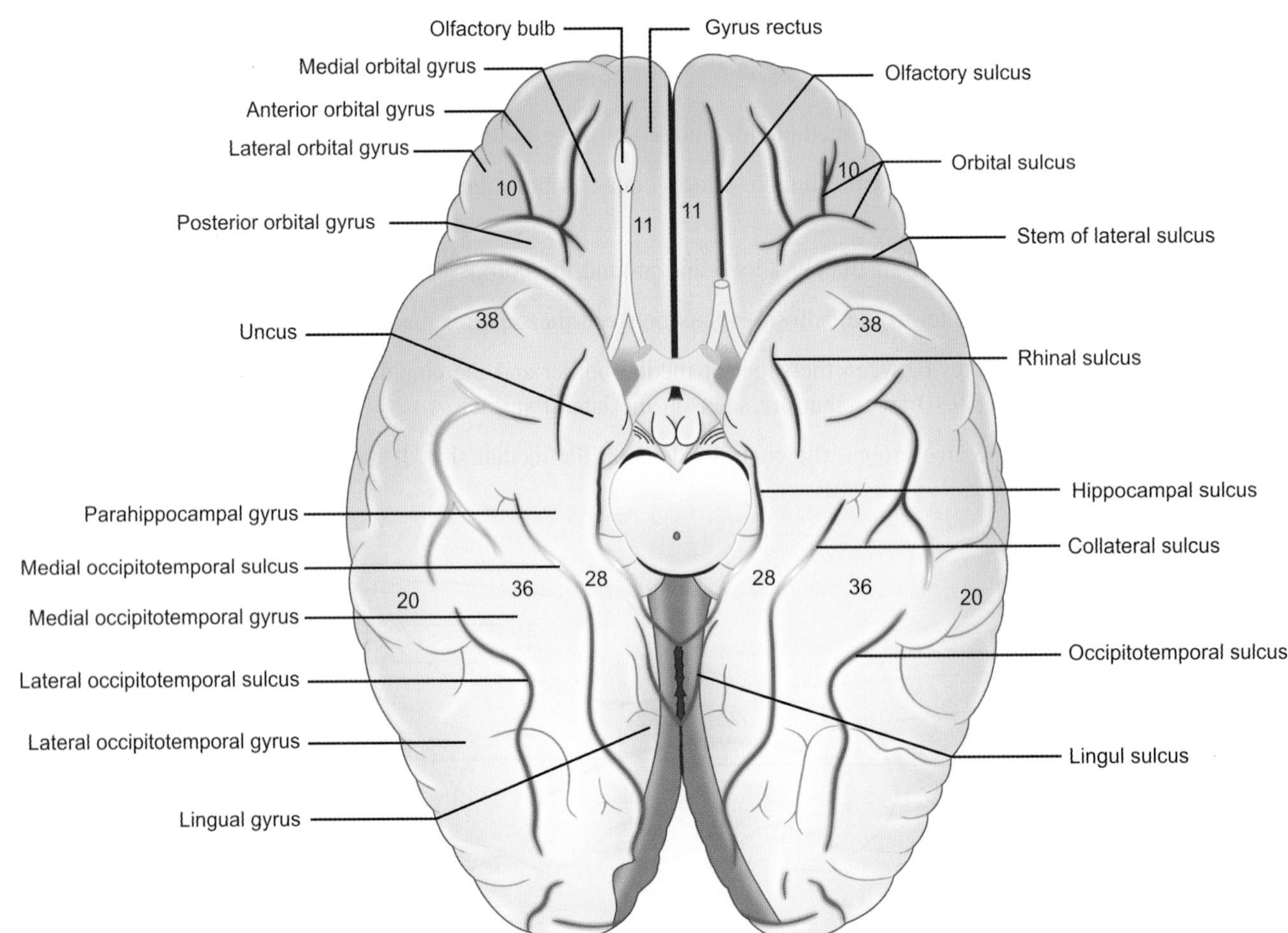

FIGURE 34: Cerebrum—inferior surface

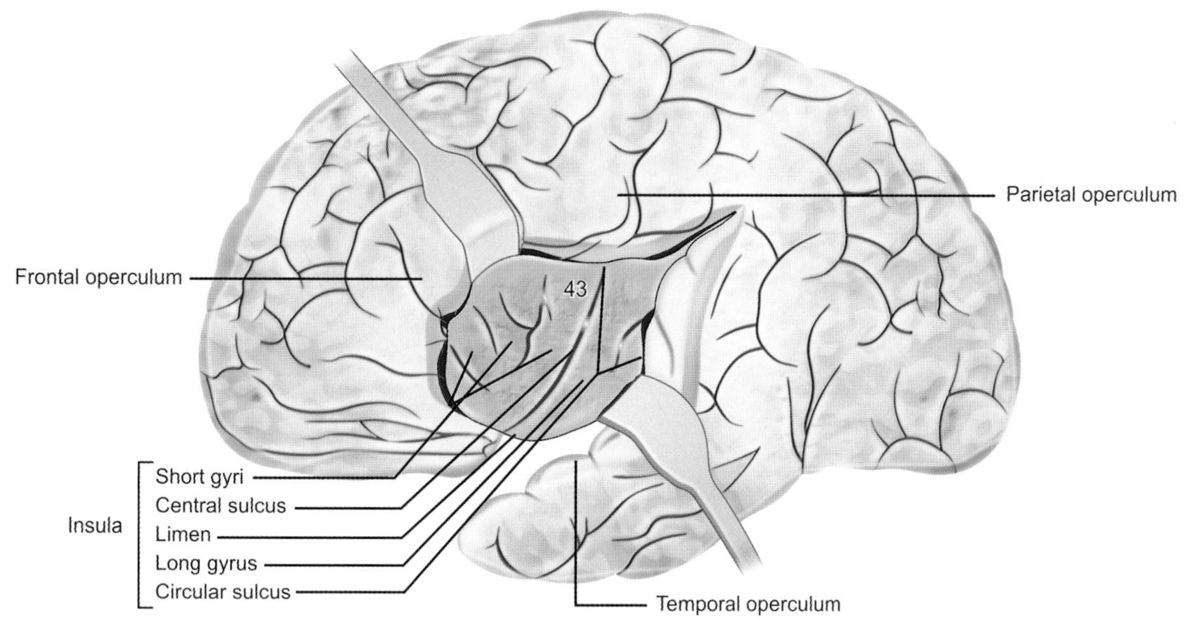

FIGURE 35: Cerebrum—insula

Temporo-occipital Surface

Rhinal sulcus: Locate this medial semilunar sulcus on the medial side.

Uncus: It is the gyrus medial to the rhinal sulcus. This is the primary olfactory area (area 38).

Parahippocampal sulcus: This is the most medial of the sulei.

Collateral sulcus: It is parallel to the parahippocampal sulcus, extends from temporal to occipital region. It is posterior to the rhinal sulcus (area 28). The gyrus medial to the collateral sulcus is parahippocampal gyrus. This is a secondary olfactory area.

Medial and lateral temporo-occipital gyri: They are on either side of the temporo-occipital sulcus. These constitute the secondary olfactory areas (area 36 and 20).

Lingual gyrus: It is posterior to the parahippocampal gyrus and lateral to the calcarine sulcus.

Insula (Fig. 35)

Insula is the submerged cortex. It is overlapped by the frontal parietal and temporal opercula. Pull these opercula and try to see the insula. The sulcus which separates the insula from the opercula is called the circular sulcus. Note the ***short and long gyri*** located within the insula. The point where the opercula meet is called the limen insulae. The Brodmann areas that are present on the operculum continue to be present on the overlapping opercula. The long and short gyri are concerned with the intestinal motility, taste and visceral sensations (area 43).

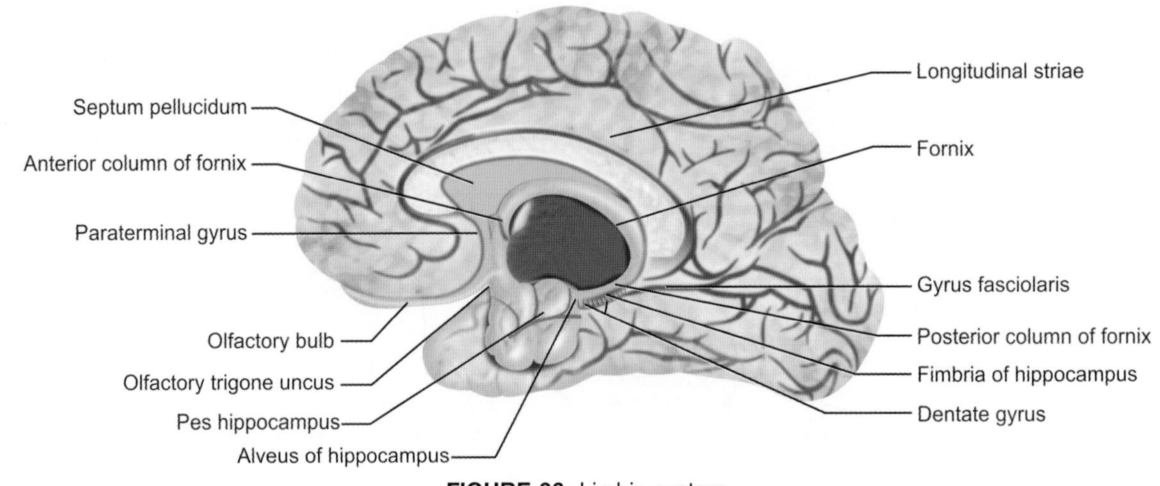

FIGURE 36: Limbic system

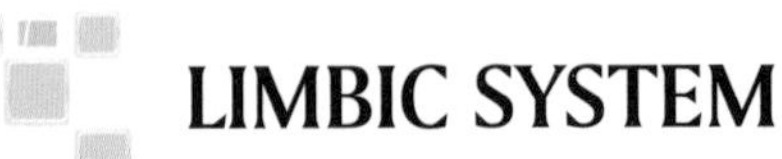

LIMBIC SYSTEM

Limbic lobe is the oldest in evolution and is located in and around the corpus callosum and thalamus **(Fig. 36).**

Turn on to the medial side and locate the following parts mostly concerned with the integration of olfactory and visceral sensations of the body.

The **olfactory bulb:** This receives the olfactory sensations from the nasal cavity through the olfactory nerves. The second order neurons traverse the olfactory tract and diverge to form the ***olfactory trigone,*** medial to it is the anterior perforated substance (already identified—the perforations are caused by the central arteries. Follow the ***medial olfactory stria*** around the gyrus rectus to the paraterminal gyrus. Trace the ***lateral olfactory striae*** along the floor of the limen insulae to the uncus, by pulling the uncus.

Identify the ***hippocampal sulcus*** medial to the uncus and parahippocampal gyrus.

Dentate gyrus: This is a thin gyrus seen in the depths of the hippocampal gyrus. Identify this gyrus by depressing the hippocampal gyrus. It shows serrations, so the name. It is continuous anteriorly with the uncus, posteriorly with the gyrus fasciolaris.

Lower the temporal lobe and identify the ***pes hippocampus,*** alveus and fimbria of hippocampus. These are inner to the dentate gyrus. The pes is enlarged paw like structure, *alveus* is the white fibres covering the hippocampus, the cell bodies of these fibres are located in the hippocampus.

Fimbria is the accumulation of these fibres on the medial side of the hippocampus between it and the dentate gyrus.

Fornix is the continuation of the fimbria. Trace the body, posterior and anterior columns of fornix. Majority of the fibres of the hippocampus from the fimbria ascend up towards the splenium and is called posterior column. ***Posterior columns*** of both sides approximate in the center to form the body. The *body* again deviates into two ***anterior columns*** for both the hemispheres. These end in the ***mammillary bodies.*** The fornix constitutes both commissural and association fibres.

Few of the fibres of the hippocampus take a different route. They are ***medial and lateral longitudinal striae:*** Trace these two striae over the corpus callosum extending from the hippocampus to the paraterminal gyrus by pulling the cingulated gyrus.

Gyrus fasciolaris: Identify this small gyrus beneath the splenium of corpus callosum.

Paraterminal gyrus: This gyrus lies in front of the lamina terminals.

Septum pellucidum: Septum pellucidum is two layered partition of the cerebral hemispheres, see it stretching between the corpus callosum and fornix. There is nuclear matter within the septum pellucidum, which is considered as a part of the limbic system. Between the two septa pellucida there is a cavity called cavity of septum pellucidum. Generally in a midline section both the layers will be seen on one side. But the layers can be pealed and the cavity can be visualized.

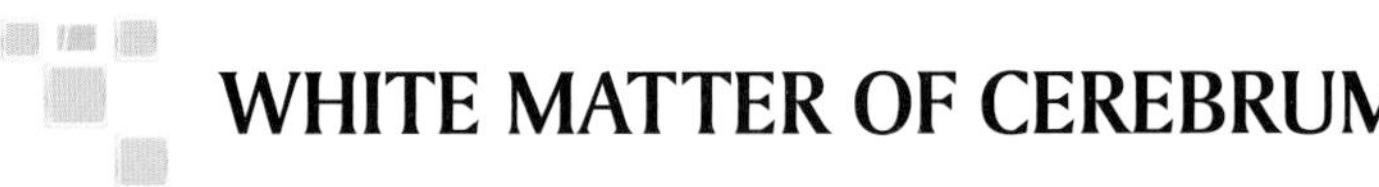

WHITE MATTER OF CEREBRUM

Cerebrum is the biggest integrating center. Billions of fibres are located here. For convenience of description they are described as the association fibres which connect one part of cerebral hemisphere with the other part. The commissural fibres connect one half of hemisphere with the other half of the hemisphere. As these cross the midline, in a midsagittal section these fibres get cut and are easily identified. The projection fibres connect the cerebral hemisphere with other parts of CNS. These form ascending and descending tracts. These are named by different names in different parts of the CNS.

COMMISSURAL FIBRES

Commissural fibres (Fig. 37): These connect the right and left halves of the cerebral hemispheres so they are best seen in the midline sagittal sections – *identify the following from front to back.*

ANTERIOR COMMISSURE: This lies in front of the lamina terminals. This connects the uncus of the temporal lobe of both the hemispheres.

CORPUS CALLOSUM: This connects the frontal, parietal, occipital and temporal lobes of one side with the other. So this is the most prominent and thickest of the commissures and presents number of parts.

The **rostrum** is the thin part of the corpus callosum connecting the genu with the anterior commissure. The fibres of this part connect the two orbital surfaces.

The **Genu** is the anterior blunt pole of the corpus callosum. The fibres from here connect the two frontal lobes. The fibres of both sides form a forceps type of arrangement, so is called forceps minor.

The **body** is the main part of the corpus callosum extending from the frontal pole to the occipital pole. The fibres arising from here connect the two frontal lobes and parietal lobes. Posterior fibres from here cross laterally, lateral to the lateral ventricle, and descend down into the occipital pole. These are called tapetal fibres. Note that the fibres of the body are cut by the descending corona radiata fibres, except for the tapetal fibres.

The **splenium** is the posterior part of the corpus callosum. Fibres from here connect the parietal occipital and temporal lobes. These fibres also give an appearance of a forceps when fibres of both sides are seen. This is called forceps major.

POSTERIOR COMMISSURE: This lies posteriorly and between the pineal body and superior colliculus connects the two superior colliculi. It lies in the lower of stalk of pineal body.

HABENULAR COMMISSURE: Identify this along the upper limb of the stalk of the pineal body. It connects the two Habenular nuclei located on the posterior aspect of the thalamus lateral to the pineal body.

At this stage it is easy to study the ventricles of the forebrain, as the structures are still undisturbed.

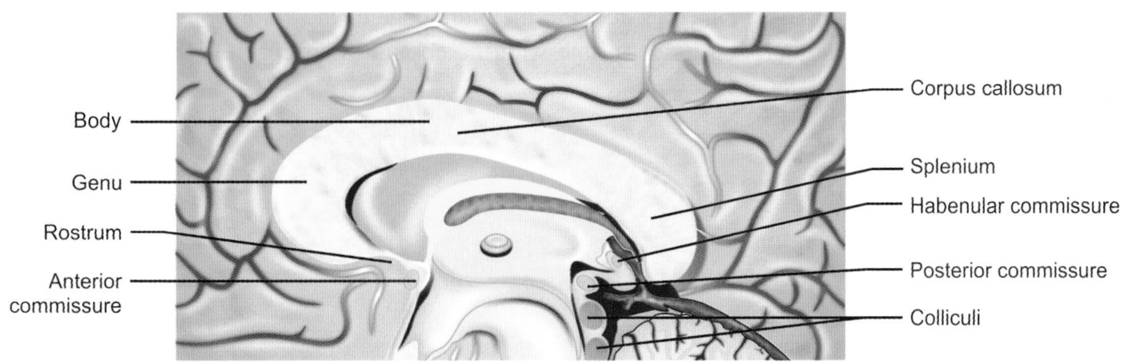

FIGURE 37: Cerebrum—white matter, commissural fibres

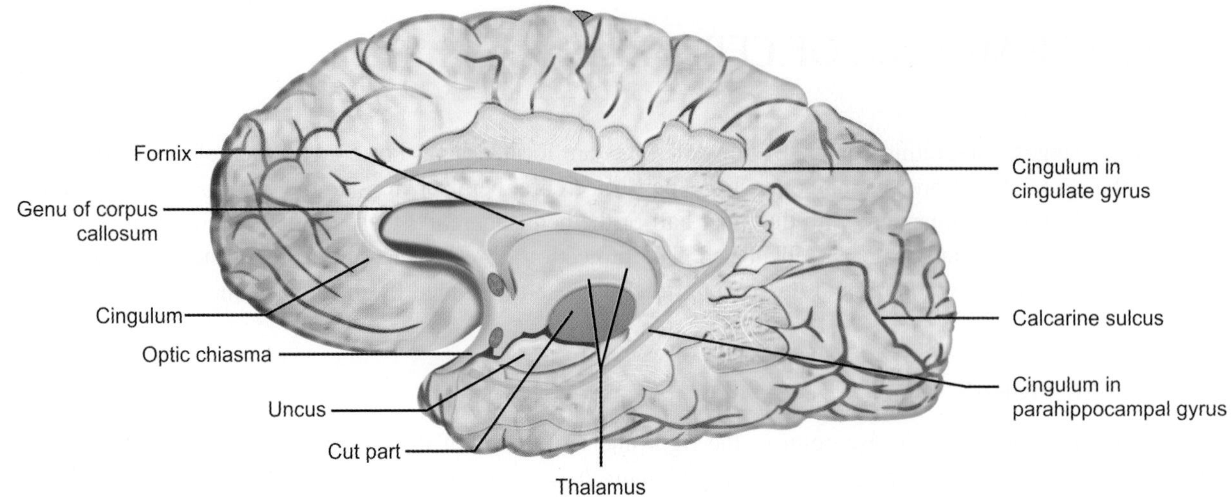

FIGURE 38: Cerebrum—white matter, medial surface

ASSOCIATION FIBRES

Association fibres connect different parts of the same hemisphere.

MEDIAL SURFACE (Fig. 38)

Short association fibres: These are the fibres which connect one gyrus to the adjoining gyrus.

Dissection: With the back of the handle of a knife or a scalpel try to scrape the superficial gray matter on the medial frontal gyrus in the paracentral lobule. Identify the curving U shaped fibres on either side of central sulcus. There are the short association fibres.

Cingulum: It is the big association fibre bundle in the cingulate gyrus. It extends down into the parahippocampal gyrus. It connects the frontal, parietal, occipital and temporal gyri on the medial side.

Dissection: Remove the gray matter of the cingulate gyrus by blunt dissection and note the fibres extending from the paraterminal gyrus along the frontal parietal, occipital lobes to the cuneus of the temporal lobe just external to the corpus callosum. Trace it down into the temporal lobe. These are the fibres of cingulum.

FORNIX: It has both association and commissural fibres. Deep to the cingulum you can trace the fibres of corpus callosum.

Dissection: Remove the cingulum on the medial side. Put the blunt edge of the knife along the upper border of the corpus callosum and remove the brain tissue in line with the corpus callosum. See the extension of fibres of corpus callosum into the gyri.

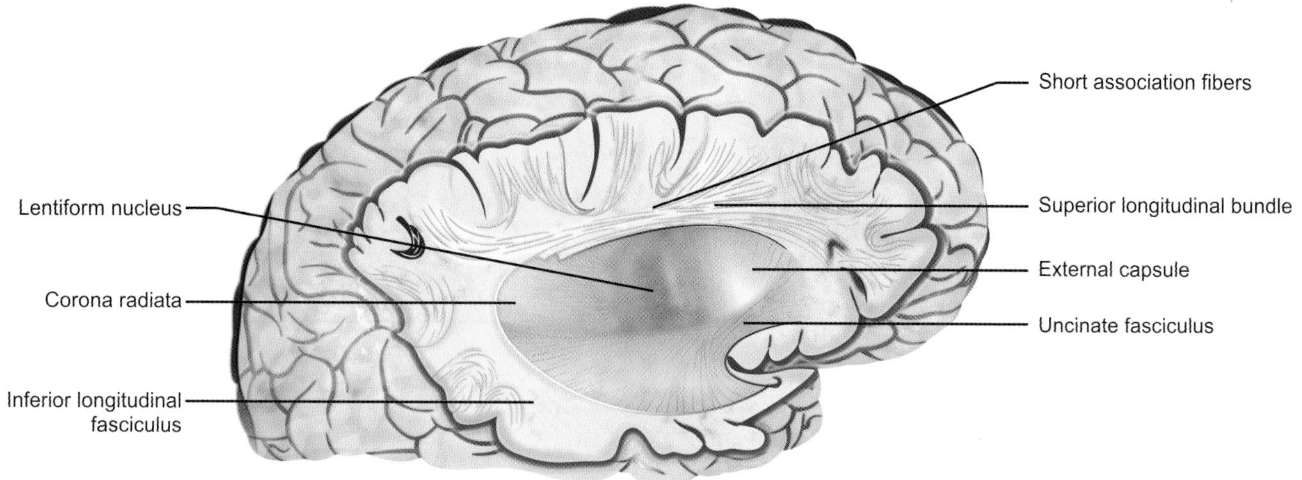

FIGURE 39: Cerebrum—white matter, lateral surface

SUPEROLATERAL SURFACE (Fig. 39)

Dissection: Turn the brain to the lateral surface, cut the opercula of the insula to reach the circular sulcus. Then proceed by blunt dissection with the back of the handle of knife into the adjoining gyri. Identify the following association fibres.

Superior longitudinal fasciculus: It is located within the inferior frontal gyrus, supramarginal, angular gyri running horizontally from frontal lobe to the occipital lobe.

Uncinate fasciculus: It arises from the orbital surfaces of the frontal lobe along the limen insulae to the uncus of the temporal lobe.

Inferior longitudinal fasciculus: It is seen in the inferior occipitotemporal gyrus. Remove the superficial gray matter and identify this gyrus.

Insula: It has got 4 layers—study it layer by layer by careful blunt dissection. The outer gray matter is the cortical gray. The outer white matter is the white matter of the cortex. This gives rise to projection fibres from here. The ***claustrum*** is a thin layer of gray matter belonging to the basal ganglia. The ***external capsule*** is the association fibre bundle connecting the frontal, parietal lobe to the temporal lobe. The fibres run vertically.

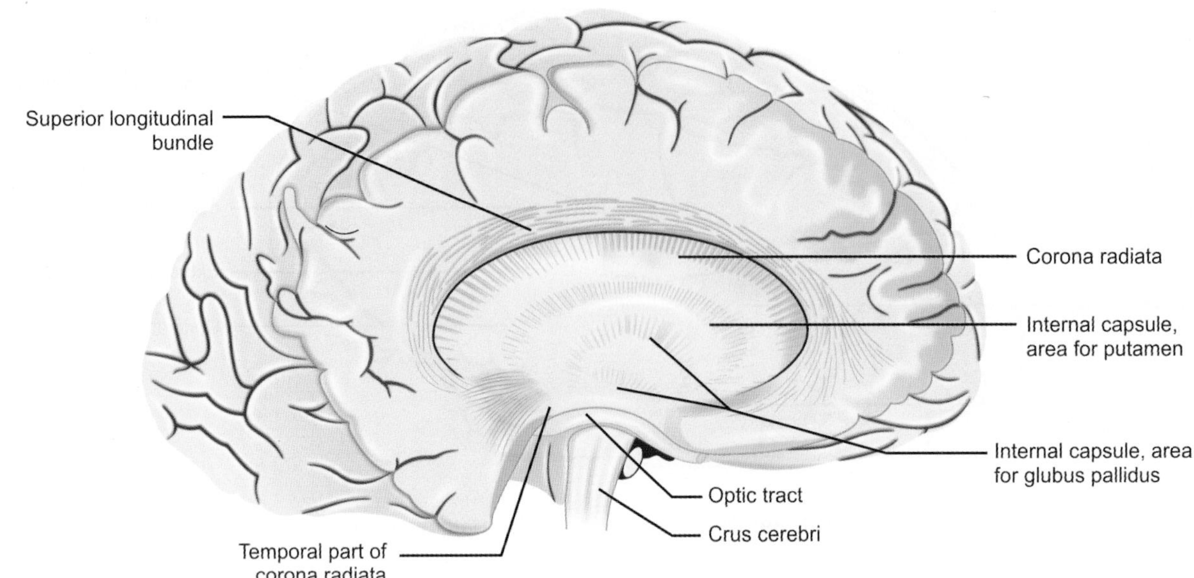

FIGURE 40: Cerebrum—projection fibres

PROJECTION FIBRES

The projection fibres **(Fig. 40)** are vertically running fibres. These are both ascending and descending fibres to the cortex. The ascending fibres constitute thalamic radiation and the descending fibres constitute corticonuclear, corticospinal and corticocerebellar fibres. They connect the different parts of the CNS. The descending fibres begin from the gray matter of the cortex, descend down as corona radiata fibres till it reaches the upper part of corpus striatum. The same fibres within the corpus striatum are called internal capsule, and below that they descend to the midbrain where they are called crus cerebri. In the pons they form the basilar part and in the medulla oblongata they form pyramidal fibres.

Dissection*:* Internal capsule—It is the big vertically running fibre bundle of projection fibres. Note that the radiation of these fibres can be seen from the periphery of the lentiform nucleus in all directions. *Scoop and remove the lentiform nucleus by the back of a blade, carefully lift it totally to see the continuation of the internal capsule fibres.*

Now trace these fibres downwards into the crus crebri. Remove the superior longitudinal fibres and trace the internal capsule fibres upwards, towards the cortex.

These are corona radiata fibres. They lie between the gray matter of the cortex to the interiorly capsule.

LATERAL VENTRICLE

Lateral ventricle in the cavity to the cerebrum. It is a C shaped cavity. *Cut the septum pellucidum and the fornix to visualize this cavity*. The thalamus and the caudate nucleus forms the inner C around which lies the cavity around which lies the corpus callosum and the hippocampus.

Look for the caudate nucleus, thalamostriate vein, stria terminalis and the upper part of the thalamus in the floor of the central part of the lateral ventricle. Trace them around and note the same structures from the roof of the inferior horn. For descriptive purposes the lateral ventricle is divided into anterior horn, body, posterior horn and interior horn. Note that it is the corpus callosum which sweeps from the roof along the lateral wall to reach the floor.

The actual details can be better appreciated in coronal sections.

DEEP NUCLEAR MATTER

The white matter of the cerebrum has buried gray matter called the basal ganglia.

Basal ganglia is made up of caudate nucleus, lentiform nucleus, amygdaloid body and claustrum. The caudate nucleus and lentiform nucleus is called the corpus striatum.

Caudate nucleus: It is a comma shaped nucleus with a wide head, tapering body and a tail. It takes the curve of the cavity of the lateral ventricle. It is continuous with the putamen of the lentiform nucleus at the anterior end. The internal capsule fibres passing at this area give it a striate appearance. So the name corpus striatum.

Lentiform nucleus: It is a biconvex lens shaped structure. It has a inner globus pallidus and a outer putamen.

Amygdaloid body: It is an enlarged gray matter attached to the tip of the caudate nucleus. This will be noted in the roof of the inferior horn of the lateral ventricle.
Claustrum is external to the external capsule (identified in the white matter dissection)

All these nuclei belong to the extrapyramidal system. They have connections to the cortex and to other parts of the extrapyramidal system. The fibres arising from here control the motor nuclei of cranial and spinal nerves.

Dissection: To study the lentiform nucleus, continue the blunt dissection of the insula without disturbing the superior longitudinal, uncinate and inferior longitudinal fascicles.

Once the thin external capsule is removed the next structure noted is the lentiform nucleus. It is lightly brownish in color the shape of a biconvex lens. Feel its periphery.

THIRD VENTRICLE (Fig. 41)

Third ventricle is the space between the two diencephalons, the right and left side. Identify the boundaries,–superiorly is the ***roof***. It is formed by the ependyma of the forebrain invaginated by the choroid plexus. The posterior choroidal artery feeds this. This extends from the pineal body posteriorly to the interventricular foramen anteriorly. Here it continues into the lateral ventricle. The ependyma is attached to the stria medullaris thalami the white matter which separates the third ventricular part of the thalamus from the lateral ventricular part. The fornix overlies this. The gap between the fornix and the ependyma forms the ***choroid fissure.***

Posterior part is formed by the epithalamus. This is constituted by the pineal gland its recess and its stalk. The pineal gland is an endocrine gland. It secretes melatonin and serotonin and influences the gonadal growth in animals. The Habenular and posterior commissures were already noted.

Anterior border in formed by lamina terminals, optic chiasma, chiasmatic recess.

Floor is formed by the chiasma, infundibulum, infundibular recess, mammillary bodies and subthalamus.

Lateral wall is divided into two parts by the hypothalamic sulcus which extends from the interventricular foramen to aqueduct of sylvius, the part above this is bounded by thalamus and below this by the hypothalamus.

Interthalamic adhesion is generally present between the two thalami.

Interventricular foramen lies between the anterior commissure and anterior end of the thalamus. The choroid plexus of the third ventricle continues into the lateral ventricle here.

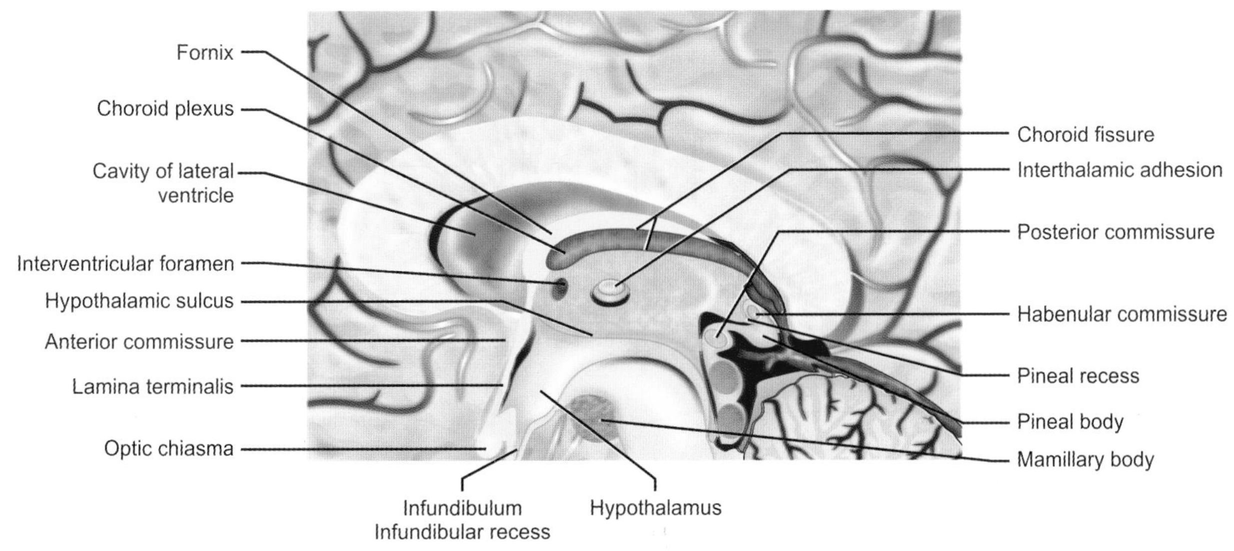

FIGURE 41: Third ventricle

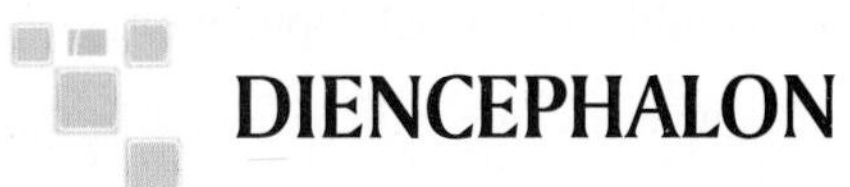

DIENCEPHALON

The diencephalon forms the submerged part of the forebrain. It is a nuclear complex and is described as having five parts—the thalamus, hypothalamus, epithalamus, subthalamus and metathalamus. It is placed around the third ventricle.

Dissection: The third ventricle is the cavity of diencephalon. It is a midline structure. In the midsagittal section the space you are seeing is the third ventricle. Identify its boundaries formed by thalamus hypothalamus and, epithalamus.

THALAMUS

Thalamus is the biggest receiving nuclear complex of the diencephalons. It is located on either side of the third ventricle. It receives all the sensory information and sends it, on to the cortex. It is divided into number of nuclear complexes, the details of which have to be studied from a textbook.

Dissection: Identify the anterior pole of thalamus behind the interventricular foramen. The body forms the lateral wall of the third ventricle. The posterior part projecting below the splenium is called the pulvinar of the thalamus. The internal medullary lamina divides the thalamus into smaller nuclear matter.

HYPOTHALAMUS (Fig. 42)

Identify the hypothalamus below the thalamus and is separated by the hypothalamic sulcus, which extends from the interventricular foramen to the aqueduct of Sylvius. It is made up of number of nuclei.

Mammillary bodies: Receive fibres through the anterior limb of fornix.

Tuber cinereum: This is the elevated part of the hypothalamus. It is connected to the pituitary gland through pituitary stalk.

EPITHALAMUS

Identify the parts of epithalamus above and posterior to the thalamus. It is formed by pineal body, habenular nucleus and its connections. ***Pineal body*** is a midline structure. It shows a central pineal recess, bounded by a stalk with a superior and an inferior limb. The superior limb lodges the ***Habenular commissure*** the inferior limb lodges the ***posterior commissure***.

SUBTHALAMUS

Subthalamus is the small area between the thalamus and the midbrain.

METATHALAMUS (Fig. 42)

Metathalamus lies lateral to the thalamus and constitute medial and lateral geniculate bodies. Turn the brain to visualize the undersurface. Here you can see the metathalamus located to the lateral side of the thalamus. It is made up of lateral and medial geniculate bodies.

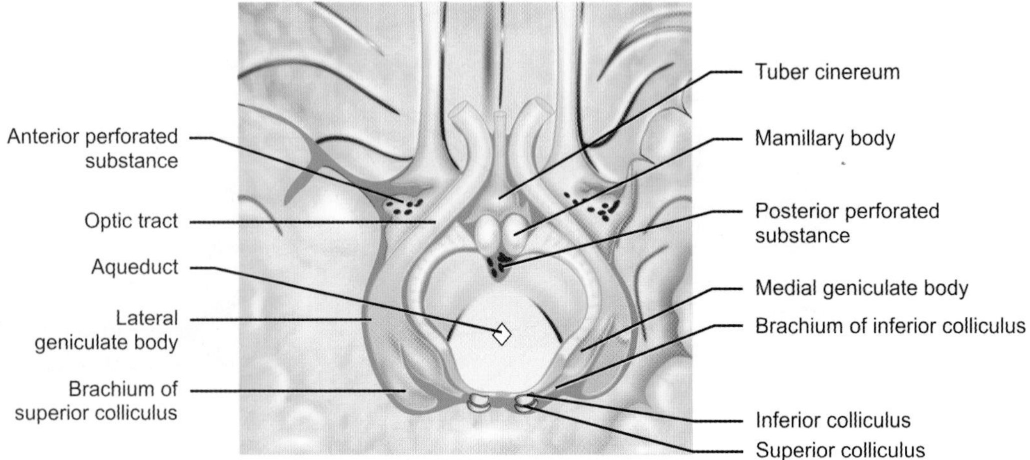

FIGURE 42: Diencephalon – Metathalamus and hypothalamus

Lateral geniculate bodies: Trace the optic tracts into the lateral geniculate bodies. Trace it further to reach the superior colliculus, it is the superior brachium. The ***optic nerves*** come from the eyeball. ***Optic chiasma*** is where the two optic nerves exchange their fibres. ***Optic tracts*** begin at the optic chiasma and wind round the thalamus end in the enlarged lateral geniculate bodies. These receive the fibres of optic nerve for relay. ***Superior brachium*** connects the lateral geniculate body to the superior colliculus. Few of the fibres from the geniculate body reach the superior colliculus to elucidate reflex movements. Majority of the fibres sweep inside as optic radiation to reach the area 17 in the occipital pole.

Medial geniculate bodies: These lie inner and more posterior to the lateral geniculate bodies. These receive the fibres from the inferior colliculus and project it to the area 41, 42, the primary auditory area in the superior temporal gyrus.

SECTIONS OF FOREBRAIN

This gives a consolidated idea of the structures within the forebrain. The knowledge of this will be very much helpful in interpreting the fibres of brain.

HORIZONTAL SECTION (Fig. 43)

Dissection: Cut the cerebral hemispheres at the level of the interventricular foramen with a brain knife by a single sharp cut and separate the two halves. Study the lower half of the cerebrum.

Identify the medial, lateral surfaces, the frontal and occipital poles and locate the following features.
- Short and broad frontal pole.
- Gray matter of frontal lobe.
- White matter of the frontal lobe.
- Short association fibres.
- Genu of the corpus callosum: This is the thick anterior part that connects the two frontal lobes. Continuation of the genu is the forceps minor, identify these fibres.
- Fibres of internal capsule.

Anterior horn of lateral ventricle: Lateral wall of the anterior horn is formed by head of caudate nucleus. Anterior wall is formed by genu of corpus callosum. Medial walls formed by the septum pellucidum and fornix.

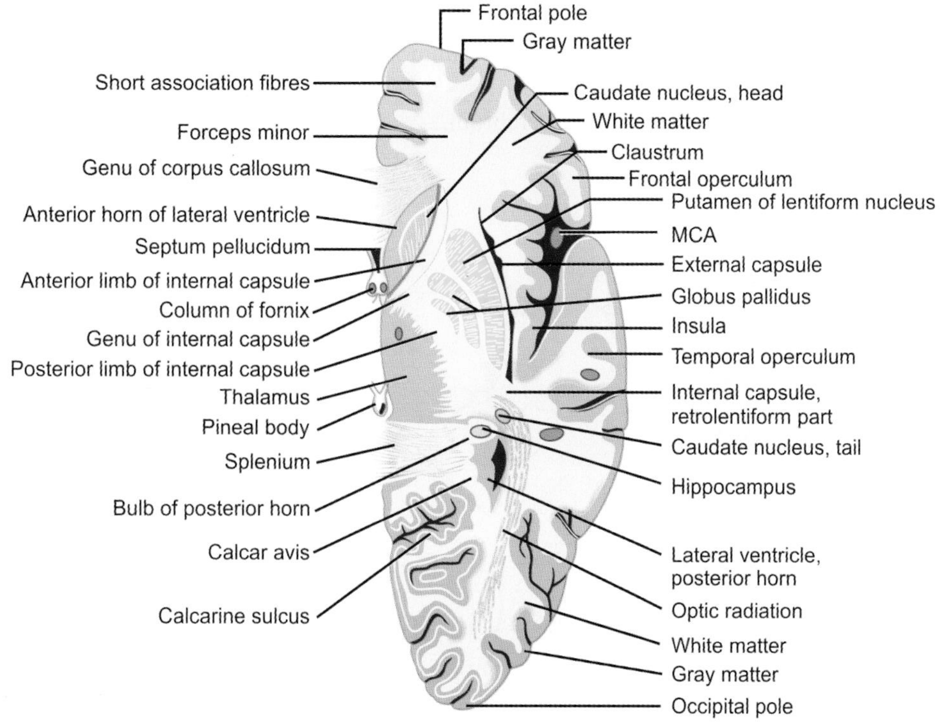

FIGURE 43: Horizontal section at the level of interventricular foramen

Thalamus: This occupies a prominent area in the central part of the medial side.

On the lateral aspect see:

- The frontal operculum: This covers insula anteriorly.
- Temporal operculum: This covers the inferior aspect of insula.
- Insula: This is the submerged cortex. It shows outer gray matter and inner white matter.
- Claustrum: This is another thin sheet of gray matter, part of basal ganglia.

External capsule: The white matter over the lentiform nucleus.

Lentiform nucleus: This presents an outer darker putamen and an inner lighter globus pallidus. This occupies the area lateral to caudate nucleus and thalamus. This is a part of basal ganglia.

Internal capsule: This is the internal white matter. It presents anterior limb between the caudate and lentiform nucleus, the genu between the caudate, lentiform nucleus and thalamus, the posterior limb, between the thalamus and lentiform nucleus.

Posterior horn of lateral ventricle

Medial wall is formed by two elevations. They are the bulb, formed by the forceps major, and the calcar avis formed by the calcarine sulcus. The roof and lateral wall are formed by the tapetum of the corpus callosum.

The optic radiation: Look for the optic radiation in continuation with the internal capsule.

Splenium of corpus callosum: Identify this and the fibres arising from this are the forceps major fibres.

Calcarine sulcus: This is a prominent sulcus extending from the medial side to the inferior horn. It lodges the visual cortex.

Occipital pole: Note the gray and white matter in this lobe.

CORONAL SECTIONS

The coronal sections give a clear idea about the lateral ventricle and its boundaries.

> **Dissection:** Take full brain if possible or at least a half a brain and cut coronal sections in the specified levels. Stain them with Mulligan stain.

CS1—THROUGH THE CENTER OF THE GENU OF CORPUS CALLOSUM (Fig. 44)

Identify the medial surface, superior, inferior and lateral sides of the section and put in anatomical position and identify the following. This shows the anterior horn of lateral ventricle.

- The anterior horn of lateral ventricle is a triangular space.
- The lateral wall forms the base and is formed by the head of the caudate nucleus.
- The genu of the corpus callosum forms the anterior limitation, superiomedial and inferomedial boundary of the triangle.
- You can note the gray and white matter of the cerebrum.

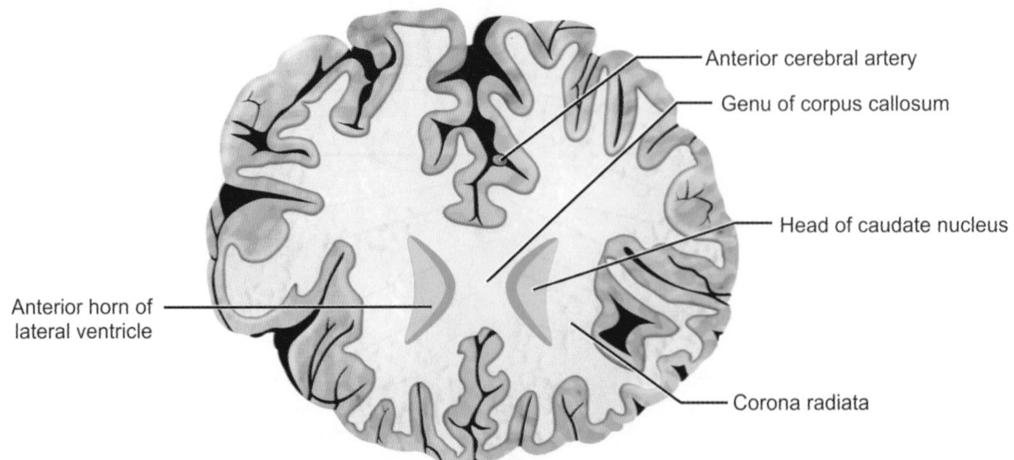

FIGURE 44: Coronal section through genu of corpus collosum

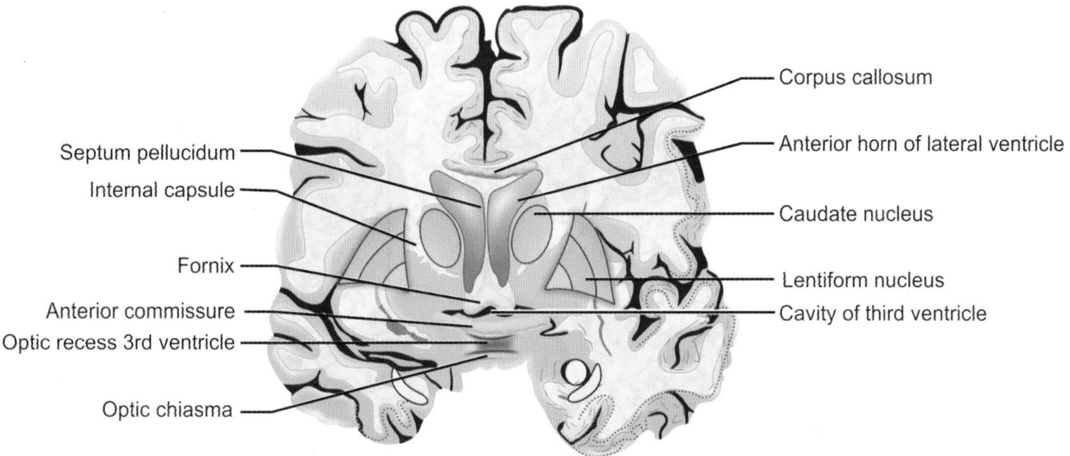

FIGURE 45: Coronal section through optic chiasma

CS2—THROUGH THE OPTIC CHIASMA (Fig. 45)

- Identify the sides of the brain and put the section on a table and identify the following structures.
- This is still in front of the interventricular foramen, so shows the anterior horn of lateral ventricle.

Anterior Horn of Lateral Ventricle

On the medial side look for the septum pellucidum. Here this forms the medial boundary of anterior horn of lateral ventricle. The roof is formed by corpus callosum and the lateral wall is formed by the head of the caudate nucleus.

Corpus striatum: In this section note that the caudate nucleus and lentiform nucleus are very closely packed and internal capsule fibres are seen crossing between them giving the appearance of a layer formation, the striatum. Note the horizontally crossing anterior commissural fibres.

Peripherally look at the gray and white matter.

Claustrum: As the section goes through the insula you can identify the claustrum, one of the basal ganglia.

Midline: In the midline the fornix, cavity of third ventricle, anterior commissure, optic recess and optic chiasma lie in this order above downwards.

CS3—THROUGH THE BODY OF LATERAL VENTRICLE (Fig. 46)

- Body of the lateral ventricle
- See the boundaries.
- Superiorly note the body of the corpus callosum
- Laterally note the body of the caudate nucleus.
- In the floor note from lateral to medial, the thalamostriate vein, the stria terminalis, the choroids plexus and the thalamus.

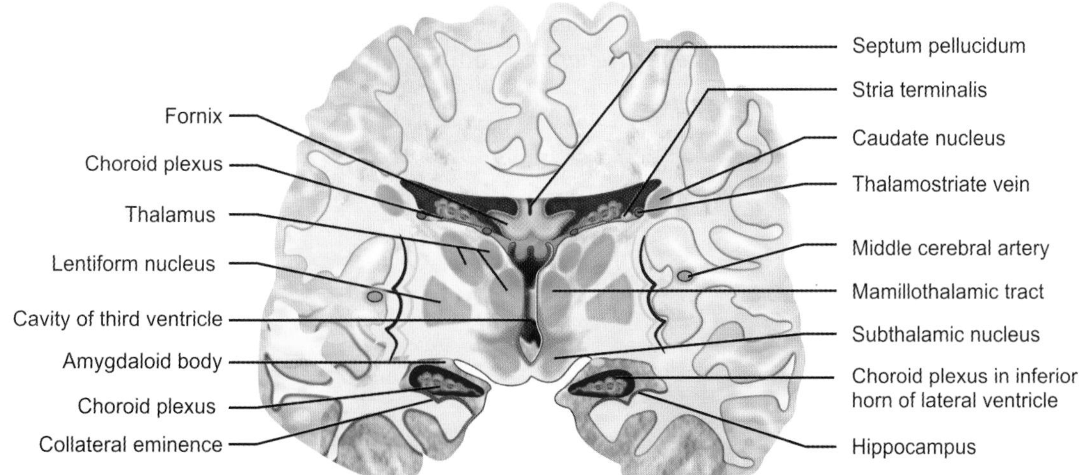

FIGURE 46: Coronal section through body of lateral ventricle

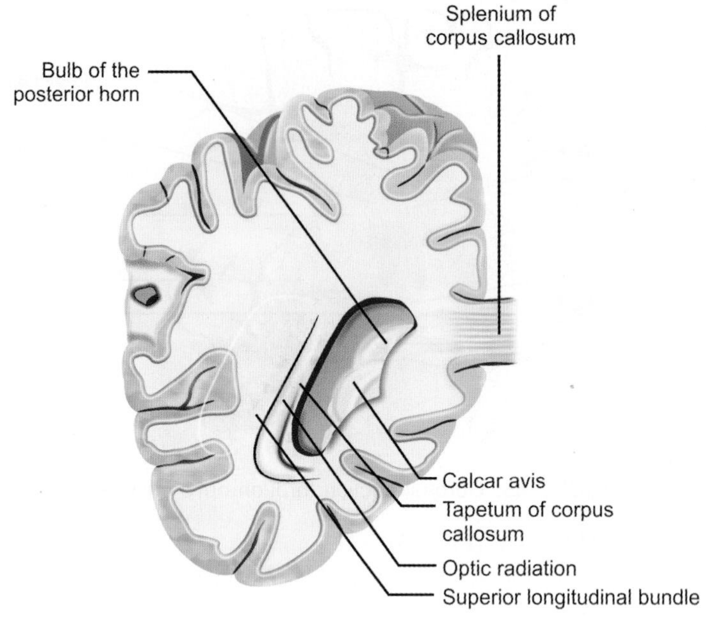

FIGURE 47: Coronal section through posterior horn of lateral ventricle

Cavity of third ventricle: Note its cavity and note the thalamus and hypothalamus forming the lateral boundary. Fornix forms the roof. Note the choroid plexus in the roof of third ventricle. It is continuous with the choroid plexus of lateral ventricle through the interventricular foramen.

The subthalamus is the nuclear matter below the thalamus.

Inferior Horn of Lateral Ventricle

Note this in the temporal lobe. Its floor is formed by the hippocampus. Note the collateral eminence formed by the collateral sulcus. This lies lateral to the hippocampus. Note the nuclear matter in the roof. It is formed by the amygdaloid body.

Identify the **insula** in the lateral aspect. Here note the parietal and temporal opercula. Note the gray matter of the insula, the white matter of the insula, claustrum, external capsule and the lentiform nucleus.

CS4—THROUGH THE SPLENIUM OF CORPUS CALLOSUM (Fig. 47)

Posterior Horn of Lateral Ventricle

Identify the oblong cavity of the lateral ventricle. Note the roof is formed by the splenium of the corpus callosum. The medial wall shows two elevations. The upper one is due to the projecting splenial fibres. It is called the ***bulb of the posterior horn***. Note the lower elevation caused by the calcarine sulcus, it is called the ***calcar avis***. Note the lateral wall is formed by fibres of ***tapetum***, fibres of ***optic radiation*** and fibres of ***superior longitudinal bundle*** in that order from inner to outer.

APPENDIX

MULIGAN STAIN

(A method of staining the brain for Macroscopic study—Journal of Anatomy 1931.65.468)

Cut a brain, well fixed in formalin, into slices and wash thoroughly in running water, overnight.

Place the sections for 2 minutes in a large volume of the following mixture at 60 degree centigrade.

Phenol	40 grams
Copper sulphate	5 grams
Con. HCl	1.2 cc
Water	1 liter

Rinse in a large volume of cold water for 1 minute.

Place in 2% solution of tannic acid for 1 minute.

Wash thoroughly for 5 minutes in running water.

Place in 2% solution of iron alum till the grey matter is purplish-black. This usually requires less than 1 minutes, and the sections should be transferred rapidly to water just before the desired depth of staining is attained.

Wash well in running water.

Caution- throughout the process avoid rough handling of the section, as the fatty layer or the stained areas may easily be rubbed off.

This method depends for its success on the production of a thin, relatively impervious fatty layer on the surface of the white matter by the action of warm phenol solution on the myelin. By this means, tannic acid in aqueous solution, which can pass into the gray matter, is prevented from entering the white matter. Treatment with a soluble iron salt then produces a purplish-black coloration on the surface of the gray matter.

Index

Page numbers followed by *f* refer to figure

F

G

H

I

J

K

L

M

N

O

P

Q

R

S

V

W

X

Z